BM

AUDIOLOGY
Science to Practice

Third Edition

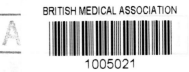

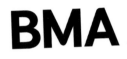

BMA

BMA Library

British Medical Association
BMA House
Tavistock Square
London
WC1H 9JP

Tel: 020 7383 6625
Email: bma-library@bma.org.uk
Web: bma.org.uk/library

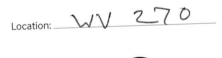

Location: ___WV 270___

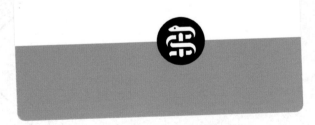

AUDIOLOGY
Science to Practice
Third Edition

Steven Kramer, PhD
David K. Brown, PhD

With contributions by
James Jerger, PhD
H. Gustav Mueller, PhD

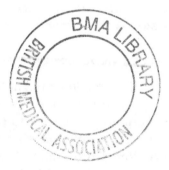

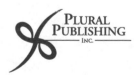
PLURAL
PUBLISHING
INC.

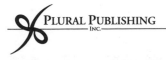

5521 Ruffin Road
San Diego, CA 92123

e-mail: info@pluralpublishing.com
website: http://www.pluralpublishing.com

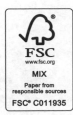

Typeset in 11/13 ITC Garamond Std by Achorn International Inc.
Printed in the United States of America by McNaughton & Gunn

For permission to use material from this text, contact us by
Telephone: (866) 758-7251
Fax: (888) 758-7255
e-mail: permissions@pluralpublishing.com

Library of Congress Cataloging-in-Publication Data

Names: Kramer, Steven J., author. | Brown, David K. (Professor of audiology), author. | Jerger, James, contributor. | Mueller, H. Gustav, contributor.
Title: Audiology : science to practice / Steven Kramer, David K. Brown ; with contributions by James Jerger, H. Gustav Mueller.
Description: Third edition. | San Diego, CA : Plural Publishing, [2019] | Includes bibliographical references and index.
Identifiers: LCCN 2017057249| ISBN 9781944883355 (alk. paper) | ISBN 1944883355 (alk. paper)
Subjects: | MESH: Hearing—physiology | Hearing Disorders | Audiology | Hearing Tests—methods
Classification: LCC RF290 | NLM WV 270 | DDC 617.8—dc23
LC record available at https://lccn.loc.gov/2017057249

Contents

Preface

This textbook provides an introductory, yet comprehensive look at the field of audiology. It is designed for undergraduate students, beginning audiology doctoral students, graduate speech-language pathology students, and other professionals who work closely with audiologists. It is expected that the knowledge obtained in this textbook will be applicable to the readers' future education or clinical practices. For some, it may help them decide to go into the profession of audiology.

From science to practice, this textbook covers anatomy and physiology, acoustic properties and perception of sounds, audiometry and speech measures, masking, audiogram interpretations, outer and middle ear assessments, otoacoustic emission and auditory brainstem responses, hearing screening, hearing aids, and cochlear and other implantable devices. Where appropriate, variations in procedures for pediatrics are presented. Beginning students also have a lot of interest in knowing about some common hearing disorders, and this book provides concise descriptions of selected auditory pathologies from different parts of the auditory system, with typical audiologic findings for many of the more commonly found ear diseases and hearing disorders to help the student learn how to integrate information from multiple tests. Also included is a separate chapter on the vestibular (balance) system, for those who wish to learn more about this important aspect of audiology. In addition, there are two chapters describing the profession of audiology, including its career outlook, what it takes to become an audiologist, as well as what audiologists do and where they practice. As a special addition, James Jerger, a legend in audiology, and University of Arizona share their perspectives on the history of audiology in the United States; these can be found throughout the various chapters as set-aside boxes (Historical Vignettes).

Although this textbook is intended for readers with little or no background in audiology, it is not a cursory overview. Instead, it presents a comprehensive and challenging coverage of hearing science and clinical audiology, but written in a style that tries to make new and/or difficult concepts relatively easy to understand. The approach to this book is to keep it readable and to punctuate the text with useful figures and tables. Each chapter has a list of key objectives, and throughout the chapter key words or phrases are italicized and included in a Glossary at the end of the textbook. In addition, most of the chapters have strategically-placed reviews (synopses) that can serve as quick refreshers before moving on, or which can provide a "quick read" of the entire text. Having taught beginning students for a number of years, the authors have learned a lot about how students learn and what keeps them motivated. After getting the students interested in the profession of audiology, information about acoustics is presented so that they have the tools to understand how the ear works and how hearing loss is assessed (which is what they really want to know) and these areas form the bulk of the text. Of course, the order of the chapters can be changed to suit any instructor.

FEATURES AND ADDITIONS TO THIS EDITION

This third edition of *Audiology: Science to Practice* has been extensively revised from the previous edition. This edition represents a collaboration with a new co-author, David Brown, whose long-time teaching experience and expertise in audiology and hearing science provided an opportunity to again update and expand the textbook in order to be useful to a wider audience. We also incorporated some of the feedback received through a survey of faculty who were current or interested users of the textbook.

This edition has four new chapters: (1) Outer and Middle Ear Assessment, that now includes a new section on otoscopy, more information on the use of different immittance probe-tone frequencies, and a well-developed section on the use of wideband acoustic immittance (reflectance); (2) Evoked Responses, with more information and examples on the use of OAEs, ABRs, and ASSRs for assessing neural pathologies and auditory sensitivity; (3) Implantable Devices, that covers cochlear implants, bone-anchored hearing aids, and other implantable devices; and (4) Vestibular System for those choosing to include a more comprehensive coverage of vestibular anatomy, physiology, disorders, and assessment. Another substantive change includes a revision of the chapter on Hearing Aids to make it more appropriate for the undergraduate student or others who want an overview of this important part of audiology. The chapter on Disorders of the Auditory System now has figures that include clinical data from a variety of audiology tests, including immittance, speech, and special tests, so that the student can begin to learn to integrate basic audiologic test results for the different disorders.

This edition has systematically reviewed each of the chapters from the previous edition to expand, update, and reorganize the material to make it even more useful to the student new to audiology, and at the same time continuing to be more comprehensive than one might find in other introductory texts on audiology. References and figures have been updated, including photos of new hearing instruments and amplification devices, and some new figures on the anatomy of the auditory and vestibular systems. This edition retains the features that worked well in previous editions, including an easy-to-read format, key learning objectives, and synopses within each chapter with bulleted highlights for review. The chapters are now organized in a more traditional sequence beginning with information about the profession of audiology, followed by acoustics, anatomy/physiology, and clinical audiology. Stylistically, this edition now has some set-aside boxes with ancillary information that are interspersed throughout the textbook, including much of Dr. Jerger's historical account of audiology in the United States. We are excited about all the improvements in this edition that will help beginning students gain an even stronger foundation about audiology concepts.

This edition also comes with a PluralPlus companion website which includes lecture outlines in slide format that can be used in teaching audiological concepts, the full text of Dr. Jerger's essay on the history of audiology, and more.

Contributors

David K. Brown, PhD
Associate Professor
Director, AUD SIMLab
School of Audiology
Pacific University
Hillsboro, Oregon

Cheryl D. Johnson, EdD
Adjunct Assistant Professor
Disability and Psychoeducational Studies
College of Education
University of Arizona
Tucson, Arizona

James Jerger, PhD
Distinguished Scholar-in-Residence
School of Behavioral and Brain Sciences
The University of Texas at Dallas
Dallas, Texas

Steven Kramer, PhD
Professor
School of Speech, Language,
and Hearing Sciences
San Diego State University
San Diego, California

H. Gustav Mueller, PhD
Professor
Department of Hearing and Speech Sciences
Vanderbilt University
Nashville, Tennessee

To the children with hearing impairments on my school bus many years ago,
who inspired me to pursue a career in audiology;
To my past, present, and future students, who have always made my work
enjoyable, challenging, and rewarding;
To my wife, Paula, for her support and sacrifices during the writing of this text;
To my colleagues who provide me with an exciting place to work, and for their
camaraderie and continued support during the revision of this textbook.

—Steven Kramer

To my mentors and teachers who spent time answering my questions,
may I spend as much time with my students as you did with me;
To my colleagues, who shared their knowledge with me;
To my students throughout the years who challenged me to learn more;
To my family and especially my wife, Dianne, who gave up and put up with so much
during the writing of this book. I promise I will be home for dinner soon!

—David Brown

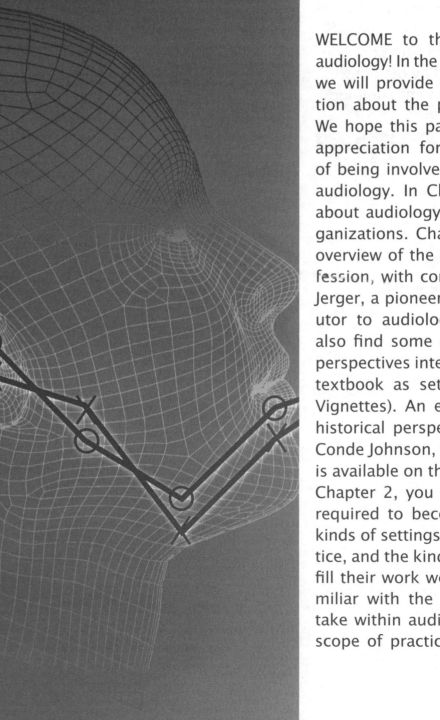

PART 1

Perspectives on the Profession of Audiology

WELCOME to the fascinating world of audiology! In the first part of this textbook, we will provide you with some information about the profession of audiology. We hope this part provides you with an appreciation for the rewarding aspects of being involved with the profession of audiology. In Chapter 1, you will learn about audiology and its professional organizations. Chapter 1 also includes an overview of the development of the profession, with contributions by Dr. James Jerger, a pioneer and continuing contributor to audiological research. You will also find some of Dr. Jerger's historical perspectives interspersed throughout the textbook as set-aside boxes (Historical Vignettes). An extended version of this historical perspective by Jerger and De-Conde Johnson, from the second edition, is available on the companion website. In Chapter 2, you will learn about what is required to become an audiologist, the kinds of settings where audiologists practice, and the kinds of activities that might fill their work week. You will become familiar with the varied paths you might take within audiology and the extensive scope of practice that defines the skills of audiologists. Chapter 2 also presents some current demographic trends in audiology, as summarized from surveys regularly conducted by our professional organizations. For those interested in speech-language pathology, nursing, optometry, rehabilitation counseling, or other related fields, we know that you will interact with people who have hearing loss and with audiologists, and the information in this textbook will, undoubtedly, be of use to you. We hope many of you will become intrigued by the possibility of joining the profession of audiology.

1

The Discipline
of Audiology

After reading this chapter, you should be able to:

1. Define audiology and understand how audiology relates to other disciplines.

2. List some professional and student organizations related to audiology.

3. Become aware of professional websites' resources to learn more about the profession.

4. Discuss how and when audiology as a profession first began, and describe key events that transpired over the years as the profession evolved.

Audiology is a discipline that focuses on the study of normal hearing and hearing disorders. Additionally, audiology includes the assessment and treatment of vestibular (balance) disorders. More precisely, audiology is a health care profession devoted to identification, assessment, treatment/rehabilitation, and prevention of hearing and balance disorders, and understanding the effects of hearing loss on related communication disorders. An *audiologist* is a professional who has the appropriate degree and license in his or her state to practice audiology, and who is, typically, certified by a professional board. Audiologists are the experts who understand the effects of hearing loss on communication and how to best improve a patient's ability to hear.

Audiologists work with many other professionals and support personnel. The medical expert in hearing disorders is the physician. The medical specialty related to the ear is called *otology*, which is practiced by appropriately trained and certified *otologists*, also called neuro-otologists, otolaryngologists, or ear, nose, and throat (ENT) specialists. Audiologists also work closely with *speech-language pathologists*, who are certified and/or licensed professionals who engage in prevention, assessment, and treatment of speech and language disorders, including those who have hearing loss. In addition, many audiologists are part of interdisciplinary teams, especially when it comes to the assessment and treatment of pediatric patients, as well as patients with implantable devices, cystic fibrosis, cleft palate, or balance problems, to name a few.

PROFESSIONAL ORGANIZATIONS

The *American Academy of Audiology (AAA)* is the professional organization for audiologists. In 1988, AAA (often referred to as "triple A") was founded in order to establish an organization devoted entirely to the needs of audiologists and the interests of the audiology profession (http://www.audiology.org). Originally, AAA focused on transitioning audiology to a doctoral level profession, which became a reality by 2007. Membership in AAA quickly skyrocketed, and, today, AAA has a membership of more than 12,000 audiologists (Amer-

ican Academy of Audiology [AAA], n.d. a). Prior to the formation of AAA, the *American Speech-Language-Hearing Association (ASHA)* was, and still remains, a professional organization for audiologists and speech-language pathologists. The ASHA was established in 1925 as the American Academy of Speech Correction, and went through several name changes including the American Society for the Study of Disorders of Speech (1927), the American Speech Correction Association (1934), the American Speech and Hearing Association (1947), and in 1978 became the American Speech-Language-Hearing Association (American Speech-Language-Hearing Association [ASHA], n.d.). In its early years, ASHA focused on speech disorders; however, during World War II, with service personnel returning with hearing losses, ASHA expanded its mission to include assessment and treatment of those with hearing disorders.

The AAA and ASHA are both strong advocates for the hearing impaired and related services by audiologists, both at the state and national levels. The AAA and ASHA each have professional certifications for audiologists: *American Board of Audiology (ABA) Certification* through AAA, and the *Certificate of Clinical Competence in Audiology (CCC-A)* through ASHA. In addition, each of these organizations can award accreditation to academic programs that meet a set of standards; the Accreditation Commission for Audiology Education (ACAE) associated with AAA, and the Commission on Academic Accreditation (CAA) associated with ASHA.

Audiologists may also choose to join other professional organizations. The Academy of Dispensing Audiologists (ADA) was established in 1977 to support the needs of audiologists who dispense (sell) hearing aids. The ADA later changed its name to the *Academy of Doctors of Audiology (ADA)* (http://www.audiologist.org), and expanded its focus to any audiologists in private practice or those who wished to establish a private practice. The *Educational Audiology Association (EAA)* (http://www.edaud.org), formed in 1983, is a professional membership organization of audiologists and related professionals who deliver a full spectrum of hearing services to all children, particularly those in educational settings. Many audiologists are also associated with the American Auditory Society (AAS) (http://www.amauditorysoc.org) and/or the Academy of Rehabilitative Audiology (ARA) (http://www.audrehab.org). Additionally, there is a national student organization for those interested in audiology, called the *Student Academy of Audiology (SAA)* (http://saa.audiology.org). The SAA is devoted to audiology education, student research, professional requirements, and networking of students enrolled in audiology doctoral programs. Undergraduate students who are potentially interested in pursuing a career in audiology may also join SAA (Undergraduate Associate). Most university programs have a local chapter of SAA that is part of the national SAA. Undergraduate programs may also have a chapter of *National Student Speech Language Hearing Association (NSSLHA)*. A wealth of information about the field of audiology and a career as an audiologist can be found on the above-mentioned websites.

DEVELOPMENT OF THE PROFESSION OF AUDIOLOGY[1]

Prior to World War II, persons with hearing disorders received services by physicians and hearing aid dispensers (Martin & Clark, 2015). Audiology in the United States established its roots in 1922 with the fabrication of the first commercial audiometer (Western Electric 1-A) by Harvey Fletcher and R. L. Wegel, who were conducting pioneering research in speech communication at Bell Telephone Laboratories (Jerger, 2009). These audiometers were used, primarily, for research and in otolaryngology practices.

Audiology as a profession began around the time of World War II, mostly because of returning service personnel who developed hearing problems from unprotected exposures to high-level noises. Initially, returning armed-service personnel were seen by otologists and speech-language pathologists, but clinical services for those with hearing loss soon evolved into a specialty practice in the United States that became known as

---

[1]Includes contributions by James Jerger and Cheryl De-Conde Johnson (adapted with permission).

Historical Vignette

The first genuine audiologist in the United States was, undoubtedly, Cordia C. Bunch. As a graduate student at the University of Iowa, late in World War I, Bunch came under the influence of Carl Seashore, a psychologist who was studying the measurement of musical aptitude, and L. W. Dean, an otolaryngologist. Together, they stimulated Bunch's interest in the measurement of hearing. Over the two decades from 1920 to 1940, Bunch carried out the first systematic studies of the relation between types of hearing loss and audiometric patterns. Bunch's pioneering efforts were published in a slender volume entitled <u>Clinical Audiometry</u>, which is now a classic in the field. In 1941, Bunch accepted an offer from the School of Speech at Northwestern University to teach courses in hearing testing and hearing disorders, as part of the education of the deaf program. While at Northwestern University, Bunch mentored a young faculty member in speech science, Raymond Carhart. In 1942, Bunch unexpectedly died at the age of 57. In order to continue the course in hearing testing and disorders, the Northwestern administration asked Raymond Carhart to teach the course. The rest, as they say, is history, as Carhart became another one of the early pioneers of the field.

the field of audiology. While the effects of excessive noise on hearing have been recognized virtually since the beginning of the industrial age, it was not until World War II that the United States military began to address the issues of hearing conservation with a series of regulations defining noise exposure as a hazard, setting forth conditions under which hearing protection must be employed, and requiring that personnel exposed to potentially hazardous noise have their hearing monitored. The introduction of jet aircraft

Historical Vignette

Attempts to exploit the residual hearing of severely and profoundly hearing-impaired persons has a history much longer than audiology. Long before there were audiometers and hearing aids, educators of the deaf were at the front lines of auditory training, using whatever tools were available. Alexander Graham Bell, inventor of the telephone and founder of the AG Bell Association, took a special interest in the possibilities of auditory training because of his wife's hearing loss. He was a strong proponent of the aural approach and lent his considerable reputation to its promulgation in the last quarter of the nineteenth century. Another early supporter of systematic training in listening was Max Goldstein, who founded the world-famous Central Institute for the Deaf in St. Louis.

into the Air Force and the Navy in the late 1940s, generating high levels of noise, was an important factor driving interest in hearing protection. Early studies of the effects of noise on the auditory system were carried out in the 1940s and 1950s at the Naval School of Aviation Medicine, in Pensacola, Florida. Similar research programs were established at the Navy submarine base in Groton, Connecticut, and at the Navy Electronics Laboratory in San Diego, California. After World War II, audiology-specific educational programs were developed in universities to prepare professionals for clinical work, as well as becoming the stage for further research efforts that would define the practice of audiology. In the early years, audiology focused on rehabilitation, including lipreading (now called speechreading), auditory training, and hearing aids.

During the late 1960s and early 1970s, there was a focus on the development of several objective measures of the auditory system: Immittance (known then as impedance) blossomed into tests called tympanometry, used for assessing middle ear disorders, and acoustic reflex thresholds, used for differentiating/documenting conductive, sensory, and neural losses. The immittance test battery is now standard in basic hearing assessments. The mid to late 1970s brought our attention to the clinical use of evoked electrical potentials, especially the auditory brainstem response (ABR), which provided an objective evaluation of the auditory system that was unaffected by sedation. The ABR continues to be used as a specialty test for neurologic function, and even more importantly for both newborn hearing screening and follow-up hearing threshold assessment. In the late 1970s, otoacoustic emission (OAE) testing was developed as another objective measure of the auditory system, and became an accepted part of clinical practice by the late 1980s. The clinical applicability of OAE testing was the primary impetus for states in the United States to adopt universal newborn hearing screening programs. Marion Downs of the University of Colorado, undoubtedly, had the greatest impact on the testing of pediatrics and, ultimately, the concept and realization of universal hearing screening of all newborns. Dr. Downs founded the first screening program in 1962 and never ceased to push for newborn hearing screening. According to the National Center for Hearing Assessment and Management (NCHAM) at Utah State University, all states and territories of America now have an Early Hearing Detection and Intervention (EHDI) program (National Center for Hearing Assessment and Management, n.d.).

The development of better-designed hearing aids and procedures for hearing aid fittings was also an important step forward in treating those with hearing loss. During the early 1950s, the transistor was developed and its value in the design of wearable hearing aids was immediately apparent. An even greater impact on hearing aid design and miniaturization was the advent of digital signal processing, and by the 1990s, digital hearing aids were becoming the standard. Other important advances in hearing aids included microphone technology and better/smaller batteries. It is interesting to point out that prior to 1977, ASHA considered it unethical for audiologists to dispense hearing aids, except in the Veteran's Hospitals. However, through the continuing interests and activities of audiologists directed toward dispensing of hearing aids throughout the 1970s, ASHA changed its perspective in 1979, and hearing aid dispensing soon became a large part of audiology practices. At the time of this writing (August 2017), the U.S. Congress passed legislation allowing hearing aids to be sold over-the-counter (OTC) for adults with mild to moderate degrees of hearing loss, and established about a three-year time window to develop regulations and implementation.

Cochlear implants (CI) were another milestone in audiology, beginning with the first implants in the 1960s. Subsequently, there was a 30-year, slow-but-steady, convincing of the profession that cochlear implants were able to produce remarkable results in adults and children, and now cochlear implants are well accepted in the audiology community. The progress of cochlear implants over the past three decades has been truly remarkable. The early CI systems were essentially aids to speechreading and few users could maintain a conversation without the aid of visual cues. However, as the number of electrodes increased and speech-coding strategies became more sophisticated, performance in the auditory-only condition improved several-fold. It is now quite reasonable to expect that a person with a cochlear implant will be able to converse, even on the telephone. Thirty years ago, few people would have predicted that this level of performance would ever be attainable.

There has also been a relatively long history in the area of vestibular disorders and testing. Bradford (1975) describes some of the early history in this area that includes the early descriptions of nystagmus (reflexive eye movements) by Purkinjie (1820), discovery of the cerebellar and labyrinthine sources of vertigo by Flourens (1828), and the development of caloric testing by Barany (1915). Pioneering work in establishing the clinical use of electronystagmography (ENG) was done by Alfred Coats (e.g., Coats, 1975), Baloh and colleagues (e.g., Baloh, Sills, & Honrubia, 1977), and Barber and colleagues (e.g., Barber and Stockwell, 1980). With advances in technology in the past decade, the electrode-based ENG method evolved to an infrared video camera method for recording eye movements (VNG)

during the vestibular exam. Other advancements include the development of rotary chair testing that rotates the whole body with head fixed in place, and posturography with a platform that allows for tilting the body in different directions. One of the more recent clinical developments is the recording of vestibular evoked myogenic potentials involving the ocular muscles (oVEMP) or the cervical muscles (cVEMP) in response to loud sounds, which have been shown to be useful for assessing the saccule and utricle, which are sensory organs of the vestibular system.

Over the last 70+ years, audiology has evolved (often in parallel) along at least the following eight distinct paths:

- Development of auditory diagnostic tests (behavioral and physiologic)
- Hearing aids and rehabilitation/treatment
- Pediatrics
- Auditory processing disorders (APDs)
- Hearing conservation
- Audiology in the educational (school) systems
- Tinnitus evaluation and therapy
- Development of vestibular tests and rehabilitation

The reader is referred to some of the comment boxes throughout this textbook for overviews of these paths. A more complete historical account of audiology in the United States has been published by Jerger (2009). In addition, Jerger and DeConde Johnson have an expanded chapter on the development of these paths in the second edition of this textbook, which is also available in this textbook's companion website. As Jerger and DeConde Johnson (2014) concluded,

. . . it is interesting to observe the degree to which these paths have interacted. We see the fruits of progress in the diagnostic path reflected in the development of APD testing, the impact of advances in electroacoustics and electrophysiology on universal screening procedures, the influence of cochlear implant advances on auditory training, and the influences of all on intervention with amplification, hearing conservation, tinnitus therapy, and audiology in the educational

SYNOPSIS 1–1

- Audiology is a discipline that focuses on the study of normal hearing and hearing disorders, as well as vestibular (balance) assessment and rehabilitation. Audiology in the United States had its beginnings around the time of World War II.
- An audiologist is a licensed professional who practices audiology, and is an expert on the effects of hearing loss on communication and psychosocial factors. Otology is the discipline primarily related to medical assessment and treatment of hearing and balance disorders, and is the specialty practiced by otologists.
- The American Academy of Audiology (AAA) and the American Speech-Language-Hearing Association (ASHA) are the two main professional organizations serving their audiologist members. The AAA was founded in 1988, and is entirely run by and for audiologists.
- The national student organization for future doctoral level audiologists is called the Student Academy of Audiology (SAA). Most doctoral audiology programs have local chapters of SAA. Many undergraduate programs encourage undergraduates to enroll in student chapters.
- Audiology became a doctoral level profession by 2007, and today the AAA has more than 12,000 members.
- Some key historical milestones in audiology include development of immittance measures (early 1970s), auditory brainstem response (ABR) measures (late 1970s), approval for audiologists to dispense hearing aids (1979), otoacoustic emission measures (1980s), digital hearing aids become the dominant type (1990s), and legislation allowing OTC hearing aids (2017).

setting. These are, we believe, hallmarks of a robust and growing profession with a remarkable history. (p. 380)

REFERENCES

American Academy of Audiology [AAA]. (n.d.). Academy Information. Retrieved from http://www.audiology.org/about-us/academy-information

American Speech-Language-Hearing Association [ASHA]. (n.d.). History of ASHA. Retrieved from http://www.asha.org/about/history

Jerger, J. (2009). *Audiology in the USA*. San Diego, CA: Plural.

Jerger, J., & DeConde Johnson, C. (2014). A brief history of audiology in the United States. In S. Kramer (Ed.), *Audiology: Science to Practice* (2nd ed.). San Diego, CA: Plural.

Martin, F. N., & Clark, J. G. (2015). *Introduction to Audiology* (12th ed.). Boston, MA: Pearson Education, Inc.

National Center for Hearing Assessment and Management (n.d.). State EDHI Information. Retrieved from http://www.infanthearing.org/states_home

2 Audiology as a Career

After reading this chapter, you should be able to:

1. Understand the academic and clinical requirements that are needed to become an audiologist: Know the basic difference between an AuD and PhD.

2. Know the legal requirements to practice audiology: List two professional certifications that are available to audiologists.

3. Describe various paths/specialties that audiologists might follow to define their careers.

4. Describe the general activities of audiologists and how they might spend their time in any given week.

5. Describe the types of settings in which audiologists typically work.

6. List four to six activities that are within an audiologist's scope of practice.

7. Discuss why some activities within an audiologist's scope of practice might diminish in importance, or disappear in the future.

8. Give an estimate of the number of audiologists there are in its professional organizations and describe the general membership demographics.

9. Access the professional websites of AAA and ASHA to find AuD programs and to learn more about the profession.

Audiology continues to gain notoriety in the labor market, and has been highly recommended as a top career choice with an excellent employment outlook. In fact, *Time Magazine* (2015) ranked audiology as the number one profession, out of 40 professions, based on job stress, salary, and job outlook. CareerCast (2015, 2017) has ranked audiology in the top four professions (out of 200 occupations) for having the least stressful job, behind medical sonographer, compliance officer, and hair stylist. The U.S. Bureau of Labor Statistics (2017) estimates that the average growth rate for all occupations between 2014 and 2022 will be 7%; however, audiology's projected job growth is estimated to be 29%. The job market outlook for audiologists is quite strong, and the need is expected to grow substantially in the future (Windmill & Freeman, 2013).

EDUCATION AND PROFESSIONAL CREDENTIALS

Today, the entry-level degree to practice clinical audiology is a professional doctorate, referred to as the *Doctor of Audiology* (*AuD*). The AuD is a 3- to 4-year graduate degree composed of a comprehensive curriculum with about 2000 to 3000 hours of clinical experiences, *precepted* (supervised) by licensed and/or certified audiologists. The AuD is the entry level clinical doctoral degree, different from the research doctorate (PhD) that has been available in audiology and hearing sciences since its inception for those interested in research and/or an academic position. The move from a clinical master's degree in audiology to a professional doctoral degree began in the late 1980s, and was a guiding force in the establishment of the American Academy of Audiology (AAA). The first AuD program became available in 1993 at Baylor College of Medicine in Houston (which subsequently closed its AuD program). In 1993, ASHA endorsed a plan to transition to the clinical doctoral degree, and by 2007 the AuD became required (a master's degree was no longer adequate) to practice audiology. As of 2017, there were 75 audiology clinical doctoral programs in the country (American Academy of Audiology [AAA], n.d.).

Students entering audiology clinical doctoral programs come from a variety of disciplines, such as speech and hearing, psychology, education, engineering, music, physics, computer science, neuroscience, medicine, nursing, and business to name a few. Audiology is a scientific discipline and requires a relatively strong science foundation and an ability to meet the challenges of a rigorous curriculum. Most AuD programs expect students to have some preparation in physical, life, social, and behavioral sciences, as well as statistics.

The curricula for AuD programs are quite similar across programs, and are partially driven by the professional accreditation standards, as well as specific requirements for professional certification. A list and links to doctoral programs can be found on the AAA website (www.audiology.org) and the American Speech-Language-Hearing (ASHA) website (www.asha.org). There are, however, differences across programs in the number of faculty, the breadth of academic courses, the variety and amount of clinical experiences, and the amount of research available to students. While most programs have a similar core of courses, a program may have strengths in one or more areas, or may provide more advanced preparation in some areas, such as hearing aids, electrophysiology, vestibular assessment, cochlear implants, tinnitus, business practice, and/or rehabilitation. As part of an AuD program, students are required to have clinical experiences that are precepted by an audiologist or other relevant professional. Some AuD programs have an on-campus clinic where students begin their clinical experiences, and then obtain additional clinical experiences in community hospitals, clinics, or other agencies. Other AuD programs may rely solely on the community resources for the clinical experiences.

The final year of the AuD program is called an *externship*, which is usually the equivalent to a year's full-time clinical experience at a clinical site approved by the AuD program. Externships are established through specific affiliation agreements developed between the externship site and the AuD program's institution. An externship site agrees to have an on-site preceptor who will take an active role in further educating and mentoring the extern during the final year of his or

SYNOPSIS 2–1

- Audiologists have been ranked as one of the top career choices with a projected need for more audiologists in the coming years. Audiology has also been ranked as one of the least stressful jobs.
- A professional doctorate (AuD) is required to practice clinical audiology. The AuD is obtained by successfully completing a 3- to 4-year clinical doctoral degree program, passing the national examination in audiology, and obtaining an audiology license from the state in which he or she resides.
- The AuD is different from the PhD; the latter being an academic, research-focused doctoral degree for those interested in an academic or research position. An externship is the final year of an AuD program, and is usually a full-time, 12-month position at a clinical site that has a formal affiliation with the university's AuD program. Externs are typically selected by the clinical site, and require site-specific applications and interviews. Externships can be from states other than the state in which the program resides.

her program, prior to entering the profession as an audiologist. Externships are located throughout the country, and in many cases the location where one completes the externship may be different than the location where the AuD program resides. Most externship placements require the student to apply for an available position, interview, and wait to see if they are offered the position. In the best-case scenario, the student may be in a position to choose among more than

one offer. Currently, the externship is part of the AuD program, and a designee of the program maintains regular contact with the extern site regarding the extern's progress, performance, and professionalism.

Upon completion of the AuD degree, including all the clinical rotations and externship requirements relevant for the state in which one chooses to practice, and upon passing a national examination in audiology (currently offered through Praxis), the student is eligible to apply for a license to practice audiology in that state. Some states may also require a separate license or exam to be qualified to dispense hearing aids. In addition to the legal requirement of having a state license, most audiologists choose to obtain professional certification through AAA and/or ASHA. But do not think that the education and training is over after obtaining a license and certification; there are mandatory continuing education hours that must be fulfilled to maintain the license and certification throughout one's professional career. For those who wish to continue their education and obtain a research doctorate (PhD), the AuD can be an excellent foundation and a valuable asset in an academic position.

WHAT DO AUDIOLOGISTS DO?

Audiologists are typically educated and clinically trained as "generalists" in the areas of diagnostic assessment of patients with hearing and balance disorders, and nonmedical treatment of hearing loss, primarily through the fitting of hearing aids or other implantable devices (e.g., cochlear implants). Although many employment settings involve a wide range of activities and populations, there are many areas within the field of audiology in which an audiologist may choose to concentrate, and many audiologists choose to be involved in more than one of these areas. Some examples of different areas within the discipline of audiology (not necessarily mutually exclusive) include:

- **Pediatric audiologist:** Interested and skilled in special audiological techniques of assessment and treatment of infants and children; good at counseling and working with families and referral agencies. Often works in a facility primarily serving children, such as a children's hospital.

- **Geriatric audiologist:** Interested and skilled in assessment and treatment of elderly patients; knowledgeable with the Medicare system; typically works in a veteran's hospital or university clinic.
- **Hearing aid dispensing audiologist:** Engages in the fitting and selling of hearing aids as part of their audiology practice; typically works in a private practice, but may also work in a medical or university setting.
- **Cochlear implant audiologist:** Part of a team that determines cochlear implant candidacy; trained in the "mapping" of the patient's device and monitoring its use. May also provide auditory rehabilitation for patients who have received an implant. An additional certification for cochlear implants is available through ABA (http://www.boardofaudiology.org/cochlear-implant-specialty-certification)
- **Auditory implant specialist:** Part of a team that determines auditory implant candidacy for patients who may benefit from this form of implantable device (i.e., transcutaneous and percutaneous implants, etc.), trains patients in the care and use of these devices, and monitors their function.
- **Educational audiologist:** Provides hearing assessment and hearing aid management of children in schools; part of a team that provides input to the child's educational plan and needs as they relate to their hearing abilities; may also engage in the evaluation of auditory processing disorders; works in a school district, often as an itinerant that services several schools.
- **Vestibular (balance) audiologist:** Provides balance system assessment and rehabilitation to children and adults. Often works in a hospital or clinic as part of a team with physicians, physical therapists, and optometrists specializing in individuals with disorders of the vestibular system including falls, imbalance, dizziness, and spatial disorientation.
- **Intraoperative monitoring specialist:** Skilled in evoked potentials in a variety of modalities; high level of knowledge in neurology and anatomy; assists surgeons in the operating room; often contracts with hospitals. Additional certification is needed through the American Board of Neurophysiologic Monitoring and/or the American Board of Registration of Electroencephalographic and Evoked Potential Technologists.
- **Military audiologist:** An enlisted audiologist (Army, Navy, or Air Force) who performs assessment and treatment of armed services personnel, recruits, and their families; establishes appropriate hearing conservation programs to monitor noise levels of enlisted personnel; works in a community-based military hospital.
- **Industrial (hearing conservation) audiologist:** Specializes in consulting with industrial companies with potentially excessive noise levels to establish appropriate hearing conservation programs to monitor noise levels, assess hearing, and educate employees and employers about protecting their hearing; contracts with companies.
- **Academic audiologist:** Clinically educated and credentialed faculty member who is part of a university audiology program; may teach, conduct research, and precept students in a university-based clinic.
- **Research audiologist:** Engages in hearing research, usually of an applied nature; often funded by grants in a university or hospital setting; may also work in private research institutes or in companies that develop test equipment or hearing aids.
- **Forensic audiologist:** Specializes in legal cases related to hearing loss and issues related to environmental or industrial noise; gives occasional depositions or testimony in legal cases; usually done outside of a regular job as an audiologist.

- **Animal audiology:** Specializes in the assessment of hearing in animals (emphasis on canines), including the use of auditory brainstem responses (ABR). Works closely with veterinarians to evaluate hearing in the more than 80 breeds with genetic hearing loss and other dogs with age- or noise-related deafness. Usually done as a portion of an audiologist's regular job. May also engage in fitting animals with hearing aids. Specialty training and certificate are available (http://www.fetchlab.org).

Audiologists provide a variety of services to meet the needs of persons with hearing and balance problems. As mentioned earlier, audiologists are involved with identification (screening), assessment, treatment, and prevention. Audiologists might wear different hats or many hats, such as those of a diagnostician, therapist, counselor, consultant, preceptor, team leader, advocate, business person, researcher, and/or teacher. An audiologist's role as a teacher might involve being an AuD student's preceptor, providing in-service training sessions, or case study presentations to other hospital staff, medical students, residents, and fellows. They might develop brochures and workshops for consumers and industry on the effects of hearing loss or its prevention and treatment. They might lead aural rehabilitation group therapy sessions with adults, or auditory habilitation therapy sessions with children who have hearing loss. They might be asked to provide input on treatment plans for those receiving cochlear implants, ototoxic medications, vestibular disorders, tinnitus, head injury, speech-language disorders, and/or a child's school-based educational plan. Audiologists must be able to assess and treat patients of all ages, including, for example, newborns and patients with a variety of disabilities, and must be culturally and linguistically sensitive in their selection of tests, counseling, and treatment.

Audiologists working in hospitals or clinics spend a good deal of their time planning, performing, and interpreting diagnostic tests; usually this is followed by some patient counseling, consulting with the physician, writing a report for the patient's chart, and filling out the billing information. In many cases, the audiologist seeks additional services for the patient. Most patients who come to an audiologist for hearing problems will receive a basic audiological assessment, including pure-tone audiometry, speech tests, immittance tests, and otoacoustic emissions. When appropriate, advanced tests may be scheduled, such as auditory brainstem response (ABR) or assessment of auditory processing disorders. In addition, audiologists are often involved with vestibular (balance) testing, tinnitus assessment, and facial nerve testing. Audiologists must keep up with technological advances and learn to incorporate new equipment and tests into their practice.

Audiologists are experts in hearing aid fittings. They determine hearing aid candidacy, perform hearing aid fittings, and verify and validate the hearing aid fitting and benefits (outcome measures). They remove ear wax (cerumen management) when appropriate, make ear impressions, order hearing aids from a selected manufacturer, handle the sales transaction, and provide the necessary orientation, counseling, and follow-up services. Audiologists also are knowledgeable about other assistive listening devices, such as FM or infrared amplifying devices, personal listening devices, amplified telephones, Bluetooth technology, and/or alarms for those who are deaf.

In many situations, audiologists are part of specialty teams consisting of physicians, nurses, and speech-language pathologists, working with patients who have cleft palate, cystic fibrosis, childhood hearing loss, or those being fit with cochlear implants or other implantable devices. Many audiologists are also involved with newborn hearing screening and work closely with pediatric nurses and trained volunteers or other hearing screening staff.

Audiologists use established and emerging technologies as tools to facilitate their patient care; however, it is important to realize that audiologists are the most knowledgeable of all professionals regarding the effects of hearing loss on communication, and how to improve the quality of life for individuals and families who are dealing with hearing loss. Counseling, treatment, and extended rehabilitation are very important and

with opportunities to work with other professionals (interprofessional practice). Audiologists in hospitals see a variety of interesting cases that need medical management, as well as audiological management, and are the perfect place to perform all those advanced audiological procedures and provide differential diagnoses. Many hospitals and university clinics also dispense hearing aids, and it is likely that this will increase in popularity.

REFERENCES

American Academy of Audiology [AAA]. (n.d.). How many audiology programs and students? Retrieved from http://www.audiology.org/news/how-many-audiology-programs-and-students

American Speech-Language-Hearing Association. (n.d.). ASHA summary membership and affiliation counts, year-end 2016. Retrieved from http://www.asha.org/uploadedFiles/2016-Member-Counts.pdf

Bureau of Labor Statistics—U.S. Department of Labor. (2017). *Occupational Outlook Handbook, 2016–2017 Edition, Audiologists.*

CareerCast. (2015). Least stressful jobs of 2015: 2. Audiologists. Retrieved from http://www.careercast.com/slide/least-stressful-jobs-2015-2-audiologist

CareerCast. (2017). Least stressful jobs of 2017. Retrieved from http://www.businessnewsdaily.com/1875-stressful-careers.html

DeBonis, D. A., & Donohue, C. L. (2007). *Survey of Audiology* (2nd ed.). Boston, MA: Pearson Allyn and Bacon.

Time Magazine. (2015). This is the best job in America. *Time Magazine, 13.*

Windmill, I. M., & Freeman, B. A. (2013). Demand for audiology services: 30 year projections and impact on academic programs. *Journal of the American Academy of Audiology, 24,* 407–416.

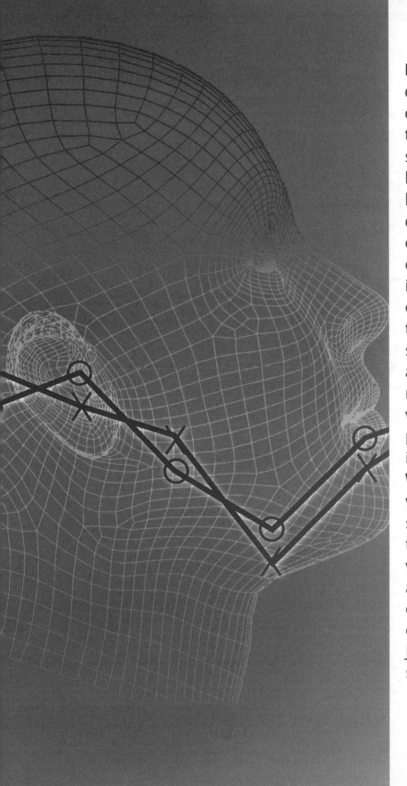

PART II

Fundamentals of Hearing Science

PART II of this textbook focuses on fundamental concepts in acoustics, and anatomy and physiology of the auditory system, as traditionally covered in hearing science courses. In Chapter 3, you will learn some important concepts regarding basic properties of sound, including frequency, amplitude, phase, physical properties of speech sounds, and an overview of some basic relations between the physical parameters of sound and their perceptions, called psychoacoustics. Chapter 4 covers the anatomy of the auditory system, with just a bit of vestibular (balance) system anatomy. For the interested reader, a more in-depth coverage of the vestibular system, including its anatomy, physiology, disorders, and common testing methods can be found in Chapter 16. While reading Chapter 4, you will find yourself eager to learn how the auditory system functions, but will have to be a little patient and wait for Chapter 5 where you will learn about the physiology of the auditory system and gain an appreciation of the intricacies and remarkable nature of how our ears process sound. The objective of Part II is to provide you with a solid foundation in hearing science that is important for understanding the clinical concepts presented in Part III of this textbook. Finally, you are encouraged to use the newly updated *Audiology Workbook* (Kramer & Small, 2019) to maximize your learning and enjoyment of the material covered in this section of the textbook.

3 Properties of Sound

After reading this chapter, you should be able to:

1. Describe how sound waves are produced, how they propagate, how fast they travel through air, and how they change with distance.

2. Define frequency, period, amplitude, starting phase, and wavelength; interpret time-domain waveforms of pure tones with different frequencies, amplitudes, and starting phases.

3. Define how intensity and pressure are related to each other; specify the minimum reference levels for intensity and pressure; specify the range of audibility for intensity (in watts/m^2) and pressure (in µPa).

4. Understand why and how to use decibels to quantify intensity and pressure; describe the range of audibility of intensity and pressure using decibels; define dB IL and dB SPL; describe the threshold of audibility across frequency.

5. Perform simple decibel calculations to compare the intensity and/or pressure of two sounds.

6. Explain the inverse square law and calculate how intensity or pressure changes with changes in distance.

7. Understand how to combine the outputs of two sounds and the resulting dB IL and dB SPL.

8. Describe periodic and aperiodic complex vibrations; interpret time-domain and spectral graphs of complex vibrations; describe the importance of Fourier analyses.

9. Describe the basic acoustic characteristics of speech and understand how to read spectrograms.

10. Understand how filtering can be used to shape the spectrum of noise; recognize commonly used filter shapes.

11. Explain what is meant by resonance; calculate resonance frequencies for simple tubes of varying length (open at both ends or only at one end); know the difference between a half-wave resonator and quarter-wave resonator.

19

12. Discuss and interpret graphs related to the psychoacoustic (perceptual) properties of loudness, pitch, temporal integration, and localization.

We live in a world of sounds, some of which are meaningful and some of which are just part of our noisy environment. We often take for granted the remarkable ability of the auditory system to extract meaningful sounds from the less meaningful so that we can sense danger, localize the source of a sound, communicate, learn, and even be entertained. Even when asleep we learn to tune out familiar sounds, but may wake up at an unfamiliar sound. At a noisy party, you can focus on a conversation with one person while ignoring the background conversations, but readily become aware when someone calls your name from across the room or your favorite song begins. When you listen to an orchestra or band you may find yourself listening to the whole song or picking out the various instruments. Our ability to hear in our everyday world requires the auditory system to process complex sounds from our environment. The process of hearing involves the generation of sounds, their travels and interactions within the environment, physiological processing by the ear, neural processing in the nervous system, and psychological/cognitive processing by the brain. The sounds we hear have basic physical properties that are processed by the auditory system into meaningful information.

Acoustics is the study of the physical properties of sounds in the environment, how they travel through air, and how they are affected by objects in their environment. As you will see in this chapter, any simple vibration can be uniquely described by its frequency, amplitude, and starting phase. Complex vibrations can be described as combinations of simple vibrations. However, not all sounds generated in the environment are audible and the audible range may be different across species; for example, dogs and cats are more responsive to higher pitched sounds than are humans. The human ear is capable of hearing a wide range of frequencies over an extensive range of amplitudes. But how does frequency relate to our perception of pitch? How does amplitude relate to our perception of loudness? How do we compare the loudness of sounds across frequencies? How do we use our two ears to localize the source of sounds? These types of questions come under the area of *psychoacoustics*, which is the study of how we perceive sound. The psychoacoustic aspects of sound covered in this chapter include some basic perceptions of pitch, loudness, temporal integration, and localization. After reading this chapter, perhaps you will be able to answer the age-old philosophical question that goes something like, "If a tree falls in the woods and there are no living creatures around, does it make a sound?"

The definitions and terminology reviewed in this chapter are necessary to be able to better understand topics that are covered in the following chapters, including the physiology of the auditory system, the clinical procedures used to evaluate hearing loss, and the function of hearing aids. A thorough understanding of acoustics requires knowledge of some mathematical concepts and formulas; however, in this introductory text, only the basic concepts are presented and every attempt is made to keep the mathematics to a minimum. The interested reader is referred to other textbooks (Gelfand, 2009; Mullin, Gerace, Mestre, & Velleman, 2003; Speaks, 2017; Villchur, 2000) for a more thorough treatment of acoustics and psychoacoustics.

SIMPLE VIBRATIONS AND SOUND TRANSMISSION

Sounds are produced because of an object being set into vibration. Some familiar examples include vibrations of tuning forks, guitar strings, other musical instruments, stereo speakers, engines, thunder, and the vocal cords while speaking. Almost any object can be made to vibrate, but some objects vibrate more easily than other objects depending on their mass and elasticity. Although most sounds in our environment are complex vibrations, we begin by looking at very simple vibrations called *pure tones*. Pure tones are used by audiologists as part of the basic hearing evaluation. In addition, an understanding of pure tones is useful because all complex vibrations can be described as combinations of different pure tones, which was mathematically proven by a man named Fourier. Today, we have electronic instruments that can perform *fast Fourier transforms (FFTs)* to determine the different pure tones that comprise any complex vibration.

The vibrating sound source sets up sound waves that travel, called *propagation* (*propagate*), through some elastic medium, such as air, water, and most solids. Propagation of sound through air occurs because of the back and forth movement of air molecules around their position of equilibrium in response to the back and forth vibration of an object. The air molecules closest to the vibrating object move back and forth first. Because of the inertial and elastic properties of the air molecules, the air molecules only move within a localized region, but as they push against adjacent air molecules the process repeats itself, which causes the *pressure* variations to propagate through the medium. When the vibrating object moves outward, the air molecules are pushed together causing an increase in the density of air molecules (more molecules per volume), called *condensation*, and this corresponds to an increase in sound pressure. When the vibrating object moves in the opposite direction, there is a decrease in the density of air molecules, called *rarefaction*, and this corresponds to a decrease in sound pressure. Figure 3–1 illustrates how these increases and decreases in the density of air molecules occur in response to a simple vibrating object such as a *tuning fork*. When the vibration repeats itself over and over, as depicted in Figure 3–1, there are continuing cycles of condensation and rarefaction that produce a continuous sound that can be measured at different points in the surrounding area. In Figure 3–1, you can see the areas in which the air molecules are more densely packed (condensations) and where the air molecules are less densely packed (rarefactions). The condensa-

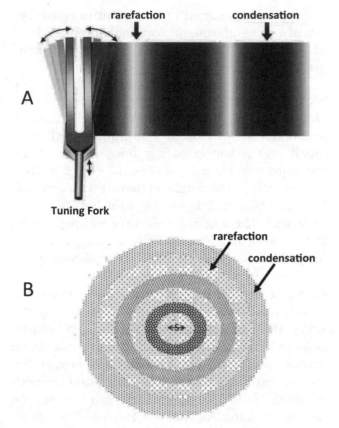

FIGURE 3–1. A and B. Illustration showing propagation of air molecules to a vibrating sound source. **A.** Tuning fork vibration producing alternating areas of increased density of air molecules (condensation) and decreased density of air molecules (rarefaction) that are propagated across the air from its source. **B.** Sound waves as they propagated spherically away from the sound source with alternating condensation and rarefaction phases. As the distance from the sound source increases, the force is distributed over a wider area.

tions and rarefactions reflect a repetitive pattern of increasing and decreasing air pressure. For unobstructed sound waves in air, the air molecules move outward in a spherical direction and the actual size of the air pressure peak (amplitude) diminishes with distance because of friction, as well as because the pressure is being radiated in an increasing spherical pattern. At some distance from the source, the pressure will no longer be measurable because the energy is spread out over a large enough spherical area. The actual amplitude of a sound at any point in space obviously depends on the original intensity level of the sound, that is, louder sounds will travel greater distances than softer sounds.

Sound propagation can also be influenced by how the waves are reflected or interfered with by objects or walls. Much of our real-world listening situations are in closed environments, whereby much of the sound energy does not penetrate the walls but instead bounces off or is absorbed by the walls. The angle at which a sound will bounce off a wall is similar to a ball bouncing off a wall. The angle of reflection will depend on the angle of incidence relative to the perpendicular. This becomes even more complicated when the encountered object is curved (convex or concave), or in a room with four walls, where the sound may bounce back and forth among the walls. How sound waves might interact with an object in its environment is also important. Some sounds will bounce off an object, whereas other sounds easily go around the object, and depends primarily on the sound's wavelength (see section on wavelength). As you will learn in the following sections, there are also areas in which the condensation phase of a wave meets up with another wave's rarefaction phase, resulting in wave cancellation (where no sound is present). In addition, materials have certain absorption characteristics that come into play in determining how sounds act in the real world. Understanding acoustics in these types of environments is especially important when designing theater or music venues (something acoustic engineers are trained to do, but it is well beyond the scope of this textbook).

Another characteristic of sound waves is the speed or velocity with which they are propagated through the medium. Sound travels faster in water and most solids than it does in air. The *speed of sound* in air is about 343 m/s or 1126 feet/s,[1] which is much slower than the 186,282 miles per second that light travels. You probably use this knowledge, maybe unknowingly, when you estimate how many miles away you are from a storm by counting the seconds between seeing the lightning (seen instantaneously) and hearing the thunder (heard later). Your estimate of how far away the storm is will be more accurate if you divide the number of counted seconds by five to take into account that the speed of sound is about one-fifth of a mile per second.

When the increases and decreases in pressure occur in the direction of the vibrating object, as for sound waves, the sound is called a *longitudinal wave*. The process of localized back and forth movement of air molecules results in the propagation of a longitudinal sound wave through the air, more precisely in a spherical pattern. When this sound wave reaches the ear, the corresponding condensations and rarefactions in air pressure cause the tympanic membrane to move in and out, thus beginning the process of hearing. You will see in the next chapter how vibrations are received by the ear and how the ear transforms the incoming vibrations into auditory information. Before that, however, we need to turn our attention to understanding the basic physical parameters of sound, frequency, amplitude, and starting phase.

FREQUENCY

Pure tones are characterized by regular repetitive movements. Imagine holding a pencil in your hand and moving it up and down on a piece of paper at a consistent height and speed. As you are moving your hand up and down, begin to move the paper from right to left; you should see a pattern that looks something like those shown in Figure 3–2. The actual separation of the peaks that are produced will depend on the speed at which you move the paper (the slower the paper, the closer the peaks). To be able to quantify the pattern of vibratory movement, the motion is displayed as a function of time along the x-axis. The y-axis represents a measure of magnitude or amplitude of the vibrations (e.g., how far up and down you moved your hand). When the pattern of movement is displayed with amplitude as a function of time, it is called a *time-domain waveform* or simply a *waveform*.

---

[1]The speed of sound in air is dependent upon both the temperature and the density. The value used in this textbook is an approximation for 68°F. The speed of sound in air slows down as temperature decreases, for example, it is about 341 m/s or 1086 feet/s at 32°F.

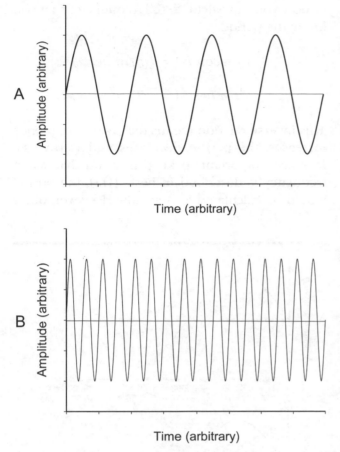

FIGURE 3–2. A and B. Representations of two different pure-tone vibration patterns as a function of time in arbitrary units. The vibration in (**A**) is slower than the vibration in (**B**) even though the time scales are equal.

A *cycle* of vibration describes the pattern of movement as the object goes through its full range of motion one time. In other words, one cycle represents the movement of an object from its starting point to its maximum peak, then to its negative peak, then back to its starting point. Figure 3–3 shows one cycle of a pure tone.

Most vibrations repeat themselves; therefore, pure tones are usually described by how many cycles occur in 1 second (s), called *frequency* of vibration. However, instead of using cycles per second as the unit of measure for frequency, the term *hertz (Hz)* is used to mean the same thing. For example, a vibration that repeats itself 100 cycles in 1 s is called a 100 Hz pure tone. Conversely, a 100 Hz pure tone would complete 100

cycles in 1 s. An 8000 Hz pure tone completes 8000 cycles in 1 second. The *frequency range of audibility for humans* is from 20 to 20,000 Hz.

Figure 3–4 shows some examples of different frequencies as they would appear on paper when graphed with a 1 s time scale. As you can notice, it is difficult to visually count the number of cycles as the frequency increases, and counting would be extremely difficult for much of the audible frequency range if graphed using a 1 s time scale. However, another way to graphically represent the different frequencies of pure tones is to change the time scale along the *x*-axis. In other words, only a few cycles (or even a single cycle) are plotted over a specified time scale. The actual frequency is calculated from knowing how long it takes to complete one cycle, called the *period* of the vibration. Figure 3–5 shows some examples of how the period is related to frequency. In Figure 3–5A, you can see that the time it takes to complete the one cycle is equal to 0.01 s (one hundredth of a second), which means it would be able to complete 100 cycles in 1.0 s (100 Hz). In Figure 3–5B, the time it takes to complete the one cycle is 0.001 s, which means this vibration would be able to complete 1000 cycles in 1 s (1000 Hz). In Figure 3–5C, the time it takes to complete the

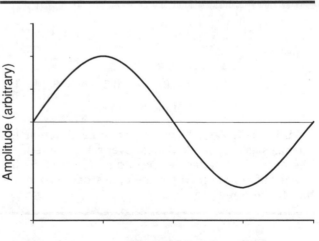

FIGURE 3–3. Time domain waveform showing one cycle of vibration. The vibration moves from its starting point to its maximum peak (amplitude), then to its negative peak, then back to its starting point as a function of time.

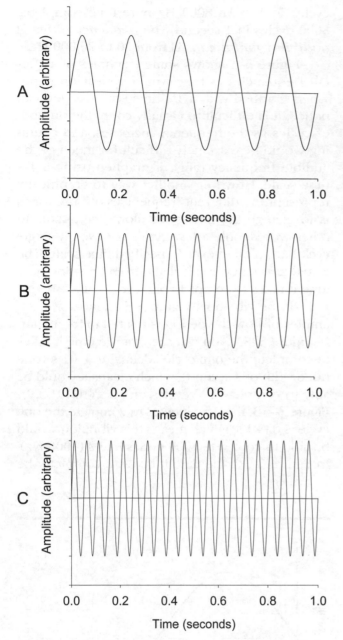

FIGURE 3–4. A–C. Examples of three different frequencies as they would appear over a 1.0 s time scale. The number of cycles per second determines the frequency of vibration. The more cycles per second, the higher the frequency.

or how you can calculate the frequency (f) if you know the period:

$$T \text{ (in seconds)} = 1/f \text{ (in hertz)}$$

$$f \text{ (in hertz)} = 1/T \text{ (in seconds)}$$

This inverse relation means that as the frequency increases, the period decreases and vice versa. It is also important to keep in mind that when frequency is described in hertz (Hz), the period would be calculated as seconds. However, other

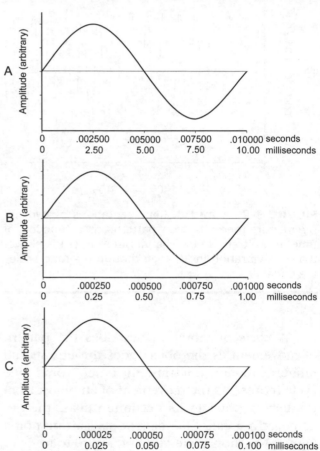

FIGURE 3–5. A–C. One cycle of vibration for three different frequencies, each plotted with a different time scale. The time it takes to complete one cycle is the period. In (**A**) the period is equal to 0.01 s (one-hundredth of a second), which means the vibrating object would be able to complete 100 cycles in 1.0 s (100 Hz). In (**B**), the period is 0.001 s, which means this vibration would be able to complete 1000 cycles in 1 s (1000 Hz). In (**C**) the period is equal to .0001 s, which means this vibration would be able to complete 10,000 cycles in 1 s (10,000 Hz).

one cycle is 0.0001 s, which means this vibration would be able to complete 10,000 cycles in 1 s (10,000 Hz). You can see that there is a reciprocal trade-off between the period and the frequency. The following equation shows how you can calculate the period (T) if you know the frequency,

TABLE 3–1. Relationship between Frequency and Period (in Seconds and Milliseconds) for Commonly Used Frequencies

Frequency (Hz)	Period (s)	Period (ms)
250	0.004	4.0
500	0.002	2.0
1000	0.001	1.0
2000	0.0005	0.5
4000	0.00025	0.25
8000	0.000125	0.125

units are often used, and you must be sure to use the appropriate units when making conversions between frequency and period. For example, frequency is often measured in units of *kilohertz* (kHz) (*kilo* means 1000), such that 1 kHz = 1000 Hz, 2 kHz = 2000 Hz, and so forth. In addition, the period of pure tones is often measured in units of *milliseconds* (ms) (milli means 1/1000), such that 1 ms = .001 s, 2 ms = .002 s, and so forth. Table 3–1 shows the relation between period and frequency for pure tones commonly used in studies of hearing and hearing tests. As the pattern in Table 3–1 shows, for each doubling of frequency, the period decreases by half; and for each halving of frequency, the period doubles. To help understand the relations in Table 3–1, try covering one column at a time and see if you can fill in the correct information by using the information in the other columns. Fortunately, there is an electronic instrument, a *frequency counter*, that can be used to measure the frequency of pure tones.

PHASE

Pure tones are also called *sine waves* or *sinusoids* because of their relationship to a sine function. As illustrated in Figure 3–6, one cycle of a pure tone is the equivalent of making a full revolution around a circle, where each point on the waveform can be described by its sine function relative to its phase angle (sin θ). You can think of a vibration starting at the object's resting (non-vibratory) state, designated as zero degrees [sin (0) = 0], then reaching its maximum positive

peak at 90° [sin (90°) = 1)], returning to its initial point at 180° [sin (180°) = 0], reaching its maximum negative peak at 270° [sin (270°) = −1], and finally returning to its starting point at 360° [sin (360°) = 0]. As Figure 3–6 shows, any point on the waveform can be found using the relationship sin θ = x/r. For example, if θ = 45°, then:

$$x = r [sin (45°)]$$

$$x = r (0.707)$$

Starting phase refers to the point along the waveform's cycle where the vibration begins, and is expressed in degrees relative to the angle around the circle. In other words, does the vibration first begin to move in the condensation direction or the rarefaction direction, and from what point does it begin? The waveforms shown in the previous figures have been plotted with a 0° starting phase, which means that the vibration begins from its equilibrium point and first moves toward the condensation peak, conventionally plotted as positive amplitude in the upward direction. Waveforms can begin at any point in their range of movement, and initially move toward the condensation peak or rarefaction peak. Figure 3–7 shows an example of a sinusoid with a 180° starting phase. In this case, the vibration

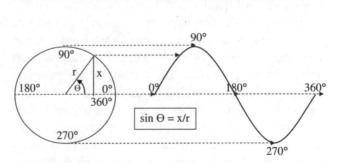

FIGURE 3–6. The projection of one cycle of a pure tone as it would appear relative to its position on a circle. One cycle of a waveform is the equivalent of making a full revolution around a circle. For example, the peak positive (condensation) point is equivalent to a 90° angle relative to the beginning point. The peak negative (rarefaction) point is equivalent to 270° (three-quarters around the circle). Equilibrium points occur at 0°, 180°, and 360°. These simple vibrations are often called sine waves because each point on the waveform can be expressed as a sine function (sin θ = x/r) relative to its angle (θ).

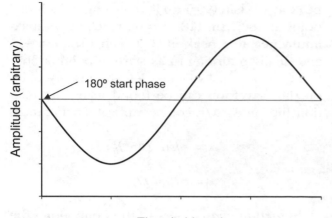

FIGURE 3–7. One cycle of a pure tone beginning at 180° starting phase. In this example, the movement begins in the direction of the rarefaction phase of vibration.

begins at its equilibrium point, but first moves toward the rarefaction peak and continues its full cycle until it ends up back in equilibrium at the 180° starting point. Figure 3–8 shows an example of two waveforms with the same frequency, but with different starting phases, one with a 90° starting phase and one with a 270° starting phase. A 90° starting phase means that the vibration begins from its point of maximum condensation, moves to its equilibrium point (amplitude = 0), continues to its point of maximum rarefaction, back to its equilibrium point, and finally ends its cycle at the point of maximum condensation (where it began). A 270° starting phase means that the vibration begins from its point of maximum rarefaction, moves to its equilibrium point, continues to its point of maximum condensation, back to its equilibrium point, and finally ends its cycle back at the point of maximum rarefaction (where it began).

Our ears are not sensitive, per se, to the starting phase; a pure tone with a starting phase of 0° will sound the same as with a starting phase of 270°. However, starting phase, or phase in general, has more relevance when two or more sounds interact with each other acoustically, before reaching the ear. For the example in Figure 3–8, can you predict what the resulting sound would be? If you answered, "no sound," you

would be correct, since in this example the two waveforms would cancel each other out due to the condensation in one wave offset by the same amount of rarefaction in the other wave. Figure 3–9 again demonstrates this phase interaction with two relatively simple examples, in which two tones of the same frequency, but with opposite starting phases, are combined. For the two examples in Figure 3–9, the two tones are 180° out-of-phase with each other. Notice that the 180° out-of-phase relation between these (or any) two pure tones of the same frequency is maintained at all points in the waveform. Again, for these examples there would be no resulting sound pressure (and no sound) generated because each condensation point would be cancelled out by an equal rarefaction point, and the net displacement would be zero. Figure 3–10 shows two examples of what happens when you combine two tones of the same frequency that are not 180° out of phase. In these examples, the phase relations of the two waves are more complicated and can produce places of cancellation when the points are in opposite phase directions or produce places of enhancement when the points are in the same phase direction. The interaction of two pure tones becomes even more complicated when they are of different frequencies as shown in Figure 3–11. In these relatively

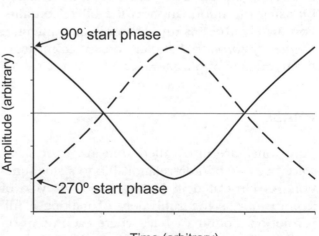

FIGURE 3–8. Two pure tones at the same frequency, but with different starting phases. In this example, the two waveforms are 180° out of phase with each other.

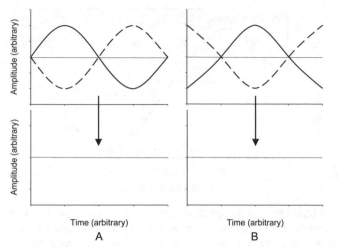

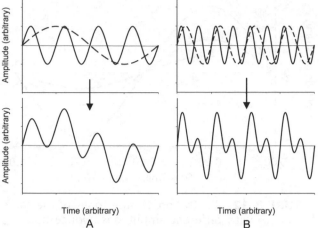

FIGURE 3–9. A and B. An illustration of how two pure tones of the same frequency, but 180° out of phase to each other, will cancel each other out. In (**A**) the *solid curve* represents a sound with a 0° starting phase and the *dashed curve* represents a sound with a 180° starting phase. In (**B**) the *solid curve* represents a sound with a 270° starting phase and the *dashed curve* represents a sound with a 90° starting phase.

FIGURE 3–11. A and B. Examples of how two pure tones with different frequencies, but with the same starting phase, combine to give different patterns of vibration resulting from the summation of the two original waveforms.

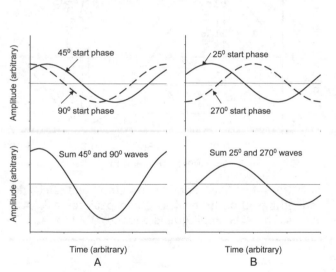

FIGURE 3–10. A and B. Examples of how two pure tones of the same frequency, but with different starting phases, can result in different patterns of vibration resulting from the summation of the two original waveforms.

resultant combination of pure tones at any point in time is called the *instantaneous phase*. When a sound is made up of more than one pure tone, the resultant waveform no longer matches the pattern of a sine wave (i.e., simple wave) and is considered to be a complex vibration. As more pure tones are combined, with or without the same starting phases, the less the waveform resembles a sinusoid (complex vibrations are discussed more in a later section of the chapter).

AMPLITUDE

Amplitude is a general term to describe the magnitude of a sound; the larger the magnitude, the higher the amplitude. Figure 3–12 shows the waveforms of pure tones with the same frequency and starting phase, but with different maximum amplitudes along the y-axis.[2] For a vibrating

simple examples, the pairs of pure tones have the same 0° starting phase, but because they are of different frequencies the phase relation between the two pure tones changes at different points in time. The phase of an individual pure tone or

[2]One can describe any sinusoidal vibration by the following equation: $a(t) = A \sin(2\pi ft + \theta)$ where $a(t)$ is the instantaneous amplitude as a function of time, A is the maximum amplitude, $2\pi f$ (also called angular velocity, ω) is a measure of revolutions around a circle, and θ is the starting phase in radians.

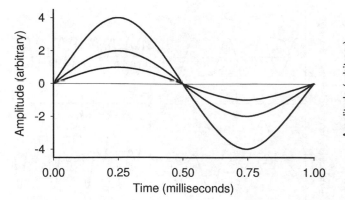

FIGURE 3–12. Illustration of pure tones of the same frequency with different amplitudes. Notice how the period of the vibration is the same for all three waveforms and only the height of the waveforms is different.

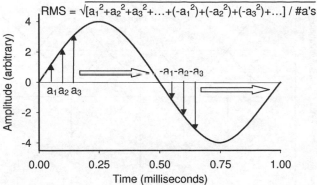

$$RMS = \sqrt{[a_1^2+a_2^2+a_3^2+...+(-a_1^2)+(-a_2^2)+(-a_3^2)+...] / \#a's}$$

FIGURE 3–13. Quantification of amplitude by the method of root mean square (RMS). The instantaneous amplitudes across the waveform are squared to remove the negative numbers, then averaged to find the mean, and finally the square root of the number is determined to get the total RMS value.

object, maximum amplitude is related to how far the object moves back and forth. For sounds propagated through air, larger amplitudes create greater amounts of condensation and rarefaction of the air molecules. The amplitude scale along the y-axis is often expressed in units of displacement, intensity, or pressure.

Amplitudes vary across the waveform; therefore, we need to have a way to specify the overall amplitude of a waveform. Because pure tones have equal positive and negative amplitudes, taking an average of the amplitudes at all points would result in zero amplitude and would not be useful at all. Instead, it is common to use the *root-mean-square* (RMS) *amplitude* (A_{rms}) to obtain an average amplitude for the waveform. As shown in Figure 3–13, to obtain the RMS amplitude: (1) square each of the instantaneous amplitudes to eliminate any negative values, (2) average the squared values, and (3) take the square root of the average. The RMS amplitude is used in many applications and, fortunately, there are electronic instruments available that directly measure the RMS amplitudes of pure tones and other sounds. Figure 3–14 illustrates two other ways to describe the overall amplitude of pure tones. One way is to take the amplitude change between the positive peak and the negative peak, called *peak-to-peak amplitude* (A_{p-p}). Another way is to measure the amplitude from baseline (zero) to one of the peaks, called *peak amplitude* (A_p). The RMS

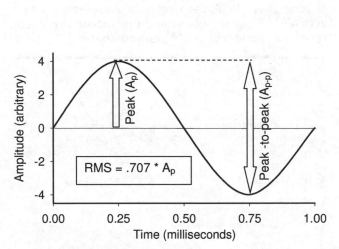

FIGURE 3–14. Illustration of how amplitude can be described based on its peak (A_p) and peak-to-peak (A_{p-p}) values. The RMS amplitude is equal to $0.707 \times A_p$.

amplitude for a pure tone is equal to 0.707 times the peak amplitude; however, this is not the case for more complex sounds.

INTENSITY AND PRESSURE

The overall amplitude of a sound wave is typically quantified and measured in units of sound pressure or sound intensity to describe how the sound

SYNOPSIS 3-1

- The back and forth vibration of a sound source sets up alternating areas where the air molecules are pushed together, called condensation, and areas where the air molecules are pulled apart, called rarefaction. The air molecules move only within a small localized area, but the condensation and rarefaction areas are passed to adjacent air molecules, which cause the waveform's pressure variations to move through the medium. Sound waves travel in air at a speed of about 343 m/s (at 68⁰ F).
- Simple vibrations, called pure tones, sine waves, or sinusoids, are characterized by their physical (acoustic) dimensions of frequency (or period), amplitude, and starting phase.
- The frequency of a sound refers to the number of vibrations that occur in 1 second and has units of hertz (Hz) or kilohertz (kHz); 1 kHz = 1000 Hz. The reciprocal of frequency is the period (T), which is the time it takes to complete one cycle of vibration and has units of seconds (s) or milliseconds (ms) (1 ms = 1/1000 s). If either the frequency or period is known, the other can be calculated ($f = 1/T$ or $T = 1/f$).
- The frequency range for human hearing is about 20 to 20,000 Hz. Other species may be sensitive to other frequency ranges.
- The starting phase of a sound refers to what position in the cycle a vibration begins its cycle, and is expressed in units of degrees around a circle (0 to 360°). For example, a vibration that begins at its equilibrium and moves toward its area of maximum condensation has a starting phase of 0°; a vibration that begins at the point of maximum rarefaction and moves toward equilibrium has a starting phase of 270°.
- For a single pure tone, humans cannot tell the difference between starting phases. Combining two or more pure tones of the same frequency, but with different starting phases, results in different phase relations at different points in time (instantaneous phase) and produces a complex waveform that is the sum of the two waveforms. Two pure tones of the same frequency that are 180° out of phase will cancel each other out and not produce any sound.
- The amplitude of a sound refers to how far an object moves back and forth and/or the amount of maximum and minimum air pressure created. The larger the movement or pressure variation, the greater the amplitude for any given frequency. A simple way to describe amplitude of a visually displayed waveform is to measure the distance or pressure between the highest point of condensation peak and the lowest point of rarefaction peak, called peak-to-peak amplitude ($A_{p\text{-}p}$). Measures can also be made between the condensation or rarefaction peak to the equilibrium point, called peak amplitude (A_p). A more practical measure is called root-mean-square (RMS) amplitude, which is the way that instruments measure a sound's overall amplitude. The RMS method averages the amplitudes across the entire waveform by squaring each value (to remove all negative values), then averaging these squared values, and finally taking the square root to bring it back into scale.

energy is distributed over some area of the propagating wave. For any given sound wave, there is a corresponding sound intensity and sound pressure. If you know either the intensity or the pressure, the other quantity can be derived. Intensity and pressure are related to each other by the following formulas:

$$I = p^2$$

$$p = \sqrt{I}$$

It should be intuitive that the farther away you are from a sound's source, the softer it will become. As the sound gets further away from the sound source (assuming there are no obstructions), it is distributed over a greater spherical area, as illustrated in Figure 3–15.

The decrease in a sound's intensity with distance is known as the *inverse square law*. The inverse square law states that the intensity (I) is inversely (decreases) related to the square of the distance between any two points (D), and is expressed by the following formula:

$$I = 1/D^2, \text{ where } D = d_1/d_2$$

For example, if the distance is doubled ($D = 2$; $d_1/d_2 = 2/1$), the intensity decreases by one-fourth ($I = 1/2^2$). Now let's see how that same sound's pressure (p) would change with distance. Because of the previously discussed relation between intensity and pressure for any given sound wave, the inverse square law for pressure is obtained by substituting p^2 for I in the above formula, which results in the following formula to describe how pressure changes with distance:

$$p^2 = 1/D^2$$

$$p = 1/D, \text{ where } D = d_1/d_2$$

This formula says that the sound pressure is inversely (decreases) related to the distance between two points (D), rather than the square of the distance that was used for intensity. For example, if the distance is doubled ($D = 2$; $d_1/d_2 = 2/1$), the pressure decreases by one half ($p = 1/2$).

Sound *intensity* is actually a measure of power that is distributed over an area, and has units of watts/m² or watts/cm² depending on the system of measurement being used (MKS or CGS). Sound pressure is a measure of force distributed over an area and has units of dynes/cm², newton/m², or micropascals (μPa) depending on the system of measurement being used. For this text, we will only use units of watts/m² for intensity and μPa for pressure. For our purposes, we are most interested in the range of sound intensities or pressures that are audible, that is, from the smallest amount needed to barely hear a sound, up to the largest amount that the ear can tolerate. Based on accepted standards derived from the lowest average levels (thresholds) obtained from young adults, the lowest average intensity needed to hear a sound, called the *reference level for intensity*, is 0.000000000001 w/m² (or 1.0×10^{-12} w/m²). The lowest average pressure needed to hear a sound, called the *reference level for pressure*, is 20 μPa (or 2.0×10^1 μPa). Remarkably, these lower levels of audition correspond roughly to a vibration about the size of a hydrogen molecule (Gelfand, 2009). The highest intensity (also called the threshold of pain) that can be tolerated is approximately 100 w/m² (or 1.0×10^2 w/m²). The highest pressure that can be tolerated is approximately 200,000,000 μPa (or 2.0×10^8 μPa). As you can see, the upper tolerated limit of sound intensity is 100,000,000,000,000 (or 10^{14}) times greater than the least audible sound (i.e., from 1.0×10^2 w/m² to 1.0×10^{-12} w/m²). For

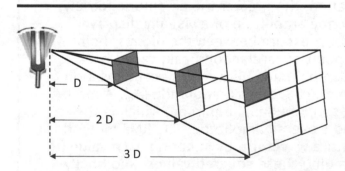

FIGURE 3–15. Illustration of how the energy of a sound is distributed over a larger area as the distance from the sound source is doubled and tripled, and is the basis for the inverse square law.

TABLE 3–2. Intensity and Pressure Ranges from the Least Audible (Reference Level) to the Upper Limit that Is Tolerated (Pain Threshold)

	Intensity (w/m²)[a]		Pressure (µPa)[b]	
Upper limit (pain)	100	or 1×10^2	200,000,000	or 20×10^7
				(or 2.0×10^8)
Lowest audible (reference level)	0.0000000000001	or 1×10^{-12}	20	or 20×10^0
				(or 2.0×10^1)

[a]Watts per square meter.
[b]MicroPascals.

pressure, the upper tolerated limit is 10,000,000 (or 10^7) times greater than for the least audible sound (i.e., from 2.0×10^1 µPa to 2.0×10^8 µPa). Recall that intensity and pressure are related by $p = \sqrt{I}$; therefore, it follows that the range of pressures (10^7) is equal to the square root of the range of intensities ($\sqrt{10^{14}} = 10^7$).

Table 3–2 summarizes the intensity and pressure ranges for the human ear. It may have struck you by now that these amplitude ranges are quite large, and it would be quite cumbersome if you were trying to graph them on a linear scale (*y*-axis). Fortunately, linear scales can be transformed into ratio scales, as described in the next section on decibels, and makes working with intensity and pressure ranges much more manageable.

DECIBELS

To avoid linear scales of intensity or pressure ranges that would require working with large numbers or scientific notation, we transform these scales into a more manageable scale called the *decibel scale*. Any decibel scale is a ratio scale in which a measured value is related to a specified reference value. For example, as was mentioned above, the most intense sound that can be tolerated is 10^{14} times greater than the lowest sound intensity that can be heard. If we consider the lowest audible sound intensity as the reference, this least audible sound could be expressed as 1 or 10^0; then the range of sound intensity can be written as a ratio of $10^{14}/10^0$. The next step

in the transformation to a decibel scale is to take the logarithm[3] (or log) of that ratio, the *Bel*. The log is the mathematical difference in the values of the exponents in the ratio. Stated another way, the log is the power to which 10 must be raised to produce the number defined by the ratio. In our example, the mathematical difference in the exponents is 14 (14-0), which means that the range for intensity, in Bels, would be from 0 (least intense) to 14 (most intense). The upper limit would be the same as saying that 10 must be raised to the 14th power (10^{14}). Because the range for Bels only goes from 0 to 14, it is considered too restrictive to effectively describe the range of audible sounds; thus, to expand the range, the Bel is multiplied by a factor of 10 and is called the *decibel* (dB). The decibel equation can be written as:

$$dB = 10 \log (X_{meas}/X_{ref})$$

where X_{meas} equals the sound that is being measured, and X_{ref} equals the reference sound to which X_{meas} is to be compared. It is important to see that when the measured value is the same as

---

[3]A logarithm of a number, in base 10 ($\log_{10}$), is the power to which 10 must be raised to obtain that number. Some simple examples are for powers of 10, in which the exponent is the log; for example, the log of 1000 or $10^3 = 3$. It is also important to remember that the log (1) = 0. Another useful example that you may want to memorize is log (2) = 0.3. Calculators can be used to find logs of other less obvious numbers. Other sources, such as Speaks (2017), should be consulted for a review of logarithms.

the reference value, that is, $X_{meas}/X_{ref} = 1$, the measured value would be equal to 0 dB because the log of 1 (or log 10^0) is equal to zero. Applying a decibel conversion to describe the range of sound intensity, the upper limit of intensity would be 140 dB greater than the least audible intensity, as determined by the following calculation:

dB intensity (at upper limit)

$= 10 \log (10^{14}/10^0)$
$= 10 \log (10^{14})$
$= 10 (14)$, where log of 10^{14} equals 14
$= 140$ dB

The formula for converting to decibels can be applied to anything that can be expressed as a ratio if the reference value is known. For example, we could calculate the decibel difference between a large bag of oranges (X_{meas}) as compared with a small bag of oranges (X_{ref}). If there are twice as many oranges in the larger bag than the smaller bag, there would be 3 dB more oranges in the larger bag than in the smaller bag, as shown in the following calculation:

dB in bag of oranges with twice as many as the reference bag:

$= 10 \log (2/1)$
$= 10 \log (2)$
$= 10 (0.3)$, where log of 2 equals .3
$= 3$ dB

Decibels of Intensity Level (dB IL)

Let's look at another example and calculate how many dB some arbitrary measured intensity is above the lowest average intensity needed to hear. In other words, how much more intense is this measured higher intensity level above the lowest possible audible intensity? Recall that the lowest average intensity needed to hear a sound, called the standard reference level for intensity, is 1×10^{-12} w/m² (or simply 10^{-12} w/m²). Let's say we measure a sound intensity to be 1×10^{-6} w/m². The calculation of dB intensity is:

dB intensity $= 10 \log (10^{-6}$ w/m²$/10^{-12}$ w/m²$)$

Whenever the standard reference value for intensity (10^{-12} w/m²) is used or implied in the denominator of the decibel formula, this is called *decibel intensity level (dB IL)*. The general equation for dB IL is:

dB IL $= 10 \log (I_{meas}$ w/m²$/10^{-12}$ w/m²$)$.

When the measured intensity is the same as the reference level for intensity (10^{-12} w/m²$/10^{-12}$ w/m²), in decibels this would be the 10 log (1), which would become 0 dB IL. By using a decibel scale, we can define the intensity range of human hearing from 0 to 140 dB IL. It is important to realize that 0 dB IL does not mean the absence of sound; it only means that the measured sound intensity is the same as the standard reference intensity. However, as you will see later, the lowest audible intensity is different depending on frequency, type of earphones, and other specified listening conditions, but all these variations are always referenced to the universally accepted standard reference intensity of 1.0×10^{-12} w/m².

Now let's look at some other examples. Suppose you make a sound measurement and find it to be 10^{-5} w/m² (0.00001 w/m²). How many dB IL is this sound? The calculation is as follows:

dB intensity level (dB IL) for a measured sound $= 10^{-5}$ w/m²

$= 10 \log (10^{-5}$ w/m²$/10^{-12}$ w/m²$)$
$= 10 \log (10^7)$
$= 10 (7)$, where log of 10^7 equals 7
$= 70$ dB

The decibel can be used to describe the ratio of any two numbers if the proper reference value is specified in the denominator. Suppose you are interested in expressing, in dB, how the intensity of one sound compares with the intensity of another sound. For example, assume that one sound has an intensity that is 10,000 times more intense than another sound. In this case, the less intense sound can be considered the reference and written as 1 in the denominator; the ratio of these two sounds would be 10,000/1 (i.e., without needing to use the 10^{-12} w/m²). The dB of the louder sound, as referenced to the softer sound, is calculated as follows:

dB intensity of a sound 10,000 times greater than another sound

= 10 log (10,000/1)
= 10 log (10^4)
= 10 (4), where log of 10^4 equals 4
= 40 dB

As another example, if the intensity of a sound is doubled, how many dB has that sound increased? In this example, the increase in intensity can be thought of as a ratio of 2/1 (the louder sound is twice as intense as the softer sound) and, therefore, would show an increase of 3 dB. The calculation is as follows:

dB intensity of a sound twice as much as another sound (increase)

= 10 log (2/1)
= 10 (0.3), where the log of 2 equals 0.3
= 3 dB

This concept and use of the formula would also apply if one were to decrease the intensity level of a sound. For example, if one sound is half the intensity of another sound, the ratio would be 1/2. The calculation is as follows:

dB intensity of a sound half as much as another sound (decrease)

= 10 log (1/2)
= 10 (–0.3), where the log of 2 equals –0.3
= –3 dB

If you find it easier, the above example could be calculated using a ratio of 2/1, but then be sure to indicate that it is negative (representing a decrease): Notice that in both cases, the answer is 3 dB (either positive or negative).

Decibels of Sound Pressure Level (dB SPL)

In audiology, decibels of sound pressure are commonly used. To derive the decibel scale for sound pressure, it is important to go back to the previous relation between pressure and inten-

sity ($I = p^2$). This relation requires that pressure squared (p^2) be substituted for intensity (I) in the general equation for decibels. The derivation is as follows:

dB sound pressure

= 10 log (p^2_{meas}/p^2_{ref})
= 10 log (p_{meas}/p_{ref})^2
= 20 log (p_{meas}/p_{ref}), where log (x)^2 equals 2 log (x)

Notice that for dB of sound pressure, the log of the pressure ratio is multiplied by 20 instead of by 10 that was used for dB of sound intensity. Using the formula for dB of sound pressure, any pressure ratio can be expressed in decibels. The decibel scale for sound pressure would also range from 0 to 140 dB because the upper limit for pressure is 10^7 times greater than the lowest pressure. The calculation is expressed as follows:

dB pressure (at upper limit)

= 20 log (10^7/10^0)
= 20 log (10^7)
= 20 (7), where log of 10^7 equals 7
= 140 dB

Recall that the standard reference sound pressure level is 20 μPa. When a measured pressure is compared to this standard reference pressure, that is, when the specific reference value for sound pressure is used or implied in the denominator of the formula for dB sound pressure, this is called decibel *sound pressure level (dB SPL)*. The formula for dB SPL is:

dB SPL = 20 log (P_{meas} μPa/20 μPa)

Whenever the measured sound pressure is equal to the standard reference level for sound pressure it would be equal to 0 dB SPL (i.e., 20 log [1] = 0). Using dB SPL, we have now defined the range of human hearing from 0 to 140 dB SPL. It is important to realize that 0 dB of sound pressure does not mean the absence of sound pressure; it only means that the measured sound pressure is the same as the standard reference sound pressure. A sound that is 0 dB SPL has the same pressure as the standard reference pressure of 20 μPa. However, as with intensity, the lowest audible pressure can depend on frequency, type of earphones, and other specified listening conditions, but these are always referenced to the universally accepted standard reference pressure of 20 μPa.

Let's look at some other decibel examples using pressure. Suppose you make a sound measurement and find it to be 200,000 μPa. What is the dB SPL of this sound? The calculation is as follows:

dB sound pressure level (dB SPL) for a measured sound = 200,000 μPa

= 20 log (200,000 μPa/20 μPa)
= 20 log (10^4)
= 20 (4), where log of 10^4 equals 4
= 80 dB SPL

What if you want to compare one sound to another sound? For example, suppose the pressure of one sound is 1000 times more than the pressure of another sound. This defines the pressure ratio of these two sounds, that is, 1000/1. In dB pressure, this is expressed using the following equation:

dB pressure of a sound 1000 times greater than another sound

= 20 log (1000/1)
= 20 log (10^3)
= 20 (3), where log of 10^3 equals 3
= 60 dB

How about the situation in which we double the pressure of a sound? How many dB greater is the louder sound? The calculation is as follows:

dB pressure for a sound twice with as much (doubling) as another sound (increase)

= 20 log (2/1)
= 20 (0.3), where the log of 2 equals 0.3
= 6 dB

As was discussed above for intensity, this would similarly apply if one were to decrease the pressure level of a sound. For example, if one sound is half the pressure of another sound, the ratio

would be 1/2 (softer sound is half the pressure level of the louder sound). The calculation is as follows:

dB pressure of a sound half as much as another sound (decrease)

= 20 log (1/2)
= 20 (–0.3), where the log of 2 equals –0.3
= –6 dB

If you find it easier, the above example could be calculated using a ratio of 2/1, but then be sure to indicate that it is negative (representing a decrease): Notice that in both cases, the answer is 6 dB (either positive or negative).

Notice that if the pressure of a sound is doubled, it increases by 6 dB, whereas if the intensity of a sound is doubled, it increases by 3 dB. However, it is important to realize that for a specific sound, the intensity and pressure must vary together ($I = p^2$), that is, one cannot double the sound's pressure and at the same time double that sound's intensity. For example, if we double the intensity of a sound, the decibel level increases by 3 dB and the pressure also increases by 3 dB because the sound's pressure would increase by the square root of two. On the other hand, if we double the pressure of a sound, the decibel level increases by 6 dB and the intensity of that sound also increases by 6 dB because the sound's intensity is squared. These comparisons can be illustrated by the following calculations (keeping in mind that $I = p^2$); (a) the pressure of a sound is doubled, and (b) the pressure of a sound is increased by a factor of 10:

(a) dB pressure increase   dB intensity increase

= 20 log (2/1)   = 10 log (2^2/1)
= 20 log (2)   = 10 log (4)
= 20 (0.3)   = 10 (0.6)
= 6 dB   = 6 dB

(b) dB pressure increase · dB intensity increase

= 20 log (10/1)   = 10 log (10^2/1)
= 20 log (10)   = 10 log (100)
= 20 (1)   = 10·(2)
= 20 dB   = 20 dB

Table 3–3 summarizes how the ranges of pressure and intensity for human hearing are related and how the linear scales are transformed into their respective decibel (ratio) scales. The decibel is defined as 10 times the log of an intensity ratio and 20 times the log of a pressure ratio. The decibel range between the least audible sound and the upper limit (threshold of pain) is 140 dB for either intensity or pressure. However, a tenfold increase in intensity results in a 10 dB increase, whereas a tenfold increase in pressure results in a 20 dB increase because of the relation between intensity and pressure ($p = \sqrt{I}$). For more information on and practice with decibels, see *Audiology Workbook* (Kramer & Small, 2019) or the textbook by Speaks (2017).

Combining Levels from Different Sound Sources

One thing to keep in mind is that decibels cannot be simply added or subtracted, that is, adding a sound of 40 dB to another sound of 40 dB does not equal 80 dB; the decibels must be converted back to intensity before being combined. Let's look at what happens to the level of a sound when you combine two or more sound sources, each producing the same or different levels. The most important thing to keep in mind is that when combining sounds, you should work with the intensity levels of the sounds that combine (not the pressures); therefore, the standard decibel formula for intensity, $10 \log (I_{meas}/10^{-12} \text{ w/m}^2)$ must be used. However, as you learned earlier "a dB is a dB," and the combined level you obtain for dB IL would be the same in dB SPL. Since we more often measure sounds in dB SPL, the following examples will have the levels in dB SPL; however, it is the actual intensity levels (not in dB) that must be added together. In the case where all the sound sources have equal output levels, you can treat this like examples discussed earlier in which the combined level can be calculated by taking the log of the number of sources (added to the level of one source). In other words, if there are three sources with equal levels, the combined output (in dB) is calculated as follows:

$$\text{Combined (dB SPL or IL)} = \text{x dB from } 1 \text{ source} + 10 \log (3/1)$$

Example: You have three fans, each with an output level of 72 dB SPL. What is the combined level of the three fans? The solution is as follows:

$$\text{dB combined} = 72 + 10 \log (3/1)$$

$$= 72 + 10 (0.48), \text{ where log of } 3 = 0.48$$
$$= 72 + 4.8$$
$$= 76.8 \text{ dB SPL (or dB IL)}$$

It is a bit more difficult when combining sound sources with different output levels. To do this, you must: (1) calculate the intensity level (not in dB) of each source; (2) add them together to get the combined numerator of the intensity ratio (I_{meas}), and; (3) calculate the dB level using the formula for intensity level. The tricky part is calculating the intensity levels of the sounds, akin to finding the antilog, i.e., that is, what is the numerator of the intensity ratio for a given dB level. The general formula for calculating the I_{meas} for each source when the dB level is specified is as follows:

$$\text{x dB (given)} = 10 \log (I_{meas} \text{ w/m}^2/10^{-12} \text{ w/m}^2);$$
$$\text{then solve for } I_{meas}.$$

Example: You have two radios, one with an output of 80 dB SPL and the other with an output of 70 dB SPL. What is the combined level of the two radios? The solution is as follows:

1) Radio 1: 80 dB SPL $= 10 \log (I_{meas}/10^{-12})$ or
$$8.0 = \log (I_{meas}/10^{-12})$$

$I_{meas} = 1 \times 10^{-4}$; determined so that the addition of exponents would $= 10^8$

2) Radio 2: 70 dB SPL $= 10 \log (I_{meas}/10^{-12})$ or
$$7.0 = \log (I_{meas}/10^{-12})$$

$I_{meas} = 1 \times 10^{-5}$; determined so that the addition of exponents would $= 10^7$

3) Convert Radio 2 so it has the same exponent as Radio 1 (10^{-4}):

TABLE 3–3. Illustration of Intensity and Pressure Ranges

Intensity					Pressure				
w/m²	Ratio (I_{meas} / I_{ref})	Scientific Notation	$\log_{10}$	dB IL[a]	μPa	Ratio (P_{meas} / P_{ref})	Sci Not.	$\log_{10}$	dB SPL[b]
1×10^2	100,000,000,000,000:1	10^{14}	14.0	140	20×10^7	$\sqrt{100{,}000{,}000{,}000{,}000}$:1	$\sqrt{10^{14}}$	7.0	140
1×10^1	10,000,000,000,000:1	10^{13}	13.0	130	$20 \times 10^{6.5}$	$\sqrt{10{,}000{,}000{,}000{,}000}$:1	$\sqrt{10^{13}}$	6.5	130
1×10^{-0}	1,000,000,000,000:1	10^{12}	12.0	120	20×10^6	$\sqrt{1{,}000{,}000{,}000{,}000}$:1	$\sqrt{10^{12}}$	6.0	120
1×10^{-1}	100,000,000,000:1	10^{11}	11.0	110	$20 \times 10^{5.5}$	$\sqrt{100{,}000{,}000{,}000}$:1	$\sqrt{10^{11}}$	5.5	110
1×10^{-2}	10,000,000,000:1	10^{10}	10.0	100	20×10^5	$\sqrt{10{,}000{,}000{,}000}$:1	$\sqrt{10^{10}}$	5.0	100
1×10^{-3}	1,000,000,000:1	10^9	9.0	90	$20 \times 10^{4.5}$	$\sqrt{1{,}000{,}000{,}000}$:1	$\sqrt{10^9}$	4.5	90
1×10^{-4}	100,000,000:1	10^8	8.0	80	20×10^4	$\sqrt{100{,}000{,}000}$:1	$\sqrt{10^8}$	4.0	80
1×10^{-5}	10,000,000:1	10^7	7.0	70	$20 \times 10^{3.5}$	$\sqrt{10{,}000{,}000}$:1	$\sqrt{10^7}$	3.5	70
1×10^{-6}	1,000,000:1	10^6	6.0	60	20×10^3	$\sqrt{1{,}000{,}000}$:1	$\sqrt{10^6}$	3.0	60
1×10^{-7}	100,000:1	10^5	5.0	50	$20 \times 10^{2.5}$	$\sqrt{100{,}000}$:1	$\sqrt{10^5}$	2.5	50
1×10^{-8}	10,000:1	10^4	4.0	40	20×10^2	$\sqrt{10{,}000}$:1	$\sqrt{10^4}$	2.0	40
1×10^{-9}	1,000:1	10^3	3.0	30	$20 \times 10^{1.5}$	$\sqrt{1{,}000}$:1	$\sqrt{10^3}$	1.5	30
1×10^{-10}	100:1	10^2	2.0	20	20×10^1	$\sqrt{100}$:1	$\sqrt{10^2}$	1.0	20
1×10^{-11}	10:1	10^1	1.0	10	$20 \times 10^{.5}$	$\sqrt{10}$:1	$\sqrt{10^1}$	0.5	10
1×10^{-12}	1:1	10^0	0.0	0	20×10^0	$\sqrt{1}$:1	$\sqrt{10^0}$	0.0	0

[a] dB IL = 10 log (I_{meas}/I_{ref})

[b] dB SPL = 20 log (P_{meas}/$P_{reference}$)

Radio 2: $1 \times 10^{-5} = .1 \times 10^{-4}$ (multiply exponent x 10; therefore, divide 1 by 10)

4) Combine the intensities from each radio:

$$(1 \times 10^{-4}) + (.1 \times 10^{-4}) = 1.1 \times 10^{-4}$$

5) Calculate the dB level from these combined levels:

$$= 10 \log (1.1 \times 10^{-4}/10^{-12})$$
$$= 10 \log (1.1 \times 10^{8})$$
$$= 10 \log (1.1) + \log (10^{8})$$
$$= 10 (0.04 + 8)$$
$$= 80.4 \text{ dB SPL (or IL)}$$

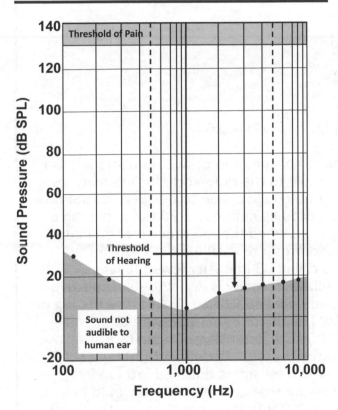

FIGURE 3–16. Thresholds and upper range of hearing as a function of frequency in humans. The variation in thresholds (in dB SPL) as a function of frequency is called the threshold of audibility curve. In this example, the closed circles represent the threshold reference levels based on American National Standards Institute [ANSI] (2010). Higher dB SPLs are needed in the low and high frequencies to reach threshold than in the middle frequencies. The threshold of pain (140 dB SPL) is also shown; although most listeners do not tolerate levels above 100 dB SPL.

AUDIBILITY BY FREQUENCY

As mentioned earlier, the human ear is responsive to frequencies from 20 to 20,000 Hz; however, the ear is not equally sensitive across the frequency range. The relation between normal thresholds (in dB SPL) and frequency is referred to as the *threshold of audibility curve*. Figure 3–16 shows an example of a threshold of audibility curve from 100 to 10,000 Hz. As you can see, humans are most sensitive to frequencies between 500 and 2000 Hz, and it takes slightly higher dB SPLs to reach threshold in the lower and higher frequencies. Also shown in Figure 3–16 is an estimate of the upper limit for hearing, called the threshold of pain. Notice that the upper limit does not vary much as a function of frequency, probably because it involves the threshold of feeling within the tympanic membrane, which is relatively constant across frequency (Durrant & Lovrinic, 1995; Kent & Read, 2002). The area between the lower threshold curve and the upper pain limit curve defines the useable range for human hearing. However, most listeners find sounds above 100 dB SPL uncomfortably loud. Many loud music venues may have sound levels on the order of 110 to 120 dB (and may damage hearing!).

WAVELENGTH

An additional acoustic parameter is the distance that pure tones travel in one cycle, the *wavelength*. The symbol for wavelength is the Greek symbol λ (lambda). The wavelength has a unit of length (e.g., feet, meters) rather than unit of time, which is used to define a pure tone's period. Wavelength is a measure of the distance between one point on the waveform to the same point on the next cycle, most easily seen as the distance between adjacent points of condensation (or rarefaction) in Figure 3–1. You should be able to surmise that higher frequencies have shorter wavelengths than lower frequencies because the cycles are closer together. Since the speed of sound is determined by the properties of the air, and is the same for all frequencies, wavelength can be defined by the following equation:

SYNOPSIS 3–2

- Intensity (w/m²) and pressure (μPa) are related to each other by the equation $p = \sqrt{I}$ (or $I = p^2$). In audiology, pressure is usually used to quantify the level (amplitude) of sounds. The minimum mean sound pressure for audibility, called the reference level for pressure, is 20 μPa. The mean upper limit of pressure that can be tolerated is 20×10^7 μPa. For intensity, the reference level is 10^{12} w/m² and the mean upper limit is 10^2 w/m². The range of hearing from the lowest to the highest is 10^7 for pressure and 10^{14} for intensity (notice the relation $10^7 = \sqrt{10^{14}}$). In either case, the range on a linear scale is too cumbersome to be very useful, so the ranges are converted to decibel (dB) scales.
- Decibel scales are based on a logarithmic (log) scale. The log of a number (x) is defined as the power to which 10 must be raised to be equal to the number (x). Stated another way, the exponent of a number is the log of that number. Most calculators can easily calculate the log of any number. Some simple examples to keep in mind are:

$$\log (10^{14}) = 14$$
$$\log (10^7) = 7$$
$$\log (10^2) = 2$$
$$\log (1) = 0$$
$$\log (2) = 0.3$$
$$\log (4) = \log (2) + \log (2) = 0.6$$

- A decibel (dB) is defined as 10 times the log of the ratio of two numbers [$10 \log (X_{meas}/X_{ref})$]. This formula is directly applicable to the ratio scale for intensity level [$10 \log (I_{meas}/I_{ref})$]; however, because $I = p^2$, the conversion to decibels for sound pressure follows basic rules of logs and becomes defined as 20 times the log of the ratio of two pressures [$20 \log (P_{meas}/P_{ref})$]. When the reference (denominator) for the ratio is 20 μPa it is called dB sound pressure level (dB SPL). When the reference for the ratio is 10^{-12} w/m², it is called dB intensity level (dB IL).
- When the measured sound pressure or sound intensity is equal to its respective reference level (giving a ratio of 1/1), it would be equal to 0 dB because the log of $1 = 0$. The range of hearing in decibels is 140 dB for either pressure or intensity as calculated for dB pressure = $20 \log (10^7)$ or dB intensity = $10 \log (10^{14})$.
- Sound pressure increases by 6 dB when the pressure is doubled [$20 \log (2/1)$]. Sound intensity increases by 3 dB when the intensity is doubled [$10 \log 2/1$]. A sound that is 100 times greater in pressure than another sound would be 40 dB greater; a sound that is 100 times greater in intensity than another sound would be 20 dB greater. However, since you cannot simultaneously double the intensity and double the pressure of the same sound (recall that $I = p^2$), the number of decibel change would be the same for pressure and intensity.
- The inverse square law defines how the intensity or pressure of a sound changes with distance. As the distance increases, the sound energy spreads out in a spherical form, and the decrease in the level of the sound can be described for intensity as $I = 1/D^2$ or for pressure as $p = 1/D$, where D is the ratio of the distance between two sounds (d_1/d_2). For example, if one doubles the distance, the intensity would decrease by 1/4 (or –6 dB) and the pressure would decrease by 1/2 (or –6 dB).

SYNOPSIS 3–2 (*continued*)

- When combining output levels from more than one source (whether specified in dB IL or dB SPL), it is the intensity levels (w/m²) that are combined; therefore, the formula 10 log (I_{meas}/10^{-12} w/m²) must be used. If sounds are unequal, first calculate I_{meas} for each sound, then combine the I_{meas} from each sound (converting exponents to be the same), then calculate the dB of the combined I_{meas} relative to 10^{-12} w/m².

$\lambda = c/f$, where c is the speed of sound and f is the frequency.

This equation shows that as frequency gets higher, the wavelength gets shorter. For example, a 2000 Hz pure tone, traveling in air ($c = 343$ m/s), has a wavelength of 0.17 m (or about 0.56 feet), whereas a 250 Hz sinusoid traveling in the same air would have a wavelength of 1.32 m (or about 4.5 feet). The same pure tones traveling in water would have wavelengths that are approximately four times longer because the speed of sound in water is about four times faster than in air. Conversely, if you know the wavelength of a sound, the frequency can be calculated by the equation:

$$f = c/\lambda.$$

The wavelength, to some extent, determines how a sound is affected as it encounters objects in its path. In a simple sense, the longer a sound's wavelength is relative to the size of the object encountered, the less likely the object will have an effect on the sound. However, if the wavelength is short (as for higher frequencies) relative to the size of an object, then the object will tend to block (and reflect) the sound. You may have noticed that it is much easier to hear drums over a greater distance than the higher frequency band instruments, like a flute; this is partly due to the higher frequencies being blocked by objects along the way, whereas the lower frequencies more easily go around the objects. As we will also see later in this chapter, part of our ability to localize sounds is related to the different amplitudes that occur between the two ears for higher frequencies, which tend to be blocked by the head because of their shorter wavelengths.

COMPLEX SOUNDS

As mentioned earlier, most sounds we listen to are complex sounds, which means that they are the result of combining two or more individual pure tones. Any complex vibration can be created or described by knowing the frequencies (or periods), amplitudes, and starting phases of the individual pure-tone components. The number of pure tones, along with their relative amplitudes and starting phases, will determine the type of sound we hear. A *spectrum* (plural = spectra) is a way to describe a complex vibration by plotting a graph that shows the amplitudes as a function of frequency, called a frequency spectrum, or the starting phases as a function of frequency, called a phase spectrum. Figure 3–17 shows an example of a complex vibration that is composed of two different pure tones with amplitudes and phases shown in the corresponding spectra. The amplitude spectra of complex periodic vibrations, as shown on the right side of Figure 3–17, show vertical lines at the discrete frequencies that make up the vibration, and this type of spectrum is called a *line spectrum*.

Vibrations are generally classified as periodic or aperiodic. A *periodic vibration* is one in which the vibratory pattern repeats at regular intervals. A pure tone (sinusoid) is an example of a *simple periodic vibration*. However, when two or more pure tones are combined into a nonsinusoidal pattern they may also be considered periodic if the wave pattern repeats itself as a function of time. These nonsinusoidal periodic vibrations are called *complex periodic vibrations* (or complex periodic tones). Complex periodic vibrations typically have a tonal or buzzing quality. The lowest frequency component in a complex periodic

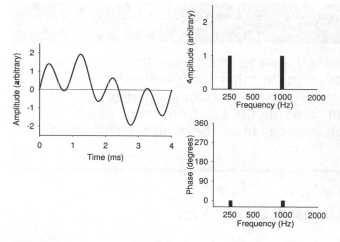

FIGURE 3–17. Example of a complex periodic waveform composed of two frequencies (*left*), which are described by their corresponding amplitude spectrum (*top right*) and starting phase spectrum (*bottom right*). These types of spectra are called line spectra.

vibration is called the *fundamental frequency* (f_0). Integer multiples of the fundamental frequency are called *harmonics*, such as $1f_0$, $2f_0$, $3f_0$, and so forth. Generally, complex periodic vibrations occur when harmonically related pure tones are combined. For example, combining 100 Hz, 200 Hz, 300 Hz, and 400 Hz will produce the complex periodic waveform shown in Figure 3–18. If additional sequential harmonics were added to those shown in Figure 3–18, the resulting waveform would smooth out the smaller bumps and, with enough harmonics, would produce what is called a *sawtooth waveform*. A sawtooth waveform is a complex periodic waveform that has more of a buzzing sound quality rather than a tonal quality. You can see in Figure 3–18 that the longest period of this complex periodic waveform is the same as the lowest frequency component (100 Hz). The fundamental frequency usually determines the primary pitch of the sound, but the other components can also be heard and will contribute to the perception/quality of the complex periodic vibration. Adding different combinations of pure tones and using different amplitudes or phases can affect the overall shape of complex periodic waveforms.

On the other hand, *aperiodic vibrations* are those in which the pattern of vibration does not regularly repeat itself over time; in other words, there is no periodicity in the wave pattern. The waveform shown in Figure 3–19 is an example of an aperiodic vibration. Aperiodic vibrations are generally called *noise*. Noise is produced by combining many pure tones with random starting phases. When there are an infinite number of frequencies with random phases and equal amplitudes over the entire frequency range it is called *white noise* (analogous to white light). The spectrum shown on the right side of Figure 3–19 is a horizontal line, rather than discrete vertical bars, to indicate that there are infinite frequencies present over the indicated range, and this type of spectrum is called a *continuous spectrum*.

Aperiodic noise-type vibrations are encountered frequently in our environment, including many speech sounds (e.g., /s/, /sh/, /f/, /th/), as well as sounds produced by things such as running water, rustling leaves, or engines. In addition, many sounds we listen to have components that give it a tonal (periodic) quality as well as a noise (aperiodic) quality, such as the speech sounds (/v/, /z/, /j/) or the different pitches associated with the buzzing of different types of

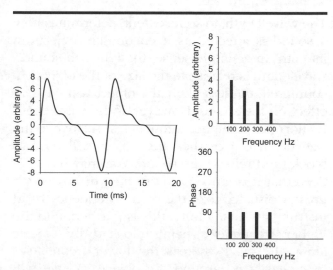

FIGURE 3–18. Example of a complex periodic waveform with a fundamental frequency of 100 Hz and its harmonics, 200 Hz, 300 Hz, and 400 Hz. With additional sequential harmonics added, the resulting waveform would be a sawtooth waveform.

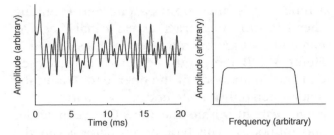

FIGURE 3–19. Example of an aperiodic noise vibration (*left*) and its corresponding amplitude spectra (*right*). These types of spectra are called continuous spectra.

motors. In some of these latter cases, the underlying periodicity or the frequency range of aperiodic combinations will determine the overall perceptions. If we know the frequencies (or periods), amplitudes, and starting phases of all the individual components of a complex periodic or aperiodic vibration, we can construct the predictable vibration pattern that would result from their combination. Instruments are available that can perform a fast Fourier transform (FFT) on complex vibrations to determine the frequencies, amplitudes, and starting phases of the individual components. Figure 3–20 shows some additional examples of complex vibrations with their corresponding amplitude spectra.

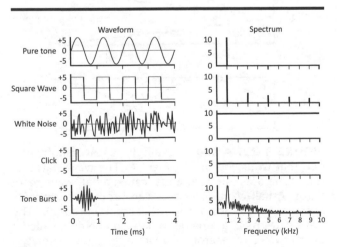

FIGURE 3–20. Examples of some continuous and transient signals with their corresponding amplitude spectra.

RESONANCE

The frequencies to which objects vibrate most easily are called *resonant* (or *resonance*) *frequencies*. You are undoubtedly familiar with this concept when you think about musical instruments, such that strings of different length vibrate best at certain frequencies, or the smaller violin's sounding board emphasizes higher frequencies compared with the much larger bass, which emphasizes the lower frequencies. In the case of a guitar string that is attached at both ends, when plucked, there are waves that move toward the ends of the strings and are then reflected back. This interaction of the two waves (incident and reflected) results in places where the displacements cancel each other, called *nodes*, and places where they combine with each other, called *antinodes*. For the guitar string, there are nodes at both ends (where the string cannot move) and an antinode at the center of the string that produces the string's primary musical note. The pattern of vibration between the nodes at the ends of the string and the antinode in the middle of the string is half of a cycle, as shown in Figure 3–21A. These patterns of displacement as a function of distance along the string are related to the frequency's wavelength (λ). The longest wavelength determines the string's primary resonant frequency (a.k.a. first mode or fundamental frequency) and is equal to half of a wavelength ($\lambda/2$). For a given length of string, the fundamental frequency can be calculated as:

$$f_0 = c/2L, \text{ where } c = \text{speed of sound;}$$
$$L = \text{length of string.}$$

The string analogy and other vibrating objects have additional modes (e.g., harmonics) of vibrations that create other possible nodes and antinodes, corresponding to f_2, f_3, f_4, and so on, as illustrated in Figure 3–21B and C. When a resonating source has a fundamental frequency that is equal to one-half of a wavelength, it is called a *half-wave resonator*, and generates a specific fundamental frequency based on its characteristics, and also generates harmonics at integer multiples of the fundamental frequency.

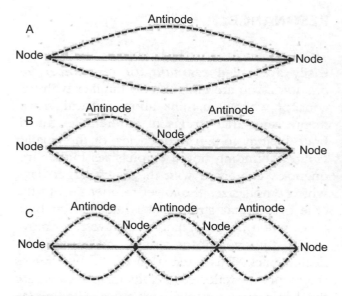

FIGURE 3–21. A–C. Examples of modes of vibration that would occur in a string that is attached at both ends showing the first mode or fundamental frequency (**A**), the second mode or second harmonic (**B**), and the third mode or third harmonic (**C**). Additional modes can occur at integer multiples of the first mode. At the nodes, the displacement is zero and creates a standing wave.

Resonance also occurs in tubes of different dimensions whereby the air molecules within the tube interact and produce regions of nodes and antinodes within the tube depending on the length of the tube. For example, blowing across a small tube produces a higher pitched tone compared with a lower pitched tone from a longer tube. The relationship of nodes and antinodes will depend also on whether the tube is open on both ends or only on one end, as illustrated in Figure 3–22. For the same-length tube, being open on both ends produces a higher-pitch tone than one open on only one end because of the different relationships of nodes to antinodes as illustrated in Figure 3–22A. As with the string example, a tube open at both ends involves half of a wavelength, and the resonant frequency can also be obtained by the formula $f_0 = c/2L$. This would also be a half-wave resonator with a fundamental frequency and harmonics at integer multiples of the fundamental frequency. Let's now look at

a tube that is open only on one end (thinking ahead to our vocal tract or ear canal that acts much like a tube open at one end). As shown in Figure 3–22B, there must be a node at the closed end and an antinode at the open end. For a tube that is open only on one end, a one-quarter wavelength can fit within the tube (between nodes and antinodes). This type of resonator is called a *quarter-wave resonator*, and generates a specific fundamental (f_0), but the harmonics are only at odd multiples of the fundamental frequency. The resonant frequency of a quarter-wave resonator is calculated as:

$$f_0 = c/4L, \text{ where } c = \text{speed of sound;}$$
$$L = \text{length of tube.}$$

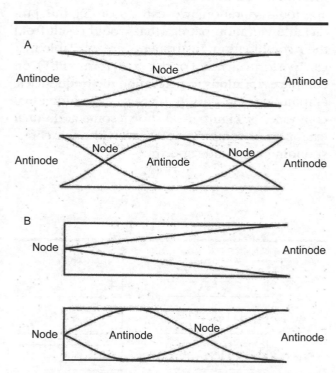

FIGURE 3–22. A and B. Examples of modes of vibration that would occur in tubes. **A.** The wave patterns for a tube open on both ends, called a half-wave resonator. A half-wave resonator can produce harmonics at integer multiples of the fundamental mode. **B.** The wave patterns in a tube open only on one end, called a quarter-wave resonator. A quarter-wave resonator can produce harmonics at odd multiples of the fundamental mode.

ACOUSTICS OF SPEECH

The primary means of producing speech is through air-flow supplied from the lungs, which passes through the vocal structures of the larynx and the oral and nasal cavities. The positioning and movements of the *articulators* (tongue, lips, velum, and jaws) alter the shape of the vocal path that results in specific resonance patterns of frequencies, amplitudes, and timing. The speech sounds are propagated into the environment, received, and ideally perceived by a listener. For example, what acoustic parameters are necessary for the listener to decide that they heard the sound /d/ in the word *day*? Or how does one perceive the word *day* differently than the words *die* or *bay*? Also, in today's world, human speech can be synthesized and digitally generated by a computer, largely based on what is known about the meaningful acoustic characteristics of the speech. Although the acoustic parameters of speech are important, keep in mind that communication involves much more than the simple production, recognition, and perception of the acoustic properties of speech.

Speech sounds can be classified into different types. On the most basic level, there are vowels, which are mostly complex periodic sounds, and consonants, which can be either complex periodic (with vocal fold vibration) or aperiodic vibrations (without vocal fold vibration). Table 3–4 lists the labels used to describe different types of sounds. When the vocal folds vibrate, there is a complex periodicity to the sound, called a *voiced sound*. When the vocal folds do not vibrate, the sound is aperiodic and called a *voiceless sound*. Vowels are voiced, but consonants can be either voiced or unvoiced. The normal average intensity level of ongoing connected speech is about 65 to 75 dB SPL (Killion & Mueller, 2010; Thibodeau, 2007), and this "volume" is primarily carried by the vowels. Consonants have less energy than the vowels during connected speech, and contribute the most to word intelligibility. Figure 3–23 shows how conversational-level speech sounds are distributed across the frequency and intensity scales. This general distribution of speech sounds is often referred to as the *speech banana* due to its general outline encompassing ranges of the vowels and consonants during ongoing speech. As you can see in Figure 3–23, there is as much as a 30 dB SPL difference between the loudest vowel (/u/) and the softest consonant (/th/). Notice also that the vowels tend to be

TABLE 3–4. Labels Used to Describe Different Types of Sounds Related to the Place of Articulation

Manner of Articulation	Voicing[a]	Bilabial	Labio-dental	Lingua-dental	Alveolar	Palatal	Velar	Glottal
Plosives (Stops)	–	p(*p*ea)			t(*t*ea)		k(*k*it)	
	+	b(*b*ee)			d(*d*id)		g(*g*o)	
Fricatives	–		f(*f*in)	θ(*th*in)	s(*s*o)	ʃ(*sh*e)		h(*h*e)
	+		v(*v*ine)	ð(*th*e)	z(*z*oo)	ʒ(lu*ge*)		
Affricates	–					tʃ(*ch*in)		
	+					dʒ(*j*ot)		
Nasals	–							
	+	m(*m*e)			n(*n*o)		ŋ(ba*ng*)	
Liquids	–				l(*l*et)			
	+					r(*r*ed)		
Glides	–				ʍ(*wh*et)			
	+	w(*w*e)				j(*y*et)		

[a]Some consonants are produced without voicing (–), and some are produced with voicing (+).

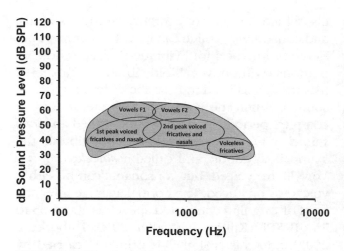

FIGURE 3–23. General distribution of speech sounds during normal conversational level of connected speech. The overall level of conversational speech is about 65 dB SPL. The outer most outlined area is called the speech banana.

plitude, and time characteristics of speech can be analyzed with some basic equipment. One of the most important pieces of equipment used to analyze speech sounds is a *spectrograph*, which measures the spectra of speech sounds, words, or sentences (in a relatively short time window) recorded through a microphone. A *spectrogram* is the graphical output from a spectrograph for a specific speech utterance. A spectrogram displays frequency (along the *y*-axis) as a function of time (along the *x*-axis). The amplitudes of the different frequencies are also represented in a spectrogram by the relative darkness of the frequency bands, that is, the more intense frequencies are seen as darker bands. Figure 3–24 shows examples of spectrograms for some vowels and consonants. As you can see in Figure 3–24A, the

lower in frequency, whereas many of the aperiodic noise-like consonants, called *fricatives*, are higher in frequency.

In the following sections, only the very basics of the acoustic properties of the different types of speech sounds are given, primarily their frequency components; however, keep in mind that amplitude and timing variations are also important acoustic properties of speech. In Chapter 8 of this textbook, you will learn about the clinical speech tests that are used to assess how well a patient is able to recognize words and sentences, and how a patient's speech recognition is altered by various disorders of the auditory system. For a more in-depth understanding of speech production, speech acoustics, and speech perception, the interested reader is referred to other sources, such as (Kent & Read, 2002; Rafael, Borden, & Harris, 2007).

Spectrogram

Speech is composed of basic periodic and aperiodic vibrations that occur in relatively short time periods, and is interspersed with short silent periods between sounds. The frequency, am-

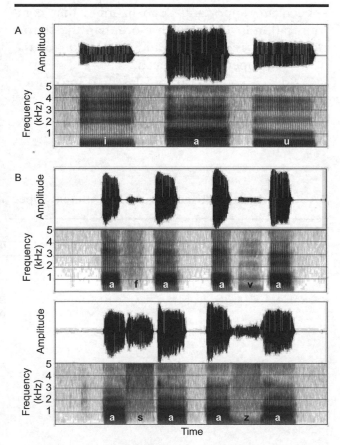

FIGURE 3–24. A and B. Spectrographic recordings for three different vowels in isolation (**A**), and some voiceless and voiced fricatives (**B**).

vowels show three or four darker frequency regions (bands). These darker frequency bands are called *formants*, beginning with the first formant (F1), the next higher F2, and so forth. Formants vary depending on the resonance properties associated with the positions of the articulators, and are similar to those harmonics seen with the example of the quarter-wave resonator. Vowels behave more like the complex periodic vibrations that we saw in the preceding section. Other speech sounds may be aperiodic, like the /s/ shown in Figure 3–24B, which does not have the discrete frequency bands like those seen with vowels, but instead shows a wider range of frequencies as expected with a noise-type sound. The following sections give a brief overview of the acoustics properties for the various vowel-like speech sounds and the various noise-like speech sounds. Although not covered in this text, keep in mind that there are also corresponding amplitude variations associated with connected speech, as well as important temporal factors such as duration of sounds and silent intervals.

Vowels

Vowels carry most of the audible energy in speech, and generally have lower frequencies and higher intensities than consonants. Vowels are complex periodic vibrations (voiced) that result from the vibration of the vocal folds. The frequency of vocal fold vibration is the fundamental frequency (f_0) which gives the sound its perceived pitch, and can vary depending on the vowel as well as the size of the larynx (which relates to males generally having a lower sounding voice). As described earlier, vowels can be characterized by their F1 and F2. In general, the F1 varies inversely with the height of the tongue, and F2 varies with the forward/backward position of the tongue. For example, /i/ is produced with the tongue in its highest position and most forward in the mouth, whereas /a/ is produced with the tongue in its lowest position and as far back as possible. Lip rounding is done for some back and center vowels and its effect is to extend the vocal tract and thus lower all formant frequencies. Keep in mind that the formant fre-

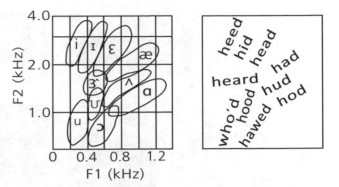

FIGURE 3–25. Distribution of F1 and F2 formants for English vowels for a variety of speakers. *Source*: From Kent and Read, 2002, p. 170, with permission of the authors.

quencies are not precise numbers, but are best considered as elliptical regions that vary depending on the speaker due to variations in size of vocal tract, articulators, and dialect. Figure 3–25 shows how the different vowels can be separated into their F1 and F2 elliptical areas, and be relatively distinct from each other.

During speech, vowels can also vary by their duration. For example, some vowels are longer in duration, like those in open syllables (e.g., "see" "so"), whereas others are shorter in duration like those in closed syllables (e.g., "sit" "sat"). Additionally, vowels that are produced in context with other consonants also have a dynamic shifting of their formant frequencies, called *formant transitions*, where there may be a rising or falling frequency transition depending on the preceding and/or target consonant. Combining vowel sounds, called *semivowels* or *diphthongs*, are characterized by formant transitions, and the shifts in F2 are the most distinguishing characteristic used to identify different semivowels and diphthongs.

Consonants

Consonants are considered the sounds that contribute most toward intelligibility as they precede and/or follow vowels to define words or parts of words. The acoustic properties of consonants are

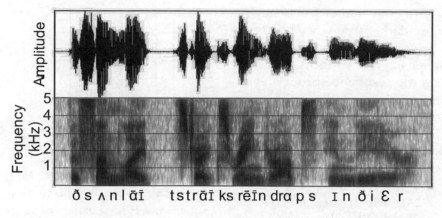

FIGURE 3–26. Sample waveform and spectrogram of the sentence, "The sunlight strikes raindrops in the air."

a bit more complicated than vowels, and one is not able to give as general a description as we were able to do with the formant structure of vowels. Consonants are divided into several different types. Some consonants are voiced, some have a noise quality, some only have a period of silence, and some may involve the nasal cavity. Only a brief description of these characteristics is given here, and only some selective examples are shown on a spectrogram. With some practice, you may be able to recognize the patterns of vowels and consonants in the complete sentence "The sunlight strikes raindrops in the air," shown in Figure 3–26.

Stops (or *plosives*) are produced by a brief period in which the airflow is blocked. The blockages can occur at the lips, alveolar area, or velum, and are referred to as *bilabial, alveolar,* or *velar stop.* Stops can be voiced or unvoiced depending on if the vocal folds are set into vibration. During the closure, air pressure is built up and when the stop is opened, there is a burst of air flow. *Fricatives* are noise-like sounds that are produced by passing air through the oral cavity in which the articulators are positioned in a way to create turbulence in the airflow. The different fricatives are produced by the location (place) of constriction from the most forward point of the oral cavity at the lips to the rearmost position at the glottal area. Fricatives can be voiced (e.g., /v/) or unvoiced (e.g., /f/) at the same place of articulation. *Affricates* are created by the transition of

a stop into a fricative. With *nasals*, the velopharyngeal port is opened so that sound energy can pass through both the nasal and oral tracts or through only the nasal tract. The formants of the nasals depend on the length of the cavity from the uvula to the nostrils, and are voiced with the vibration of the vocal folds.

FILTERING

Filtering is a means by which certain frequencies are excluded and certain frequencies are allowed to pass. Filtering can be used to generate a sound that is composed of a specified range of frequencies by filtering out some portion of a wider range of frequencies. For example, one can start with white noise and then filter out some of the frequencies so that a more restricted range of frequencies is passed.

Figure 3–27 shows the spectra for different types of commonly used filters. The band of frequencies that is passed is represented under the curve, and those outside the curve are the frequencies that are filtered out. The point where frequencies begin to be filtered out is called the *cutoff frequency* and is usually defined at the point that is 3 dB less than the peak (called 3 dB *down-points* or *half-power point*). The extent to which the frequencies are excluded is determined by the slope of the curve, called *attenuation rate* or *rejection rate*, which is usually

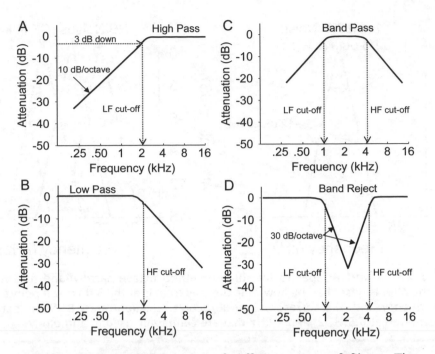

FIGURE 3–27. A–D. Examples of different types of filters. The region under the curves shows those frequencies that are heard (passed). The places where the filter begins to reject frequencies are called cutoff frequencies, which are at the 3 dB down points. The filter's rate of frequency rejection is indicated by the dB/octave. **A.** High-pass filter with 2000 Hz cutoff with 10 dB/octave rejection rate. **B.** Low-pass filter with 2000 Hz cutoff with 10 dB/octave rejection rate. **C.** Band-pass filter with 1000 Hz low frequency cutoff and 4000 Hz high frequency cutoff, with 10 dB/octave rejection rates. **D.** Band-reject filter with 1000 and 4000 Hz cutoff points, with 30 dB/octave rejection rates.

specified in dB per octave (dB/octave). An *octave* means a doubling or halving of the frequency. As an example (see Figure 3–27A), a *high-pass filter* passes frequencies higher than the cutoff frequency and rejects frequencies lower than the cutoff frequency at a specified dB/octave slope toward the lower frequencies. In this example, the filter would be called a high-pass filter with a 2000 Hz low frequency cutoff and a rejection rate of 10 dB/octave. The other examples in Figure 3–27 include a *low-pass filter* that passes all the frequencies lower than the cutoff frequency and rejects frequencies higher than the cutoff frequency at a specified dB/octave slope directed toward the higher frequencies. A *band-pass filter* passes a band of frequencies as defined by the high and low cutoff frequencies and rejects fre-

quencies above and below the cutoff at the specified rejection rates toward the higher and lower frequencies. The *band-reject filter* (also known as a notched filter) specifies a range of frequencies in the middle of a wider range of noise that is rejected, and the frequencies on both sides of the specified band-reject area are passed.

A special type of band-pass filtered noise is called *narrowband noise*, where there is a relatively restricted range of frequencies. These frequencies are often described by the width of the curve as measured across the 3 dB down points from the *center frequency*. A commonly used narrowband noise is called a *one-third octave* narrowband noise, which means the filter is one third of an octave wide at the 3 dB down points. Figure 3–28 shows the spectra for some one-third

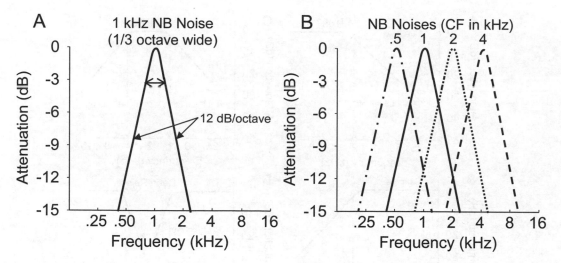

FIGURE 3–28. A and B. Spectra for some one-third octave narrowband noises. **A.** The width of the filter is described by how wide the spectrum is at the 3 dB down points from the center frequency, with the corresponding dB/octave rejection rates. **B.** Some narrowband noises, centered at 0.5, 1, 2, and 4 kHz that are commonly used in audiology.

SYNOPSIS 3–3

- Humans are capable of hearing sounds from 20 to 20,000 Hz; however, we are most sensitive to frequencies in the 500 to 2000 Hz range, and it takes slightly greater amounts of sound pressure (or intensity) for lower and higher frequencies to be just audible (threshold). The variation threshold as a function of frequency is referred to as the threshold of audibility curve.

- The wavelength of a sound (λ) describes how far a pure tone travels in one cycle. The wavelength can be calculated by the equation $\lambda = c/f$, where c is the speed of sound and f is the frequency. Conversely, if you know the wavelength, the frequency can be calculated from $f = c/\lambda$.

- Complex sounds are much more typical in our environment than pure tones; however, any complex sound is the result of some combination of pure tones with specific amplitudes and starting phases. The individual sinusoidal components of complex sounds can be determined using equipment that can perform a fast Fourier transform (FFT).

- A spectrum describes a sound's amplitude or starting phase (along the y-axis) as a function of frequency (along the x-axis). A line spectrum is used when discrete (and usually limited) frequencies contribute to the complex vibration. A continuous spectrum is used when a range of frequencies (all inclusive) contributes to the complex vibration.

- A periodic vibration repeats itself at regular time intervals. Complex vibrations can be periodic if the combined waveform repeats itself over time; periodic complex vibrations occur when the combined pure tones are harmonically related as integer multiples of the lowest frequency, called the fundamental

SYNOPSIS 3–3 (*continued*)

frequency (f_0). A sawtooth waveform results when all harmonics ($1f_0 + 2f_0 + 3f_0 + 4f_0$ . . .) are included and a square wave results when only the odd harmonics ($1f_0 + 3f_0 + 5f_0 + 7f_0$ . . .) are included.

- An aperiodic complex vibration (often called noise) does not repeat itself at regular time intervals and typically results from a range of pure tones with random starting phases. White noise (analogous to white light) has an infinite number of frequencies present with random phases.
- Most vibrating objects (except for a pure tone), including air molecules in tubes, have a fundamental frequency and additional harmonics. The vocal tract and ear canal are similar to a tube that is open at one end, called a quarter-wave resonator. A quarter-wave resonator produces vibrations at a fundamental frequency and at odd integer harmonics. The resonance frequencies are dependent on the wavelengths associated with the length of the tube.
- Speech has specific acoustic properties generated by airflow passing through the vocal fold, oral cavity, and nasal cavity, resulting in complex periodic and aperiodic acoustic waveforms. The articulators modify the airflow depending on the targeted speech sound.
- Vowels are more intense than consonants in connected speech and produce the perception of voice loudness. The long-term average level of conversational speech is about 65 dB SPL.
- Vowels are complex periodic vibrations with a fundamental frequency (giving rise to the pitch of the voice), and additional bands of energy called formants. The F1 and F2 formants are most important for vowel differentiation.
- Consonants can be periodic if accompanied by vocal fold vibration (voicing) or aperiodic if entirely noise-like (unvoiced). There are many types of consonants depending on the manner and place of articulation. Consonants are generally less intense than vowels and contribute most to intelligibility when in connected speech.
- Filtering is a way to exclude certain frequencies and allow other frequencies to pass through. Filters are used to shape the spectra of noise stimuli and/or to focus on a specific frequency range that is to be analyzed. Common types of filters include high-pass, low-pass, band-pass, and band-reject as defined by their cutoff frequencies and rejection rates. Narrowband noises, used extensively in hearing testing, are filtered noises that are typically one-third of an octave wide.

octave narrowband noises. Narrowband noises are used frequently as noise maskers during basic hearing tests. Filtering can also be used when analyzing or measuring a complex wave pattern to exclude frequencies that you are not interested in analyzing or measuring, and instead focuses only on those frequencies that are of interest. This type of filtering is used in many of the physiological measures from the auditory system.

PSYCHOACOUSTICS

The study of how humans perceive the acoustic properties of sound is called psychoacoustics.

The following sections will present basic information on how frequency and intensity translate into our perception of loudness and pitch; how our thresholds change as the duration of a sound is shortened, called *temporal integration*, and, finally, how we use acoustic information to determine where sounds are coming from, called *localization*. The introductory material covered in this chapter only touches the surface of this fascinating area and only covers how normal hearing humans perceive simple sounds. For more advanced coverage of this topic for a variety of simple and complex sounds, the interested reader is referred to other texts (Durrant & Lovrinic, 1995; Gelfand, 2009; Moore, 2013; Zwicker & Fastl, 2013).

Loudness

Loudness is generally considered the psychological correlate of intensity. Most of us have a general idea that soft and loud sounds are related to low and high intensities (or pressures) of sounds. As discussed earlier, the ear responds to a wide range of intensities (or pressures); the minimum level is perceived as threshold and the upper limit is perceived as being uncomfortably loud. As we learned from the threshold of audibility curve, it takes a different amount of intensity to reach threshold for different frequencies. So, an obvious question is what intensities are needed to maintain equal loudness across frequencies? To answer this question, a loudness-matching procedure is typically used in which the dB SPL for different frequencies are adjusted until they sound equally loud to a 1000 Hz reference tone (Fletcher & Munson, 1933; Robinson & Dadson, 1956). The scaling unit used to compare loudness across frequencies is called a *phon*. Figure 3–29 shows a series of phon curves. The phon equates loudness across frequencies (also called *equal loudness contours*). The level of each phon curve is defined as the dB SPL of a given level of a 1000 Hz tone. For example, a loudness level of 30 phons is equal to a 1000 Hz tone presented at 30 dB SPL, and a loudness level of 60 phons is equal to a 1000 Hz tone presented at 60 dB SPL. Different phon curves are established for differ-

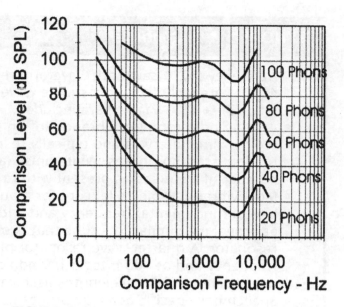

FIGURE 3–29. Phon scales of loudness (or equal loudness contours). A phon is defined as the loudness associated with a 1000 Hz reference tone. Each line represents frequencies that are perceived as equally loud for the given phon level. *Source*: From Yost, 2013, p. 190. Copyright 2013 by Koninklijke Brill.

ent levels of the 1000 Hz reference tone. The dB SPLs needed for other frequencies to sound equally loud to the 1000 Hz tone, at a specified phon level, are measured to establish the corresponding phon curve across the frequency range. In other words, all frequencies at the given phon level (along the same phon curve) are judged to be equally loud even though their actual SPLs are different. As you can see from Figure 3–29, the general shape of the phon curves follows the threshold of audibility curve; however, they tend to flatten out across frequency as the phon level increases, especially in the lower frequencies. This means that at higher sound levels it does not take as much increase in dB SPL in the lower frequencies to sound equally loud to the mid frequencies.

The phon scale does not tell us much about how our perception of loudness is related to the continuum of sound pressures. Another question of interest is how does a scale of loudness relate to a range of sound pressures? For example, if the dB SPL of a sound is doubled, does the perceived loudness also double? Or how much increase in dB SPL is needed to achieve a doubling of the perceived loudness? The relationship of loudness to pressure (or intensity) is generally determined by using magnitude estimation or scaling method (Stevens, 1956). This type of loudness scale uses *sones* as the unit of loudness, where one sone is defined as the loudness of a 1000 Hz tone at 40 dB SPL. In these types of experiments, the subject is asked to adjust the dB SPL of the tone until the loudness is judged to be half, double, triple, and so on, of the loudness of the reference value. In other words, how many dB SPL corresponds to 2 sones or 0.5 sones? The data are typically presented for a 1000 Hz tone; however, similar data can be obtained for different frequencies by making the reference value equal to the loudness in phons for the frequency being measured. Figure 3–30 shows the relationship that occurs between the loudness in sones and the dB SPL of a 1000 Hz tone (or loudness level in phons). As you can see, the sone scale for loudness (on a log-log plot) shows a relatively straight line above 30 dB SPL for a 1000 Hz tone. In this region, a doubling of loudness corresponds to a 10 dB increase in sound pressure and approximates a power function, where the slope of the line is the exponent of the power function; in this case, loudness = pressure[6]. For

levels between threshold and 30 dB SPL, the loudness function is much steeper and does not fit the simple power function. Notice also that the entire range of sound pressures (10^7) is compressed into a range of only around 100 sones.

Pitch

Pitch is generally considered the psychological correlate of frequency. Most of us have a sense that low and high-pitch sounds are related to low and high frequencies. Although we can detect a wide range of frequencies and can attribute a general perception of pitch to these frequencies, the question of interest here is how does a scale of pitch relate to a scale of frequency, that is, if we double the frequency of a sound, does the pitch also double? In other words, how much of a frequency increase is needed for a doubling of the perceived pitch? As you will see, there is not a one-to-one correspondence between pitch and frequency. The relationship of pitch to frequency was first described by Stevens and Volkmann (1940). The pitch scale is typically presented in units called *mels*. The mel scale assigns a standard reference value of 1000 mels to the pitch associated with 1000 Hz. The subject then adjusts the frequency of a tone until the pitch is judged to be half, double, triple, and so on, of the pitch of the 1000 Hz reference tone. In other words, what frequency best corresponds to 500, 2000, or 3000 mels? Figure 3–31 shows the relationship that occurs between pitch (linear scale) and frequency (logarithmic scale). As you can see, the mel scale for pitch does not show a one-to-one relation to frequency. For example, a doubling of frequency from 1000 to 2000 Hz corresponds to a 1.5 increase in pitch (from 1000 to 1500 mels). Conversely, a doubling of pitch from 1000 to 2000 mels corresponds to about a threefold increase in frequency (from 1000 to 3000 Hz). Notice also that the entire range of frequencies (20 to 20,000 Hz) is compressed into a range of only 3500 mels, and that the data follow a curvilinear function in a semi-log plot across the frequency range.

Pitch also changes with intensity, as shown in Figure 3–32, for a variety of frequencies (Stevens,

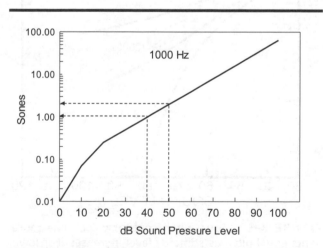

FIGURE 3–30. Sone scale of loudness for 1000 Hz. One sone equals the loudness associated with a 1000 Hz tone at 40 dB SPL. A doubling of loudness occurs for tenfold increases in stimulus level.

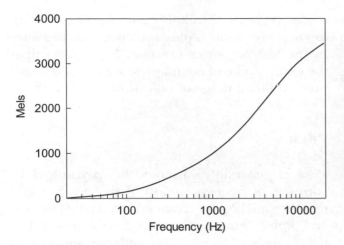

FIGURE 3–31. Mel scale of pitch. The pitch associated with 1000 Hz is defined as 1000 mels. The range of audible frequencies (20 to 20,000 Hz) is compressed into about 3500 mels.

1935). These pitch versus intensity data are called *equal pitch contours*. In general, increasing intensity results in an increased pitch for the higher frequencies and a decreased pitch for the lower frequencies (Durrant & Lovrinic, 1995; Gulick, Gescheider, & Frisina, 1989). It should be pointed out that these increases and decreases in pitch with intensity are relatively small and not generally noticeable except under controlled laboratory conditions (Cohen, 1961).

Temporal Integration

Temporal integration describes how the threshold of audibility for a sound changes with the duration of the sound. In general, as the duration of a sound is shortened to less than 200 ms, the level of the sound must be increased in order for the sound to be audible (Durrant & Lovrinic, 1995; Watson & Gengel, 1969). Figure 3–33 shows how the threshold changes as a function of duration. As you can see, there is about a 10 dB increase in level (threshold shift) for a tenfold decrease in duration. In other words, as the duration is shortened from 200 to 20 ms, the sound level must be increased by 10 dB to remain audible. Similarly, as the duration is shortened from 20 to 2 ms, an additional 10 dB increase in the level of the sound is needed to remain audible. It should

also be pointed out that for tones less than 10 ms in duration, the quality of the sound also changes significantly, such that the tonality is lost and it is perceived as a brief click (transient) type sound. These brief transients also spread their energy across a wider frequency range called *spectral splatter*. You can also see from Figure 3–33 that for sounds with durations greater than 200 ms, the threshold remains constant.

Localization

Localization refers to the ability to determine the direction from which a sound is coming. In gen-

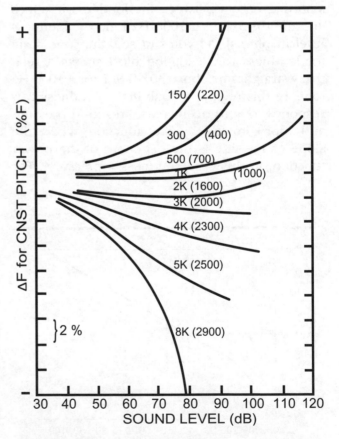

FIGURE 3–32. Equal pitch contours. Each line represents equal pitch as stimulus level increases. For lower frequencies, as stimulus level is increased, the frequency tends to decrease. For higher frequencies, as stimulus level is increased, the frequency tends to increase. *Source*: From Durrant and Lovrinic, 1995, p. 279. Copyright 1995 by Williams and Wilkins.

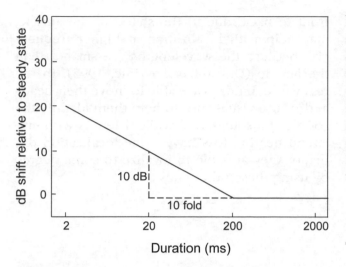

FIGURE 3–33. Temporal integration function. This shows how the threshold for a pure tone changes as a function of duration. As the duration is shortened by a factor of 10 (e.g., from 200 to 20 ms), the sound level must be increased by 10 dB to remain audible.

eral, our ability to localize is greatly dependent on the use of both ears, called *binaural hearing*. Most animals have a keen sense of localization, and many animals are able to move their pinnae to help them localize. Humans, on the other hand, do not move their auricles as a means of localizing. Instead, humans rely (unconsciously) on different arrival times and/or intensities of sounds at the two ears to determine from where sounds are coming. These mechanisms are referred to as *interaural time differences* or *interaural intensity differences*. These two mechanisms can explain localization of simple sounds that come from one side of the head. For localization, clearly two ears are better than one, and a typical complaint of people with hearing loss in one ear is that they have some difficulty localizing sounds.

Figure 3–34 shows how interaural time and interaural intensity mechanisms operate when listening with two ears to a sound presented to one side of the head. As shown in Figure 3–34B, higher frequencies (>1500 Hz) have shorter wavelengths as compared to the size of the head, and these frequencies tend to be blocked by the head (Fedderson, Sandel, Teas, & Jeffress, 1957). In this case, the sound at the ear farther away

from the sound source is less audible, called *head shadow*. For lower frequencies, shown in Figure 3-34C, the wavelength is larger than the size of the head and wraps around the head due to diffraction and does not create interaural intensity differences; however, it does take slightly more time for the sound to get to the ear farther away from the sound source. These interaural time differences appear to be important for lower frequency localization as long as

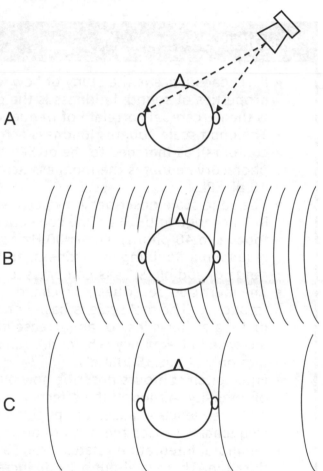

FIGURE 3–34. A–C. Illustrations showing factors important for sound localization in the horizontal plane. **A.** Interaural time differences between the two ears; varies as a function of azimuth. **B.** Interaural intensity differences between the two ears resulting from sound shadow area that occurs at the ear farther away from the sound source when wavelength is short, which may explain some localization at high frequencies. **C.** Sound shadow does not occur when wavelength is at least as long as the width of the head.

the wavelength is larger than the distance between the two ears; however, this simple model has been shown to have some discrepancies in more recent studies (Kuhn, 1977) and these are beyond the scope of this textbook. As the direction of the sound source moves more toward the center, localization based on interaural time and intensity differences becomes more difficult. In those situations, and in vertically directed localization, spectral differences in the sound from front to back, due to the shape of the auricle, may help with localization at higher frequencies because the wavelengths are smaller than the auricle (Durrant & Lovrinic, 1995). In the real world, humans are able to move their heads and/or use visual cues to help them identify the source of a sound; and while listeners with unilateral hearing loss have some localization difficulty, they are able to localize to some degree by using these other cues.

SYNOPSIS 3–4

- Psychoacoustics is the study of how we perceive the different acoustic properties of sound; loudness is the perceptual correlate of intensity and pitch is the perceptual correlate of frequency.
- The phon scale equates loudness across frequencies (also called equal loudness contours), as matched to the dB SPL of a 1000 Hz tone: For example, a 40 dB phon curve equates the loudness across frequencies to a 1000 Hz tone at 40 dB SPL.
- The sone scale describes how perceived loudness of a tone relates to changes in its change in dB SPL. One sone equals the loudness of a 40 dB SPL 1000 Hz tone (also 40 phons). For 1000 Hz above 30 dB SPL, an increase of 10 dB SPL results in a doubling in loudness, and is described as a power function. The range of audible SPLs is compressed into a range of only about 100 sones.
- The mel scale describes how changes in pitch correspond to changes in frequency. The mel scale is based on the pitch of 1000 Hz = 1000 mels. The mel scale shows less of an increase in perceived pitch for a corresponding increase in frequency. The entire range of audible frequencies is compressed into only about 3500 mels.
- Equal pitch contours describe how pitch of a specific tone changes as a function of intensity. Although the effects are quite small, increasing the intensity of high frequencies causes the pitch to increase; increasing the intensity of low frequencies causes the pitch to decrease.
- Temporal integration relates a tone's threshold to changes in the tone's duration. There is about a 10 dB increase in threshold for each tenfold decrease in duration below 200 ms (e.g., 200 to 20 ms). For durations longer than 200 ms, threshold remains constant (complete integration).
- Localization of a sound's source is easiest with binaural hearing. Localizing the source of a sound from the sides is facilitated by the interaural intensity differences for higher frequencies (due to head shadow effect), and interaural time differences for lower frequencies. Localizing from front/back and in the vertical plane are facilitated by spectral differences due to the auricle.

REFERENCES

American National Standards Institute [ANSI] (2010). Specifications for audiometers ANSI S3.6-2010. New York, NY: Author.

Cohen, A. (1961). Further investigations of the effects of intensity upon the pitch of pure tones. *Journal of the Acoustical Society of America, 33,* 1363–1376.

Durrant, J. D., & Lovrinic, J. H. (1995). *Bases of Hearing Science* (3rd ed.). Baltimore, MD: Williams & Wilkins.

Fedderson, W. E., Sandel, T. T., Teas, D. C., & Jeffress, L. A. (1957). Localization of high-frequency tones. *Journal of the Acoustical Society of America, 29,* 988–991.

Fletcher, H., & Munson, W. A. (1933). Loudness, its definition, measurement, and calculation. *Journal of the Acoustical Society of America, 5,* 82–105.

Gelfand, S. A. (2012). *Hearing: An Introduction to Psychological and Physiological Acoustics* (6th ed.). Bingley, United Kingdom: Emerald Group Publishing Ltd.

Gulick, W., Gescheider, G., & Frisina, R. (1989). *Hearing: Physiological Acoustics, Neural Coding, and Psychoacoustics*. New York, NY: Oxford University Press.

Kent, R. D., & Read, C. (2002). *Acoustic Analysis of Speech*. Toronto, Canada: Thomson Learning.

Killion, M. C., & Mueller, H. G. (2010). Twenty years later: A new count-the-dots method. *The Hearing Journal, 63,* 10–17.

Kramer, S. J., & Small, L. (2019). *Audiology Workbook*. San Diego, CA: Plural.

Kuhn, G. F. (1977). Model for the interaural time differences in azimuthal plane. *Journal of the Acoustical Society of America, 62,* 157–167.

Moore, B. C. J. (2013). *Introduction to the Psychology of Hearing* (6th ed.). Leiden, Netherlands: Koninklijke Brill.

Mullin, W. J., Gerace, W. L., Mestre, J. P., & Velleman, S. V. (2003). *Fundamentals of Sound with Applications to Speech and Hearing*. Boston, MA: Allyn and Bacon.

Rafael, L. J., Borden, G. J., & Harris, K. S. (2007). *Speech Science Primer: Physiology, Acoustic, and Speech Production* (5th ed.). Baltimore, MD: Lippencott Williams & Wilkins.

Robinson, D. W., & Dadson, R. S. (1956). A redetermination of the equal loudness relations for pure tones. *British Journal of Applied Physiology, 7,* 166–181.

Speaks, C. E. (2017). *Introduction to Sound Acoustics for the Hearing and Speech Sciences* (4th ed.). San Diego, CA: Plural.

Stevens, S. S. (1935). The relation of pitch to intensity. *Journal of the Acoustical Society of America, 6,* 150–154.

Stevens, S. S. (1956). The measurement of loudness. *Journal of the Acoustical Society of America, 7,* 815–829.

Stevens, S. S., & Volkmann, J. (1940). The relation of pitch to frequency: A revised scale. *American Journal of Psychology, 53,* 329–353.

Thibodeau, L. (2007). Speech audiometry. In M. Roeser, M. Valente, & H. Hosford-Dunn (Eds.), *Audiology Diagnosis* (2nd ed.). New York, NY: Thieme.

Villchur, E. (2000). *Acoustics for Audiologists*. San Diego, CA: Singular Press.

Watson, C. S., & Gengel, R. W. (1969). Signal duration and signal frequency in relation to auditory sensitivity. *Journal of the Acoustical Society of America, 46,* 989–997.

Yost, W. (2013). *Fundamentals of Hearing* (5th ed.). Leiden, Netherlands: Koninklijke Brill.

Zwicker, E., & Fastl, H. (2013). *Psychoacoustics: Facts and Models* (2nd ed.). New York, NY: Springer-Verlag.

4

Anatomy of the Auditory System

After reading this chapter, you should be able to:

1. Visualize the location of the auditory (and some basic vestibular) structures/organs in your own head and be able to describe the locations of these structures within the temporal bone.

2. Divide the auditory system into five major divisions based on anatomy, and identify the primary parts within each division.

3. Identify the parts of the outer ear and middle ear, and the major landmarks observed in an otoscopic view of a normal tympanic membrane.

4. Describe the relationship of the bony and membranous labyrinths within the inner ear and their different fluids.

5. Sequence different anatomical views progressing from a general view to more detailed views of the inner ear labyrinths and sensory structures.

6. Identify and name the parts of the cochlea and the organ of Corti.

7. Describe several differences between the inner hair cells (IHCs) and the outer hair cells (OHCs) within the organ of Corti.

8. Define and describe the afferent and efferent neural systems within the auditory system as they relate to the hair cells, brainstem auditory nuclei, and primary auditory cortex.

The ear is a fascinating structure! Relatively few people come to appreciate the intricacies of the sensory structures and neural connections responsible for hearing (auditory system) and balance (vestibular system). You are in for an enjoyable journey through these sensory structures no matter what your background or where your career interests lie. For some, this glimpse into the anatomy of the auditory and vestibular systems becomes a pivotal moment that propels them to pursue audiology as a career. This chapter will give you a detailed look at the different parts of the ear, their orientations to each other, and how they are interconnected. The approach taken in this chapter is to present the anatomy with very little discussion on the function of the different structures: The functions of the auditory system are covered in Chapter 5. The vestibular anatomy and functions, along with common vestibular disorders and assessments are covered in more detail in Chapter 16.

This chapter is filled with diagrams and photos. As the adage goes, "a picture is worth a thousand words." The text in this chapter is meant primarily to orient you to the figures, with the expectation that you will navigate through the figures to learn the anatomy and the unique vocabulary associated with these sensory systems. As you progress through this anatomy chapter, keep looking back at previous figures to establish how the different structures relate to each other. Eventually, you will come to mentally visualize these structures in your own head. So, for now, sit back and enjoy a pictorial presentation and description of the anatomy of the auditory and vestibular systems.

GENERAL ORIENTATION TO THE ANATOMY OF THE AUDITORY AND VESTIBULAR SYSTEMS

When discussing the anatomy of the human body, you need to be able to orient yourself to the different viewing angles and planes of reference so that you can more easily locate the parts and pieces and gain a better understanding of how they relate to each other. Figure 4–1 shows the three anatomical planes of reference that are commonly used to divide the body into sections. The *sagittal* plane divides the sturcture into right and left parts/sections. The *coronal* (or frontal) plane divides the structure into anterior (front) and posterior (back) parts/sections. The *transverse* (or horizontal) plane divides a structure into superior (upper) and inferior (lower) parts/sections. These anatomical planes of reference and their commonly used anatomical directions are listed in Table 4–1.

A general orientation of the auditory and vestibular structures as they would appear within the skull when looking from the front of the head is shown in Figure 4–2A. Although this figure

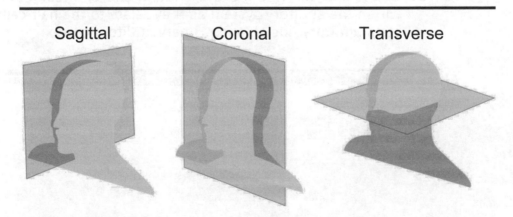

FIGURE 4–1. Anatomical planes of reference. The sagittal plane divides the head or organ into right and left sections. The coronal plane divides the head or organ into anterior and posterior sections. The transverse plane divides the head or organ into superior and inferior sections. *Source*: Illustration by Tatiana Piatanova.

TABLE 4–1. Commonly Used Terms for Anatomic Planes of Reference and Related Directions Used in Reference to Humans and Four-Legged Animals

Planes of Reference	Result in Humans	Related Directions in Humans	Result in Four-Legged Animals	Related Directions in Four-Legged Animals
Coronal	Front/Back	Anterior/Posterior	Head/Tail	Rostral/Caudal
Sagittal	Left/Right	Lateral/Medial	Left/Right	Lateral/Medial
Transverse	Top/Bottom	Superior/Inferior	Top/Bottom	Superior/Inferior

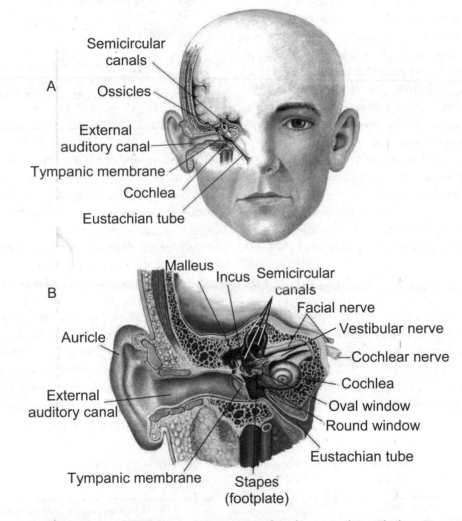

FIGURE 4–2. A and B. A. Orientation of auditory and vestibular structures in the human skull. **B.** Coronal view of the auditory and vestibular structures. See Table 4–2 in order to relate the various structures seen here to the general divisions of the auditory and vestibular systems. *Source*: From Seidel, Ball, Dains, & Benedict, 2003, p. 314. Copyright 2003 by Mosby, Inc.

only shows the details for the right ear, the same structures occur on both sides. As you can see, there are structures that run from the side of the skull (lateral direction) to a location toward the middle of the skull (medial direction). Figure 4–2B is a closer view of these structures in a coronal/frontal section.

Each ear is divided into five general divisions based on their location. The five general divisions of the auditory system are the *outer ear, middle ear, inner ear, 8th cranial nerve*, and the *central auditory nervous system*. Table 4–2 lists the five general divisions of the ear, along with some of the primary structures that are identified in Figure 4–2. Although these divisions are convenient, they are connected and work together to receive and process sounds. Obviously, we have two ears and each ear has the same anatomical and neural components; therefore, in this textbook most of the anatomical descriptions are given only for one ear. The term *central auditory* (or *vestibular*) *nervous system* is used to refer to the related neural pathways in the brainstem and cortical areas; the term *peripheral auditory* (or *vestibular*) *system* is used to refer to the auditory or vestibular structures that are outside of the central nervous system. The peripheral sensory structure for hearing is called the *cochlea*. The peripheral sensory structures of the vestibular system include three *semicircular canals*, a *saccule*, and a *utricle*. The utricle and saccule are collectively referred to as the *otolith organs* and are located within the *vestibule*. For more details on the anatomy of the vestibular system, see Chapter 16 in this textbook.

The auditory and vestibular structures are attached or embedded in the part of the skull

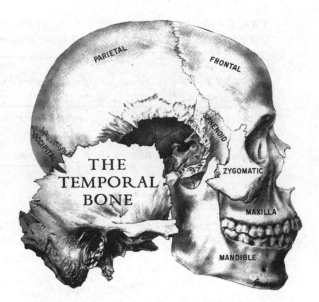

FIGURE 4–3. The temporal bone and its relation to the other parts of the human skull. *Source*: From Anson & Donaldson, 1967, p. 1. Copyright 1967 by W.B. Saunders.

called the *temporal bone*, shown in Figure 4–3. Not shown in Figure 4–3 is the part of the ear easily seen on the side of your head, called the auricle. The auricle is composed primarily of cartilage that also extends into the initial part of the ear canal. Details of the temporal bone are shown in Figure 4–4, as seen from two different directions. In the top part of Figure 4–4, you can see the opening of the bony part of the *external auditory canal* or ear canal (also called the external acoustic meatus). The bony part of the ear canal is a continuation of the cartilaginous part of the ear canal that has been removed in Figures 4–3 and 4–4. The temporal bone is divided into four main parts, tympanic, mastoid,

TABLE 4–2. Five Major Divisions of the Auditory/Vestibular Systems with Primary Structures that Correspond to Those Shown in Figure 4–2B

Outer Ear	Middle Ear	Inner Ear	Cranial Nerve (CN)	Central Nervous System
Auricle	Tympanic membrane	Cochlea (with oval and round windows)	Cochlear nerve (8th CN)	Brainstem
External auditory canal	Ossicles (malleus, incus, stapes)	Semicircular canals	Vestibular nerve (8th CN)	Cortices
	Eustachian tube	Saccule, utricle (not shown)	Facial nerve (7th CN)	

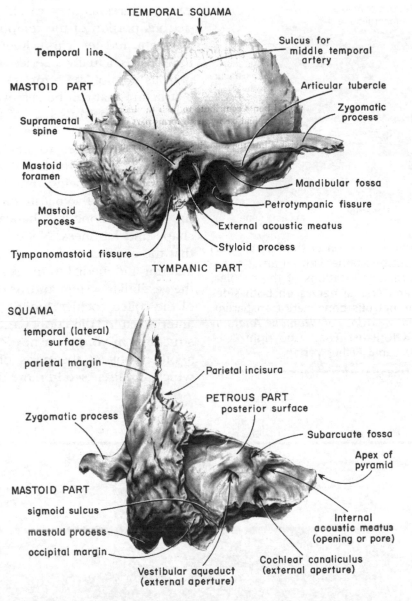

FIGURE 4–4. Anatomic details of the temporal bone. The top part of the figure shows the lateral surface of the temporal bone as viewed from the side of the head. The bottom part of the figure shows the temporal bone as viewed from the top of the head, and reveals the petrous portion of the temporal bone. *Source*: From Anson & Donaldson, 1967, p. 4. Copyright 1967 by W.B. Saunders.

squamous, and petrous. The temporal bone also has two small processes, the zygomatic process that forms the contour of the cheek bone and articulates with the zygomatic bone, and the styloid process to which muscles associated with the tongue and the larynx are connected. The ear canal runs through the tympanic part of the tem-

poral bone, whereas the middle ear and inner ear structures are housed in the petrous part of the temporal bone.

Figure 4–5 shows a transverse view of the skull looking down on the petrous parts of the temporal bones on each side of the skull. The artist's rendition shows the locations of the inner

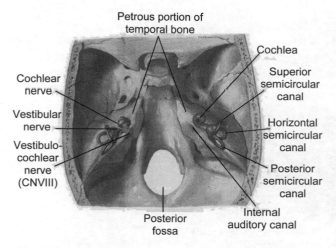

Petrous portion of
temporal bone

Cochlear
nerve

Vestibular
nerve

Vestibulo-
cochlear
nerve
(CNVIII)

Cochlea

Superior
semicircular
canal

Horizontal
semicircular
canal

Posterior
semicircular
canal

Internal
auditory canal

Posterior
fossa

FIGURE 4–5. Transverse section of the human skull at the level of the petrous bone with an artist's rendition showing the relative locations of the cochlea, vestibular organs, and cranial nerves on both sides of the head as if the petrous bone were transparent. *Source*: From *Sobotta Atlas of Human Anatomy* (15th ed.). R. Putz & R. Pabst (Eds.). Copyright 2011 by Elsevier GmbH, Urban & Fisher Verlag.

ear structures as they would appear within the petrous portion of the temporal bone (for both the right and left ears). Keep in mind that the inner ear is actually a series of canals within the petrous part of the temporal bone, rather than a structure that can be removed. As seen in Figure 4–5, the petrous part of the temporal bone is located medially in the skull; this allows the inner ear structures to be located away from the lateral surface of the skull for greater protection. Besides being internally located in the skull, the protective nature of the petrous part of the temporal bone is enhanced by its pyramidal shape and hardness. Notice also in Figure 4–5 that the cochlea of the auditory system is more anterior and medial to the semicircular canals of the vestibular system and, as one can see, the tip of the coiled cochlea "points" horizontally in an anterior–lateral direction. Can you visualize these structures in your own head? Figure 4–6 shows another look at the parts of the ear, each of which are discussed in more detail in the follow-

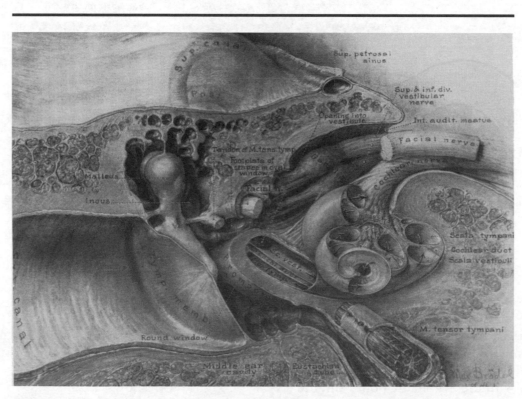

FIGURE 4–6. A drawing of auditory and vestibular structures from a coronal view. *Source*: From Brodel, 1946. Copyright 1946 by W.B. Saunders.

ing sections. You should periodically look back at this figure, and others, so you have a good anatomical orientation of the auditory system.

OUTER EAR

The outer ear is the most visible, but least important, of the auditory structures. The visible portion of the outer ear that is attached to the lateral surface of the temporal bone is primarily a cartilaginous structure called the *auricle*. There are several ridges and indentations in the auricle. Although there are some variations among individuals, the primary features of the auricle are labeled in Figure 4–7. To get a better sense of the auricle's anatomy, use your own auricle as an example. Begin by touching your earlobe with your finger. The *earlobe* is the lower portion of the auricle where earrings are often attached; it is primarily fatty tissue and is not cartilaginous as is the rest of the auricle. Immediately superior and anterior to the earlobe you can place your finger in an indentation that separates the *tragus* anteriorly and the *antitragus* posteriorly. The tragus

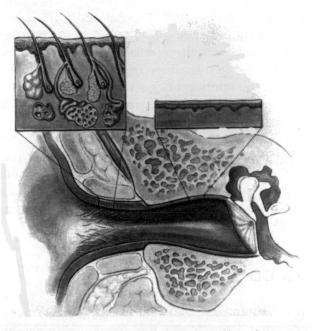

FIGURE 4–8. A drawing of the external auditory canal. The insets illustrate how the various parts differ in the presence or absence of hair follicles and cerumen glands. *Source*: From Office of Visual Media, Indiana University School of Medicine, 1994. Copyright 1994 Indiana University School of Medicine.

is the flap of cartilage that you have undoubtedly used in closing off your ear by pushing this flap in with your finger. Do you feel those landmarks? Now, run your finger superiorly from the antitragus along the ridge of cartilage called the *antihelix*, which ends at an indentation called the *triangular fossa*. If you move your finger to the outer rim of the ear, you can trace the ridge of cartilage that is called the *helix*, which runs around the outer border of the auricle. The relatively large bowl-shaped indentation just before the entrance (meatus) to the external auditory canal is called the *concha*.

The *external auditory canal* is the other part of the outer ear. The external auditory canal is the canal that leads from the auricle to the *tympanic membrane* (ear drum) of the middle ear. Figure 4–8 shows a coronal/frontal section of the *external auditory canal*. The external auditory canal is approximately 25 mm in length and has a somewhat curved route. As mentioned earlier,

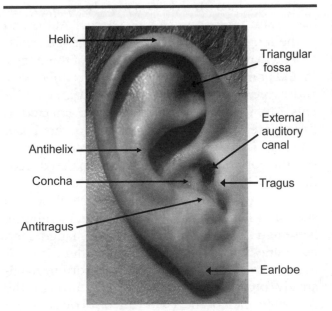

FIGURE 4–7. A picture of an auricle with key landmarks identified.

the lateral half of the external auditory canal is formed by cartilage and is continuous with the auricle, whereas the medial half of the auditory canal is formed by bone from the tympanic portion of the temporal bone and covered with skin. The outer half of the external auditory canal can be straightened by pulling up and back on the auricle (as is done during a clinical examination of the outer ear). Along the cartilaginous portion of the ear canal are small hairs, as well as glands that produce earwax, called *cerumen*. The hairs and cerumen help protect and clean the external auditory canal.

MIDDLE EAR

The middle ear is a small air-filled cavity that is bounded laterally by the tympanic membrane (eardrum) and medially by the cochlea. The upper portion of the middle ear cavity is called the *epitympanic recess*. The middle ear cavity houses the *ossicles,* a series of three bones named *malleus*, *incus*, and *stapes*, which are the smallest bones in the human body. The ossicles are connected to each other as synovial joints and form the *ossicular chain*. Details of the ossicular chain are shown in Figure 4–9, as viewed from inside the middle

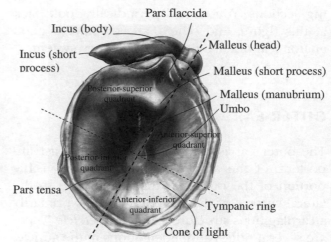

FIGURE 4–10. Drawing of a tympanic membrane and related middle ear structures. The superimposed *dotted lines* divide the tympanic membrane into four quadrants. *Source*: Adapted from Anson & Donaldson, 1967, p. 54. Copyright 1967 by W.B. Saunders.

ear cavity looking toward the inner surface of the tympanic membrane (not shown). The malleus has a *manubrium* (handle), a lateral process, a neck, and a head. The manubrium of the malleus attaches to the tympanic membrane. The head of the malleus articulates (united by joints) with the body of the incus. In addition to its body, the incus has a short process and a long process. At the end of the long process of the incus is the *lenticular process* that articulates with the head of the stapes. In addition to the head, the stapes has a *footplate* and two *crura*, an anterior crus and a posterior crus. The footplate of the stapes is connected to the inner ear through the membrane-covered *oval window*. There is another window into the inner ear, the *round window*, which is separated from the oval window by the *promontory*.

A drawing of the tympanic membrane is shown in Figure 4–10. The tympanic membrane is semi-translucent, slightly cone shaped, and pearl gray in color. Some of the middle ear landmarks can be seen through the eardrum. A relatively prominent landmark seen through the tympanic membrane (with an otoscope) is the manubrium of the malleus, which runs upward from the center of the tympanic membrane. The

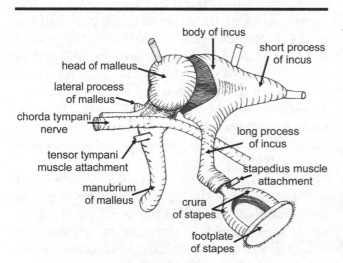

FIGURE 4–9. Drawing of an ossicular chain, composed of the three bones, malleus, incus, and stapes. *Source*: From Tos, 1995. Copyright 1995 by Thieme-Verlag.

lower attachment point of the manubrium at the middle of the tympanic membrane is called the *umbo*. In addition, the lateral process of malleus is readily visible through the upper part of the tympanic membrane. Notice also that the upper portions of the malleus and incus lie above the superior border of the tympanic membrane and would not be visible with an otoscope. There is often a *light reflex* (also called cone of light) that can be seen bouncing off the tympanic membrane. This is a reflection of the light from the otoscope, and the characteristic appearance and location of the light reflex in a normal ear is due to the curved shape of the tympanic membrane. As seen in Figure 4–10, the tympanic membrane can be described by quadrants as visualized by an imaginary line running along the manubrium and a bisecting perpendicular line. These quadrants allow one to describe where different structures or pathologies are located; for instance, the cone of light normally appears in the anterior-inferior quadrant.

Most of the tympanic membrane has a fibrous tissue layer, the *pars tensa*, that lies between the skin lining the external ear canal wall and the mucous tissue that lines the middle ear space. The pars tensa provides strength to the membrane. In the anterior part of the tympanic membrane just above the lateral process, there is a small area that does not have the fibrous tissue layer; this thinner area of the tympanic membrane is called the *pars flaccida* or *Shrapnell's membrane*. The outer rim of the tympanic membrane is called the *tympanic ring* (or tympanic annulus). The tympanic ring is embedded into the *tympanic sulcus*, an indentation in the tympanic portion of the temporal bone that holds the tympanic membrane in place. Figure 4–11 shows actual photos of tympanic membranes for the left and right ears. Can you identify the main landmarks? The orientation of the observed landmarks appears differently for the two ears, as seen in Figure 4–11. However, one can keep this straight by looking for the light reflex in the anterior–inferior part of the tympanic membrane; or the lateral process appears on the right when looking at the right tympanic membrane and on the left when looking at the left tympanic membrane.

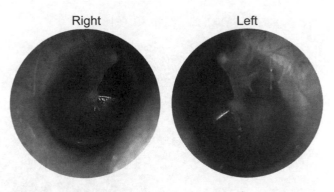

Right   Left

FIGURE 4–11. Photos of the tympanic membranes for the right and left ears as they would appear when viewed through an otoscope.

The middle ear has a tube, the *eustachian tube*, that connects the middle ear to an opening into the *nasopharynx*, an area above the tonsils in the upper part of the oral cavity/throat. Figure 4–12 shows the anatomy of the eustachian tube and its relationship to the nasopharynx. The eustachian tube is composed of a bony (osseous) portion that originates in the middle ear cavity and a cartilaginous portion that extends to the back of the nasopharynx. The cartilaginous portion of the eustachian tube is normally closed, but is opened by action of the *tensor veli palatini* muscle during chewing or swallowing. The periodic opening of the eustachian tube allows the middle ear to maintain its air-filled environment at atmospheric pressure, since it connects to the outside world through its opening in the nasopharynx. Figure 4–12C shows that the adult eustachian tube is longer than in a young child, and is oriented at about a 45° angle from the middle ear to the nasopharynx compared with a shallower angle in the young child (Bluestone & Klein, 1988). These developmental differences in the eustachian tube make it more difficult for the infant to maintain a normal air-filled environment of the middle ear, and is a primary reason why infants and toddlers have more middle ear problems than adults.

The middle ear also has two small muscles, the *stapedius muscle* and the *tensor tympani muscle*, that attach to the ossicular chain by their corresponding tendons (refer back to Figure 4–9). The stapedius muscle arises from

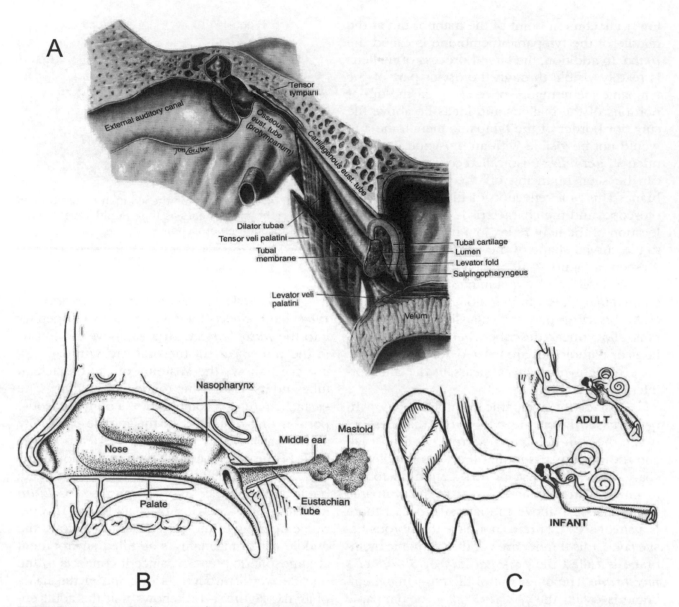

FIGURE 4–12. A–C. The eustachian tube. **A.** Anatomy of the eustachian tube with its bony and cartilaginous parts. The eustachian tube is normally closed, and is opened briefly by the tensor veli palatini muscle during chewing or swallowing. **B.** Illustration showing the eustachian tube from the middle ear to an opening in the nasopharynx. **C.** Illustration showing the differences in the angle of the eustachian tube between adults and infants. *Source*: Adapted from Bluestone & Klein, 1988, pp. 5–7. Copyright 1988 by W.B. Saunders.

the posterior wall of the middle ear cavity and attaches to the head of the stapes. The stapedius muscle is innervated by the stapedial branch of the *facial nerve* (7th cranial nerve). The tensor tympani muscle arises from the bony wall above the eustachian tube and attaches to the upper part of the manubrium of the malleus. The ten-sor tympani muscle is innervated by a branch of the *trigeminal nerve* (5th cranial nerve). These middle ear muscles are involved in a reflexive response to loud sounds, called the *acoustic reflex*. Evaluation of the acoustic reflex is one of the basic audiological clinical procedures that will be described in more detail in Chapter 10.

SYNOPSIS 4–1

- Each ear is divided into five general divisions:
  - Outer ear
  - Middle ear
  - Inner ear
  - 8th cranial nerve
  - Central auditory nervous system
- The peripheral auditory and vestibular structures are located in the temporal bone of the skull. The parts of the temporal bone include the tympanic, mastoid, squamous, and petrous, as well as two processes, the zygomatic and styloid.
- The organs for hearing and balance are within the petrous portion of the temporal bone, which affords them good protection due to the more medial location, dense composition, and pyramidal shape.
- The cochlea is anterior and medial to the semicircular canals, and the tip of the cochlea points horizontally in an anterior–lateral direction.
- The main components of the outer ear are:
  - Auricle
    - Helix
    - Antihelix
    - Tragus
    - Antitragus
    - Earlobe
    - Triangular fossa
    - Concha
  - The external ear canal, which is irregularly shaped with cartilaginous and bony parts, has an adult length of about 25 mm. There are cerumen glands and hair follicles in the cartilaginous part.
- The middle ear is a small air-filled cavity that begins with the tympanic membrane at the end of the external ear canal. The main components and their parts are:
  - Tympanic membrane (pars tensa, pars flaccida, umbo, tympanic ring): Semi-translucent and pearl gray in color. Notable landmarks of a normal tympanic membrane, when viewed with an otoscope, include the manubrium of malleus, lateral process of malleus, umbo, and a light reflex (from the otoscope).
  - Ossicular chain: Malleus (manubrium, lateral process, neck, head); incus (body, short process, long process, lenticular process); stapes (head, anterior and posterior crura, footplate). The footplate is attached to the inner ear at the oval window.
  - Two small muscles: Stapedius muscle connects to the stapes; tensor tympani muscle connects to the malleus. Stapedius muscle is innervated by a branch of the 7th cranial nerve; tensor tympani muscle is innervated by a branch of the 5th cranial nerve. The stapedius muscle is involved in the human acoustic reflex that is useful for clinical assessments (see Chapter 10).
  - Eustachian tube: Cartilaginous tube from the middle ear space to the nasopharynx that maintains atmospheric pressure in the middle ear. Normally closed, but opens (by tensor veli palatini muscle) with chewing and swallowing. Infants and young children have developmental differences in shape and function of the eustachian tube, which is a primary reason for ear infections in young children.

INNER EAR

The inner ear is a series of canals and cavities within the petrous portion of the temporal bone, called the *bony labyrinth*. The bony labyrinth is carved out of the bone; whereas if one were to make a cast of the bony labyrinth it would look something like that shown in Figure 4–13. Keep in mind that the entire inner ear is smaller than the end of your little finger. The coiled structure on the right of Figure 4–13 is the cochlea, which houses the sensory organ for hearing. The cochlea spirals about 2¾ turns to save space within the skull, because if uncoiled it is about 35 mm long (Yost, 2013). The wider part of the cochlea is called the base, and the tip of the cochlea is called the apex. The height of the cochlea from base to apex is only about 5 mm. On the left side of Figure 4–13, you can see the three semicircular canals of the vestibular system. These three semicircular canals are oriented in three orthogonal planes and respond primarily to angular accelerations of the head. The vestibule is the area of the bony labyrinth that lies between the cochlea and the semicircular canals. Inside the vestibule is where two other vestibular organs, the saccule and utricle, are located. The saccule and utricle are often referred to as the *otolith* organs, and respond primarily to linear accelerations of

the head (see Chapter 16 for a more detailed look at the vestibular system). The vestibule is also the location of the oval window, through which the stapes footplate of the ossicular chain connects to the cochlea. The *round window* is another membrane-covered small opening in the cochlear portion of the bony labyrinth between the middle ear cavity and the cochlea. As you will learn in Chapter 5, the inner ear is filled with fluid and if vibrations are to occur within the cochlea there must be reciprocal movements (in and out) of the stapes in the oval window with movements (out and in) of the round window membrane.

Suspended within the bony labyrinth of the inner ear is a *membranous labyrinth*. The membranous labyrinth has the same general shape of the bony labyrinth. The membranous labyrinth is where the auditory and vestibular sensory cells are located. Figure 4–14 shows a drawing of a coronal cross-section of the bony and membranous labyrinths. The entire inner ear is filled with fluids; however, the fluid within the membranous labyrinth is different from the fluid within the bony labyrinth (surrounding the membranous labyrinth) as described in Table 4–3. The bony labyrinth is filled with fluid called *perilymph*, which is similar to cerebral spinal fluid. Perilymph has a high sodium (Na+) concentra-

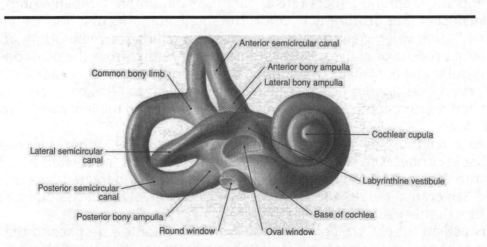

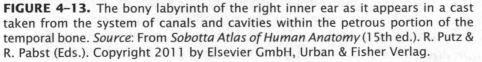

FIGURE 4–13. The bony labyrinth of the right inner ear as it appears in a cast taken from the system of canals and cavities within the petrous portion of the temporal bone. *Source*: From *Sobotta Atlas of Human Anatomy* (15th ed.). R. Putz & R. Pabst (Eds.). Copyright 2011 by Elsevier GmbH, Urban & Fisher Verlag.

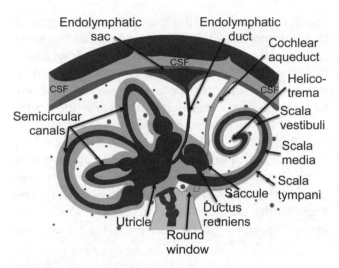

FIGURE 4–14. Cross-section of the petrous portion of the temporal bone showing the bony labyrinth (*unfilled areas*) and the membranous labyrinth (*filled areas*). The membranous labyrinth is suspended within the bony labyrinth and is mostly filled with endolymph, whereas the bony labyrinth is filled with perilymph. *Source*: Illustration by Tatiana Piatanova.

tion and low potassium (K+) concentration. Most of the membranous labyrinth is filled with fluid called *endolymph*. Endolymph has high potassium (K+) concentration and low sodium (N+) concentration. Endolymph is similar to fluids found inside cells (intracellular); therefore, in the cochlea endolymph is unique because it is found outside of cells (extracellular). Notice, in Figure 4–14, that the membranous labyrinth (and its endolymph) is continuous between the cochlea and the vestibular organs by way of a small channel called the *ductus reuniens*. The membranous

labyrinth also has an extension to the dural area of the brain through the *endolymphatic duct*, which ends in the *endolymphatic sac*. The perilymph of the bony labyrinth connects to the cerebral spinal fluid through a narrow bony canal called the *cochlear aqueduct*.

THE SENSORY ORGAN OF HEARING

Now let's take a more detailed look at the fine structure of the cochlea. Figure 4–15 shows a drawing of the bony labyrinth of the inner ear, but with a transverse section that runs through the center of the cochlea so we can see inside the cochlea (upper half of the cochlea is removed). The central bony core of the cochlea is called the *modiolus*, which is a porous area of bone that forms the inner wall of the cochlea. The modiolus is where the nerve fibers from the sensory cells of the cochlea come together and form the auditory portion of the 8th cranial nerve. Because the top half of the cochlea has been removed in Figure 4–15, we can see circular-looking cross sections of the coiled cochlea at different locations. Figure 4–16 shows photomicrographs of a cochlea from a chinchilla. Figure 4–16A shows the modiolus after a portion of the bony wall was chipped away and the membranous labyrinth removed. As you can see, the modiolus (inner core of the cochlea) resembles a screw with the bony shelf, *osseous spiral lamina*, that spirals around the shaft (modiolus) as the "threads of a screw." Figure 4–16B shows a cross-section through the middle of the modiolus of the cochlea with the membranous

TABLE 4–3. Ionic Composition of the Fluids in the Inner Ear and Cerebral Spinal Fluid (CSF)

Fluid Type	Potassium (K) (mEq/liter)	Sodium (Na) (mEq/liter)	Protein (mg %)
Cerebral Spinal Fluid	4 (K)	152 (Na)	20–50
Endolymph	144 (K+)	5 (Na+)	126
Perilymph	10 (K+)	140 (Na)	200–400

Source: Based on Baloh & Honrubia (2001).

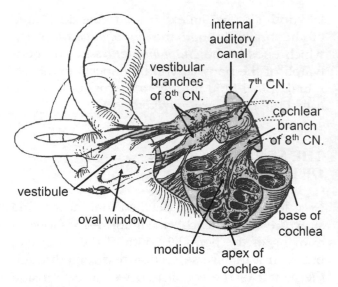

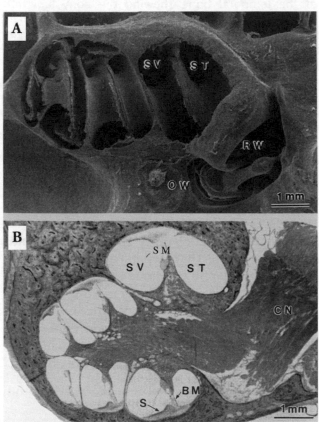

FIGURE 4–15. A drawing of the bony labyrinth with a transverse section through the cochlea (midmodiolar view) revealing the modiolus and cochlear chambers (scalae). *Source*: Republished with permission of Oxford University Press, from Baloh, R. W., & Honrubia, V. H. (2001). *Clinical Neurophysiology of the Vestibular System*. New York, NY: Oxford University Press. p. 11; permission conveyed through Copyright Clearance Center, Inc.

labyrinth in place (and resembles the cross-section of the cochlea seen in Figure 4–15). Notice that the osseous spiral lamina partially divides the bony labyrinth into different sections (called scalae). Actually, coming off the osseous spiral lamina is a small triangular-shaped part of the membranous labyrinth, called the *scala media*, that attaches to the outer wall of the bony labyrinth. Thus, the scala media separates the bony labyrinth into two other sections, one called *scala tympani* and the other called *scala vestibuli*. As we will see in more detail, the sensory organ of hearing, *organ of Corti*, lies within scala media along one side of its membranous surface, the *basilar membrane*. The basilar membrane is the portion of the membranous labyrinth that is attached from the osseous spiral lamina to the outer wall of the bony labyrinth. The other surface of the membranous labyrinth in the cochlea, *Reissner's membrane*, is attached from the modiolus part of the bony labyrinth to the outer wall of the bony labyrinth. You can identify each of these scala by remembering that the scala tympani is the part of the bony lab-

yrinth next to the basilar membrane and organ of Corti. It may also help to remember that the scala tympani terminates at the round window membrane which is like a drum (hence, "tympani"), whereas the scala vestibuli is the part of the bony labyrinth next to Reissner's membrane and terminates at the oval window in the vestibule (hence, "vestibuli"). The scala tympani and scala vestibuli are filled with perilymph, whereas scala media is primarily filled with endolymph (except in portions of the organ of Corti, as described later). The scala media does not quite go all the way to the end of the apex of the cochlea, which leaves an

FIGURE 4–16. A and B. Two views of the cochlea from a chinchilla model. **A.** Chinchilla cochlea with bony labyrinth opened to show the coiled modiolus. **B.** Midmodiolar cross-section through cochlea. SV, scala vestibuli; ST, scala tympani; SM, scala media; BM, basilar membrane; S, stria vascularis; CN, cochlear nerve; OW, oval window; RW, round window. *Source*: Reprinted with permission from Harrison, R. V. (1988). *The biology of hearing and deafness*, p. 12. Courtesy of Charles C Thomas Publisher, Ltd., Springfield, Illinois.

area called the *helicotrema*. At the helicotrema, the scala tympani and scala vestibuli are continuous with each other. The cochlea, including the scala media, spirals from base to apex, as shown in Figure 4–17. The basilar membrane also spirals from base to apex; however, the width of the basilar membrane is narrower at the base and gets wider as it spirals to the apex. The width changes of the basilar membrane are important to the processing of sounds, as will be covered in Chapter 5. To account for the changing width of the basilar membrane, the osseous spiral lamina is wider at the base than at the apex (look back at Figure 4–16B) and looks like the "threads of a screw."

We are now ready to take a look at the fine structure of the organ of Corti. Figure 4–18 is a drawing of a "slice" (cross-section) through a part of the spiraling cochlea, and shows an expanded view of the three scalae. Be sure to look back at earlier figures to get a perspective on how this drawing relates to the entire cochlea. As you will see, many of the following figures will zoom further and further into this cross-section of the cochlea, especially the scala media to view the details of the organ of Corti. In Figure 4–18, you can again see how the membranous labyrinth (bounded by the basilar membrane and Reissner's membrane) divides the cochlea into its three scalae with their attachments from the osseous spiral lamina to the outer wall of the bony labyrinth. Scala media is the "pie-shaped" portion formed by the membranous labyrinth of

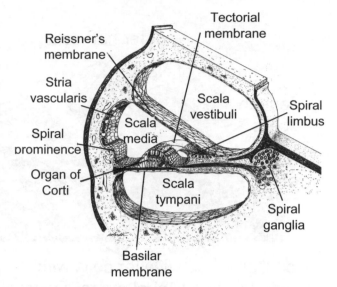

FIGURE 4–18. Cross-section of the cochlea showing the three scalae and the organ of Corti in the scala media. *Source:* From Fawcett, D. W. (1994). *Bloom and Fawcett: A Textbook of Histology* (p. 929). New York, NY: Chapman and Hall. Reproduced by permission of Taylor & Francis Books UK.

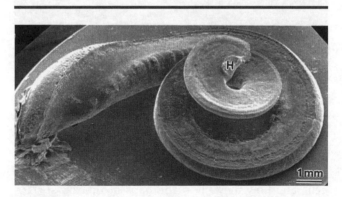

FIGURE 4–17. A plastic cast of the human cochlea showing the different turns. H, helicotrema. *Source:* Reprinted with permission from Harrison, R. V. (1988). *The biology of hearing and deafness*, p. 13. Courtesy of Charles C Thomas Publisher, Ltd., Springfield, Illinois.

the cochlea. Scala tympani is next to the basilar membrane and scala vestibuli is next to Reissner's membrane. Recall that scala tympani and scala vestibuli contain perilymph (and join each other at the helicotrema), whereas scala media contains mostly endolymph. Along the outer surface of the scala media is the *stria vascularis*, a highly vascularized system of cells that maintains the ionic charge of the endolymph that is very important for the biological function of the organ of Corti.

The organ of Corti is a collection of different specialized cells found within the scala media along the basilar membrane. You should now be even more impressed by how small the organ of Corti is when you think of where it is in relation to the entire inner ear, which itself is smaller than a dime. The details of the organ of Corti are shown in Figure 4–19. When describing some of the structures of the organ of Corti, keep in mind that "inner" is toward the modiolus and "outer" is toward the stria vascularis. Figure 4–19 shows a two-dimensional "slice" through the organ of Corti; however, as you have come to appreciate, these cells are laid out, one next to the

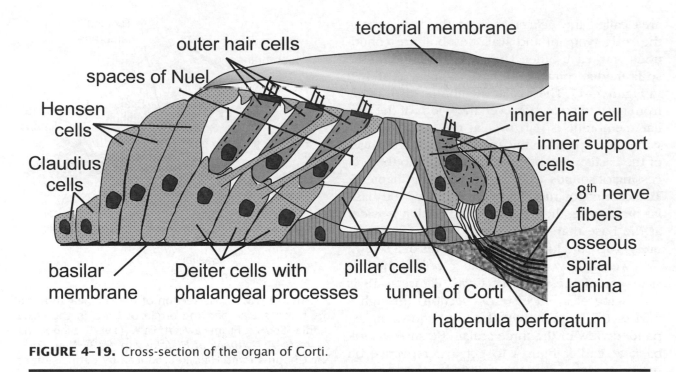

FIGURE 4–19. Cross-section of the organ of Corti.

other, along the entire length of the coiled co-chlea from the base to the apex. The cells of the organ of Corti consist of two types of function-ally relevant cells, the *inner hair cells* (IHCs) and the *outer hair cells* (OHCs). Spiraling from the base to the apex of the cochlea are about 3500 IHCs arranged in a single row and about 12,000 OHCs arranged in three rows (Yost, 2013). The tops of the IHCs and OHCs have bundles of tiny "hairs" called *stereocilia*. Above the stereocilia of the hair cells is another membrane, the *tectorial membrane*. The tectorial membrane is attached to the *spiral limbus*, a cell that curves up from the osseous spiral lamina (seen best on Fig-ure 4–18) and outward to the upper surface of the *Hensen cells*, which are next to and supported by the *Claudius cells*. Notice that the stereocilia of the OHCs are attached to the underside of the tectorial membrane, whereas the stereocilia of the IHCs are not attached to the tectorial mem-brane. The other cells of the organ of Corti pro-vide structural support and shape for the organ of Corti. The IHCs are supported by the *inner support (*phalangeal*) cells*. The OHCs and IHCs are separated by the *tunnel of Corti*, a space in the center of the organ of Corti that is formed by

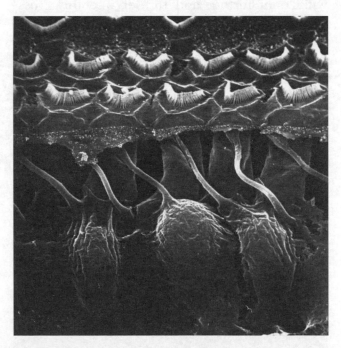

FIGURE 4–20. Close-up view within the organ of Corti showing the phalangeal processes of the Deiter cells and how they fill in the gaps at the top surface of the adjacent outer hair cells, forming part of the reticular lamina. *Source*: From Bagger-Sjöback, Anniko, & Lundquist, 1984, p. 15. Copyright 1984 by Butterworths and Company Ltd.

the inner and outer *pillar cells*. The OHCs (unlike the IHCs) are surrounded by spaces, called *spaces of Nuel*. Each OHC sits on top of a support cell, called a *Deiter cell* (also called outer phalangeal cell). Each Deiter cell has a *phalangeal process* that reaches up to the upper surface of an adjacent OHC and fills in what would have been a space between the tops of the OHCs. Figure 4–20 is a close-up of the OHCs, where you can see how the phalangeal processes of the Deiter cells extend to the upper surface of the organ of Corti.

Figure 4–21 shows a photomicrograph looking down on the top surface of the organ of Corti after pulling back the tectorial membrane. Notice that the tops of all the cells are tightly

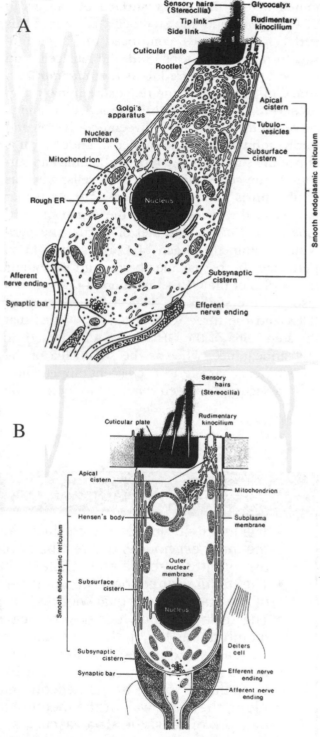

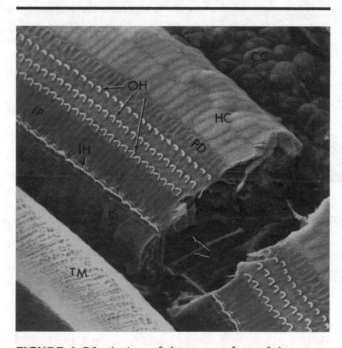

FIGURE 4–21. A view of the top surface of the organ of Corti with the tectorial membrane (TM) pulled back to reveal the reticular lamina and the stereocilia of the three rows of outer hair cells (OH) and the single row of inner hair cells (IH). The top surface of the tunnel of Corti is defined by the top plates of the inner pillar cells (IP) and separates the inner hair cells from the outer hair cells. A section is opened up to view below the reticular lamina. OP, outer pillar cells; PD, phalangeal processes of Deiter cells; HC, Hensen cells; CC, Claudius cells. *Source*: From Kimura, 1984, p. 102. Copyright 1984 by Butterworths and Company Ltd.

FIGURE 4–22. Drawings of inner hairs cells (**A**) and outer hair cells (**B**) that illustrate their different shapes, location of the nucleus, and organization of the cell's cytoplasm. Notice also that the stereocilia are connected by tip links and side links. *Source*: Adapted from Lim, 1986, pp. 75 & 76. Copyright 1986 by W.B. Saunders.

joined across the upper surface of the organ of Corti, and only the stereocilia are above this surface. This surface, comprised of a tight mosaic formed by the tops of all the hair cells and support cells, is referred to as the *reticular lamina*. Can you identify the reticular lamina in Figures 4–18, 4–19, and 4–20? The reticular lamina serves as the boundary between endolymph and perilymph within the scala media: Endolymph is above the surface of the reticular lamina and surrounds the stereocilia of the hair cells, whereas perilymph is below the surface of the reticular lamina in the spaces within the organ of Corti (spaces of Nuel and tunnel of Corti). The perilymph within the organ of Corti is thought to permeate the basilar membrane and surrounds the bodies of the OHCs. In Figure 4–21, you can also see the stereocilia from the single row of IHCs and the three rows of OHCs. Notice that the stereocilia of the OHCs have a characteristic "W" appearance, whereas the stereocilia of the IHCs have a characteristic "crescent" appearance. Also, a section has been removed to look inside

the organ of Corti, where you can see the tunnel of Corti and some of the cell bodies of the organ of Corti.

Figure 4–22 shows more detailed drawings of an IHC and an OHC. Besides differences in the overall number of cells and the number of rows of IHCs and OHCs, other differences are seen between IHCs and OHCs. The IHCs are flask shaped, have a centralized nucleus, and the cytoplasmic organelles are distributed throughout the cell body. The OHCs are more cylinder shaped, have a nucleus closer to the base of the cell, and the organelles are more organized along the cell's outer wall, which has important physiological relevance, as discussed in Chapter 5. The stereocilia on each hair cell are arranged in three to four rows with increasing heights, and many of the stereocilia of a single hair cell are joined to each other by small microfilaments, called *tip links* that join the tips of the stereocilia from the different rows of stereocilia on each individual hair cell, and *cross links* (or side links) that join the adjacent stereocilia within each row of stereocilia.

SYNOPSIS 4–2

- The inner ear houses the cochlea, the sensory organ for hearing. In addition, the inner ear houses the vestibular organs with its three semicircular canals and two otoliths (saccule and utricle).
- The middle ear connects to the inner ear membranous labyrinth at the footplate of the stapes in the oval window.
- The scala media divides the cochlea into three chambers: (a) scala media (the membranous labyrinth), (b) scala tympani (next to the basilar membrane), and (c) scala vestibuli (next to Reissner's membrane).
- Because the scala media ends just before the apex, the scala vestibuli and scala tympani are joined at the helicotrema.
- Along the outer wall of the membranous labyrinth is a highly vascularized network of cells, the stria vascularis, which maintains the ionic composition of the endolymph.
- The organ of Corti is found within the scala media along the basilar membrane. The cells of the organ of Corti (in order from modiolus toward the outer wall) include:
  - Inner support (phalangeal) cells
  - Inner hair cells (IHCs)
  - Inner and outer pillar cells (which form the tunnel of Corti)

SYNOPSIS 4–2 (*continued*)

- ○ Outer hair cells (OHCs): The OHCs sit on top of the supporting Deiter cells which have phalangeal processes that extend to the tops of the hair cells to fill in any spaces between the tops of the OHCs
  - ○ Hensen cells
- Claudius cells
- Each cochlea has about 3500 IHCs (arranged in one row) and about 12,000 OHCs (arranged in three rows). Each hair cell has small hair-like bundles of tiny hairs, called stereocilia, arranged in three to four rows with increasing height toward the outer wall of the cochlea, and are connected by cross-link and tip-link filaments. The stereocilia on each IHC appear as a shallow crescent shape and the stereocilia on each OHC appear as a W shape.
- OHCs differ from IHCs in their overall number, arrangement, shape, and organization of their internal cellular organelles.
- The organ of Corti has a membrane, the tectorial membrane, that attaches from the spiral limbus on the modiolus side to the Hensen cells across the organ of Corti. The stereocilia of the OHCs are imbedded within the underside of the tectorial membrane, whereas the stereocilia of the IHCs do not directly contact the tectorial membrane.
- The OHCs are surrounded by spaces of Nuel and contain perilymph.
- The reticular lamina is a mosaic comprised of the tops of the inner support cells, IHCs, pillar cells, OHCs, and phalangeal processes of the Deiter cells. In this way, the upper surfaces of all the cells of the organ of Corti (below the tectorial membrane) are tightly butted against each other with only the stereocilia of the hair cells sticking out above the reticular lamina. The reticular lamina serves as the boundary between the endolymph above and perilymph below (in the spaces of the organ of Corti).
- Endolymph is similar to fluids typically found within cells (high K+, low Na+) and is unique as an extracellular fluid in the inner ear. The bony labyrinth (surrounding the membranous labyrinth) is filled with a fluid called perilymph (high Na+, low K+), which is similar to cerebral spinal fluid.

AUDITORY NEURAL PATHWAYS

Referring back to Figures 4–2, 4–6, and 4–15, you can see the location of the 8th cranial nerve, *vestibulocochlear* (or *cochleovestibular*) *nerve*, which, as the name implies, has a cochlear branch and a vestibular branch. The 8th cranial nerve exits the petrous part of the temporal bone through an opening in the posterior wall, the *internal auditory canal*. Notice that the 7th cranial nerve (facial nerve) also exits the petrous portion of the temporal bone through the internal auditory canal. In the following sections, the auditory neu-

ral pathways are described in more detail. For the vestibular neural pathways, see Chapter 16.

Auditory Nervous System Pathways

Most of the nerve fibers in the cochlear nerve are *afferent neurons* (approximately 30,000) that carry impulses from the organ of Corti to the brainstem; however, there are a small number of *efferent neurons* (about 1200) that carry impulses from the brainstem to the organ of Corti.

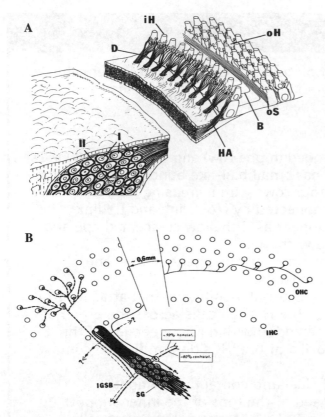

FIGURE 4–23. A. Illustration showing the afferent neurons entering the cochlea through the habenula perforata (*HA*) with multiple synapses with the inner hair cells (*iH*). The cell bodies of the cochlear neurons (I, type I neurons; II, type II neurons) are shown in Rosenthal's canal along the spiral lamina of the modiolus. oH, outer hair cell; oS, outer spiral bundle; B, basilar fibers; D, dendrites. *Source*: From Spoendlin, 1984, p. 133. Copyright 1984 by Butterworths and Company Ltd. **B.** Innervation pattern of cochlear neurons in the organ of Corti. *Solid lines* indicate afferent neurons; *dashed lines* indicate efferent neurons. SG, spiral ganglion; IGSB, intraganglion spiral bundle; IHC, inner hair cell; OHC, outer hair cell. *Source*: Reprinted with permission from Spoendlin, H. (1988). Neural Anatomy of the Inner Ear. In A. F. Jahn & J. Santos-Sacchi (Eds.), *Physiology of the ear*. Philadelphia, PA: Wolters Kluwer, p. 204.

Figure 4–23 shows the connections of the auditory neurons (both afferent and efferent) to the hair cells in the organ of Corti. Keep in mind that the auditory neurons are distributed from/to hair cells along the entire length of the coiled organ of Corti. Most of the afferent nerve fibers (*inner radial fibers*) come from connections with the

IHCs. In fact, approximately 95% of the 30,000 afferent neurons are connected to the 3500 IHCs, that is, many afferent neurons connect to each IHC (Spoendlin, 1978). The remaining afferent neurons (*outer spiral fibers*) come from OHCs that are located approximately 0.6 mm basally from where they cross the tunnel of Corti. Each outer spiral fiber has collaterals coming from several OHCs distributed across their three rows.

The efferent auditory nerve fibers within the organ of Corti are much fewer in number and more difficult to trace. A greater proportion of the efferent nerve fibers connect to the OHCs than to the IHCs, and are more prevalent in the basal end of the cochlea than the apical end (Gelfand, 2009). Figure 4–24 shows that the efferent fibers have different types of connections to the IHCs and OHCs. For the OHCs, both the efferent neurons and the afferent neurons synapse directly with the body of the hair cell. This suggests that the efferent nerve fibers can have a direct influence on the OHCs. However, for the IHCs only the afferent neurons synapse directly with the body of the hair cell, whereas the efferent neurons synapse with the afferent nerve

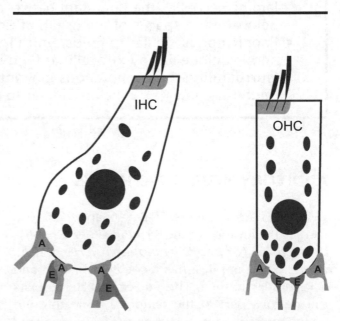

FIGURE 4–24. Illustration showing the different synapse of afferent and efferent neurons with an inner hair cell (IHC) and an outer hair cell (OHC). *Source*: Illustration by Tatiana Piatanova.

dendrites after they leave the IHC, and do not have direct connections with the IHC (Spoendlin, 1978).

The afferent and efferent auditory neurons exit and enter the organ of Corti through tiny holes, *habenula perforata* (see Figure 4–23A), in the osseous spiral lamina. The cell bodies of the afferent auditory neurons are located in the modiolus near the osseous spiral lamina within a bony canal, *Rosenthal's canal*. The afferent auditory nerve cell bodies are called *spiral ganglia* (singular = spiral ganglion) and are distributed along the spiraling cochlea. The cell bodies for the efferent nerve fibers are located in the pontine region of the brainstem near the *superior olivary complex* (SOC), and their axons travel as the *olivocochlear bundle* (OCB) in the 8th cranial nerve, following the same route to the organ of Corti as the afferent nerve fibers through the modiolus, habenula perforata, and to the corresponding hair cells. The efferent nerve fibers that connect to the OHCs originate from the area around the *medial superior olive* (MSO) on both sides of the brainstem, with the majority coming from the contralateral side. The efferent nerve fibers that connect to the IHCs originate from the area around the lateral superior olive (LSO) on both sides of the brainstem, again with the majority coming from the contralateral side.

The afferent nerve fibers of the cochlear branch of the 8th cranial nerve exit the internal auditory canal and travel a short distance to enter the brainstem at the junction of the pontine (pons) and medullary (medulla) regions of the brainstem. The term *nucleus* is used to identify a location within the brainstem where there is a collection of specialized cell bodies. This is similar to the use of ganglion to describe a collection of specialized cell bodies in the peripheral sensory systems (e.g., spiral ganglion in the cochlea). Connections and pathways in the brainstem and cortical regions of the brain are considered to be part of the central nervous system. As shown in Figure 4–25, the primary auditory nuclei, in ascending order, are the *cochlear nucleus*, superior olivary complex, *lateral lemniscus*, *inferior colliculus*, and *medial geniculate body* (in the thalamus). Each of these auditory nuclei is present on both sides of the brainstem. The central auditory

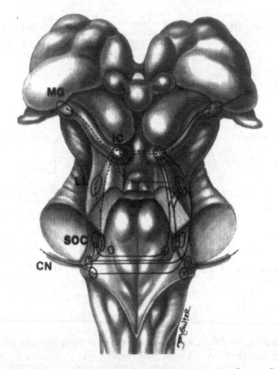

FIGURE 4–25. Drawing of the posterior surface of the brainstem, with superimposed pathways and nuclei of the central auditory system. Nuclei include cochlear nuclei (CN), superior olivary complex (SOC), lateral lemniscus (LL), inferior colliculus (IC), and medial geniculate body (MG). *Source*: From Møller, 2000, p. 131. Copyright 2000 by Academic Press.

afferent pathway involves multiple synapses with multiple cells within multiple brainstem nuclei.

The neural connections of the central auditory system within the brainstem are relatively complex, are not easy to document, and may vary slightly among species. A complete description is beyond the scope of this introductory text. However, a relatively simplified schematic representation of the afferent auditory pathways is shown in Figure 4–26, representing auditory input to the brainstem from the cochlea on one side of the head (the pathways would be duplicated from the other ear). The nerve fibers of the cochlear portion of the 8th cranial nerve enter the brainstem at the lateral side of the pontine region of the brainstem. All of the cochlear 8th nerve afferent neurons synapse with cells in the cochlear nucleus on the same side (ipsilateral) as the ear. Upon entering the cochlear nucleus, each afferent

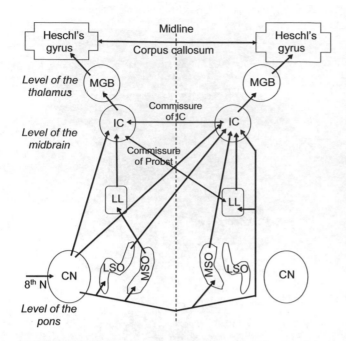

FIGURE 4–26. Central auditory neural pathways from one ear through the brainstem to the auditory cortex. The *dotted line* represents the midline of the brainstem. There are multiple pathways coursing along an ipsilateral route and a more dominant contralateral route. 8th N, 8th cranial nerve; CN, cochlear nucleus; LSO, lateral superior olivary complex; MSO, medial superior olivary complex; LL, lateral lemniscus; IC, inferior colliculus; MGB, medial geniculate body.

superior olivary complexes. To add to the complexity, there are *commissures* (interconnections) across the brainstem between the lateral lemnisci and inferior colliculi, commissure of Probst, and between the inferior colliculi, commissure of the inferior colliculus. From the medial geniculate body on each side of the brainstem, the neurons travel to the ipsilateral primary auditory reception area (AI) of the cortex. The primary auditory reception area of the cortex is located along the upper surface of the *temporal lobe* in *Heschl's gyrus* (Figure 4–27). The primary auditory cortex is not the final stop for auditory information; within the primary AI there are projections that transverse to other areas of the auditory cortex and associated cortices. The secondary auditory cortex (AII) is located below the AI and provides connection to other parts of the brain. This is where auditory information is integrated with information from parts of the CNS, including other sensory information. The two hemispheres of the cortex, including the temporal lobes, are interconnected through the *corpus callosum*.

auditory nerve fiber sends collaterals to different areas of the cochlear nucleus. The afferent (ascending) outputs from the cochlear nucleus take different paths depending on the location of the cells. The primary neural output of the cochlear nucleus comes from the anterior–ventral part of the cochlear nucleus (AVCN) and travels to the other side of the brainstem (contralateral). However, even these neurons can take different paths, for example, some neurons from the AVCN cross the midline and synapse with cells in the contralateral lateral lemniscus or inferior colliculus, while others synapse in cells of either the ipsilateral or contralateral superior olivary complex. The primary afferent pathways consist of connections to the contralateral side of the brainstem; however, there is also an ipsilateral ascending representation from the superior olivary complex. Notice that the first location where there would be connections from both ears is at the

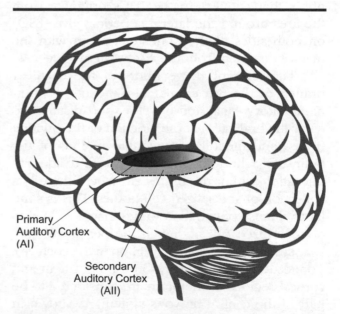

FIGURE 4–27. Diagram of the left side of the human brain. The primary auditory area (Heschl's gyrus) is on the upper surface of the temporal lobe. The secondary auditory cortices are located below the AI. There is an auditory reception area on the temporal lobe on both sides of the brain. *Source*: Illustration by Tatiana Piatanova.

SYNOPSIS 4–3

- The 8th cranial nerve or vestibulocochlear nerve, has branches from the cochlea and each semicircular canal, the saccule and the utricle. The 8th cranial nerve exits the petrous portion of the temporal bone through the internal auditory canal. It is also joined in the internal auditory canal by the 7th cranial nerve.
- There are about 30,000 afferent neurons from each cochlea that send information from the cochlea to the brainstem. There are also about 1200 efferent auditory neurons that send information from the brainstem to each organ of Corti.
- Approximately 95% of afferent auditory neurons originate from IHCs as inner radial fibers. Several inner radial fibers are attached to each IHC. The remaining 5% of afferent neurons, called outer spiral fibers, come from collaterals originating from a more basal location from multiple OHCs across all three rows, and then cross the tunnel of Corti to exit with the inner spiral fibers through the habenula perforata in the osseous spiral lamina.
- Cell bodies for the auditory afferent neurons are called spiral ganglia. The spiral ganglia are distributed from base to apex within the modiolus of the cochlea in Rosenthal's canal (near the osseous spiral lamina).
- The neurons of the efferent auditory pathway, called the olivocochlear bundle, originate in the SOC. More of the efferent neurons connect to the OHCs than the IHCs. Those neurons connecting to the OHCs originate in the MSO region of the SOC from both sides of the brainstem, but more from the contralateral side; those connecting to the IHCs originate in the LSO region of the SOC from both sides of the brainstem, also with more from the contralateral side.
- OHCs have both afferent and efferent synapses with each hair cell body allowing direct efferent control to OHCs. The IHCs have only afferent synapses with each hair cell body, but the efferent neurons synapse on the afferent neurons associated with the IHC.
- The cochlear and vestibular portions of the 8th cranial nerve enter the brainstem at the level of the pontine–medulla junction.
- The afferent auditory neurons send collaterals to synapse with cells in three different regions of the cochlear nucleus. From the cochlear nucleus, central auditory neurons take several paths, which include both ipsilateral and contralateral auditory brainstem nuclei. The auditory nuclei within the brainstem (one on each side of the brainstem) are (in ascending order):
  - Cochlear nucleus (CN)
  - Superior olivary complex (SOC)
  - Lateral lemniscus (LL)
  - Inferior colliculus (IC)
  - Medial geniculate body (MGB)
- From each cochlea, there is a predominance of contralateral neural pathways for the auditory system in the brainstem; however, there are also other pathways, some of which do not synapse in each of the nuclei, and there are interconnections between the nuclei on each side of the brainstem.

SYNOPSIS 4–3 (continued)

- From each MGB, the neurons proceed to the ipsilateral temporal lobe and terminate in the primary auditory reception area (AI), called Heschl's gyrus. There is also a secondary auditory cortex (AII) located below the AI where auditory information is integrated with information from other parts of the CNS. The temporal lobes from each side of the brain are connected through the corpus callosum.

REFERENCES

Anson, B. J., & Donaldson, J. A. (1967). *The Surgical Anatomy of the Temporal Bone and Ear*. Philadelphia, PA: W.B. Saunders.

Bagger-Sjoback, S., Anniko, M., & Lundquist, P. G. (1984). Techniques in ultrastructural anatomy. In I. Friedman & J. Ballantyne (Eds.), *Ultrastructural Atlas of the Inner Ear* (p. 15). Boston, MA: Butterworths and Company.

Bluestone, C. D. (1991). Physiology of the middle ear and eustachian tube. In M. M. Paparella, D. A. Shumrick, J. L. Gluckman, & W. L. Meyerhoff (Eds.), *Otolaryngology* (3rd ed., pp. 163–197). Philadelphia, PA: W.B. Saunders.

Bluestone, C. D., & Klein, J. O. (1988). *Otitis Media in Infants and Children*. Philadelphia, PA: W. B. Saunders.

Brodel, M. (1946). *Three Unpublished Drawings of the Anatomy of the Human Ear*. Philadelphia, PA: W. B. Saunders.

Fawcett, D. W. (1994). *Bloom and Fawcett: A Textbook of Histology* (p. 929). New York, NY: Chapman and Hall.

Gelfand, S. A. (2009). *Hearing: An Introduction to Psychological and Physiological Acoustics* (5th ed.). Boca Roton, FL: Taylor & Francis.

Harrison, R. V. (1988). *The Biology of Hearing and Deafness*. Springfield, IL: Charles C. Thomas.

Kimura, R. S. (1984). Sensory and accessory epithelia of the cochlea. In I. Friedman & J. Ballantyne (Eds.), *Ultrastructureal Atlas of the Inner Ear* (p. 102). Boston, MA: Butterworths and Company.

Lim, D. J. (1986). Effects of noise and ototoxic drugs at the cellular level in the cochlea: a review. *American Journal of Otolaryngology, 7*, 73–99.

Moller, A. R. (2013). *Hearing: Anatomy, Physiology, and Disorders of the Auditory System*. San Diego, CA: Plural.

Office of Visual Media, & Indiana School of Medicine (1994). [Personal communication].

Putz, R., & Pabst, R. (2011). *Sobotta Atlas of Human Anatomy* (15th ed.). Munchen, Germany: Elsevier GmbH, Urban & Fisher Verlag.

Seidel, H. M., Ball, J. W., Dains, J. E., & Benedict, G. W. (2003). *Mosby's Guide to Physical Examination*. Saint Louis, MO: Mosby.

Seidel, H. M., Ball, J. W., Dains, J. E., Benedict, G. W., & Louis, M. O. (2003). *Mosby's Guide to Physical Examination*. St. Louis, MO: Mosby, Inc.

Spoendlin, H. (1978). *The Afferent Innervation of the Cochlea*. San Diego, CA: Academic Press.

Spoendlin, H. (1984). Primary neurons and synapses. In I. Friedman & J. Ballantyne (Eds.), *Ultrastructural Atlas of the Inner Ear* (p. 133). Boston, MA: Butterworths and Company.

Spoendlin, H. (1988). Neural anatomy of the inner ear. In A. F. Jahn & J. Santos-Sacchi (Eds.), *Physiology of the Ear*. New York, NY: Raven Press.

Tos, M. (1995). *Manual of middle ear surgery, Vol. 2, Mastoid surgery and reconstructive procedures*. Stuttgart, Germany: Thieme-Verlag.

Yost, W. (2013). *Fundamentals of Hearing* (5th ed.). Leiden, Netherlands: Koninklijke Brill.

5 Functions of the Auditory System

After reading this chapter, you should be able to:

1. Understand why there is a need for the outer ear and middle ear to amplify pressures at the oval window.

2. Describe the amplifying mechanisms of the outer ear and middle ear, and how the predicted gains in pressure relate to the measured transfer functions.

3. Draw the ipsilateral and contralateral acoustic reflex pathways, and describe the functions of the acoustic reflex.

4. Understand how traveling waves occur along the basilar membrane and what is meant by basilar membrane tonotopic arrangement. Draw traveling wave envelopes for low, mid, and high frequency pure tones.

5. Discuss the different roles of the inner and outer hair cells relative to the passive and active processes that occur in the cochlea.

6. Describe tuning curves for the passive and active cochlear processes. Describe what happens to the tuning in a cochlea with damage to the active process (or outer hair cells).

7. Describe the different stages of transduction that sounds undergo from the environment through the level of the 8th cranial nerve.

8. Discuss how frequency and intensity may be coded in the peripheral auditory system.

Our sense of hearing is truly remarkable. Close your eyes for a moment and think about all the different types of vibrations in your environment that your ears are processing into useful and meaningful information; people talking, birds chirping, sound of cars in the distance, air conditioner, and/or music that may be playing. Think back to what you learned in Chapter 4 about the different parts of the auditory system, and imagine how the different components must somehow work together to allow you to hear and extract relevant information. As you will see in this chapter, the primary function of the ear is to receive vibrations from the environment and convert them into neural information that the brain can use. The changes that occur in the sound energy through the different parts of the auditory system are referred to as the *transduction* process. The different parts of the auditory system transduce the sound energy from one form into another form. This chapter will detail the transduction process through the peripheral auditory system.

AIR-TO-FLUID IMPEDANCE MISMATCH

To begin with, acoustic vibrations from the environment must be converted by the outer and middle ears into something usable by the inner ear. If we did not have our outer and middle ears, the acoustic vibrations would impinge directly on the oval and round window membranes: This would be analogous to talking directly into the fluid-filled cochlea. However, when two types of media (e.g., air and water) have different properties, they have an inherent opposition to the efficient flow of energy. The total opposition to the flow of energy is called *impedance*. The flow of energy is most efficient when the impedance is low or when two systems have equal impedances. When two systems have different impedances, they are said to have an *impedance mismatch*. If we were to try to talk directly into the cochlea, the air-to-fluid impedance mismatch would result in a loss of energy to the cochlea. You have, undoubtedly, experienced an analogous situation where you try to talk from the deck of a pool to someone who is under water. In the pool analogy, about 99.9% of the sound

energy would be reflected off the water's surface due to the air-to-fluid impedance mismatch, and only 0.1% would be transmitted into the water. The estimated loss of energy can also be expressed in decibels if you consider the ratio of the reflected energy to the transmitted energy to be approximately 1000/1 (i.e., 99.9%/0.1% = 999/1). In decibels, this could be expressed as:

$$dB = 10 \log (1000/1)$$

$$dB = 10 \ (3), \text{ where log of } 1000 = 3$$

$$= 30 \ dB$$

In other words, you would predict that there would be about a 30 dB loss of sound energy due to the impedance mismatch when going from air to fluid. While this analogy is useful as a basic understanding of the problem, the actual impedance mismatch would depend on knowing the precise impedance characteristics of the cochlear fluids at the oval window, something that has not yet been determined (Durrant & Lovrinic, 1995).

Obviously, a significant air-to-fluid impedance mismatch in the ear would not be an efficient way to transduce the sound energy through the ear. Therefore, one of the important functions of both the outer ear and middle ear is to overcome this impedance mismatch so that there is a more efficient transfer of energy to the fluid-filled cochlea; in other words, to create a situation whereby the predicted 30 dB loss of sound energy does not occur during the transduction process to the inner ear. The ways in which the outer ear and middle ear overcome this impedance mismatch are discussed in the following sections.

FUNCTIONS OF THE OUTER EAR

The outer ear serves as the primary connection between the sounds in the environment and the middle ear. The auricle and external canal of the outer ear have only modest contributions to the overall processing of sound, and most pathologies affecting the outer ear do not cause much hearing loss. The outer ear is important, however, in protecting the more important middle and inner ear structures by allowing them to be embedded further into the skull, away from potentially damaging events or foreign objects. Even the cerumen of the ear canal keeps debris and bugs away from the tympanic membrane.

The outer ear also modifies the incoming sound prior to arrival at the tympanic membrane. As mentioned in Chapter 4, many animals can move their pinnae to help localize the source of a sound. Humans, on the other hand, do not have (or seem to need) the ability to move their auricles. The auricle, even without moving, can alter the spectra of sounds due to its shape and irregular series of depressions and ridges. These spectral variations affect primarily the higher frequencies, and these variations may provide some cues for sound localization, especially from the front, back, or overhead (Yost, 2013).

The outer ear also amplifies, through the mechanism of resonance, the sound pressure delivered to the tympanic membrane. Resonance is what makes different-sized jars produce different pitches when struck, or when one blows air into cavities with different sizes. As you learned in Chapter 3, the size (and shape) of a cavity (or tube) will be most responsive to certain frequencies, such that smaller sizes resonate better to higher frequencies and larger sizes resonate better to lower frequencies. The external ear canal acts like a tube-shaped cavity that is closed on one end. The resonant frequency of this type of tube is dependent on the relationship of the wavelength of the sound to the length of the tube. For this type of tube, enhancement of the sound pressure occurs maximally (resonant frequency) for a frequency that is equal to one-quarter the length of the tube (quarter-wave resonator). If the average adult ear canal length is 0.025 m (Ballachanda, 1995), then the resonant frequency (f_{res}) can be calculated as:

$$f_{res} = c/4L, \text{ where c is speed of sound (m/s)}$$
$$\text{and L is length of the tube (m);}$$

$$f_{res} = 343/4 \times 0.025$$

$$f_{res} = 3430 \text{ Hz}$$

Remember, however, that the ear canal is also irregular in shape and is preceded by the concha, both of which contribute to the resonance characteristics of the outer ear and will enhance certain frequencies. In order to verify the actual resonance frequencies of the outer ear, measurements have been made to document the changes in sound pressure that occur at the tympanic membrane compared to the sound pressure entering the outer ear. These types of measurements are referred to as *transfer functions*. The interested reader is referred to Shaw (1974) and Ballachanda (1995) for more detailed data on the outer ear transfer function. These empirical data have shown that the ear canal is most important for enhancement of frequencies between 1500 and 3000 Hz, whereas the concha provides enhancement for frequencies between 4500 and 6000 Hz (Shaw, 1974). Other parts of the outer ear also make small contributions to the resonance characteristics. In general, the combined effect of resonances from all parts of the outer ear provides an increase in amplitude (*gain*) of about 15 to 20 dB at the tympanic membrane in the frequency range 1500 to 7000 Hz (Ballachanda, 1995), and this gain contributes to overcoming the loss of energy that would occur due to the impedance mismatch. The frequency range amplified by the outer ear is, somewhat remarkably, matched to those frequencies most important for understanding speech. Our auditory system is already performing some important processing at the level of the external ear that contributes to our ability to use speech for communication.

FUNCTIONS OF THE MIDDLE EAR

The middle ear is a mechanical system that transduces the acoustic vibrations (rarefactions and condensations) that impinge on the tympanic membrane into *mechanical vibrations* (in and out) of the ossicular chain. The ossicular chain delivers the vibrations received at the tympanic membrane directly to the oval window. Without the ossicles, acoustic vibrations would strike both the oval and round window membranes at essentially the same time, and this would not allow reciprocal back-and-forth movements of these membranes that are necessary for vibrations to occur in the incompressible fluid-filled cochlea. In other words, in order for the vibrations of the ossicular chain to move the oval window in and out, the round window membrane must also respond such that an inward movement of the oval window corresponds to an outward movement of the round window membrane; and an outward movement of the oval window corresponds to an inward movement of the round window membrane. Figure 5–1 summarizes the transduction process thus far: Up to this point, the energy has been transduced from acoustic vibrations (condensations and rarefactions) in the ear canal, to mechanical vibrations (in and out) of the tympanic membrane and ossicular chain, and then to *hydromechanical vibrations* that are delivered to the fluid filled cochlea from the reciprocal in-and-out movements of the oval and round window membranes. As you will see in a later section, the vibrations delivered to the fluid in the cochlea cause a hydromechanical reaction of the basilar membrane in the organ of Corti.

Middle Ear Amplifier

As mentioned earlier, one of the primary functions of the outer and middle ears is to overcome the potential loss of energy that would occur due to a potential air-to-fluid impedance mismatch in order to allow a more efficient transfer of sound energy to the inner ear. In addition to directing the mechanical vibrations to the oval window, the middle ear is designed to function as a mechanical amplifier, whereby the sound pressures at the oval window are greater than those striking the tympanic membrane. There are three ways that the middle ear amplifies sound at the oval window. The largest amplification through the middle ear occurs as a result of the size (area) difference between the tympanic membrane and the oval window, referred to as the *area ratio advantage*. An estimate of the effective area of the tympanic membrane is about 55 mm², whereas the area of the oval window is about 3.2 mm² (Yost, 2013). Since pressure is equal to force per area

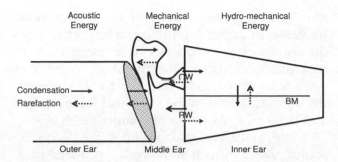

FIGURE 5–1. Overview of the transduction process from acoustic to hydromechanical, whereby the acoustic energy that enters the ear canal is converted into mechanical energy in the middle ear and then to hydromechanical energy in the fluid-filled inner ear. The *arrows* represent the vibration phase (rarefaction or condensation). Notice that there is a reciprocal relationship in the movement of the oval window (OW) and the round window (RW) that is necessary for the vibrational energy to occur in the incompressible fluid-filled cochlea. BM, basilar membrane; RW, round window; OW, oval window.

(p = F/A), for a given amount of force applied to the larger area (tympanic membrane), there will be an increase in pressure on the smaller area (oval window). As an analogy, think of yourself standing on snow with snow shoes on (or standing flat-footed on sand at the beach); then think about what would happen if you took the snow shoes off (or when you stand on your toes in the sand). When the force of your body is applied over a smaller area, more pressure is applied and you sink deeper into the snow (or sand). In the middle ear, because the force that is exerted on the larger tympanic membrane is transferred by the ossicular chain to the smaller oval window, there is an increase in pressure at the oval window. Given an area ratio of 17 to 1 (55 mm²/ 3.2 mm²), there would be an increase (gain) of about 25 dB in sound pressure at the oval window due to the area ratio advantage [dB = 20 log (17/1)]. The second mechanical amplifying mechanism of the middle ear is called the *curved membrane advantage*. This curved membrane advantage is related to the cone shape of the tympanic membrane, which tends to focus its movement in such a way that it moves the malleus with more force than if the tympanic membrane were a flat disk. The curved membrane advantage increases the pressure about twofold (2/1), which would be equivalent to about a 6 dB increase in pressure at the oval window [dB =20 log (2/1)]. The third middle ear amplifying mechanism is called the *lever advantage*. The lever advantage of the ossicular chain occurs because of the longer length of the manubrium of the malleus relative to the length of the long process of the incus. This acts like a fulcrum, where the force applied to the longer arm results in more pressure being exerted at the shorter arm. For the lever advantage, the pressure at the oval window is predicted to be about 1.3 times greater than at the tympanic membrane, which would be equivalent to about a 2.2 dB increase (gain) in pressure at the oval window [dB = 20 log (1.3/1)]. When all three of the middle ear's mechanical advantages are considered, there would be a predicted increase (gain) of about 33 dB in pressure at the oval window compared with the pressure at the tympanic membrane [dB = 20 log (17 × 2 × 1.3)].

As you can see from the above predictions/ calculations, the loss in sound pressure that would occur due to the air-to-fluid impedance mismatch is effectively overcome by the mechanical amplifying effects of the middle ear. However, to empirically determine the actual amount of amplification and over what range of frequencies the middle ear amplifier is effective, a transfer function can be measured (mostly in animals) between the tympanic membrane and the oval window as a function of frequency. The transfer function for the middle ear has been shown to provide approximately 20 to 25 dB increase (gain) in pressure at the oval window across a fairly wide frequency range, but is especially effective in the middle frequencies (Békésy, 1960; Møller, 1983; Nedzelnitsky, 1980), with a resonance frequency of about 1000 Hz (Hamill & Price, 2014). When the middle ear amplification is combined with the amplification from the outer ear, there is an effective transfer of sound pressure to the cochlea for a fairly wide frequency range, especially for those frequencies most important for the perception and recognition of speech sounds. Working together, the outer ear and middle ear overcome the loss of sound pressure that would occur due to the air-to-fluid impedance mismatch.

Acoustic Reflex

The middle ear has two small muscles, stapedius and tensor tympani, that attach to the ossicular chain by their corresponding tendons. The middle ear muscles are known to contract involuntarily when stimulated by loud sounds, for example, above 80 dB SPL, and this response is called the *acoustic reflex*, *middle ear reflex*, or *stapedial reflex*. In this textbook, we will use the term acoustic reflex to refer to the middle ear reflex. The stapedius muscle is innervated by a branch of the *facial nerve* (7th cranial nerve) and the tensor tympani muscle is innervated by a branch of the *trigeminal nerve* (5th cranial nerve). In humans, it is the stapedius muscle that is primarily involved in the acoustic reflex. Figure 5–2 shows the components of the facial nerve. The facial nerve has a variety of motor and sensory functions not related to hearing; however, there is a small branch, called the *stapedial branch*, that innervates the stapedius muscle. Because the middle ear muscles are oriented perpendicular to the direction of movement of the ossicular chain, their contractions reduce (stiffen) the movement of the ossicular chain, which lowers the sound pressure to the oval window.

A popular theory on the role of the acoustic reflex is that it affords some protection to the ear from loud sounds. However, this role has been questioned, and may only be a factor in certain situations. The acoustic reflex can reduce the pressure delivered to the oval window by as much as 10 to 20 dB SPL, but only for low frequencies and does not give any appreciable reduction in the mid to high frequencies (Møller, 1965; Reger, 1960); therefore, the acoustic reflex may not provide much help in the mid to higher frequencies that are typically damaged by exposure to excessive noise. Another problem with the protection theory is that the middle ear muscles take about 20 to 100 ms to contract and they fail to maintain contraction during continuous exposures

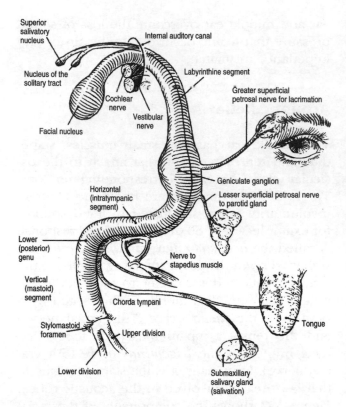

FIGURE 5–2. A diagram of the facial nerve that originates in the facial nucleus of the brainstem and has various motor and sensory nerve branches. The motor nerve branch that innervates the stapedius muscle, the stapedial branch, is involved in the acoustic reflex. *Source*: Republished with permission of Oxford University Press, from Baloh, R. W. (1998). *Dizziness, Hearing Loss, and Tinnitus*. Philadelphia, PA: F. A. Davis. p. 9; permission conveyed through Copyright Clearance Center, Inc.

(Møller, 1958); therefore, the acoustic reflex may not have much of a protective role, especially for impulsive type sounds like gunshots, explosions, or loud banging sounds. An additional problem for the protection theory is that hearing loss due to excessive continuous exposure to loud noises is quite prevalent, and if the acoustic reflex was designed for protection, it does not do a very good job in today's society. A more tenable theory for the role of the acoustic reflex is that it may reduce distortion within the movement of the ossicular chain that may occur at high sound intensities. This reduction in distortion may be important during your own vocalizations, especially if talking loudly in the presence of other

background sounds (Borg & Counter, 1989). Bats have a well-developed use of the acoustic reflex to protect their ears from their echo-location sounds; however, the precise role of the acoustic reflex in humans is still to be defined and better understood.

The acoustic reflex pathway is illustrated in Figure 5–3. The acoustic reflex has a sensory component (auditory) and a motor component (contraction of stapedius). The acoustic reflex involves a bilateral neural pathway in which a loud sound to one ear results in a contraction of the stapedius muscle in both ears. The acoustic reflex pathway that is involved with the contraction of the stapedius muscle on the same side as the stimulus is called the *ipsilateral acoustic reflex* pathway. The acoustic reflex pathway that is involved with the contraction of the stapedius muscle on the side opposite to the stimulus is called the *contralateral acoustic reflex* pathway. The ipsilateral and contralateral acoustic reflex

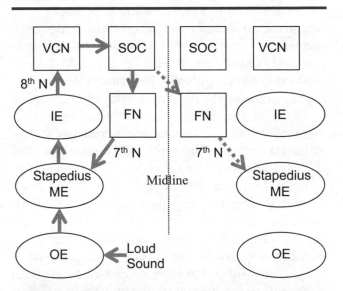

FIGURE 5–3. Block diagram of the acoustic reflex pathway for sound stimulation to one ear. The acoustic reflex is a bilateral response in which the stapedius muscles in both ears are stimulated through the ipsilateral (solid arrows) and contralateral pathways (dashed arrows). OE, outer ear; ME, middle ear; IE, inner ear; 8th N, 8th cranial nerve; VCN, ventral cochlear nucleus; SOC, superior olivary complex; FN, facial nucleus; 7th N, 7th cranial nerve (stapedial branch).

pathways include the sensory input through the outer ear, middle ear, inner ear, 8th cranial nerve, and ipsilateral cochlear nucleus. From the ipsilateral cochlear nucleus, there are connections to specialized neurons around the superior olivary complexes on both sides of the brainstem. The motor portion of the acoustic reflex pathway involves neurons from the areas around the superior olivary complexes that then connect to the facial nerve nucleus on each side of the brainstem and then to the stapedial branch of the 7th cranial nerve on each side, resulting in contraction of the stapedius muscle in each ear. As you will see in later chapters, the acoustic reflex is very useful as a diagnostic audiology test and shows characteristic patterns that are associated with disorders in different parts of the ear, as well as the neural integrity of the 7th and 8th cranial nerves.

Equalizing Middle Ear Pressure

Another function of the middle ear involves the eustachian tube to equalize air pressure in the middle ear to that in the environment. The middle ear is normally an air-filled cavity. In order for the tympanic membrane and ossicles to vibrate effectively, the air pressure in the middle ear must be equal to the air pressure in the outer ear canal (impedance matched). This pressure equalization is accomplished by the eustachian tube that connects the bottom of the middle ear cavity to the nasopharynx. The eustachian tube is mostly a cartilaginous tube that is normally closed, but is periodically opened during normal physiological activities like swallowing or yawning. When the eustachian tube opens, it allows the air pressure to equalize with the environment. You have, undoubtedly, experienced this event when you "pop" your ears.

The eustachian tube is normally opened by contraction of the *tensor veli palatini muscle* and closes when the muscle relaxes. Failure of the eustachian tube to equalize the air pressure in the middle ear can lead to middle ear infections and related hearing loss. As described in Chapter 4, the anatomy and function of the eustachian tube are not fully developed in young children,

Ear Troubles on a Plane?

Some of you may have experienced problems with your ears during an airplane flight. This occurs if you are unable to equalize the cabin pressure changes through your eustachian tubes. As the airplane takes off, there is a gradual decrease in cabin air pressure, and the pressure inside the middle ear becomes more positive than inside the cabin. During this part of the flight, the eustachian tubes can open relatively easily, even without any conscious effort because the positive pressure helps open the tubes and the middle ear pressure equalizes due to the decreased cabin pressure. However, during the descent for landing, the cabin pressure is increased and the pressure inside the middle ear is more negative than inside the cabin, and the eustachian tube may resist being opened. Most of us can still periodically open our eustachian tubes to equalize the changes in pressure by chewing, swallowing, or popping of ears during descent; however, some individuals are unable to open their eustachian tubes during descent, and may experience some ear discomfort or pain, and the negative middle ear pressure may subsequently lead to an ear infection.

which is a primary reason why young children are more prone to middle ear infections than adults.

FUNCTIONS OF THE INNER EAR

The processing of sound in the inner ear begins with the in and out movements of the stapes footplate in the oval window (with reciprocal movements of the round window membrane) that deliver the vibrational energy to the fluids of the cochlea (refer back to Figure 5–1). In other words, the mechanical pressure variations of the

SYNOPSIS 5-1

- The outer and middle ears connect to the inner ear located deep within the skull where it is better protected.
- The tympanic membrane and ossicles transduce the acoustic vibrations into mechanical vibrations and channel them to the oval window. Because the fluid in the inner ear is incompressible, there is a reciprocal movement of the stapes footplate in the oval window and the round window membrane that allows for vibrational energy to occur in the inner ear.
- The outer and middle ears compensate for a theoretical 30 dB loss of energy that would occur due to an air-to-fluid impedance mismatch between airborne sounds and the fluid of the inner ear, thus improving our hearing sensitivity.
- The outer ear amplifies acoustic energy through resonance of its various cavities and the shape/length of the external ear canal. Measurements of the outer ear transfer function shows about a 15 to 20 dB increase in sound pressure at the tympanic membrane, especially in the middle to high frequencies.
- The mechanical amplifying effects of the middle ear include:
  - The area ratio between tympanic membrane and oval window provides a gain of about 25 dB.
  - The curvature of the tympanic membrane produces more force than if it was a flat membrane and provides a gain of about 6 dB.
  - The lever ratio between the length of the manubrium and the incus acts like a fulcrum and provides a gain of about 2.2 dB.
  - Collectively, the above three mechanical advantages produce a gain of about 33 dB in pressure at the oval window, which effectively overcomes the loss of energy that would occur due to the air-to-fluid impedance mismatch. Actual measures comparing pressure at the tympanic membrane to those at the oval window indicate an increase of 20 to 25 dB SPL, especially in the low and middle frequencies.
- The middle ear stapedius muscle contracts in response to loud sounds (greater than 80 dB SPL), called the acoustic reflex or middle ear reflex. The acoustic reflex neural pathways include the 8th cranial nerve from the cochlea, the lower brainstem auditory nuclei, the facial nucleus, and the stapedial branch of the 7th cranial nerve. The acoustic reflex pathway is bilateral, whereby input to one ear results in contraction of the stapedius muscle in both ears through an ipsilateral pathway and a contralateral pathway.
- Acoustic reflex measures are very useful in assessment of a variety of auditory disorders.
- The purpose of the acoustic reflex is not fully understood. When stimulated, there is a short onset delay, and it only reduces the level of lower frequencies. A more tenable theory is that the reflex reduces distortion through the middle ear during vocalizations.
- The eustachian tube of the middle ear extends to the nasopharynx to allow equalization of air pressure on the outside of the tympanic membrane with the air pressure inside the middle ear so that the proper transmission of sound vibrations can occur. It is regularly opened by the tensor veli palatini during chewing, swallowing, or speaking. Young children are prone to more middle ear disorders because their eustachian tubes are not yet fully developed.

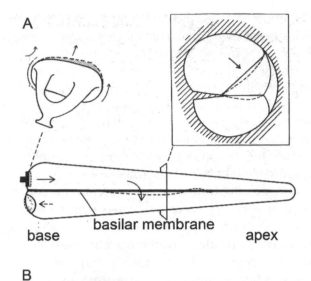

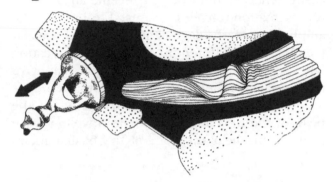

FIGURE 5–4. A. Demonstration of how movement of the stapes imparts pressure variations into the scala vestibuli, which in turn leads to displacement of the basilar membrane in the scala media. It is common to show the cochlea and/or basilar membrane uncoiled from its base to its apex for ease of illustration. *Source*: From Durrant & Lovrinic, 1995, p. 150. Copyright 1995 by Williams & Wilkins. **B.** A snapshot of how a traveling wave appears on the basilar membrane in response to the pressure variations occurring in the scala media. *Source*: From Dallos, 1988, p. 51. Copyright 1988 by American Speech-Language-Hearing Association.

stapes in the oval window sets up pressure variations in the fluid. This is the beginning of the hydromechanical events in the cochlea. Figure 5–4 shows how the mechanical vibrations of the stapes footplate are transduced into hydromechanical vibrations within the membranous labyrinth. You will notice in Figure 5–4A that the cochlea is shown uncoiled, a common/convenient practice when discussing the physiology of the inner ear. The cochlea is quite small and the cochlear fluids

are incompressible; therefore, the pressure variations delivered to the inner ear are felt instantaneously throughout the entire cochlea, as if it was a solid object. It is important to realize that the fluid is not pushed through the cochlea from the oval window to the round window; instead, the pressure variations are received instantaneously throughout the cochlea, including within the membranous labyrinth that is suspended in the bony labyrinth. It is the reactions of the basilar membrane, called the *traveling wave*, to these pressure variations within the membranous labyrinth that are most important in the hydromechanical transduction process (see Figure 5–4B) as you will see in the next section.

Traveling Waves in the Cochlea

The pressure variations in the cochlea cause the basilar membrane to react in a characteristic way, resulting in a traveling wave. Much of the pioneering work in this area was done by George von Békésy in the 1950s and is summarized in Békésy (1960). Békésy's remarkable work formed the foundation of auditory theory for the next 20 years. Békésy's traveling wave occurs because of the basilar membrane's physical characteristics. As you recall from Chapter 4, and as shown in Figure 5–5, the basilar membrane is narrower at the base of the cochlea and systematically widens toward the apex of the cochlea. In addition, the basilar membrane is stiffer at the base of the cochlea and systematically becomes less stiff toward the apex of the cochlea. These physical characteristics determine how different parts of the basilar membrane respond to the different frequencies. The relationship between frequency and a specific place is called *tonotopic* arrangement. On the basilar membrane, the tonotopic arrangement is such that the higher frequencies are processed toward the base of the cochlea and the lower frequencies are processed primarily toward the apex of the cochlea. You might think of the simple analogy of a musical harp, where the shorter/tighter strings produce the higher frequencies and the longer/looser strings produce the lower frequencies.

So, how does a traveling wave occur? First of all, keep in mind that all locations along the

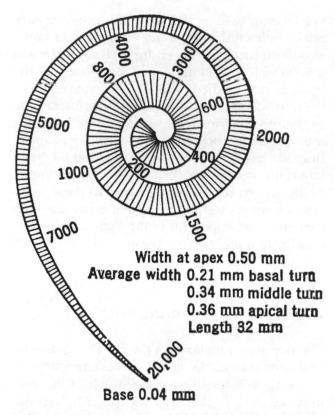

Width at apex 0.50 mm
Average width 0.21 mm basal turn
0.34 mm middle turn
0.36 mm apical turn
Length 32 mm

Base 0.04 mm

FIGURE 5–5. Tonotopic arrangement along the basilar membrane; high frequencies at the base and low frequencies at the apex. The tonotopic arrangement is related to the physical properties of the basilar membrane: narrower and stiffer at the base; wider and less stiff at the apex. *Source*: From Stuhlman Jr., 1943, p. 286. Copyright 1943 by John Wiley & Sons/ Chapman & Hall.

a fraction of a second later (phase lag) than the more basal locations. This causes some parts of the membrane to move up while other areas are moving down (refer back to Figure 5–4D). The amplitude (amount of displacement) of the traveling wave is relatively small at the base and progressively increases until it reaches its peak amplitude at the place that responds best to the stimulating frequency; after that, the amplitude quickly declines in regions more apical.

Figure 5–6 illustrates a convenient way to show where the traveling wave stimulates different parts of the basilar membrane by showing the *envelope* (outline) of the traveling wave's motion. In other words, because a diagram cannot easily reflect a time-varying event, an artificial representation (envelope) is used to indicate the amplitudes of displacements along the basilar membrane for different frequencies. The location where the maximum amplitude (displacement) of the basilar membrane occurs for any given pure tone is called the *traveling wave peak* (or the peak of the traveling wave). The traveling wave peak occurs near the base of the basilar mem-

basilar membrane receive the same vibrational input at the same time due to the incompressible nature of the fluid-filled cavity; however, because of the changes in the basilar membrane's physical characteristics from base to apex, different areas of the basilar membrane move up and down at different times (phases). In other words, the narrower/stiffer basal end of the basilar membrane begins to move up and down sooner than the more wide/less stiff apical parts of the basilar membrane because there is less inertia to overcome (less mass) at the basal end of the membrane: The more apical parts of the basilar membrane take a little longer to overcome the inertia and, therefore, begin to move

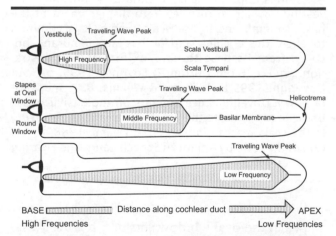

FIGURE 5–6. Displacement patterns (envelopes) of traveling waves showing high frequencies with peak displacements at the base, mid-frequencies further toward the apex, and low frequencies near the apex. Notice that for all frequencies, the traveling wave begins at the base, reaches peak amplitude at its preferred location, and then quickly declines in amplitude for more apical area. *Source*: From Gelfand, 2015, p. 56. Copyright 2015 by Thieme.

brane for high frequency sounds and progressively more toward the apex for lower frequency sounds (tonotopic arrangement). Békésy did an interesting experiment in which he introduced vibrations into the cochlea by placing a piston in a small hole at the apex of the cochlea, and found that the traveling wave still began at the base, moved in an apical direction, and reached its peak at the appropriate location dependent on the frequency of stimulation. In other words, regardless of how the vibrations enter the cochlea, there is a characteristic traveling wave that moves from the base of the cochlea and peaks at a location that is determined by the tonotopic arrangement of the basilar membrane. You will notice in Figure 5–6 that the traveling wave for the high frequency sound only stimulates the base of the cochlea, whereas middle and lower frequency sounds result in a wider part of the basilar membrane that is involved in the traveling wave. Keep in mind that the up and down movement (displacement) of the basilar membrane, regardless of frequency, always begins near the base and "travels" (very quickly—within milliseconds) toward the apex until it reaches its peak amplitude at a location based on its frequency.

Bone Conducted Sounds also Induce Traveling Waves

As you will see in later chapters, one of the clinical tests of hearing involves directly sending vibrations through the skull by placing a small mechanical vibrator on the mastoid portion of the temporal bone. These bone-conducted vibrations initiate the same hydromechanical events (basilar membrane traveling wave) in the cochlea as those that occur when vibrations are delivered to the cochlea through the ossicular chain in the oval window. Bone-conducted sounds are part of our everyday listening experience when sounds are loud enough to cause vibrations in the skull, and are especially apparent when you hum or talk.

Transduction Through the Inner Hair Cells

In addition to the traveling waves, the hydromechanical part of the transduction process within the cochlea also includes mechanical displacements of the stereocilia of the inner hair cells (IHCs) and the outer hair cells (OHCs). During this part of the transduction process, in those regions where there is enough displacement of the basilar membrane from the traveling wave, there are mechanical displacements of the stereocilia, commonly referred to as bending or shearing of the stereocilia as a result of their contact with the tectorial membrane. Figure 5–7 illustrates bending of the stereocilia due to contact with the tectorial membrane for up and down movements of the basilar membrane during actions of the traveling wave. When the basilar membrane moves up and down, the stereocilia of the hair cells bend back and forth when contacting the tectorial membrane. As the basilar membrane and the tectorial membrane move together or apart, they bend the stereocilia one way or the other due to the differences in the relative pivot points of the two membranes.

The next phase of the transduction process is the *biochemical transduction process*, which describes what happens within the IHCs. Bending of the stereocilia toward the tallest row of stereocilia (away from the modiolus) triggers the *depolarization (excitatory) phase* of the biochemical transduction process within the hair cells; bending of the stereocilia away from the tallest row (toward the modiolus) triggers the *hyperpolarization (inhibitory) phase* of the biochemical transduction process.

Figure 5–8 shows how the bending of the stereocilia causes a change in the flow of ions into the hair cell during excitation that alters its *intracellular potential*, which is about –40 mV for IHCs and –60 mV for OHCs (Dallos, 1986). The endolymph surrounding the stereocilia has a relatively high K+ concentration. Although similar biochemical events occur in the IHCs and OHCs, it is the IHCs that initiate the neural activity through their synapses with the afferent nerves (the role of the OHCs will be discussed in a subsequent section). It is also important to

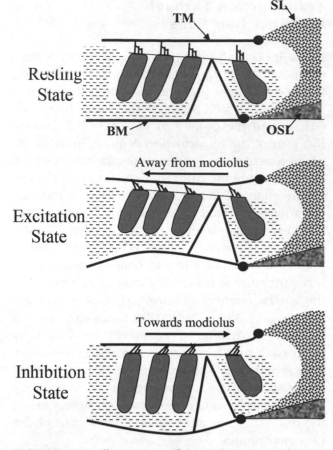

FIGURE 5–7. Illustration of how the stereocilia are displaced by the action of the basilar membrane and the tectorial membrane. During the resting state, the stereocilia are not actively displaced. As the basilar membrane moves up and down, the stereocilia bend back and forth due to the different pivot points of the basilar membrane and the tectorial membrane. Bending of stereocilia away from the modiolus is excitation; bending toward the modiolus is inhibition. TM, tectorial membrane; SL, spiral limbus; OSL, osseous spiral lamina; BM, basilar membrane.

often known as the *Davis Battery Theory*, the 120 to 140 mV electrical potential acts like the voltage of a battery that serves as the force that drives ionic current (K+) into the hair cell when the stereocilia bend in an excitatory direction. The amount of ionic current that flows into a hair cell is modulated by changes in resistance that occur when the stereocilia bend in different directions. When the stereocilia bend in the excitatory direction, away from the modiolus and toward the tallest row, the tip-links of the stereo-

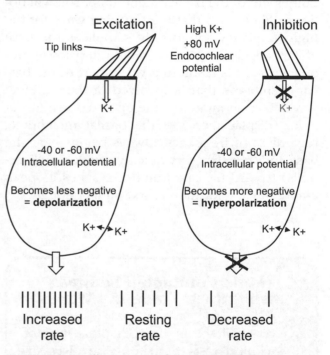

FIGURE 5–8. Illustration of the transduction process going from hydromechanical activity of the stereocilia to neural activity in the afferent neurons attached to the hair cells. During excitation, the stereocilia bend toward the tallest row causing tip links to open up the potassium (K+) channels and allowing an influx of potassium ions (K+) into the cell body, which depolarizes the intracellular potential. During inhibition, the stereocilia bend away from the tallest row causing tip links to close potassium channels (K+), which hyperpolarizes the intracellular potential. The excitation (depolarization) phase results in an increase in the neural discharge rate of the neurons relative to its spontaneous resting discharge rate. This is followed by the inhibition (hyperpolarization) phase that results in a decrease in the discharge rate relative to its spontaneous resting discharge rate.

know that within the endolymph of the scala media there is a +80 mV electrical potential (charge), the *endocochlear potential* (EP). The EP is the highest resting electrical potential in the body and is maintained by the stria vascularis, often called the "biological battery" for the scala media. The +80 mV EP and the –40 mV (or –60 mV) intracellular potential provide an electrical difference (potential) of about 120 to 140 mV between the scala media and the inside of the hair cells. As Davis (1965) first proposed, cilia open up K+ channels within the stereocilia allowing an influx (increased flow) of K+ into the hair cell. The intracellular potential becomes less negative during the influx of K+ (excitatory phase). When the stereocilia bend in the inhibitory direction, away from the modiolus and away from the tallest row, the tip-links of the stereocilia close the K+ channels within the stereocilia and reduce the K+ flow into the hair cell; the intracellular potential becomes more negative (inhibitory phase) as the biochemical cell activity removes K+ across the membrane. Through this series of events, the frequency of the incoming sound is being transduced from hydromechanical energy into biochemical energy.

To summarize events up to this point: The incoming condensations and rarefactions of the acoustic vibrations cause in-and-out movements of the tympanic membrane, in-and-out movements of the ossicular chain, up-and-down movements of the basilar membrane (producing a traveling wave), back-and-forth bending of the stereocilia at locations where the basilar membrane displacement is adequate, increases and decreases of ions (K+) flowing into the hair cells, and finally increases (depolarization) and decreases (hyperpolarization) of the respective hair cell intracellular potentials.

Auditory Nerve Fibers

The final stage in the transduction process is to convert the biochemical events within the hair cells into neural events along the afferent 8th cranial nerve fibers. Since at least 95% of the afferent neural information of the 8th cranial nerve comes from the IHCs, the activation of the stereocilia of the IHCs is the primary route for sensory transduction through the cochlea. For now, we will focus primarily on the activity that occurs in the IHCs (hopefully, you are anxiously anticipating learning about the role of the OHCs that will be discussed in a later section). The *neural transduction* process occurs at the chemical synapses that lie between the base of each IHC and the peripheral processes of the afferent auditory neurons that synapse with the IHC. Figure 5–8 illustrates how the transduction of energy

changes from biochemical (within the hair cells) to neural (within the 8th cranial nerve fibers). During the excitatory phase of the intracellular potential (*depolarization*), there is an increase in the release of neurotransmitter substance at the synapse. During the inhibitory phase of the intracellular potential (*hyperpolarization*), there is a reduction in the release of neurotransmitter substance at the synapse. The connections of the bipolar afferent nerve fibers react to the amount of available neurotransmitter substance and carry this synaptic information, called *graded potential*, to the neuron's cell body located in the spiral ganglion. If there is enough graded potential within a cell body to reach its criterion level for excitation, then the myelinated axon of the nerve fiber, beginning in the modiolus, sends out an all-or-none discharge, that is, the cell "fires." Once the cell fires, there is a chain reaction along the axon, through the internal auditory canal, and then to the connecting cells in the cochlear nucleus of the brainstem.

The all-or-none discharges, called *spikes*, from an auditory nerve fiber are all of the same amplitude and duration. Because there are no differences in the size of the discharges, the only neural information that is available is in the pattern of the neural discharges, for example, how many spikes occur per second, *discharge rate*, or the time intervals between spikes, *interspike interval*. How the brain codes this information to determine the frequency and intensity of a sound is briefly covered later in this chapter.

TUNING CURVES

The basilar membrane acts like a series of interconnected and overlapping filters. Each location along the basilar membrane responds best to a specific frequency, its *characteristic frequency* (CF). However, these filters are not precise (sharp) enough to only respond to a single frequency, as might be implied by the analogy to strings on a harp. Instead, each location on the basilar membrane can respond to a range of frequencies around its CF if the intensities are sufficient. The combinations of frequencies and intensities that produce a response for a particular

---

SYNOPSIS 5-2

- The basilar membrane is narrower and stiffer at the basal end of the cochlea and becomes wider and less stiff toward the apex of the cochlea. These physical characteristics result in a tonotopic arrangement, whereby high frequencies stimulate the basal end of the membrane and low frequencies stimulate the apical end of the membrane.

- The traveling wave always begins with small displacements at the base and proceeds to a location of maximum displacement based on the tonotopic arrangement, and then rapidly declines more apically.

- The basilar membrane and tectorial membrane move at different pivot points that results in bending of the stereocilia away from the modiolus when the basilar membrane moves in one direction and toward the modiolus when the basilar membrane moves in the other direction.

- The transduction process through the inner ear involves hydromechanical events (traveling wave and bending of stereocilia on the hair cells), chemical events (changes in the hair cell potentials), and neural events (activation of the afferent nerve fibers, primarily from the IHCs). The transduction process in the inner ear can be summarized by the following events:
  - In and out movement of the stapes footplate creates pressure variations in the fluid that are transmitted instantaneously along the entire basilar membrane.
  - The basilar membrane reacts with a traveling wave that moves from the base of the cochlea and peaks at a location based on the tonotopic arrangement (highs toward the base, lows toward the apex).
  - Up and down movements of the basilar membrane in the vicinity of the traveling wave peak bend the stereocilia of the IHC back and forth.
  - Back and forth bending of the stereocilia opens and closes the ion channels by the tip links so that the K+ concentration increases or decreases relative to the normal intracellular resting level.
  - Increases and decreases of K+ into the hair cell makes the intracellular potential less negative (excitatory) or more negative (inhibitory) relative to the normal resting potential.
  - Excitatory and inhibitory stages of the intracellular potential cause increases and decreases in the neurotransmitter substances deposited in the synaptic cleft. Almost all of the afferent neural activity is associated with the IHCs.
  - Excitatory and inhibitory stages of the afferent auditory neurons from the spiral ganglia result in increases and decreases in the all-or-none (spike) discharges, and these spikes travel to the awaiting dendrites of neurons in the cochlear nucleus.

---

location on the basilar membrane provide an estimate of the shape of the filter associated with that location, and this is referred to as a measure of *frequency selectivity* or *tuning*. *Tuning curves* are a useful way to describe the frequency selectivity or tuning characteristics of the audi-tory system. Figure 5–9 shows some examples of tuning curves. In essence, a tuning curve is obtained by defining a minimum criterion response for the measure of interest, and then sweeping through a series of frequency-intensity combinations to find those that meet or exceed the minimum criterion; the lowest level of those combinations defines the threshold tuning curve. The tuning curve is defined by its CF, which is the lowest frequency-intensity combination that produces the minimum criterion response. However, as you can see, frequencies other than the CF can also produce the criterion response when presented at higher stimulus levels. For frequencies close to the CF, the tuning curve rises fairly steeply on both sides of the CF, called the *tip region* of the tuning curve. For frequencies considerably lower than the CF, the tuning curve flattens out for a wide range of lower frequencies presented at moderate intensity levels, called the *low frequency tail*. For frequencies higher than the CF, the steep slope continues, called the *high frequency slope*. A tuning curve with a relatively narrow tip region is considered to be *sharply tuned*, which is expected for normal functioning ears. Figure 5–9B illustrates what happens to an ear with damaged hair cells. In this case, the tip (threshold) of the tuning curve is elevated and is also more *broadly tuned*; this type of cochlear damage produces a hearing loss as well as more difficulty in frequency selectivity causing the person to have greater difficulty in processing speech, especially in a background noise.

Tuning curves can be generated for many levels of the auditory system, including the basilar membrane, auditory neurons, and psychoacoustic (perceptual) measures; however, in a normal auditory system, tuning curves from different levels are very similar in shape as those shown in Figure 5–9A. A basilar membrane tuning curve is obtained by measuring the range of frequency–intensity combinations that produce a criterion amount of displacement for a particular location on the basilar membrane. A neural tuning curve is obtained by measuring the range of frequency–intensity combinations that produce a criterion increase in the discharge rate for a particular neuron. A psychoacoustic tuning curve is obtained by measuring the range of frequency–intensity combinations that can interfere with (mask) the perception of a target tone near the CF.

Békésy (1960) was the first to demonstrate tuning curves from the basilar membrane, and found them to be much broader than the normal

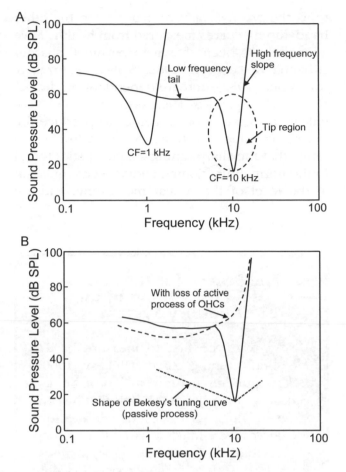

FIGURE 5–9. A AND B. Examples of tuning curves. **A.** Normal tuning curve illustrated for 1 kHz characteristic frequency (CF) and 10 kHz CF. The most sensitive point (lowest dB SPL), called the tip region of the tuning curve, occurs at CF. Each tuning curve shows that it is responsive to other frequencies (but with higher dB SPLs), especially those lower than the CF, the low frequency tail, whereas the frequencies above the CF continue to show a steep high frequency slope. **B.** Illustration showing how damage to the active process of the outer hair cells elevates the tip region of the tuning curve and leaves only a broader tuning curve representing the passive process. Also shown is a representation of a relatively broad tuning curve originally found by Békésy (1960).

tuning curves shown in Figure 5–9. The relatively broad basilar membrane tuning curves found by Békésy in models and cadavers are, as now known, due to the physical characteristics of the basilar membrane (width and stiffness), referred to as the *passive cochlear process*. On the other hand, tuning curves measured from healthy alive animals have been shown to be much sharper (Khanna & Leonard, 1982; Sellick, Patuzzi, & Johnstone, 1982), and are dependent on the *active cochlear process*. The passive and active cochlear processes work together to produce the normal cochlear reactions to sound. Today, we know that the sharp tuning characteristics found in the normal functioning auditory system begin at the level of the basilar membrane, and are

---

The Search for the Source of Sharp Tuning in the Auditory System

Békésy was the first to measure basilar membrane tuning curves (Békésy, 1960). Békésy's tuning curves were done in human cadavers or in physical models that he constructed. Békésy's basilar membrane tuning curves were much broader than tuning curves that others had found from nerve fibers of the 8th nerve and in psychoacoustic experiments. During the 1970s to 1980s, Békésy and many others engaged in an abundance of auditory research directed at finding another filter ("second filter") that might be responsible for sharpening the tuning between the basilar membrane and the auditory nerve fibers. Was it in the hair cells, the neurons, or something in the central auditory system? This issue, however, was finally resolved with advances in technology, especially laser methods, that allowed measurements of basilar membrane tuning curves to be performed in live animal specimens without compromising the integrity of the cochlea (Khanna & Leonard, 1982; Sellick et al., 1982). With the newer methods, in live animals, the basilar membrane was shown to be as sharp as 8th cranial nerve fibers and psychoacoustic tuning curves, and there was no need of a second filter in the cochlea.

---

present in the hair cell, 8th cranial nerve fibers, and a variety of psychoacoustic measures. Moreover, as you will see in the next section, it is the OHCs that play an important role in the active process that is responsible for the sharp frequency tuning and good sensitivity.

ROLE OF THE OUTER HAIR CELLS

As you recall from Chapter 4, there are about three times as many OHCs as there are IHCs in each human cochlea, and less than 5% of the OHCs have afferent nerve connections (Spoendlin, 1978). This discovery suggests that the OHCs may not have the same function as the IHCs. So what is the role of the more numerous OHCs? This paradox set off another important wave of research in the late 1970s to early 1980s during which time not only was the role of the OHCs determined, but the foundation was laid for a very important physiological test called *otoacoustic emissions* (OAEs). The OAE test is now a routine part of the audiology test battery and is used in many newborn hearing screening programs.

About 70 years ago, even before we knew about the tuning paradox of the basilar membrane and differences between IHCs and OHCs, a British physicist named Thomas Gold (1948) concluded that some active energy process would be needed in the cochlea in order to have sharp frequency tuning. Gold suggested that this process would have to involve an active feedback loop that would generate some vibratory energy in the cochlea. Thirty years later, another British physicist named David Kemp (1978) gave credence to this theory by actually recording sounds that were coming out of the ear, now known as OAEs. Kemp postulated that these emissions were from some active cochlear process that generates additional mechanical activity on the basilar membrane that travels back out through the middle ear and generates very low level acoustic sounds in the ear canal that can be measured with a very sensitive microphone.

Soon after Kemp's discovery, a neuroscientist named William Brownell (1983) demonstrated that OHCs were able to elongate and contract in response to electrical currents. These elongations and contractions are generally referred to as the *motility* of the OHCs. The motility of the OHCs was subsequently confirmed by many investigators. Recall that OHCs have a unique organization along their outer wall consisting of structural and contractile proteins, as well as enzymes, and these elements have been shown to be partly responsible for the rigidity and motility of the OHCs. The motility of the OHCs is unique in that they can elongate and contract, rather than just contract like muscles. The stria vascularis is thought to provide the external energy source that allows the OHCs to elongate and contract indefinitely, and can even occur at high frequencies without getting tired. The complete biochemistry of OHC motility is beyond the scope of this textbook. The biochemical transduction process can be considered to include a chemical-mechanical (motor) transduction within the OHCs and a chemical-neural transduction within the IHCs.

So, how does the OHC motility influence cochlear mechanics? Recall that the stereocilia of the IHCs are not imbedded into the underside of the tectorial membrane and that it is the stimulation of the IHCs that is necessary for afferent neural transduction. At low to moderate intensities, the traveling wave displacements of the basilar membrane are not sufficient to make the stereocilia of the IHCs contact the tectorial membrane to initiate bending of their stereocilia; this would only occur at much higher intensities, and our ears would not be nearly as sensitive to sounds. There must be some other mechanism that causes the stereocilia of the IHCs to bend to initiate the afferent neural activity. As it turns out, it is the active cochlear process of the OHCs that amplifies the displacement of the basilar membrane through their motility. At low to moderate intensities, the elongations and contractions of the OHCs in the vicinity of the CF are in phase with the frequency of basilar membrane displacements, resulting in sort of a resonance/amplification of the displacements. In other words, the motility of the OHCs works with the passive process of the traveling wave motion of the basilar membrane, and this additional activity causes the greater displacement of the basilar membrane sufficient to initiate bending of

the IHC stereocilia. This is often explained with a swing analogy, where the amplitude of the swing's height can be increased by having someone push (adding energy) at the proper time (in resonance) with the swing's motion. You can also increase the amplitude of the swing on your own by pumping your legs (adding energy) in resonance with the swing's motion. In other words, because the OHC stereocilia are firmly embedded into the tectorial membrane, the motility of the OHCs causes the basilar membrane and tectorial membrane to be pulled together and pushed apart in resonance with the displacements of the basilar membrane. This active process in the cochlea serves to amplify the traveling wave motion of the basilar membrane enough to allow the stereocilia of the IHCs to make contact with the tectorial membrane even at low to moderate stimulus intensities. This active cochlear process is necessary for our good hearing sensitivity and frequency tuning (Kiang, Liberman, Sewell, & Guinan, 1986).

At high stimulus intensities, it is believed that the displacement of the basilar membrane from the passive cochlear process is sufficient to allow the stereocilia of the IHCs to make contact with the tectorial membrane. Looking back at Figure 5–9B, the elevated tip region of the tuning curve occurs because there is damage to the active process of the OHCs; the remaining broadly-tuned tuning curve results from the passive cochlear process (Liberman, Dodds, & Learson, 1986). When damage occurs to the OHCs, the active process in the cochlea is compromised and mild-to-moderate degrees of hearing loss occur. For greater degrees of hearing loss, there is additional damage to the IHCs that would also compromise the output from the passive cochlear process. An important point to realize is that when damage occurs to the OHCs, OAEs are not generated. On the other hand, if OAEs are present, it can be inferred that there is good auditory function up to at least the level of the OHCs. The absence of OAEs suggests some abnormality of auditory function, either in the OHCs, middle ear, or outer ear. As discussed in Chapter 13, OAEs are widely used as a screening measure for newborns, and those who do not pass the OAE screen are referred for diagnostic follow-up.

FREQUENCY CODING

As you might imagine, given that there is much to learn and understand about how the normal ear functions, the field is only beginning to scratch the surface on how we make use of the auditory neural information that ultimately is processed at the cortex, and how sounds are perceived; again, there is much more to learn through future research. At this introductory level, only some general theories of perception are presented.

There are two general principles used to explain how we determine (code) the frequency of the incoming sound, the place theory and the frequency theory. The *place theory* of hearing refers to the tonotopic arrangement along the basilar membrane. The tonotopic arrangement of the auditory system is present along the basilar membrane, but is also a characteristic of the auditory neurons, auditory nuclei in the brainstem, and auditory reception areas of the cortex. The place theory assumes that the frequency information is first coded where the peak of the traveling wave occurs along the basilar membrane, high frequencies near the base and low frequencies near the apex, and this frequency information is preserved as the neural information ascends through the auditory neural pathways.

An alternative theory of frequency coding, the neural *frequency theory*, is based on the processing of the pattern of discharges in the afferent auditory nerve fibers. Let's look at some patterns of discharges that occur in response to simple sounds to see if they could be a viable means to code frequency. One method is to measure the time intervals between the discharges, called *interspike interval* (ISI). As Figure 5–10 shows, a neuron responds with a preferred ISI; however, it also responds with other ISIs, and these can be seen to follow a specific temporal pattern. For example (see Figure 5–10 panel D), the 1000 Hz tone has a preferred ISI of 1 ms (highest number of intervals), which corresponds to the period for 1000 Hz. However, other ISIs also occur for the 1000 Hz tone, but notice that they occur only at multiples of the period of the 1000 Hz tone.

Using this strategy, a neuron does not have to discharge every cycle of the stimulus; it can skip some cycles of the stimulus due to its need for

A Problem for the Place Theory

As nice as the place theory sounds, there are some limitations. One problem for the place theory comes from psychoacoustic experiments that have demonstrated that the perception of frequency does not always relate to the place predicted by the tonotopic arrangement. For example, when listening to multiple pure tones that are harmonically related the perceived pitch is determined by the lowest fundamental frequency. For example, when presented simultaneously with 1200, 1400, and 1600 Hz, the perceived pitch would be 200 Hz, even though it is not even presented to the ears. However, this 200 Hz pitch will still be perceived even when the low frequency areas are masked by a noise or have some type of damage. In other words, the place theory would predict that the 200 Hz is perceived because it generates a traveling wave at the 200 Hz location, when in fact the 200 Hz is still perceived when the apical area of the basilar membrane is unable to respond to the tone due to the noise or damage. Somehow, the pitch of this missing fundamental is still perceived because of information coming from the activity in the high frequency area of the cochlea; thus, the place theory does not explain all types of frequency coding.

neural recovery time, but when the neuron does respond it always responds at some multiple of the preferred interval. Different frequencies have different patterns of ISIs that are related to the period of the stimulus. As you may have noticed in Figure 5–10, the relation between ISIs and the period of the stimulus gets weaker at mid frequencies (see Figure 5–10, panel J), and at higher frequencies (above 2000 Hz) a preferred interval no longer can be recorded.

If, however, recordings from a neuron are displayed as a function of the period of the stimulus, called a *period histogram*, it can be observed

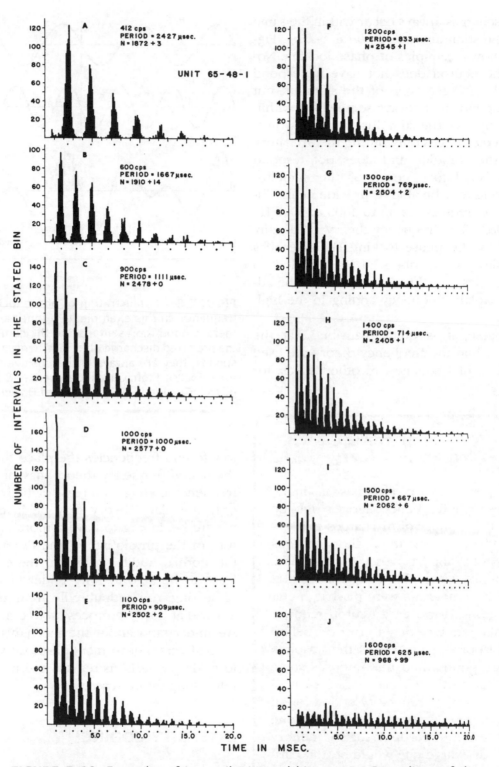

FIGURE 5–10. Examples of interspike interval histograms. Recordings of the intervals between discharges are plotted as a function of stimulation time. Notice how the peaks in the histograms are related to the periods of the different frequencies up to about 1500 Hz. *Source*: From Rose, Hind, Anderson, & Brugge, 1967, p. 772. Copyright 1967 by The American Physiological Society.

that the discharges always occur within the same phase of the stimulus, called *phase locking*. Figure 5–11 shows examples of phase locking. Notice that the neuron does not have to respond at the peak of every cycle of the stimulus, but when it responds it is always somewhere within the same phase of the stimulus. In other words, the neuron discharges only during the excitatory phase of the stimulus and does not respond during the inhibitory phase of the stimulus. Phase locking may be able to provide neural information for frequencies up to 4000 to 5000 Hz (Møller, 1983). The frequency theory is partially supported by the phase locking characteristics of the auditory nerve fibers, at least for low to mid frequencies, but this theory may not be adequate to explain frequency coding in the high frequencies.

Of course, it is quite plausible that the place theory and the frequency theory are used in the coding of frequency. In other words, for

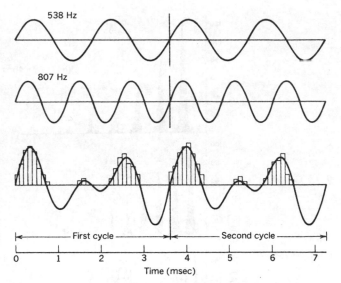

FIGURE 5–11. Illustration of phase locking code for frequency. In this example, two tones are played and there is good representation of the combined tone in the preferred discharge pattern. Whenever the nerve responds, they are always in the positive phases of the tone. *Source*: From Gulick, Gescheider, & Frisina, 1989, p. 183. Copyright 1989 by Oxford University Press.

low to mid frequencies the place theory and/or the neural frequency theory may be involved in frequency coding, whereas for high frequencies only the place theory may be involved. While we are beginning to have a more complete picture of the physiology of the different parts of the normal auditory system, there is much to learn to be able to fully understand our sense of hearing. You undoubtedly are finding yourself amazed at how we process sound and how little we understand about the mechanisms, even in normal ears, not to mention those with hearing loss. Many questions remain and make for some interesting future research.

INTENSITY CODING

How does the auditory system provide information that we use to code for stimulus intensity? One theory for coding intensity has to do with how much of the basilar membrane is stimulated. In other words, as intensity increases, the tails of tuning curves from more basal locations are also stimulated. Figure 5–12 illustrates how a spread

A Problem for the Frequency Theory

The frequency theory also has its limitations. A simple frequency theory would be to have the number of discharges per second (discharge rate) in the auditory neurons correspond to the frequency of the sound. For example, we would perceive a 2000 Hz tone because neurons were discharging at 2000 times/s. However, a neuron requires a minimal period of time to recover before it can respond again, called the absolute refractory period, and this imposes some restrictions on the discharge rate of neurons. The absolute refractory period for an auditory neuron is about 1.0 ms; therefore, the theoretical upper limit for an auditory neuron's discharge rate would be 1000 discharges per second. In fact, it is actually more typical for an auditory nerve fiber to respond up to a maximum of only 200 discharges per second, regardless of the stimulus frequency. Clearly, the discharge rate per se is not useful for coding frequency.

of activity could occur across more of the basilar membrane by crossing the tails of the tuning curves from higher frequency regions as the intensity of a sound increases (Evans, 1975). The activation of more neurons from a wider area of the basilar membrane could code for intensity, while the activity of neurons at the tip (CF) of the tuning curve could code for the frequency.

Can a single auditory neuron code intensity? In other words, could one fiber from a single place keep increasing its discharge rate as a function of stimulus intensity? We can begin to answer this question by looking at an *input–output* (I/O) *function*, which is a measure of how

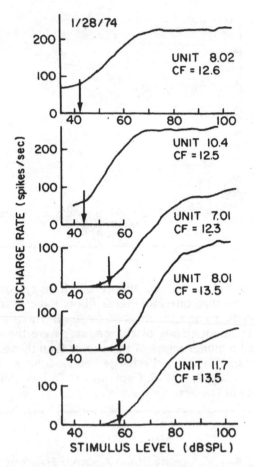

FIGURE 5–13. Input-output functions for some auditory nerve fibers. Most nerve fibers tend to plateau (saturate) in their discharge rates within 40 dB above threshold and, therefore, cannot explain the much wider intensity range of hearing. *Source*: Reprinted with permission from Sachs & Abbas, 1974, p. 1837. Copyright 1974 by Acoustic Society of America.

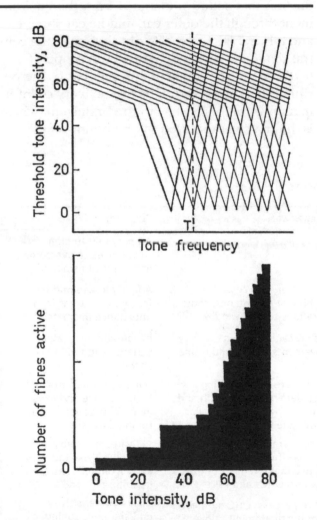

FIGURE 5–12. A theory of intensity coding postulated by Evans (1975). In this theory, more nerve fibers are recruited at higher intensities because they are activated by crossing the low frequency tails of higher frequency nerve fibers. *Source*: From Evans, 1975, p. 436. Copyright 1975 by Taylor & Francis.

the number of discharges per second changes as a function of stimulus intensity. As Figure 5–13 shows, most auditory nerves increase their discharge rates over a limited intensity range of only 20 to 40 dB above threshold (Kiang, 1965; Sachs & Abbas, 1974). This immediately suggests a problem in coding intensity over the entire 140 dB range, since neurons can only increase a maximum of 40 dB above their threshold; however, Liberman (1978) suggested that the range of intensity coding based on the discharge rate could be expanded by staggered thresholds for different neurons attached to each IHC. As Figure 5–14 shows, neurons have been shown to have a range of thresholds, some of which do

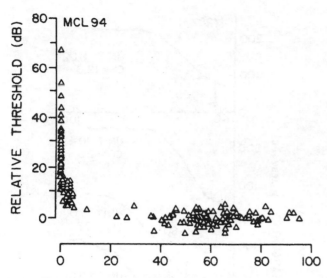

FIGURE 5–14. Another theory of intensity coding. Data show that different nerve fibers have different thresholds, some as high as 60 to 70 dB. Those fibers with low spontaneous discharge rates were the ones that had a higher range of thresholds than those with higher spontaneous discharge rates. *Source*: From Liberman, 1978, p. 448. Copyright 1978 by American Institute of Physics.

not begin to respond until 60 to 70 dB above the threshold of the most sensitive neurons attached to the IHC. Liberman (1978) showed that the staggered thresholds of neurons were related to the spontaneous discharge rates; high spontaneous rate neurons had low thresholds, and low spontaneous rate neurons had higher thresholds.

SUMMARY OF THE AUDITORY TRANSDUCTION PROCESS

This chapter provided an overview of how sound is processed in the peripheral auditory system. Table 5–1 summarizes the different stages of transduction that sound undergoes from the environment through the outer ear, middle ear, inner ear, and 8th cranial nerve. The physiology of the central nervous system is beyond the scope of this textbook. of the transduction process of the peripheral auditory system is the delivery of information (from both ears) to the brainstem, which is, ultimately, processed by the brain.

TABLE 5–1. Summary of the Auditory Transduction Processes

Process	Part of Ear	Structures	Mechanism	Function
Acoustic	Outer	Auricle, ear canal	Resonance	Amplify mid to high frequencies to overcome impedance mismatch
Mechanical	Middle	Tympanic membrane, ossicles, oval window	Area, lever, and curved membrane advantages; route vibrations to oval window	Amplify low to mid frequencies to overcome impedance mismatch
Hydromechanical	Cochlea	Oval and round windows, scalae	Reciprocal in-and-out movements of oval and round windows	Instantaneous pressure variations in fluid-filled cochlea
		Basilar membrane	Passive process: traveling wave dependent on width and stiffness gradients of basilar membrane	Tonotopic place principle; highs at base and lows at apex; produces broad tuning curves
		Tectorial and basilar membranes, stereocilia	Bends stereocilia back and forth due to different pivot points of the two membranes; controls K^+ flow into OHCs and IHCs	Activates hair cells: toward modiolus = excitation; away from modiolus = inhibition
Chemical-motoric	Cochlea	OHCs	Active process: OHC motility, from fluctuation in K^+ flow, adds displacement to traveling wave to allow direct bending of IHC stereocilia	Increases sensitivity and sharpens tuning; responsible for sharp-tip region of tuning curves

continues

TABLE 5–1. Summary of the Auditory Transduction Processes (*continued*)

Process	Part of Ear	Structures	Mechanism	Function
Chemical-neural	Cochlea	IHCs	Increase and decrease of intracellular potential resulting from fluctuation in K+ flow	Controls release of neurotransmitter substance
Neural	8th Nerve	Auditory nerve fibers	Uptake of neurotransmitter substance; if adequate, cells initiate all-or-none discharges down 8th nerve axons to cells in cochlear nucleus	Neural discharge patterns provide intensity and frequency information to central nervous system

Note. IHC, inner hair cells; *OHC*, outer hair cells.

SYNOPSIS 5–3

- The auditory system's excellent frequency selectivity (sharp tuning) and sensitivity originate along the basilar membrane only when the cochlea is physiologically healthy. Earlier measures in cadavers using compromised cochleae showed much broader tuning than had been demonstrated in the tuning of 8th cranial nerve fibers and in psychoacoustic experiments.
- The additional mechanical energy exerted by the motility (elongations and contractions) of the OHCs at low to moderate intensities increases the displacements of the basilar membrane, much like pushing someone on a swing. The motility of the OHCs allows the stereocilia of the IHCs to be directly stimulated by the tectorial membrane in response to the basilar membrane's enhanced displacement.
- The motility of the OHCs in a healthy, normal functioning ear is responsible for the ear's remarkable sensitivity and sharp frequency selectivity. Damage to the OHCs may lead to a mild to moderate hearing loss and a loss of frequency tuning/resolution (broader tuning curves). The OHC motility is referred to as the active cochlear process, whereas the process of traveling waves that occur along the basilar membrane due to its physical characteristics is called the passive cochlear process.
- The cochlear transduction process has both a chemical-neural mechanism involving the IHCs and a chemical-motor mechanism involving the OHCs. See Table 5–1 for a summary of the transduction process through all parts of the peripheral auditory system.
- Otoacoustic emissions, which are predictable consequences of the OHCs' motility, travel from the cochlea, back out the middle ear, and are transduced into acoustic vibrations by the tympanic membrane. OAEs can be recorded with a sensitive microphone placed in the ear canal and have become a popular auditory physiological screening test.
- Because most auditory neurons respond with rates less than 200 discharges, the number of discharges per second is not a viable method to code for frequency. A more plausible explanation is by analyzing the interspike intervals

SYNOPSIS 5–3 (*continued*)

or phase locking of neurons. Coding frequency by phase locking may be possible up to about 4000 Hz. An alternate theory for frequency coding is the place that is maximally activated along the basilar membrane. The place theory has limitations in explaining some psychoacoustic phenomena, especially coding low frequencies, but may be plausible for higher frequencies where the phase locking is inadequate.

• Intensity coding is also not fully understood. A single auditory nerve fiber can only increase its discharge rate over a maximum range of about 40 dB. Possible explanations for intensity coding include (a) activation of more nerve fibers at higher intensities as they cross the low frequency tails of other neurons, and/or (b) different nerve fibers may become activated at different stimulus levels.

REFERENCES

Ballachanda, B. B. (1995). *The Human Ear Canal*. San Diego, CA: Singular.

Baloh, R. W. (1998). *Dizzyness, Hearing Loss, and Tinnitus*. Philadelphia, PA: F. A. Davis.

Békésy, G. (1960). *Experiments in Hearing*. New York, NY: McGraw-Hill.

Borg, E., & Counter, S. A. (1989). The middle ear muscles. *Scientific American, 260*, 74–80.

Brownell, W. E. (1983). Observations on a motile response in isolated outer hair cells. In W. R. Webster & L. Aitken (Eds.), *Mechanisms of Hearing* (pp. 5–10). Clayten, Australia: Monash University Press.

Dallos, P. (1986). Neurobiology of cochlear inner and outer hair cells: Intracellular recordings. *Hearing Research, 22*, 185–198.

Dallos, P. (1988). Cochlear neurobiology: Revolutionary developments. *ASHA, 30*(6–7), 50–56.

Davis, H. (1965). A model for transducer action in the cochlea. *Cold Spring Harbor Symposia on Quantitative Biology, 30*, 181–190.

Durrant, J. D., & Lovrinic, J. H. (1995). *Bases of Hearing Science* (3rd ed.). Baltimore, MD: Williams & Wilkins.

Evans, F. (1975). The sharpening of cochlear frequency selectivity in the normal and abnormal cochlea. *Audiology, 14*, 436.

Gelfand, S. A. (2009). *Hearing: An Introduction to Psychological and Physiological Acoustics* (5th ed.). Boca Roton, FL: Taylor & Francis.

Gelfand, S. A. (2015). *Essentials of Audiology* (4th ed.). New York, NY: Thieme.

Gold, T. (1948). The physical basis of the action of the cochlea. *Proceedings of the Royal Society of London, Series B: Biological Sciences, 135*, 492–498.

Hamill, T., & Price, L. (2014). *The Hearing Sciences* (2nd ed.). San Diego, CA: Plural.

Kemp, D. T. (1978). Stimulated acoustic emissions from within the human auditory system. *The Journal of the Acoustical Society of America, 64*(5), 1386–1391.

Khanna, S. M., & Leonard, D. G. (1982). Basilar membrane tuning in the cat cochlea. *Science, 215*, 305–306.

Kiang, N. Y. (1965). Discharge patterns of single fibers in the cat's auditory nerve. *Research Monographs, 35*. Cambridge, MA: MIT Press.

Kiang, N. Y., Liberman, M. C., Sewell, W. F., & Guinan, J. J. (1986). Single unit clues to cochlear mechanisms. *Hearing Research, 22*, 171–182.

Liberman, M. C. (1978). Auditory-nerve response from cats raised in a low-noise chamber. *The Journal of the Acoustical Society of America, 63*(2), 442–455.

Liberman, M. C., Dodds, L. W., & Learson, D. A. (1986). Structure-function correlation in noise-damaged ears. In R. J. Salvi, D. Henderson, R. P. Hamermik, & V. Colletti (Eds.), *Basic and Applied Aspects of Noise Induced Hearing Loss*. New York, NY: Plenum Press.

Møller A. R. (1983). *Auditory Physiology*. New York, NY: New Academic Press.

Møller, A. R. (1958). Intra-aural muscle contraction in man examined by measuring acoustic impedance of the ear. *Laryngoscope, 68*, 48–62.

Møller, A. R. (1965). An experimental study of the acoustic impedance and its transmission properties. *Acta Otolaryngology, 60,* 129–149.

Nedzelnitsky, V. (1980). Sound pressures in the basal turn of the cat cochlea. *The Journal of the Acoustical Society of America, 68*(6), 1676–1689.

Reger, S. (1960). Effect of middle ear muscle action on certain psycho-physical measurements *Annals of Otology, Rhinology, & Laryngology, 69,* 1179–1198.

Rose, J. E., Hind, J. E., Anderson, D. J., & Brugge, J. F. (1967). Phase-locked response to low-frequency tones in single auditory nerve fibers in the squirrel monkey. *Journal of Neurophysiology, 30*(4), 769–793.

Sachs, M. B., & Abbas, P. J. (1974). Rate versus level functions for auditory-nerve fibers in cats: tone-burst stimuli. *The Journal of the Acoustical Society of America, 56*(6), 1835–1847.

Sellick, P. M., Patuzzi, R., & Johnstone, B. M. (1982). Measurement of basilar membrane motion in the guinea pig using the Mössbauer technique. *The Journal of the Acoustical Society of America, 72*(1), 131–141.

Shaw, E. A. (1974). Transformation of sound pressure level from the free field to the eardrum in the horizontal plane. *The Journal of the Acoustical Society of America, 56*(6), 1848–1861.

Spoendlin, H. (1978). *The Afferent Innervation of the Cochlea.* San Diego, CA: Academic Press.

Yost, W. (2013). *Fundamentals of Hearing* (5th ed.). Leiden, Netherlands: Koninklijke Brill.

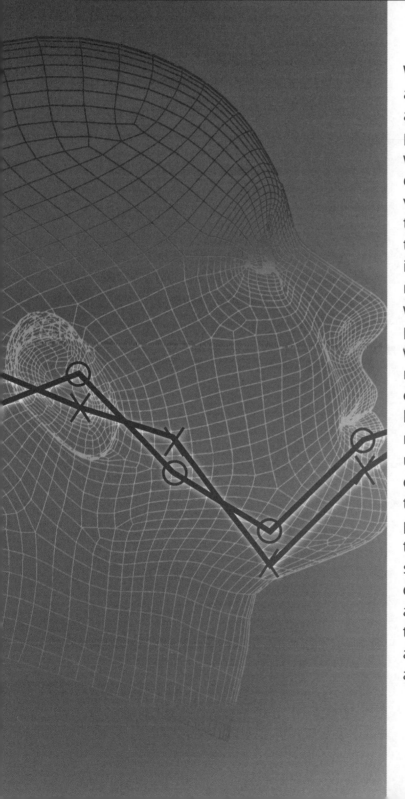

PART III

Clinical Audiology

WE now switch our focus to the clinical assessment of hearing and the rewarding aspects of interacting with and helping patients. In the following chapters, you will learn about several tests used by audiologists to diagnose hearing loss and vestibular function, and you will be introduced to hearing aids as one of the treatments used by audiologists to help improve communication of patients with nonmedically treatable hearing loss, as well as cochlear implants and other implantable hearing devices. In this book, we prefer to use the terms patient, diagnosis/assessment, and treatment in the context of providing audiologic services; however, in some settings audiologists may prefer to use the terms client, evaluation, and management. While audiologists do not use the audiologic results to diagnose auditory diseases, they often provide information to physicians about the hearing loss that is useful to the physician in making a medical diagnosis and deciding on the medical treatment. The audiologic results do bear directly on the treatment, including fitting hearing aids, aural rehabilitation, tinnitus management, and/or vestibular rehabilitation.

Some of the tests covered in this book are behavioral measures, which require the patient to make a judgment and perform a task, like push a button when he or she hears a sound or repeats words. Some examples of behavioral tests include pure-tone audiometry and speech measures as described in Chapters 6 through 9. Other audiologic tests are physiologic measures, which do not require subjective judgments or responses by the patient; however, the patient must be cooperative and sit quietly or, in some cases, can even be asleep. Some examples of physiologic tests include tympanometry, acoustic reflexes, wideband acoustic immittance, otoacoustic emissions, and auditory brainstem responses, which are described in Chapters 10 and 11. Behavioral measures are generally referred to as *subjective tests*, whereas physiologic measures are generally called *objective tests*. It is important to keep in mind, however, that many of the objective tests require the audiologist to make subjective decisions during the testing, and in most cases the audiologist is required to make subjective interpretations about the objective test data.

The audiologist needs to be keenly aware of when to refer the patient to a physician for medical management. Chapter 12 provides descriptions of some common hearing disorders and how they relate to the audiologic measures. Also covered in this part of the textbook are hearing screening (Chapter 13), hearing aids (Chapter 14), and implantable devices (Chapter 15). And lastly, in Chapter 16, you will learn more about the vestibular anatomy, physiology, common vestibular disorders, and assessment of vestibular disorders. One of the enjoyable aspects of audiology is the symbiotic relationships that can be established among audiologists, physicians, and other health care providers. Working together with mutual respect provides the most complete care possible to those with hearing and vestibular problems. In many cases, there is no underlying medical condition related to the patient's hearing or vestibular problems and the patient is referred to or seeks services directly from the audiologist, who then takes primary responsibility for diagnosing and treating the patient regarding the hearing loss and its effects on communication and/or vestibular rehabilitation. The audiologist is the most knowledgeable and appropriate professional to deal with the sensory and psychosocial aspects associated with hearing loss and vestibular problems.

6 Audiometric Testing

After reading this chapter, you should be able to:

1. Discuss why pure tones are useful for assessing hearing and hearing loss.

2. Describe different types of audiometers and the functions of their basic components.

3. Describe the types of transducers used in audiometry and the advantages of each type.

4. Describe what is meant by air conduction and bone conduction audiometry and how these types of testing are used to determine which parts of the auditory system are affected.

5. Describe the audiometric testing environment and how the patient is positioned.

6. Describe the steps used to obtain pure-tone thresholds, including the up-5-down-10 (modified Hughson–Westlake) bracketing procedure.

7. Determine thresholds from hypothetical examples of threshold searches.

8. Discuss the variables that can affect thresholds and what can be done to accommodate and/or account for this variability.

9. Describe the methods for testing infants and toddlers using behavioral types of tests.

Now that you are equipped with the knowledge from previous chapters about basic acoustics and the anatomy/physiology of the normal ear, you can begin to learn how these principles are applied to the clinical assessment of a person's hearing ability. The measurement of a person's ability to hear different sounds is called *audiometry*. The term *audiometric* is used to describe different aspects pertaining to audiometry, such as audiometric results or audiometric testing. A basic hearing test, called *pure-tone audiometry*, involves finding the lowest sound pressure levels for different pure tones that a person is barely able to hear. The lowest sound pressure level of a pure tone to which a person reliably responds at least 50% of the time is called his or her *threshold* for that frequency. In pure-tone audiometry, pure-tone thresholds are obtained in a quiet environment for a range of frequencies between 250 and 8000 Hz, which is most relevant for speech sounds. In some specialized cases, thresholds in the 10,000 to 16,000 Hz range are measured. Keep in mind that most activities in the real world do not involve listening to barely audible pure tones in quiet test environments. Everyday sounds are much more complex, occur at moderate intensity levels, and are usually surrounded by background sounds. Although one's ability to hear depends on the processing of frequency, intensity, and temporal parameters of sounds, it can also be influenced by a variety of other non-acoustic factors, including maturation, cognition, motivation, and context.

Pure tones are used for basic testing for a variety of reasons. First of all, pure tones are relatively easy to produce and calibrate. In addition, since many types of hearing losses do not affect frequencies equally, the pattern of hearing loss as a function of frequency is often characteristic of certain types of hearing loss. For example, high frequencies are more affected than low frequencies for older persons with hearing loss due to aging. Pure-tone thresholds may also be useful when discussing how a patient's hearing loss might relate to his or her ability to hear different frequencies of speech sounds such as /f/, /s/, or /th/, which have relatively higher frequency components than other speech sounds.

It is important to keep in mind that while pure tones are relatively easy to generate, the actual testing of a patient requires considerable skill and experience in order to be able to recognize and adapt to different patient response abilities and patterns. The testing of an 8-month-old child, a mentally disabled young adult, an elderly person with dementia, or someone who is purposefully exaggerating a hearing loss are only some of the challenges that make audiometry interesting. An audiologist's ability to incorporate and integrate the pure-tone results and other test results with information from the patient, and then make appropriate interpretations, impressions, and recommendations, are competencies that develop with time and experience.

Pure-tone audiometry is almost always part of the basic audiologic assessment with cooperative patients, and has been a key element in hearing testing since audiology's modern beginnings in the mid-1900s (Jerger, 2009). Pure-tone audiometric thresholds are used by audiologists to: (a) describe the amount of the patient's hearing loss; (b) determine which parts of the auditory system are involved; (c) determine if a medical referral is needed, and (d) predict how the patient's hearing loss may relate to his or her ability to listen and communicate.

THE AUDIOMETER

The audiologist uses an instrument called an *audiometer* for many of the hearing tests. There are different types of audiometers that are classified based on their capabilities and use. Although the appearance and operation of audiometers may differ depending on the manufacturer or model, they all have similar functions and components.

Types of Audiometers

One class of audiometer is called a *diagnostic* or *clinical audiometer*. Some examples of diagnostic audiometers are shown in Figure 6–1. A diagnostic audiometer is an instrument capable of performing a variety of hearing tests, including pure-tone audiometry, and must conform to certain standards of operations, as specified by the *American National Standards Institute (ANSI)* for diagnostic audiometers. The ANSI standards

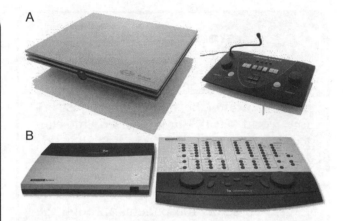

FIGURE 6–2. A and B. Two examples of computer-based audiometer systems. **A.** Interacoustics Equinox with instrument panel. **B.** Madsen Astera with instrument panel. Interfacing computers are required but not shown. *Source*: Photos courtesy of Interacoustics (**A**) and Otometrics/Audiology Systems (**B**).

are periodically updated, the most current being ANSI (2010). Diagnostic audiometers are available from a variety of manufacturers and come in a variety of shapes and sizes, including some that are designed for limited space and/or for portability. Many diagnostic audiometers have the option to save the patient response information through a computer interface cable for storage and printing.

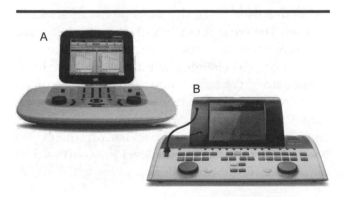

FIGURE 6–1. A and B. Some examples of two-channel diagnostic audiometers used for comprehensive clinical evaluations. **A.** Grason-Stadler Inc. Model AudioStar Pro. **B.** Interacoustic Model AC40. Source: Photos courtesy of Grason-Stadler Inc. (**A**) and Interacoustics (**B**).

Computer-based audiometry is now becoming more widely used for clinical testing. With the more sophisticated computer-based audiometers, the audiologist can control the testing with the computer keyboard and/or mouse. The audiometry software generates and controls the delivery of the sounds (pure tones and speech materials), and allows for direct storage of the patient's response, viewing and printing the results, and tracking patient data. Other software is available that allows audiometric data to be stored on the Internet in a secure program, and allows integration of data from other tests, templates for report writing, and keeps track of patient billing and services. Some of the computer-based audiometry systems may also interface with a more traditional audiometer instrument panel, thereby giving the audiologist the flexibility of testing with the instrument panel, the keyboard, and/or the mouse. Some examples of computer-based audiometry systems are shown in Figure 6–2.

Another type of audiometer is called an *automatic audiometer*. An automatic audiometer has the capability of changing the signal level based on the response of the patient. Today, automatic audiometry usually refers to the use

Historical Vignette

The automatic audiometer was invented by Georg von Békésy during his time in Stockholm after he fled Hungary just before World War II. But it received little clinical attention until the Grason-Stadler Co., in the late 1950s, produced a commercial instrument, the venerable E-800. Northwestern bought one of the first units, and Jerger ran some 400 patients through the procedure in which the patient tracked his or her thresholds to a continuous tone and then a pulsed tone that swept across the frequency range. This type of testing resulted in four Békésy types; Type I, in which the continuous and pulsed tone thresholds were similar, as found in normal listeners and conductive losses; Type II, in which the size of the excursions for the continuous tone was much smaller than those of the pulsed tone, as found in ears with recruitment (cochlear losses); and Types III and IV, in which the threshold for the continuous tone was dramatically worse than for the pulsed tone, as found in 8th nerve disorders. Later, Gilbert Herer added a Type V, in which the threshold to the pulsed tone was poorer than to the continuous tone, contrary to the relationship seen in the other four types, and was found in patients with functional (feigned) losses.

of computer-based systems that can be set-up/programmed to test one or more people at the same time, and is commonly used as an efficient way to assess a group of workers in industrial settings. The original automatic audiometer, called a Békésy audiometer, allows the patient to control the level of the signal using a handheld response button while the tones are automatically changed from low to high frequencies. In Békésy audiometry, the patient holds down a button to increase the intensity of the tone until it is just barely audible, then releases the button to decrease the intensity until it is inaudible. The printout produces a tracing in one direction when the button is held down and then reverses direction when it is released. The patient's threshold is taken as the midpoint of the excursions. Békésy audiometry has some useful diagnostic patterns when tracings are done for pulsed versus continuous tones. Békésy audiometry was popular through the 1970s, but is not used much today for clinical testing. However, Békésy audiometry is still an available option on some audiometers, and is used in some laboratory settings. For more information on Békésy audiometry, see Jerger (1960) and Johnson (1977).

Another type of audiometer is called a *screening audiometer*. A screening audiometer is usually smaller, portable, and has very limited capability. A screening audiometer typically tests over a limited range of frequencies and intensities. A hearing screening is usually done only at a single intensity level, and the patient either passes or fails. A screening audiometer is typically used for hearing screenings in schools, hospital rooms, or other situations in which a patient cannot be tested in the audiology clinic. Speech-language pathologists, nurses, or those with an Audiometrist Certificate typically use screening audiometers.

Basic Components of Pure-Tone Audiometers

Table 6–1 lists the basic components of an audiometer. The basic functions of an audiometer are to: (a) produce pure tones at selected frequencies (oscillator), (b) change the intensity of the signal (attenuator), (c) select how the signal is delivered to the ear (transducer), and (d) direct the signal to a desired location (router). For example, a tester would set the oscillator frequency to 1000 Hz, set the attenuator level to 40 dB[1], select earphones as the transducer, and route the signal

---

[1]You are probably thinking, "What is the reference value for this dB?" You will learn more about the decibel hearing level (dB HL) scale used in audiometry in

TABLE 6–1. Basic Functions and Components of a Pure-Tone Audiometer

Function	Component
Selects the frequency of the pure tone	Frequency selector
Changes sound pressure level of signal	Attenuator dial
Selects how the signal is delivered	Transducer selector
Directs signal to desired location	Router switch
Presents the signal to the patient	Interrupter switch
Indicates whether patient responded	Patient response indicator
Monitors/calibrates input level	VU meter

to the right ear. When ready, the tester pushes the interrupter switch to deliver the signal to the patient and then observes the patient to see if he or she responds. The patient can indicate that he or she heard the signal by either raising a hand or by pushing a response button that activates a patient response indicator on the audiometer. Audiometers also have a *volume unit (VU) meter* that allows for monitoring and calibrating the signal level, and this important component will be discussed in more detail in the chapter on speech audiometry.

Diagnostic audiometers must always have two separate channels with all of the functions duplicated, since many of the hearing tests require that two different signals be presented at the same time to one ear or to each ear. There are other functions and components of diagnostic audiometers that are specific for other diagnostic tests, many of which are discussed in later chapters. It is highly recommended that the tester develop a habit of reviewing the instrument manual that accompanies each audiometer in order to learn the specific details of the audiometer's operation and to become familiar with all of its components and functions.

the following chapter: To simplify some of the concepts in this chapter, the dB reference will be omitted.

TRANSDUCERS

The pure tones (or other test signals) are delivered to the patient through *transducers*, such as earphones. An audiometric transducer is a device that is capable of vibrating when activated by an electrical signal from the oscillator, thus converting (*transducing*) electrical signals into vibrations that can be heard. The transducers are connected to the audiometer, and the tester selects the desired transducer to which the signal is to be routed. Table 6–2 lists the different types of transducers commonly used in audiometry. Earphones are color-coded to indicate which ear is being tested; the red earphone should be used for the right ear (Red = Right) and the blue earphone should be used for the left ear. It is very important to be sure that the correct earphone is on the appropriate ear so that the audiometer routing switch corresponds to the ear to which you are actually sending the signal.

Insert Earphone

Insert earphones, such as the Etymotic ER-3A or EARTone-3A, are the recommended transducers for most clinical testing today. The insert earphones were developed in the mid-1980s (Killion, Wilber, & Gugmundsen, 1985) to improve on the supra-aural earphones that have been around much longer in clinical practice (see below for description of supra-aural earphones).

TABLE 6–2. Types of Transducers Used in Pure-Tone Audiometry

Transducer	Common Models	Corresponding Figure
Insert earphones	ER-3A, ER-5A, EARTone-3A	6–3
Supra-aural earphones	TDH-39, 49, 50P	6–4
High frequency earphones	Sennheiser HDA200	6–5
Speakers	Various models	6–6
Bone conduction vibrator	B-71, B-81	6–7

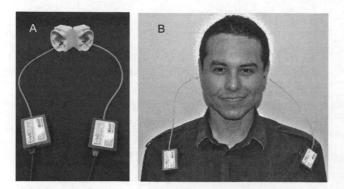

FIGURE 6–3. A. A set of insert earphones (ER-3A). **B.** Insert earphones properly placed for testing.

Figure 6–3 shows photographs of insert earphones, along with a patient being tested with the insert earphones. Each of the insert earphones has the electroacoustic diaphragm housed in a small case that is attached by a clip to the patient's clothing. The signal is sent from the case to the ear through a small tube that is inserted into the ear canal and held in place with a disposable foam cuff. The foam cuff is compressed by hand prior to insertion into the ear canal, and it expands after insertion to conform to the shape of the patient's ear canal. For sanitary purposes, the disposable foam cuffs are replaced for each patient. The proper placement of the insert earphone into the ear canal is important, and it should be inserted so that the outer edge of the foam cuff is just within the first bend of the ear canal. This type of earphone prevents the possibility of temporary ear canal collapse that can occur with supra-aural earphones, reduces background noise, and reduces the need for masking the other ear (see Chapter 9), making the task of pure-tone audiometry much easier and faster.

Supra-Aural Earphones

Supra-aural earphones, such as the Telephonics TDH series (TDH-39, 49, 50P), were the standard earphones used in audiometry until the insert earphones were developed, but are still used in many situations. Figure 6–4 shows photographs of supra-aural earphones, along with a patient

being tested with the supra-aural earphones. Each of the supra-aural earphones has its electroacoustic diaphragm surrounded by a rubber cushion that rests on the auricle. Supra-aural earphones are held in place with a headband designed to produce a specific tension. For sanitary purposes, the supra-aural earphone cushions are covered with disposable paper covers (or cleaned with an appropriate sanitary wipe) between each patient. The proper position of the supra-aural earphones is to align the center of the earphone diaphragms with the openings of the ear canals. An off-centered earphone can affect the delivery of higher frequencies, which have small wavelengths relative to the ear canal. In some patients, a supra-aural earphone can temporarily collapse (close off) the cartilaginous part of the ear canal due to the pressure of the earphone resting on the ear, and the tester must be aware of this possibility when using this type of transducer. Inaccurate hearing thresholds due to temporarily collapsing the ear canal when using supra-aural earphones is discussed in Chapter 7.

Supra-aural earphones and insert earphones are designed to test frequencies from 125 to 8000 Hz and up to a maximum output level of 120 dB HL; however, insert earphones have about a 5–10 dB lower maximum output level than supra-aural earphones. Supra-aural earphones are still used in situations where insert earphones are not available or when a patient is unwilling or unable to complete testing with the insert ear-

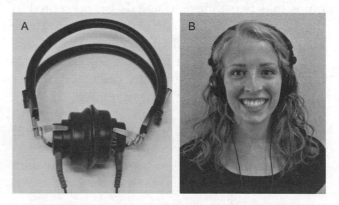

FIGURE 6–4. A. A set of supra-aural earphones (TDH-39). **B.** Supra-aural earphones properly placed for testing.

phones. Supra-aural earphones must be used in patients who do not have ear canals (called atresia), patients who have profound hearing loss, or those with active drainage from the ears.

Extended High-Frequency Earphone

Another type of earphone is an *extended high-frequency (EHF)*, or *circumaural earphone*, such as the Sennheiser HDA200. Circumaural earphones are used in special situations where the frequencies above 8000 Hz need to be evaluated (e.g., monitoring the effects of some drugs). The diaphragm of the circumaural earphone is housed in a larger cushioned cavity, which is designed to be positioned around the auricle so that it is less likely to move. Since the extended high-frequencies have shorter wavelengths, proper position of the circumaural earphones is critical to avoid any effects related to the size of the ear canal. Figure 6–5 shows photographs of circumaural earphones, along with a patient being tested with the circumaural earphones.

Sound-Field Speakers

Speakers (or loudspeakers) are another type of transducer sometimes used in audiometry. The speaker is usually positioned in the corner of

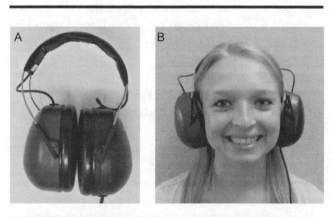

FIGURE 6–5. A. A set of extended high-frequency earphones (Sennheiser HDA200). **B.** Extended high-frequency earphones properly placed for testing.

the test room a few feet away from the patient. When speakers are used for testing, it is referred to as *sound-field* or *free-field* testing. Speaker models vary by audiometer manufactures; there is not a standard model number. Speakers may be needed for testing the occasional patient who does not tolerate keeping the earphones on his or her head, such as some young children. Speakers may also be used if testing a patient with hearing aids or cochlear implants in a sound field, since earphones are not able to be positioned over the ears while the patient is wearing most amplification. A limitation of testing in a sound field is that both ears will receive the sounds, so the response is based on the better hearing ear and, therefore, it is not possible to get ear-specific information. Whenever possible, it is recommended that hearing testing be done with earphones so that each ear can be tested separately. Even difficult patients and young children can often be convinced to wear the earphones with some encouragement and demonstration. Figure 6–6 shows a photograph of a sound-field speaker positioned in a hearing test room.

Bone Conduction Vibrator

Another important type of transducer used in audiometry is called a *bone conduction vibrator* (or bone oscillator), such as the Radioear B-71 or B-81. Figure 6–7 shows photographs of a bone conduction vibrator, along with a patient being tested with the bone conduction vibrator. The bone conduction vibrator has a plastic casing that is set into vibration by the pure tone stimulus. The bone conduction vibrator delivers the pure-tone vibrations mechanically to the skull, and these bone conducted vibrations stimulate the inner ears that are embedded within the temporal bones of the skull. The bone conduction vibrator is placed against the skull usually behind the ear (on the mastoid bone) and held in place with a headband designed with a specific tension to produce a specific force on the skull. The bone conduction vibrator should not touch the auricle and should be placed under the hair. The headband of the bone conduction vibrator is placed across the top of the head. The bone conduction

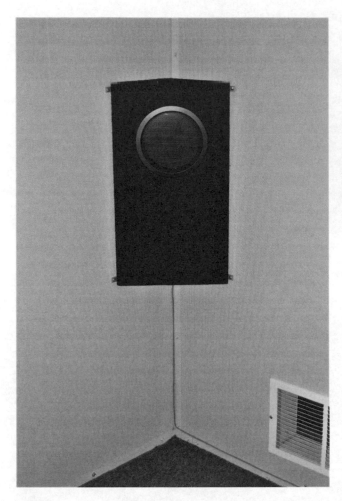

FIGURE 6–6. A sound field speaker shown placed in the corner of a hearing test room.

vibrator can also be placed on the forehead with a specially designed headband, but most audiologists use a mastoid location for bone conduction testing. Notice in Figure 6–7 that the bone conduction vibrator is a single transducer placed at one location on the skull rather than a transducer for each ear. The bone conduction vibrator is not color coded and is switched from one side to the other. It is important to realize that when the bone conducted vibrations are delivered anywhere on the skull, both ears will receive these vibrations simultaneously because the bones of the skull act like a solid object. In order to obtain bone conduction thresholds from one ear at a time, a noise sound, called a *masker*, needs

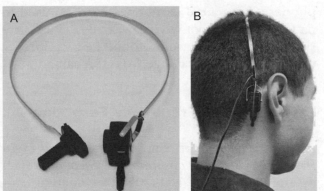

FIGURE 6–7. A. A bone conduction vibrator (B-71). **B.** Bone conduction vibrator properly placed on the right mastoid and held in place with the headband to allow for testing. Note that the bone conduction vibrator is placed on one side at a time and switched from side to side.

to be delivered by an earphone to the other ear to keep it busy so that it cannot hear the test tone being presented by the bone conduction vibrator. The specific clinical situations that require masking and the procedures for obtaining thresholds with masking are covered in subsequent chapters. The bone conduction vibrator output is more limited than earphones; threshold testing is generally restricted from 250 to 4000 Hz, and only up to levels as high as 70 to 80 dB because of the distortion that can occur with the bone conduction vibrator at higher frequencies and at higher intensities. Also, at lower frequencies patients can sometimes feel the vibrations, something that needs to be considered when doing bone conduction testing.

AIR CONDUCTION VERSUS BONE CONDUCTION TESTING

When earphones are used to deliver sounds to the patient, this is referred to as *air conduction* (AC) testing. When the bone conduction vibrator is used to deliver sounds to the patient, it is called *bone conduction* (BC) testing. Figure 6–8 illustrates how the use of AC and BC testing helps identify if and where there is any hearing problem

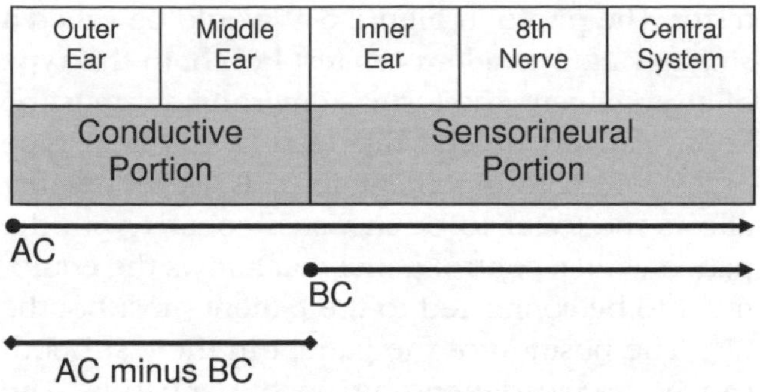

Outer Ear	Middle Ear	Inner Ear	8th Nerve	Central System
Conductive Portion		Sensorineural Portion		

AC

BC

AC minus BC

FIGURE 6–8. Illustration of the auditory pathways involved with air conduction (AC) and bone conduction (BC) testing. Testing with AC involves all parts of the ear, whereas the testing with BC only involves the sensorineural portion of the ear. A hearing loss in the sensorineural portion of the ear affects thresholds obtained by AC and BC by the same amount. A hearing loss in the conductive portion affects AC thresholds, but does not affect BC thresholds. The difference in thresholds between AC and BC is called the air–bone gap, and is the amount of the conductive involvement.

in the auditory pathway. Testing by AC stimulates the entire auditory system, whereas testing by BC delivers the vibrations through the skull and are picked up by the inner ears; BC testing essentially bypasses the conductive (outer and middle ear) portions of the auditory pathway. The difference in thresholds between AC and BC is referred to as the *air-bone gap*. If a patient has a hearing loss due to a problem in the sensorineural part of the auditory system (inner ear, 8th nerve, and/or central) he or she would have the same amount of hearing loss when tested by AC and by BC, since both of these types of testing include the sensorineural part of the ear. For example, a hearing loss in the inner ear would show an elevated (poorer than normal) threshold when tested by AC, and the same amount of threshold elevation when tested by BC: This type of hearing loss is called a *sensorineural hearing loss*. As we will see in later chapters, there are additional diagnostic tests that allow us to determine if a sensorineural hearing loss is due to problems in the inner ear (sensory loss), 8th cranial nerve (neural loss), or central pathways (central loss). If a patient has a hearing loss due to a problem in the conductive portion of the auditory system (outer and/

or middle ear) he or she would have normal BC thresholds because BC testing bypasses the outer ear and middle ear, and elevated AC thresholds because AC testing includes the outer and middle ear. This type of hearing loss is called a *conductive hearing loss*. It is important to keep in mind that AC testing includes all parts of the auditory system and, therefore, the AC thresholds are not a measure of the conductive hearing loss per se. In order to determine the amount of hearing loss from the conductive portions of the ear, you must look at the air–bone gap. A conductive hearing loss would have normal BC thresholds and air–bone gaps. Of course, a patient could have more than one type of hearing problem at the same time; there could be concomitant involvement of both the sensorineural and conductive portions of the auditory system. In that case, the patient would have an elevated threshold by BC (reflecting a problem in the sensorineural portion) and a greater elevation in threshold by AC, hence an air–bone gap, that reflects the additional involvement of the conductive portion. This type of hearing loss is called a *mixed hearing loss*. As you may already have surmised, theoretically BC thresholds should not be worse than AC thresholds because any changes in threshold due to the sensorineural portions of the ear, as reflected in the BC thresholds, would also be reflected in the AC thresholds. However, in clinical practice the BC thresholds may be slightly poorer (e.g., 5 to 10 dB) than the AC thresholds, but this does not have any clinical significance and is not called an air–bone gap. Instead, it is simply due to an inherent testing variability, as well as the fact that the calibrated equipment levels are based on average BC thresholds (Studebaker, 1967).

THE TEST ENVIRONMENT

Diagnostic hearing testing must be done in a specially designed sound-attenuating test room (also called a "sound booth" or "test suite") that meets standards for permissible background noise levels suitable for audiometric testing (American National Standards Institute [ANSI], 1999). Figure 6–9 shows a picture of an audiometric test room. The test room walls are about 4 inches

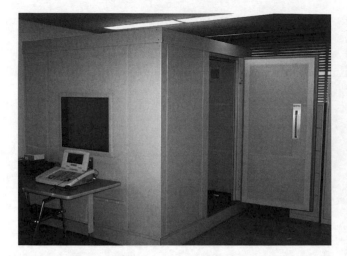

FIGURE 6–9. A single-room audiometric test environment. The patient sits inside the room and the tester and equipment are outside the room. The tester's equipment is connected to the room through a connector (jack) panel, and there is a window to maintain visual contact. In many clinics, the tester is also in another similarly treated test room that is connected to the patient's test booth, called a double-room test environment.

thick with sound absorption material and small holes in the inside wall to absorb the sounds and reduce reflections. The test room can be single-walled or double-walled (a room within a room for more attenuation). In addition, test rooms can be arranged so that the equipment/tester is outside of the patient test booth, or as a two-room test suite that has one room for the patient and a separate room for the equipment/tester. The photo in Figure 6–9 would be called a single-walled, single-room test booth. In this type of arrangement, the tester's environment must be kept relatively quiet while testing. In either type of test booth arrangement, there is a window that allows the tester to be in visual contact with the patient, and a control panel that allows the equipment to be connected to the patient's test booth.

The position of the patient in the test booth can be varied depending on the situation. The arrangement must be such that the patient is unable to discern any inadvertent cues by the tester, such as hand, head, or eye movements, facial expressions, or visible reflections. In order to reduce the possibility of inadvertent cues, the typical orientation would have the patient facing 45° to 90° away from the observation window. For some patients, the audiologist might prefer to have more direct eye contact to better read some of the patient's signs of confusion or to provide visual reinforcement. In this case, the tester should be careful to cover/disguise anything that could be taken as a visual cue. If conducting the test in the sound field, the orientation of the patient would depend on what is needed. For example, if pure-tone testing requires the patient to respond by turning toward the sound (e.g., when testing some toddlers), then the patient should be oriented 45° to 90° away from the speaker so that a noticeable head-turn is observable. This can be done with one speaker on one side of the room (the patient turns toward the speaker when he or she hears a sound) or with a loudspeaker on each side of the room (the

SYNOPSIS 6–1

- A variety of audiometers are available with different functions. The most common audiometer is a two-channel clinical audiometer capable of performing a comprehensive battery of audiometric tests. Clinical audiometers can be stand-alone instruments with or without computer storage capability, or can be entirely computer-based.
- Basic features of an audiometer include an oscillator to generate the pure tones, an attenuator to adjust the intensity, and switches to select the type of transducer for the ear to be tested, and to present the signal to the patient.

SYNOPSIS 6–1 (continued)

- Audiometry transducers convert the electrical stimuli from the audiometer to something that the patient can hear. These include insert earphones (e.g., ER-3A) that are inserted part way into the ear canals, supra-aural earphones (e.g., TDH-39) that rest on the auricles, and speakers that present the pure tones in the sound-field. These earphones are used to test frequencies from 250 to 8000 Hz. Special earphones are needed for testing frequencies above 8000 Hz, called extended high-frequency audiometry.
- Insert earphones avoid the problem of supra-aural earphones that potentially can temporarily collapse the ear canals during testing. Insert earphones also reduce some of the background noise, and have some advantages when there is the need to mask the other ear (discussed in later chapters).
- Another transducer routinely used in audiometry is called a bone conduction vibrator (e.g., Radioear B-71) that delivers the pure tones to the inner ear through vibrations of the bones of the skull. Since both cochleae are embedded in the skull, both ears receive the vibrations from a single bone vibrator placed anywhere on the skull. When vibrations occur in the skull it is often necessary to use a masking noise in the non-test ear so that it cannot hear the test tone.
- Thresholds obtained with insert or supra-aural earphones are called air conduction (AC) thresholds and those obtained with a bone vibrator are called bone conduction (BC) thresholds.
- Testing by AC sends the sounds through the entire auditory pathway, whereas testing by BC sends sounds to the inner ear, thus bypassing the outer and middle ears. A difference in the threshold by AC and the threshold by BC, called the air–bone gap, will indicate hearing loss that is due to the conductive parts of the auditory system (outer or middle ear).
  - A sensorineural hearing loss is characterized by equal threshold elevations by AC and BC (no air–bone gap).
  - A conductive hearing loss is characterized by a normal BC threshold and elevated threshold by AC (an air–bone gap).
  - A mixed hearing loss is characterized by an elevated threshold by BC and an even greater elevated threshold by AC (loss by BC and an air–bone gap). A mixed hearing loss indicates that the hearing loss is from two sources, the sensorineural portion and conductive portion.
- Clinical pure-tone hearing testing should be performed in a sound-attenuating test room that meets the most current ANSI standards. Test rooms can be single room or double room suites.
- In order to reduce the possibility of inadvertent cues from the tester, such as hand, head, or eye movements, facial expressions, or visible reflections, the typical orientation would have the patient facing 45° to 90° away from the tester. Should direct eye contact with the patient be needed, then care must be taken to avoid giving cues to the patient.

patient localizes the source of the sound by turning to the correct side). If interested in knowing whether the patient hears a sound without turning the head, the patient can be oriented toward the speaker to avoid direct visualization of the tester. Likewise, if testing a patient with hearing aids, the patient should face the speaker to have the sound directed into the microphone of the hearing aid.

PROCEDURES FOR OBTAINING PURE-TONE THRESHOLDS

In pure-tone audiometry, there are guidelines for how to determine thresholds. The most current guidelines for establishing pure-tone thresholds are found in documents from the American National Standards Institute [ANSI] (2004) and the American Speech-Language-Hearing Association [ASHA] (2005), both of which are in general agreement with each other. It is important for audiologists to use the same procedures so that a patient's thresholds are reasonably consistent when obtained by different audiologists or from the same audiologist at different times. The generally accepted procedures for establishing pure-tone thresholds are based on what is called the modified Hughson–Westlake technique, first described by Carhart and Jerger (1959). Today, the modified Hughson–Westlake procedure for establishing clinical pure-tone thresholds is also commonly referred to as the "*up-5-down-10*" (or "down-10-up-5") procedure, and is discussed in more detail below. While there are some variations among audiologists in how they apply the procedures, the following steps are typically followed:

1. Provide some clear instructions to the patient, such as: "We are interested in finding the faintest level at which you are able to hear sounds of different pitches. Listen carefully and be sure to press the response button (or raise your hand) as soon as you think you hear a sound and release the button (or lower your hand) as soon as the sound goes away. We will be testing each ear separately. Do you have any questions?"

2. Place the appropriate transducer on the patient in the proper position (remember Red = Right). Do not allow the patient to put the transducer on or move it. Improper placement will result in inaccurate thresholds. Test AC before BC, and begin AC testing in the better ear if known or as reported by the patient.

3. Begin testing with a familiarization phase. This involves presenting a 1000 Hz pure tone at a relatively easy level to hear (e.g., 30 to 40 dB above the estimated threshold of the patient), in order to allow the patient to become familiar with the task and to show the tester that the patient understands the task. If the patient does not hear the pure tone at the initial level, the level is increased in 20 dB steps until a response is obtained. Often, the familiarization phase is continued by decreasing the level of the pure tone in 10 dB steps until the patient no longer responds; this then marks the beginning of the threshold search phase (see below). An alternate familiarization method is to present a continuous tone at the lowest intensity level and gradually increase the level of the tone until the patient responds, and then decrease the level by 10 dB to mark the beginning of the threshold search phase.

4. Select the desired frequency: Testing usually begins with 1000 Hz because it is a mid-range tone that is generally easier to perceive, and is the frequency used for the familiarization phase. The order of frequencies tested is not critical; however, the order suggested by ASHA (2005) is 1000, 2000, 3000, 4000, 6000, 8000, 500, 250 Hz. Retesting 1000 Hz in the first ear is recommended in order to account for improvement due to practice effects with the other frequencies. The inclusion of 125 Hz for AC testing is recommended in cases when there is a low frequency hearing loss or when interested in better characterizing residual low frequency hearing. In addition, 750 and 1500 Hz should be tested if there is more than a 20 dB difference in thresholds between the adjacent octave frequencies. For BC testing, the recommended testing sequence is 1000, 2000, 3000, and 4000 Hz, retest 1000 Hz, 500, 250 Hz.

5. Present the pure tone by pressing and releasing the interrupter button. Most diagnostic audiometers have a pulse tone option that presents a series of short tones when the interrupter switch is activated. A series of pulsed tones is often used because they are easier to perceive and are more distinguishable from any ringing sounds the patient may have in the ears. The presentations of the tones or series of pulses should be 1 to 2 s in duration. There should be variable pauses (1 to 4 s) between presentations so that the patient is not able to predict the rhythm of the presentations.

6. Begin the threshold search phase using the up-5-down-10 procedure. This means that when the patient does not respond, the level of the pure tone is increased in 5 dB steps until he or she does respond, and decreased by 10 dB (presumably below threshold) until the patient does not respond. These bracketing steps are repeated until a threshold for that frequency is established. The recommended threshold search procedure (after the familiarization phase) is an *ascending threshold procedure* whereby you increase the level of the stimulus from a level that the patient does not hear the tone (below threshold) up to a level in which the patient barely hears the tone. The tester usually keeps mental track of "response" or "no response" in relation to the ascending trials. Keeping track of the patient's responses mentally may seem complicated; however, this ability becomes routine with practice.

7. Continue the tone presentations, using the up-5-down-10 procedure, until the threshold is established based on the following definition: A pure-tone threshold is defined as the lowest intensity level that the patient responds to *at least 50%* of a series of ascending presentations, with at least two responses out of at least three trials for a single level (ANSI, 2004; ASHA, 2005).

Generally, the implementation of the procedure is that up to four presentations may be required, and that at least 50% be heard. Since the guidelines state that there be at least three trials at a level, two out of three is about 67%, which meets the definition of *at least* 50%. Some audiologists, in some situations, may modify the procedures: For example, the threshold may be taken as the level in which there were two correct responses out of only two presentations (2/2); this would require that there were no responses to two presentations at 5 dB lower (0/2). If the standard procedures are modified, such as with young children or the disabled, then these modifications should be documented with the test results.

EXAMPLES OF HOW TO ESTABLISH THRESHOLDS

Let's examine more closely the process of how to determine an accurate threshold based on the recommended professional guidelines (ANSI, 2004; ASHA, 2005). Let's say that after two ascending series (following the up-5-down-10 procedure) the patient has responded 0% (0/2) at 35 dB and 100% (2/2) at 40 dB. At this point, you might be tempted to select 40 dB as the threshold, since 40 dB is the lowest level that the patient responded to at least 50% of the presentations (and at 35 dB it was less than 50%). However, this would not be an accurate threshold based on the recommended guidelines, which say that the patient must respond to at least two out of a minimum of three ascending series (and up to four ascending series). In this example, the patient could respond to the next two ascending series at 35 dB and, therefore, the threshold would be 35 dB (2/4 responses). On the other hand, if the patient does not respond at 35 dB in the third ascending series (0/3), the threshold would be 40 dB (3/3). Keep in mind that the threshold is the lowest level in which the patient gives at least two correct responses out of at least three presentations, that is, if the patient does not respond to the third presentation at 35 dB, you would not have to give the fourth presentation because the best that he or she could do at 35 dB would be 25% (1/4). In some cases, it might take four presentations to eliminate the possibility of 50% (1/4). This is what is meant by four possible (or theoretical) presentations, but the threshold could be established with two out of three (2/3) correct responses. For this example, in either case, a third ascending series was necessary.

Let's look at some more examples of the steps used to establish threshold. Figure 6–10 shows three examples demonstrating how the presentation level was varied, using an up-5-down-10 procedure, until an acceptable threshold was established following the guidelines. In Figure 6–10A, the testing started at 30 dB (Trial 1) and the patient responded (+). Because the patient responded, the level was lowered to 20 dB (down 10) for Trial 2 and the patient again responded (+). Again, the level was lowered to 10 dB (down 10) for Trial 3 and now the patient did not respond (–). You should now be thinking that the threshold is somewhere between 10 dB and 20 dB. The first ascending series began from 10 dB by increasing the level in 5 dB steps; first to 15 dB for Trial 4 where the patient did not respond (–), and then to 20 dB for Trial 5 where the patient did respond (+). At this point, there has been one ascending series with a response at 20 dB, and no response at 10 dB or 15 dB. Trials 6 through 8 showed a similar response pattern following the rule of lowering the level by 10 dB following a response (+) and increasing the level by 5 dB when there was no response (–); this second ascending series ended with a second response at 20 dB (2/2) and no response at 10 dB (0/2) or 15 dB (0/2). However, there was still the possibility that 15 dB could be the threshold if two more trials were to be given at that level to satisfy the criterion that the patient had the opportunity to obtain at least 50% of the presentations out of a possible four presentations. So, Trials 9 through 11 show the third ascending series in which the patient did not respond at 15 dB (0/3) and did respond at 20 dB (3/3). Trial 11, technically, would not have been required because it would have already been determined that the best score out of a theoretical four presentation that the patient could achieve at 15 dB would be 25% (1/4), and even if he or she did not respond at 20 dB in the third trial, he or she would have satisfied the criterion of two out of three at this level. However, this last trial (Trial 11) at 20 dB would usually be included to complete the series and in this example the patient again responded at 20 dB (3/3); thus, the patient's threshold would be 20 dB.

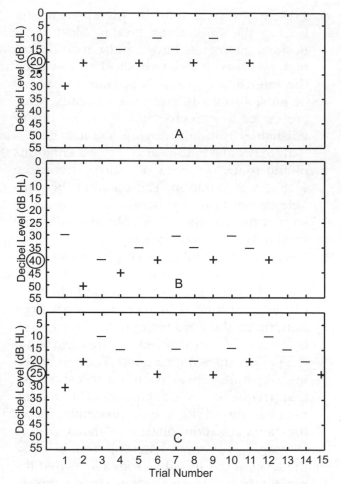

FIGURE 6–10. A–C. Hypothetical examples demonstrating the modified Hughson–Westlake (up-5-down-10) method to establish thresholds. A plus sign (+) indicates that the patient responded to (heard) the tone, and a minus sign (–) indicates that the patient did not respond to (did not hear) the tone. In these three examples, the threshold was based on the lowest level in which the patient responded to at least 50% of ascending series of trials; with a minimum of two responses out of three trials (2/3) or two responses out of four trials (2/4). After each trial in which the patient responded, the intensity of the signal was decreased by 10 dB, and after each trial in which the patient did not respond, the intensity was increased by 5 dB. For each of the three examples, the threshold is indicated by the *circled dB value*. See text for a detailed explanation for each of these examples.

The example shown in Figure 6–10B started at the same level as in Figure 6–10A; however, this patient did not hear (–) the initial 30 dB presentation level, so the level was raised to 50 dB in order to find a level that is above the threshold for the familiarization phase of the procedure. At 50 dB (Trial 2) the patient responded (+). At this point, you suspect that the threshold would be somewhere between 30 and 50 dB. In Trial 3, the level was lowered to 40 dB (down 10) and the patient did not respond (–). In Trial 4, the level was raised to 45 dB (up 5) and the patient responded (+). In Trial 5, the level was lowered to 35 dB and the patient did not respond (–). In Trial 6, the level was raised to 40 dB and the patient responded (+). You now have one out of two (1/2) responses at 40 dB, so additional trials are needed. The level was then lowered to 30 dB for Trial 7 and the patient did not respond. The sequence continued until Trial 12, where it was determined that there was more than 50% at 40 dB (3/4) and that at least 50% would not be possible at lower levels even if a fourth presentation were given (already had 0/3 at 35 dB).

The example shown in Figure 6–10C needed more trials because the patient was not as consistent as in the other two examples. In this case, the patient responded twice at 25 dB during ascending trials (Trials 5 and 8), but after a third ascending trial at 20 dB (Trial 11) the patient had 1/3, so a fourth ascending series was needed since there was still the possibility of obtaining 2/4. In this case, however, the patient did not respond to the fourth presentation at 20 dB (Trial 14); therefore, the threshold was 25 dB. Notice how the threshold is not always 50%. In Figure 6–10A, the threshold was based on responses showing 100% of three ascending presentations at 20 dB (3/3) and 0% at 15 dB (0/3). In Figure 6–10B, the threshold was based on responses showing 75% of four ascending presentations at 40 dB (3/4) and 0% at 35 dB (0/3). In Figure 6–10C, the threshold was based on responses showing 100% of three ascending presentations at 25 dB (3/3) and only 25% of four ascending presentations at 20 dB (0/4).

VARIABLES INFLUENCING THRESHOLDS

There is no absolute physiologic minimum response level that defines threshold, even for the same patient on different occasions (test-retest variability). There is some inherent variability when determining thresholds in a clinical setting, and this variability is related to a variety of factors. Remember, the thresholds you obtain in pure-tone audiometry are determined by monitoring the responses that the patient is willing to provide. All patients operate with some perceptual criterion that determines when to respond, and this criterion may be different across patients or even in the same patient on different days. Some patients may not want to make any mistakes and, therefore, choose to respond only when the auditory sensation is obvious. Other patients may not want to miss any of the sounds, so they tend to respond to questionably audible sounds. Thresholds can, in fact, be manipulated by the costs and rewards associated with a response. For example, if a person is told that he or she will earn one dollar for every tone detected, he or she will tend to respond more often and will end up with a lower threshold. On the other hand, if a person (or the same person) is told he or she will have to pay one dollar every time he or she responds when a signal was not presented, he or she will tend to respond less often and will have a higher threshold.

It would be nice if all patients were highly cooperative and consistent in their responses. The fact is, however, that most patients occasionally respond when a signal is not presented (false positives) and fail to respond to signals that they may have really heard or you expect them to hear (false negatives). Some of this lack of consistency is inherent in the concept of determining threshold. However, you should become cognizant of situations in which there are too many false positive or false negatives and learn to adjust your testing strategy. The most important strategy is to be sure not to present the tones in a predictable pattern, so that the patient responds to an audible sensation instead of anticipating when you are going to present a tone. In addition, it is a good strategy to intersperse some longer (and variable) pauses between the presentations to get a sense of whether the patient has a tendency toward false positives. Most of the time, just giving patients some feedback and reinstructing them on what is expected of them may be sufficient. However, if there are too many false positives you might say, "Make sure you only push the button when you hear a tone," or for too many false negatives you might say, "Listen carefully and push the button even for the faintest sounds." In some cases, you might use a varying number (1, 2, or 3) of tone pulses instead of a continuous tone and ask the patient to push the button the same number of times that correspond to the number of pulses heard. If there is a difference between the number of times the patient pushes the button and the number of pulses presented, that trial should be considered a false positive and treated the same as no response to that presentation trial.

You will, undoubtedly, observe other interesting response behaviors from your patients. For example, it is not uncommon to observe patients who give a "partial" response, for example, they cock their head and/or have an expression that conveys, "I think I hear something." This may be accompanied by holding their hand part-way up or "hovering" their thumb over the response button, not quite ready to push it. In most cases, the patient will produce the full response when the pure tone is raised 5 dB. It may be useful to reinstruct the patient with something like, "Go ahead and raise your hand all the way up (or push the button) even if you think you hear the sound." Of course, in some cases this may lead to increased false positives and one would need to revise the instructions again. You will also see some patients who keep their hand up or the button pushed while listening for the next sound. This behavior is usually extinguished with the next presentation or by giving them more instructions. A competent audiologist learns quickly to recognize and adjust for the nuances of the patient's behavior.

Pure-tone thresholds must represent a reliable and valid picture of the patient's hearing loss across frequencies and must be obtained in a reasonable amount of time. To be clinically useful, the goal of pure-tone audiometry is to obtain good estimates of the lowest levels the patient is willing to respond to consistently. To account for the inherent variations in thresholds, standardized procedures are used with 5 dB step sizes, and test-retest variability of +/− 5 dB is acceptable and expected. The fact that pure-tone thresholds are repeatable within +/− 5 dB using the recommended procedures, even in different settings, makes them clinically robust. Pure-tone audiometry is highly effective at establishing reliable and valid thresholds in a relatively short period of time when performed by a competent audiologist using standardized procedures.

TECHNIQUES FOR TESTING INFANTS AND TODDLERS

For children under the age of 4 or 5 years, there are special considerations and procedures that are required when conducting pure-tone audiometry. While most of the auditory system is fully developed at birth, infants and toddlers undergo developmental changes in their ability to respond to sounds; accounting for these changes is critical in order to obtain valid measures of hearing thresholds. Equally important is the child's interest in the task and how well the audiologist can keep the child motivated through a lot of verbal praise and/or other means of providing positive reinforcement. In many cases, having an assistant who interacts with the child in the test booth makes testing more efficient. It is also recommended that whenever possible, for all ages, testing should be attempted with earphones so that information can be obtained from each ear separately. When earphones are not tolerated, testing can be done with speakers in the sound field. Some audiologists prefer to use frequency-modulated tones, called *warble tones*, or narrow bands of noises centered at different audiometric frequencies, called one-third octave narrowband noises, because these stimuli have been shown to have greater attention-getting ability, especially with children (Madell, 2014; Thompson & Thompson, 1972). A relatively new test stimulus that combines, in a sense, narrow bands of noise with tone characteristics is called *FRESH (FREquency Specific Hearing) noise*, created by filtering the noise with much steeper cutoffs than the standard narrowband noises (Lantz, n.d.). FRESH noise has been shown to have a better correspondence to pure-tone thresholds than narrowband noises (Norrix & Anderson, 2015). Warble tones, FRESH noises, or narrowband noises should be used when testing in the sound field in order to avoid the effects from sound reflections off the walls of the test booth.

The following sections briefly describe some of the techniques used to behaviorally test pediatric patients from 6 months to 4 years of age. Behavioral hearing testing is not effective for infants less than 5 to 6 months of age; for these younger infants, physiologic measures are more appropriate to evaluate auditory function. For more complete coverage of auditory development and testing of young children, you should consult other more comprehensive books on pediatric audiology (Madell, 2014; Northern & Downs, 2014; Seewald & Tharpe, 2016).

Conditioned-Play Audiometry (Ages 2 to 4 Years)

Children between the ages of 2 and 4 years are very receptive to the task of listening and responding to sounds when they are incorporated into structured play-like activities. Testing children in this age range is usually very successful with an experienced audiologist who can engage the child in the task and can keep the child happy and motivated. It cannot be overemphasized how important it is for the audiologist to be enthusiastic and offer lots of positive reinforcement to the child, while at the same time being able to discern false positive or false negative responses, and to be able to quickly change activities as needed to keep the attention going. With an experienced audiologist, children in this age range can be tested by AC and BC, and they can respond with thresholds similar to adults.

The technique for testing this age group is typically called *conditioned-play audiometry* (CPA). The child is asked to perform a fun activity whenever he or she hears the sound. Usually, the audiologist or assistant demonstrates what he or she wants the child to do. The play activities might be something like putting rings on a pole, putting blocks in a box, and/or flying toy airplanes into the hanger. This technique is a straightforward conditioning paradigm. The demonstration by the audiologist serves as the conditioning phase, familiarizing the child with what he or she will hear and teaching him or her what to do when a sound is heard. During the conditioning phase, the child should also demonstrate that he or she understands the task by correctly doing the activity when a *suprathreshold* tone is presented. If needed, the audiologist should help the child with the task (modeling the behavior) when the tone is clearly audible and then have the child do it on his or her own when he or she hears the tone. Be sure not to allow the child to do the activity when the tone is not presented. The activity serves as a reinforcer to the child and is an indication of the child's response to the tone. Once the audiologist is confident that the child understands the activity, then the test phase begins. During the test phase, the sound intensity is varied using the standard bracketing procedure based on the child's response until a valid threshold is obtained. In some cases, modification of the bracketing procedure to an up-10-down-20 procedure can be used to save time. You have to work quickly with children of this age in order to obtain as much information as possible before they lose interest in the task. It is usually best to try to obtain a couple of thresholds in each ear, such as 2000 Hz then 500 Hz, and then add other frequencies back and forth between ears as time permits. Remember to document any modifications of procedures on the audiogram. For some children, usually those with other disorders, wearing the earphones and/or conditioning to the task may not be successful in the clinic. In those cases, the parents might be taught to familiarize the child with the earphones and to the conditioning phase of the task while at home.

Visual Reinforcement Audiometry (Ages 6 Months to 2 Years)

For children as young as 6 months of age and toddlers who are not successfully conditioned to perform conditioned-play audiometry, visual reinforcers have been found to be effective for obtaining thresholds to pure tones and/or narrowband noises (Moore, Wilson, & Thompson, 1977; Widen, 2011). When visual reinforcers are used in a conditioning paradigm, it is called *visual reinforcement audiometry* (VRA). As shown in Figure 6–11, the visual reinforcers are presented

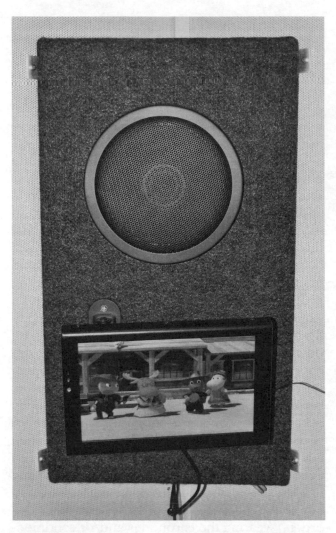

FIGURE 6–11. A sound-field speaker and a flat screen for projecting visual images when performing visual reinforcement audiometry (VRA). The VRA device allows the audiologist to pair the sound with the response when the child looks toward the speaker.

method of VRA only requires a *unilateral head turn*; the child only has to look in one direction for the reinforcer regardless of the ear to which the sound is presented. For children older than 12 months, it is possible to test localization to sounds by placing the visual reinforcers on both sides of the child and teaching him or her to look to the side that corresponds to the sound he or she heard.

The conditioning procedure used for VRA is similar to that used in conditioned-play audiometry. It is best to try testing with earphones first in order to get ear-specific information, but testing can also be conducted in the sound field. Bone conduction testing can be performed if time permits. The VRA procedure begins by pairing an audible sound with the visual reinforcer and getting the child to look at the visual reinforcer (see Figure 6–11). Often the visual stimulus itself will get the child to turn the head, but in some cases an assistant may be needed to direct (with enthusiasm) the child's attention to the visual reinforcer. The child's attention is then taken off the visual reinforcer by directing attention to other objects or another visual stimulus in front of him or her, often called "centering." When the child is not looking for the visual reinforcer, conditioning can continue by pairing the audible stimulus with the visual reinforcer until (usually after two or three times) the child is able to turn the head to look for the reinforcer when he or she hears the conditioning sound. Once the audiologist is confident that the child is performing the desired head turn in response to the sound, then the test phase begins. During the test phase, the reinforcer should only be activated after the child turns his or her head in response to a sound that was presented. Head turns without a sound presented should not be reinforced with the visual stimulus. During the test phase, the sound intensity is varied based on the child's responses, preferably using the bracketing procedure, until a valid threshold is obtained. When testing a young child with VRA, it is often a good strategy to try to obtain a couple of thresholds in each ear, such as 2000 Hz then 500 Hz, and then add other frequencies back and forth between ears as time permits. In some cases, modification of the standard threshold search procedure

on flat screen monitors in the sound booth, and/ or by activating mechanical toys (e.g., animals) sitting on a shelf or enclosed in tinted plastic enclosures adjacent to the speakers. With flat screen monitors, different pictures are available to keep the child's attention if needed; or with mechanical visual reinforcers there are usually at least two that can be switched in order to keep the child's interest longer. The visual reinforcer is usually placed at a 45° to 90° angle away from the child's forward-facing position. The common to an up-10-down-20 procedure can be used to save time.

For VRA and CPA, the audiologist must learn to make decisions about whether the child might have a hearing loss or whether the child was unable to be conditioned to perform the task. In other words, was the child just not interested in the task or was it too difficult to perform? With a skilled tester and cooperative children, thresholds obtained using unilateral head-turn VRA are similar to those of adults (Diefendorf & Gravel, 1996; Madell, 2014; Widen, 2011; Wilson & Thompson, 1984). Other tests in the audiological test battery can be used as a cross-check to the responses so that the audiologist is not relying on just a single test result.

SYNOPSIS 6–2

- Proper and clear instructions to patients are important. Be sure to let them know you are trying to find the faintest level of the tones that they can hear. Giving the patients feedback when they are doing the task correctly or reinstructing them when they are giving too many false positives or false negatives may reduce the false positives or false negatives.
- Thresholds are obtained using established guidelines (ANSI, 2004; ASHA, 2005) referred to as the modified Hughson–Westlake procedure or the up-5-down-10 procedure, where the level of the tone is increased 5 dB when the patient does not respond and decreased 10 dB when the patient does respond. Using this procedure, thresholds are established in the ascending direction.
- Each threshold is defined as the lowest level in which the patient responds to at least 50% of a theoretical four presentations (2/4), with a minimum of two out of three responses (67%) to ascending series of presentations.
- Thresholds can be affected by a patient's motivation or response criterion, which may be different across patients or even in the same patient on different days. A skilled audiologist must be aware of these patient variables and be able to adapt the testing strategy in ways that will produce valid and reliable thresholds.
- False positives (responding when tone is not presented) and false negatives (not responding to a tone that should be audible) are common response modes from many patients. Some variations in tone presentation rate and/or having them count pulses may be useful test modifications to help determine true response.
- To be clinically useful, the goal of pure-tone audiometry is to obtain good estimates of the lowest levels the patient is willing to respond to consistently. When standardized test procedures are used, test-retest variability of ±5 dB for thresholds is expected and acceptable as valid measures of hearing sensitivity.
- Infants and toddlers who are 6 months to 4 years of age require special techniques to obtain behavioral thresholds. Conditioned-play audiometry (CPA), such as putting blocks into a bucket in response to hearing a sound, can be used for children 2 to 4 years of age. Visual reinforcement audiometry (VRA), using a unilateral head turn in response to hearing a sound and then rewarding that behavior with a picture presented on a monitor or animated and/or lighted toy, can be used for children as young as 5 to 6 months of age.

SYNOPSIS 6–2 (*continued*)

- The use of warble tones, FRESH noise, or narrowband noise may provide more attention-getting characteristics than pure tones, and are often recommended when testing young children or testing in sound field.
- When successful, behavioral thresholds of children in these age ranges are similar to those of adults. However, careful decisions must be made by the audiologist to differentiate between whether the child actually has a hearing loss or whether he or she is only having difficulty performing the task.
- Children less than 6 months of age must be tested with physiologic measures. Several of these physiologic measures of auditory function are described in later chapters.

REFERENCES

American National Standards Institute [ANSI]. (1999). Maximum permissible ambient noise levels for audiometric test rooms *ANSI S3.1-1999*. New York, NY: Author.

American National Standards Institute [ANSI]. (2004). Methods for manual pure-tone threshold audiometry, *ANSI S3.21-2004*. New York, NY: Author.

American National Standards Institute [ANSI]. (2010). Specifications for audiometers, *ANSI S3.6-2010*. New York, NY: Author.

American Speech-Language-Hearing Association [ASHA]. (2005). Guidelines for manual pure-tone threshold audiometry. Retrieved from http://www.asha.org/policy.

Carhart, R., & Jerger, J. (1959). Preferred method for clinical determination of pure-tone thresholds. *Journal of Speech and Hearing Disorders, 24*, 330–345.

Diefendorf, A. O., & Gravel, J. S. (Eds.) (1996). *Visual Reinforcement and Behavioral Observation Audiometry*. Washington, DC: Gallaudet University Press.

Jerger, J. (1960). Békésy audiometry in analysis of auditory disorders. *Journal of Speech and Hearing Disabilities, 3*, 275–287.

Jerger, J. (2009). *Audiology in the USA*. San Diego, CA: Plural.

Johnson, E. W. (1977). Auditory test results in 500 cases of acoustic neuroma. *Archives of Otolaryngology, 103*, 152–158.

Killion, M. C., Wilber, L. A., & Gugmundsen, G. I. (1985). Insert earphones for more interaural attenuation. *Hearing Institute, 36*, 34–36.

Lantz, J. (n.d.). FRESH noise [White Paper]. Retrieved from http://www.otometrics.com/Knowledge-Center/Hearing%20Assessment%20resources.

Madell, J. R. (2014). Using visual reinforcement audiometry to evaluate hearing in infants from 5 to 36 months. In J. R. Madell & C. Flexer (Eds.), *Pediatric Audiology: Diagnosis, Technology, and Management* (2nd ed., pp. 79–88). New York, NY: Thieme.

Moore, J. M., Wilson, W. R., & Thompson, G. (1977). Visual reinforcement of head-turn responses in infants under 12 months of age. *The Journal of Speech and Hearing Disorders, 42*(3), 328–334.

Norrix, L. W., & Anderson, A. (2015). Audiometric thresholds: Stimulus considerations in sound field and under earphones. *American Journal of Audiology, 24*, 487–493.

Northern, J., & Downs, M. P. (2014). *Hearing in Children* (6th ed.). San Diego, CA: Plural.

Seewald, R., & Tharpe, A. M. (2016). *Comprehensive Handbook of Pediatric Audiology* (2nd ed.). San Diego, CA: Plural.

Studebaker, G. A. (1967). Intertest variability and the air-bone gap. *Journal of Speech and Hearing Disorders, 32*, 82–86.

Thompson, M., & Thompson, G. (1972). Response of infants and young children as a function of auditory stimuli and test methods. *Journal of Speech and Hearing Research, 15*(4), 699–707.

Widen, J. E. (Ed.) (2011). *Behavioral Audiometry with Infants*. San Diego, CA: Plural Publishing Inc.

Wilson, W. R., & Thompson, G. (Eds.). (1984). *Behavioral Audiometry*. San Diego, CA: Plural.

7 Audiogram Interpretation

After reading this chapter, you should be able to:

1. Describe the parameters of an audiogram and why decibel hearing level (dB HL) is used for audiograms.

2. Identify, from ANSI standards, the corresponding calibration reference values for different transducers.

3. Convert among dB hearing level (dB HL), dB sound pressure level (dB SPL), and dB sensation level (dB SL).

4. Identify unmasked and masked air conduction (AC) and bone conduction (BC) thresholds for each ear from symbols on audiograms.

5. Explain and use three different ways to record pure-tone thresholds.

6. Understand why and when masking of the non-test ear might be needed for AC and BC testing.

7. Know how to apply common terminology for describing degree, type, and shapes (configurations) of hearing losses.

8. Describe a variety of audiograms relative to type, degree, and shape of hearing loss.

9. Recognize audiograms that show thresholds at the limits of the equipment, tactile responses, or collapsed ear canals.

10. Calculate a pure-tone average (PTA) from the audiometric thresholds.

Proper documentation of information about a patient's hearing sensitivity is an integral part of the audiologist's evaluation. Understanding the results from a hearing evaluation is also important for other professionals so they can understand a patient's hearing ability to plan/provide appropriate services. This chapter focuses your learning on how to document pure-tone thresholds and how to describe and interpret the results of pure-tone audiometry. In addition, the concept of masking (putting noise into the non-test ear) is introduced in this chapter so that you can understand what the different unmasked and masked symbols used on an audiogram represent. A more complete discussion of masking, including how to perform masking, is covered in Chapter 9.

THE AUDIOGRAM

The patient's pure-tone thresholds are typically recorded on a graph called an *audiogram*. Figure 7–1 shows an example of an audiogram.

While the actual size of an audiogram can vary, the *aspect ratio* (the size relationship between the y-axis and the x-axis) should be maintained so that a 20 dB change along the y-axis corresponds to a doubling of frequency (*octave*) along the x-axis. For example, the distance from 20 to 40 dB along the y-axis should equal the distance from 2000 to 4000 Hz along the x-axis (American National Standards Institute [ANSI], 2004; American Speech-Language-Hearing Association [ASHA], 2005).

Frequency is represented along the x-axis of the audiogram (either at the top or the bottom), typically beginning at 250 Hz, and at equally spaced successive octave intervals (doubling of frequencies) up to 8000 Hz. Usually the inter-octave frequencies 3000 Hz and 6000 Hz are also represented on the audiogram. Testing at 125 Hz is recommended in cases of low frequency residual hearing, for example, when there is a severe hearing loss in the mid to higher frequencies. If you need to test above 8000 Hz, an extended high-frequency audiogram or numerical audiogram is used to document the thresh-

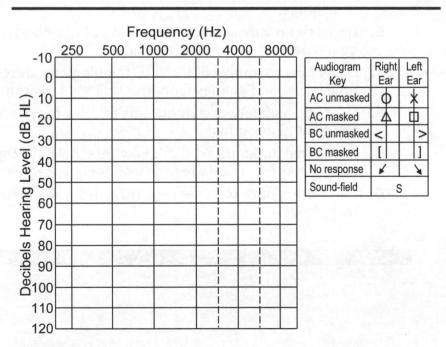

FIGURE 7–1. An example of an audiogram used to record pure-tone thresholds. An audiogram key, as shown on the right, is usually included with an audiogram to identify the symbols. AC, air conduction; BC, bone conduction.

The Upside-Down Audiogram

Two-dimensional line graphs typically have the axes' scales arranged so that low to high values go from left to right (*x*-axis) and from bottom to top (*y*-axis). The audiogram, however, has the *y*-axis scale (dB HL) reversed. James Jerger, a pioneer in the field of audiology, gives an historical perspective on why the audiogram is "upside down" (Jerger, 2013). According to Jerger, the origination and orientation of the audiogram was established in the early 1900s through collaboration/discussions among Edmund Fowler, an otolaryngologist, and physicists Harvey Fletcher and R. L. Wegel, all of whom were involved with early research in the developing fields of hearing sciences and audiology. Their early collaboration involved the development of the audiometer for AT&T just after World War I, and had to come up with a way to standardize documentation of pure-tone thresholds. Initially, they used a more traditional scale of dB SPL that went from low to high as one went from bottom to top of the graph (see threshold of audibility curve in Chapter 3); however, as they began to think about how to clinically document changes in hearing levels as a function of frequency, Fowler began to think in terms of describing hearing loss as a fraction/percentage of normal hearing for each frequency. Graphically, this would have 0% at the bottom (most amount of hearing loss) and 100% at the top (normal hearing), and a person with hearing loss would have different percentages as a function of frequency. Fowler found this useful clinically, as a way to tell his patients how much hearing they had left. Although Fletcher argued for a *y*-axis scale in actual physical units of hearing loss rather than percentages of normal hearing, he left the 0 dB line at the top, which ultimately became the 0 dB HL line on an audiogram. As Jerger states, "The audiogram was doomed to be upside down forever" (p. 4).

olds for frequencies in specific increments, such as 10,000, 12,000, 14,000, and 16,000 Hz; and as you learned previously, this would require circumaural earphones. The intensity levels of the test sounds are represented along the *y*-axis of the audiogram. You will notice that the intensity scale has the lowest intensity at the top of the graph and the highest intensity at the bottom of the graph.

Decibels of Hearing Level (dB HL)

The *y*-axis of the audiogram represents the decibel level of sounds, in units of dB hearing level (dB HL). The dB HL scale is different than the dB SPL scale discussed in Chapter 3. As you recall from Chapter 3, the threshold of audibility curve for normal hearing listeners shows that air-conducted pure tones have different amounts of dB SPL (re: 20 µPa) as a function of frequency (see Figure 3–16). For clinical purposes, it would be somewhat cumbersome to use a dB SPL scale for the audiogram, since the same amount of hearing loss at different frequencies would be represented by different values of dB SPL, and the lines on the audiogram would not be linear. To simplify the representation of hearing loss across frequencies, the threshold of audibility curve is normalized; in other words, the threshold of audibility curve is "straightened out" by creating a 0 dB HL for each frequency that is equal to the average amount of dB SPL needed for normal hearing listeners to hear each frequency when presented by air-conduction. For bone conduction, the concept is the same, such that 0 dB HL for each frequency is the average amount of force (re: 1 µN) needed for normal hearing listeners to hear each frequency when presented by bone conduction. The actual amount of dB SPL or dB force needed for 0 dB HL at each frequency is specified in standards developed by the American National Standards Institute (ANSI) or by the International Standards Organization (ISO). The ISO standards are used in countries other than the United States, but they are very similar to the ANSI standards. Table 7–1 shows the reference levels for 0 dB HL for each of the audiometric

TABLE 7–1. Air Conduction and Bone Conduction Reference Values Corresponding to 0 dB HL for Commonly Used Transducers. Also called "Audiometric Zero." Based on ANSI S3.6 (2010). Air Conduction Reference Values Are in dB SPL re: 20 µPa. Bone Conduction Reference Values for Mastoid Placement and Are in dB Force re: 1 µN

Frequency (Hz)									
Transducer	**125**	**250**	**500**	**1000**	**2000**	**3000**	**4000**	**6000**	**8000**
Supra-aural[a] (TDH-49)	47.5	26.5	13.5	7.5	11.0	9.5	10.5	13.5	13.0
Insert[b] (ER-3A)	28.0	17.5	9.5	5.5	11.5	13.0	15.0	16.0	15.5
Bone[c] (B-71)	NA	67.0	58.0	42.5	31.0	30.0	35.5	(40.0)	(40.0)
	4000	**6000**	**8000**	**9000**	**10,000**	**11,200**	**12,500**	**14,000**	**16,000**
Circumaural[d] (HDA-200)	9.5	17.0	17.5	19.0	22.0	23.0	27.5	35.0	56.0

[a]Calibrated with 6-cc coupler.

[b]Calibrated with an occluded ear simulator. Values slightly different for HA-1 or HA-2 couplers.

[c]Calibrated with artificial mastoid. Although bone calibration levels are provided for 6000 and 8000 Hz, testing at these frequencies is not in common practice and should be used with caution (ANSI, 2005).

[d]Calibrated with Type 1 Adaptor.

frequencies and transducers based on the most current standards (American National Standards Institute [ANSI], 2010). As you may recall, all decibel scales need a reference level; the reference levels for dB HL are the most current ANSI specified values. The ANSI and ISO periodically update or reaffirm the standards for pure tone reference values; however, the reference levels do not change appreciably for existing transducers, but may include updates for newer transducers or for updated models of existing transducers when necessary. Whenever new standards become available, any changes from previous standards should be incorporated into the calibration values of the audiometer and the new ANSI references are usually included on the audiogram. For the audiograms in this textbook, the reference year of the ANSI standards has not been included along the *y*-axis for convenience.

The definition of 0 dB HL can also be illustrated with the basic formula used for decibel calculations: As you recall, whenever a sound is the same as its reference value, by definition it would be equal to 0 dB. The following calculation illustrates how the decibel formula would apply for a 500 Hz tone presented using insert earphones at 9.5 dB SPL, the corresponding ANSI (2010) reference value for 0 dB HL at 500 Hz.

$$n \text{ dB HL} = 10 \log (P_{meas} / P_{ref})$$

$$n \text{ dB HL} = 10 \log (9.5 \text{ dB SPL} / 9.5 \text{ dB SPL})$$

$$n \text{ dB HL} = 10 \log (1)$$

$$n \text{ dB HL} = 10 (0)$$

$$n = 0 \text{ dB HL}$$

Converting from dB HL to dB SPL, and vice versa, is a matter of adding or subtracting the ANSI reference values. For example, if a 500 Hz pure tone is presented at 40 dB HL using supra-aural earphones, how many dB SPL is that sound? The answer would be found in the following way:

$$n \text{ dB SPL} = \text{dB HL (dial reading)} + \text{the ANSI reference value}$$

$$n \text{ dB SPL} = 40 + 13.5$$

$$n \text{ dB SPL} = 53.5 \text{ dB SPL}$$

Going the other way, if a 500 Hz pure tone is presented at 53.5 dB SPL, how many dB HL is that sound? The answer would be found in the following way:

n dB HL = dB SPL – the ANSI reference value

n dB HL = 53.5 – 13.5

n dB HL = 40

Knowing how to do these conversions is useful because sometimes audiologists work in dB SPL, such as when making some measures during hearing aid fittings, and may need to relate these dB SPL values to a patient's audiogram in dB HL. Also, when making dB SPL measurements of different sounds, like speech or background noise, you may be interested in describing how those sounds relate to the patient's audiogram in dB HL.

Documentation of Thresholds

Let's now see how to properly document the patient's thresholds on the audiogram. Figure 7–2 shows an audiogram with air conduction (AC) thresholds plotted for the right and left ears

using symbols recommended by ASHA (2005). Audiograms are usually accompanied by a key (legend) that specifies what each symbol represents. In Figure 7–2, AC thresholds (unmasked) are denoted with a circle for the right ear and an X for the left ear. While not required, these symbols may also be color coded to match the appropriate ear; red for the right ear and blue for the left ear. The AC thresholds are centered on the vertical lines of the appropriate frequencies and the symbols are usually joined by solid lines. There are other symbols included in the key shown in Figure 7–2 that will be explained as we go along.

After obtaining AC thresholds, the bone conduction (BC) thresholds are obtained. Figure 7–3 shows the same AC thresholds as in Figure 7–2, but now the BC thresholds have been plotted for each ear. The BC symbols are usually not connected by lines. The BC symbols are placed to the side of the vertical line for each frequency. Notice from the audiogram key that the right ear BC symbol (<) is placed on the left side of the line and the left ear BC symbol (>) is placed on

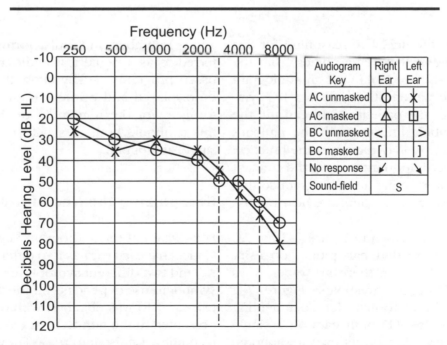

FIGURE 7–2. An audiogram with unmasked air conduction (AC) thresholds plotted for the right and left ears. Note that the AC thresholds are plotted on the corresponding frequency lines and are usually connected with a solid line.

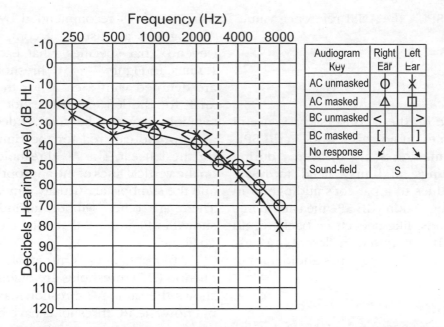

FIGURE 7–3. An audiogram with unmasked air conduction (AC) and bone conduction (BC) thresholds plotted for the right and left ears. Note that the BC symbols are plotted to the right side of the frequency line when testing is done with the bone vibrator placed on the left mastoid bone, and plotted on the left side of the frequency line when testing is done with the bone vibrator placed on the right mastoid bone. The BC thresholds are usually not connected with a line.

the right side of the line. The reasoning for this BC symbol placement scheme comes from the idea that when you are looking at an audiogram while facing the patient, the right ear BC symbols line up with the patient's right ear and the left ear BC symbols line up with the patient's left ear. This strategy may require some practice; however, it is very important to keep the concept straight when interpreting an audiogram so that you are sure you are describing the hearing loss for the appropriate ear.

The audiogram shown in Figure 7–3 has AC and BC thresholds for both ears plotted on a single audiogram. However, there are other ways to record audiometric thresholds. Figure 7–4 shows three different formats for documenting pure-tone thresholds: (1) both ears on a single audiogram; (2) each ear on its own audiogram, often referred to as a two-panel audiogram or side by side audiogram (notice that the right ear is displayed on the left and left ear on the right);

and (3) numbers in tabular form, sometimes referred to as a numerical audiogram. Computer-based programs usually allow the thresholds to be displayed and printed in any of these three formats. For the remainder of the examples in this textbook, both ears will be displayed on a single audiogram.

Recognizing the Need for Masking

Look again at the audiogram key in Figure 7–4. Notice that each ear has two different symbols for AC and two different symbols for BC. The proper symbol to use depends on if the threshold in the test ear (TE) was obtained with or without noise presented to the non-test ear (NTE). The process of putting a noise into the NTE while measuring a pure-tone threshold in the TE is called *clinical masking*. For clinical masking, the noise presented in the NTE is called the *masker* and the

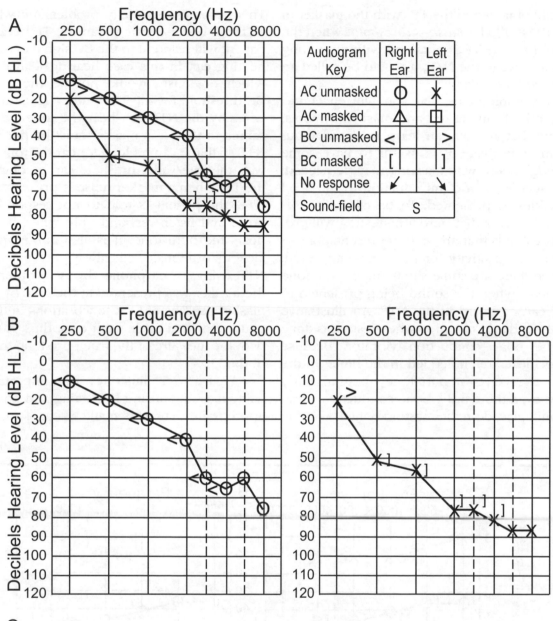

FIGURE 7-4. A-C. Illustrations of three different ways to record pure-tone thresholds. In **A**, thresholds for both ears are plotted on a single-panel audiogram. In **B**, a two-panel (or side by side) audiogram is shown, where thresholds for each ear are plotted on a separate audiogram arranged side by side; the audiogram on the left side is used to display thresholds for the patient's right ear, and the audiogram on the right side is used to display thresholds for the patient's left ear. In **C**, the pure-tone thresholds are plotted in tabular or numeric format.

threshold obtained in the TE (with the masker in the NTE) is called a *masked threshold*. When the threshold for the TE is obtained without putting masking noise in the NTE, it would be called an *unmasked threshold*.

Many audiograms that you will encounter will have both unmasked and masked symbols; therefore, before you can learn to describe audiograms effectively, it is useful to have some knowledge about why masking may be needed. In this section, a brief introduction to the need for masking is presented. To be clinically useful, it is expected that pure-tone testing will produce thresholds that are valid representations of the hearing sensitivity for the ear being tested. However, there are some situations in pure-tone audiometry when the sound being presented to the TE can be heard in the NTE. An illustrative example of this problem is when testing is done with the bone conduction vibrator. Because both cochleae are embedded in the bones of the skull, both receive the pure-tone vibrations fairly equally, even though the bone conduction vibrator is only placed on the mastoid behind one ear.

This becomes especially problematic when the NTE has better hearing than the TE because the patient will respond to the BC signal in the better hearing ear, in this case hearing it in the NTE, which obviously would not be the true/valid BC threshold for the TE. When a situation arises whereby the NTE can hear the tone being presented to the TE, a masker must be put into the NTE so that it can no longer hear the tone. In this way, the true/valid threshold can be obtained in the TE. When a masker noise is presented to the NTE, the patient is told to not respond to the noise and listen/respond only when he or she hears the pure tone. It is also important to realize that the masker is always presented to the NTE using an earphone (by AC); otherwise, if the masker was presented to the NTE by BC, the masker itself would cause vibrations in the skull that are picked up in both ears, thus interfering with the measure of the true pure-tone threshold in the TE.

Figure 7–5 illustrates the importance of using masking during BC testing and how an inappropriate diagnosis could occur if BC testing

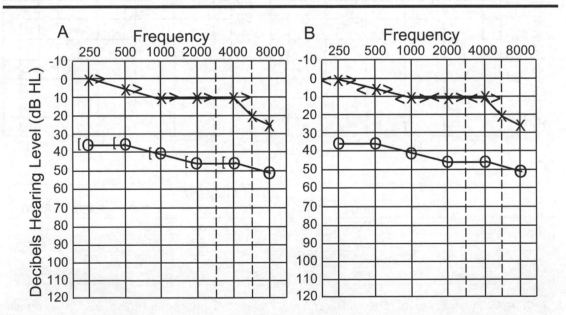

FIGURE 7–5. A and B. An example of why masking for bone conduction (BC) is important for proper diagnosis. In **A**, the patient's right ear *true* (masked) BC thresholds reveal a sensorineural hearing loss (AC = BC). In **B**, the same patient's BC for the right ear are shown as they would appear if masking was not used in the left ear, and indicate an *invalid* conductive loss (AC > BC) due to the responses coming from the left (better hearing) ear by BC that stimulates both cochleae. See the audiogram key in Figure 7–1 for definitions of the audiometric symbols.

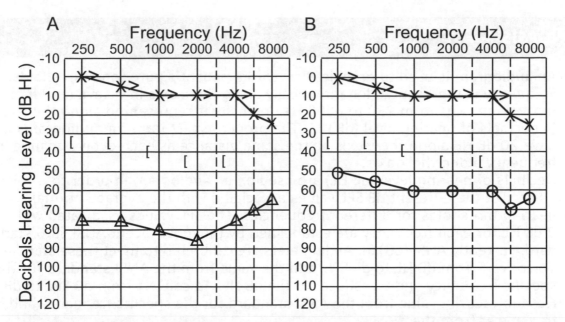

FIGURE 7–6. A and B. An example of why masking for air-conduction (AC) is important for proper diagnosis. In **A**, the patient's right ear *true* (masked) AC thresholds are around 75–85 dB HL. In **B**, the same patient's AC thresholds for the right ear are shown as they would appear without masking, and *incorrectly* show thresholds to be at better hearing levels than the true hearing thresholds due to the responses coming from the BC of the left (better hearing) ear. See the audiogram key in Figure 7–1 for definitions of the audiometric symbols.

was done without masking. In Figure 7–5A, the patient's right ear masked BC thresholds (masker in the left ear) reveal that the patient has a sensorineural hearing loss, since the AC thresholds are the same as the masked BC thresholds (as you learned in Chapter 6). However, as you can see in Figure 7–5B, when the BC thresholds are obtained without masking, the right ear shows an erroneous air–bone gap (and a critical mistake) suggesting a problem in the conductive portions of the ear, when the patient actually has a sensorineural hearing loss. Recognizing when to use masking is, therefore, very important in order to obtain the true thresholds for the ear being tested and not make any misdiagnoses.

You may be wondering why masking would be needed for AC testing since the earphones are not on the mastoid as for BC testing. As it turns out, since the AC transducer is also near the skull, at high enough intensities (40 to 60 dB HL and higher) the pure tones from the AC transducers can actually set up vibrations in the bones of

the skull and, therefore, stimulate both cochleae. Figure 7–6 illustrates the importance of using masking for AC testing, and how an inappropriate diagnosis could occur if done without masking. Figure 7–6A shows the patient's masked (true/valid) AC thresholds. However, if masking had not been used, the patient would have responded to the AC tones at the levels indicated by the circles (shown in Figure 7-6B) because they were loud enough to cause vibrations of the skull, which were able to be heard by the left ear through BC. Again, failure to mask when needed would lead to an erroneous result. The general guideline is that masking is needed for AC testing, when using supra-aural earphones, if the presentation level of the signal in the TE is 40 dB or higher than the BC threshold of the NTE. For insert earphones, due to less surface area in contact with the skull, masking is needed when the presentation level of the signal in the TE is 55 dB or higher than the BC threshold of the NTE. For more on how to decide when to

SYNOPSIS 7–1

- An audiogram is used to graphically record a patient's pure tone thresholds. Frequency is represented logarithmically along the *x*-axis in octave (and inter-octave) intervals from 250 to 8000 Hz. Intensity is represented along the *y*-axis in decibels of hearing level (dB HL). The proper aspect ratio for audiograms is to have 20 dB HL along the *y*-axis be the same distance as each octave change in frequency along the *x*-axis.
- Decibels of hearing level (dB HL) are used on an audiogram in order to normalize the different dB SPL values associated with the average normal hearing thresholds for different frequencies. The SPL values associated with 0 dB HL for each frequency are established by the most recent ANSI S3.6 standard, currently ANSI (2010). Audiometers are calibrated to meet these standards.
- To convert from dB HL to dB SPL, add the value from the ANSI standard for the specific frequency and transducer to the dB HL. To convert from dB SPL to dB HL, subtract the value from the ANSI standard for the specific frequency and transducer from the dB SPL.
- There are recommended symbols used on an audiogram that are found in the audiogram key (see any of the audiogram figures in this chapter).
- Pure-tone thresholds can be documented using a single-panel audiogram (data for both ears on the same graph), a two-panel audiogram (data for each ear on a separate graph), or in tabular form.
- Testing by BC at any level, and by AC at moderate to high levels, produces vibrations in the skull that can be heard through BC in both cochleae.
- Masking of the NTE with a noise (masker) is needed in those conditions where there is the possibility that the tone presented to the TE may be heard through BC in the NTE.
- When masking is performed, masked symbols are required on the audiogram to represent the true TE thresholds. Masked thresholds imply that masking noise was delivered (by AC) to the NTE.

mask and how to perform masking, see Chapter 9. For now, these introductory concepts on masking are meant to give an understanding of why there may be masked symbols on an audiogram. When masked thresholds are obtained, typically the unmasked thresholds are not included on the audiogram.

DESCRIBING AUDIOGRAMS

We will now turn our attention to describing hearing losses based on examples of audiograms. In this section you will learn how to succinctly describe a person's hearing loss based on the pure-tone audiometric results. When describing the pure-tone audiogram, the following three types of information should be conveyed:

- Degree (amount) of hearing loss
- Type of hearing loss
- Shape of hearing loss

It is common practice to summarize, in brief sentences, the general characteristics of the pure-tone thresholds that are plotted on the audiogram. The sentences should be able to generate a mental picture of the audiogram, but not be so detailed as to be a repetition of all the audiometric thresholds. Information about each ear should be provided and significant differences across the frequency range should be noted. Although there are different ways to describe audiograms, the information presented in this chapter is generally accepted and commonly used in clinical practice. There is considerable leeway in the details and format that might be used to describe the same audiogram, thus there are many possible correct descriptions of a patient's audiogram. In a sense, this might be considered the "art of audiometry." However, there are also incorrect descriptions that you will want to avoid. You will learn to circumvent these mistakes as you go through the examples in this chapter.

Degrees of Hearing Loss

The *degree* (amount) *of hearing loss* is based on the AC thresholds, since this would include hearing loss from all parts of the auditory system. Describing the degree of hearing loss from the audiogram means to apply some general descriptive term (e.g., mild) that corresponds to a range of dB HL associated with the patient's thresholds. The generally accepted classification scheme used to describe the degree of hearing loss is based on a continuum from normal to profound and, to a certain extent, reflects how those degrees of loss may affect communication (Clark, 1981; Goodman, 1965). The categories commonly used to describe degree of hearing loss (or hearing sensitivity) are given in Table 7–2. Notice that the range 16 to 25 dB HL has different terms depending on whether the patient is an adult or a child. This is because children are still acquiring language and are in educational environments, so even a slight (small amount) degree of hearing loss might have a greater impact than it would for an adult. It is also important to be cautious in assuming that these categories accurately portray a patient's actual communication difficulty; they are merely a conventional and convenient way to describe the thresholds on an audiogram. This is particularly true of children where the above descriptive terms may not accurately re-

TABLE 7–2. Common Descriptive Categories Used for Degree of Hearing Loss

dB HL Range	Descriptive Category
–10 to 15 dB HL	Normal
16 to 25 dB HL	Normal for adults; slight[a] for children
26 to 40 dB HL	Mild
41 to 55 dB HL	Moderate
56 to 70 dB HL	Moderately severe
71 to 90 dB HL	Severe
91+ dB HL	Profound

[a]Some use the term minimal or educationally significant.

flect the extent of a child's problems or the parents' perceptions (Haggard & Primus, 1999). As you will see, each patient has a unique set of circumstances, perceptions, and underlying cause of his or her hearing loss. The pure-tone thresholds are only part of the puzzle that audiologists use in the overall evaluation of a patient.

It is quite common for the degree of hearing loss to change across the audiogram; therefore, the description should provide a general sense of how the degree of hearing loss changes across frequency. It is not required that each frequency be assigned a specific category. As you work through some of the examples, you will see that these categories are sometimes loosely applied over a range of frequencies and/or even cascaded. For example, a hearing loss may be described as being moderately-severe to severe over a specified frequency range. Remember, the goal is to provide a summary description of the pure-tone thresholds, knowing that the details are available in the audiogram.

Type of Hearing Loss

To describe the *type of hearing loss* from the audiogram means to determine whether the hearing loss involves the conductive and/or sensorineural portions of the auditory pathways. Recall, from Chapter 6, that the sensorineural portion of the auditory system refers to the cochlea, 8th cranial nerve, and central pathways, whereas the

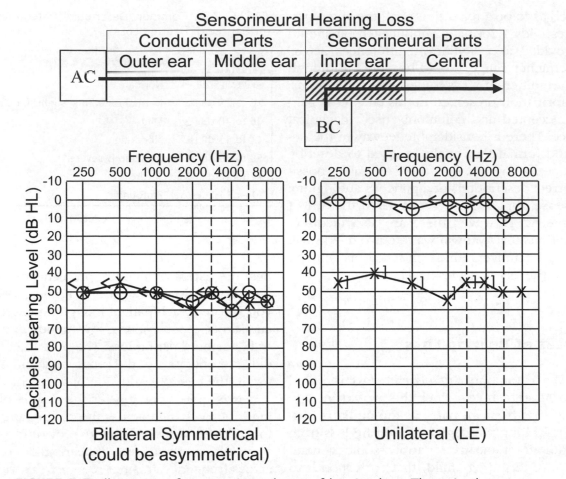

FIGURE 7–7. Illustration of a sensorineural type of hearing loss. The striped area represents a pathology in the cochlea (could also occur in the 8th cranial nerve). Air-conduction (AC) testing assesses the entire auditory system and bone-conduction (BC) testing assesses the sensorineural parts of the auditory system, bypassing the outer and middle ears. Sample audiograms are shown for a bilateral and a unilateral sensorineural hearing loss. For the unilateral loss, the left ear AC thresholds shown in this audiogram were obtained with insert earphones, thus masking was not needed; however, if supra-aural earphones had been used, masked AC thresholds would have been obtained. See the audiogram key in Figure 7–1 for definitions of the audiometric symbols.

conductive portion refers to the outer ear and middle ear. A hearing problem in the sensorineural portions of the auditory pathways would have essentially the same hearing loss when tested by AC as when tested by BC. An audiogram example of a sensorineural hearing loss can be seen in Figure 7–7. On the other hand, a hearing problem in the conductive parts of the ear would show an air–bone gap, that is, normal hearing by BC and poorer hearing by AC. An audiogram example of a conductive hearing loss can be seen in Figure 7–8. Because of inherent testing variability, small air–bone gaps may occur, which are of no real clinical significance; therefore, an abnormal air–bone gap is generally considered to be greater than 10 dB (> 10 dB). Although theoretically, BC thresholds should not be poorer than AC thresholds, small reverse air–

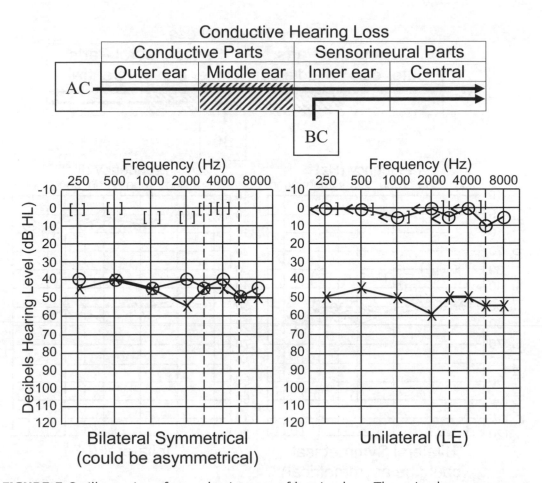

FIGURE 7–8. Illustration of a conductive type of hearing loss. The striped area represents a pathology in the middle ear (could also occur in the outer ear). Air-conduction (AC) testing assesses the entire auditory system and bone-conduction (BC) testing assesses the sensorineural parts of the auditory system, bypassing the outer and middle ears. Sample audiograms are shown for a bilateral and a unilateral hearing loss. For the unilateral loss, the left ear AC thresholds shown in this audiogram were obtained with insert earphones, thus masking was not needed; however, if supra-aural earphones had been used, masked thresholds would have been obtained. See the audiogram key in Figure 7–1 for definitions of the audiometric symbols.

bone gaps (BC thresholds 5-10 dB poorer than AC thresholds) may occur due to normal testing variability within a patient, as well as the fact that calibration standards are based on averages with some standard variation (Studebaker, 1967). Small reverse air–bone gaps do not have any clinical significance. And finally, a hearing loss that occurs in both the sensorineural and conductive parts, called a mixed hearing loss, would have a hearing loss by BC and an abnormal air–bone

gap. An audiogram example of a mixed hearing loss can be seen in Figure 7–9. Table 7–3 summarizes the definitions of the three types of hearing loss based on the AC and BC thresholds.

As you look at an audiogram, the type of hearing loss should be considered at each frequency. In other words, there could be a different type of hearing loss in different frequency areas of the audiogram. For example, there may be a conductive hearing loss in the lower frequencies

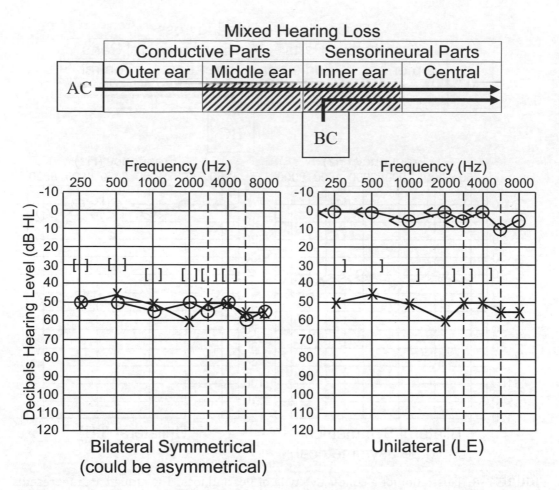

FIGURE 7–9. Illustration of a mixed type of hearing loss. The striped areas represent a pathology in the cochlea and a pathology in the middle ear. Air-conduction (AC) testing assesses the entire auditory system and bone-conduction (BC) testing assesses the sensorineural parts of the auditory system, bypassing the outer and middle ears. Sample audiograms are shown for a bilateral and a unilateral hearing loss. For the unilateral loss, the left ear AC thresholds shown in this audiogram were obtained with insert earphones, thus masking was not needed; however, if supra-aural earphones had been used, masked thresholds would have been obtained. See the audiogram key in Figure 7–1 for definitions of the audiometric symbols.

and a sensorineural hearing loss in the higher frequencies; how the type of hearing loss changes across the audiogram should be included in the description. On a final note, you may sometimes encounter audiogram descriptions in which the term mixed hearing loss is used when there are two different types of hearing loss across the audiogram, such as a conductive loss in the low frequencies and a sensorineural hearing loss in the higher frequencies. The authors prefer not to use that definition of mixed hearing loss, and instead will only use the definitions in Table 7–3 and apply them as needed across the audiogram.

As you can see, pure-tone audiometry can only grossly localize the problem to the conductive and/or sensorineural parts of the auditory system. Information from a battery of audiologic

TABLE 7–3. Common Audiometric Definitions of Types of Hearing Loss

Type of Hearing Loss	Audiometric Definition
Sensorineural	Abnormal AC, abnormal BC, ABG ≤ 10 dB
Conductive	Abnormal AC, normal BC, ABG > 10 dB
Mixed	Abnormal AC, abnormal BC; ABG > 10 dB

Note. AC = Air conduction thresholds; BC = Bone conduction thresholds; ABG = Air–bone gap (>10 dB difference between the thresholds by AC and BC).

tests (covered in later chapters) can be used to better define the location and/or cause of the hearing loss.

Shape of Hearing Loss

Describing the *shape (configuration) of hearing loss* from the audiogram means that you point out significant characteristics that convey a mental picture of how the thresholds look/change across the frequency range or across the two ears. For example, a hearing loss that is the same in both ears and the degree of hearing loss changes across the frequency range might be described as "a bilateral sensorineural hearing loss, sloping from mild in the low frequencies to severe in the high frequencies." The term *bilateral* refers to both ears and "sloping" refers to the downward (left to right) slope of the threshold curve on the audiogram. Figure 7–10 illustrates some general shapes of audiograms and the terms commonly used to describe those shapes. Although not exhaustive, a list of terms and generally accepted definitions for describing the shape of a hearing loss are given in Table 7–4.

The term *unilateral* is sometimes used in reference to a hearing loss if it is only in one ear, and the term *asymmetric* is sometimes used when there is a significant difference in the hearing loss between the two ears. The use

of unilateral in the description of an audiogram may not be very useful since you would need to indicate which ear it was anyway; and the term asymmetric may not be too useful since each ear would need its own description. There is considerable variability in how different audiologists convey the shape of the audiogram, and even greater variability in how words are combined to convey degree, type, and shape of hearing loss (the "art of audiology"). Undoubtedly, you will develop your own style for summarizing and describing audiograms. Conversely, when you are given a summary description of a person's hearing loss, you should have a good mental picture of the audiogram.

SAMPLE AUDIOGRAMS WITH DESCRIPTIONS

In this section, there are four sample audiograms (Figures 7–11, 7–12, 7–13, and 7–14). For each audiogram, there are two examples provided in the legends on how the audiograms might be described. Remember, there are many correct ways to describe audiograms, some lengthier than others, and many different possibilities of word order. When describing an audiogram, the goal is to convey a summary of the audiogram (degree, type, shape) for each ear and how these change across the frequency range. The description of the audiogram should conjure up a reasonably accurate mental picture of the audiogram. As you read the descriptions included with the sample audiograms you will notice that some descriptions include only the areas of the audiogram where there is a hearing loss; this generally implies that the parts left out of the description are normal.

ADDITIONAL FACTORS TO CONSIDER

Tactile Responses

Tactile (or *vibrotactile*) *responses* are a result of the patient feeling the vibrations rather than

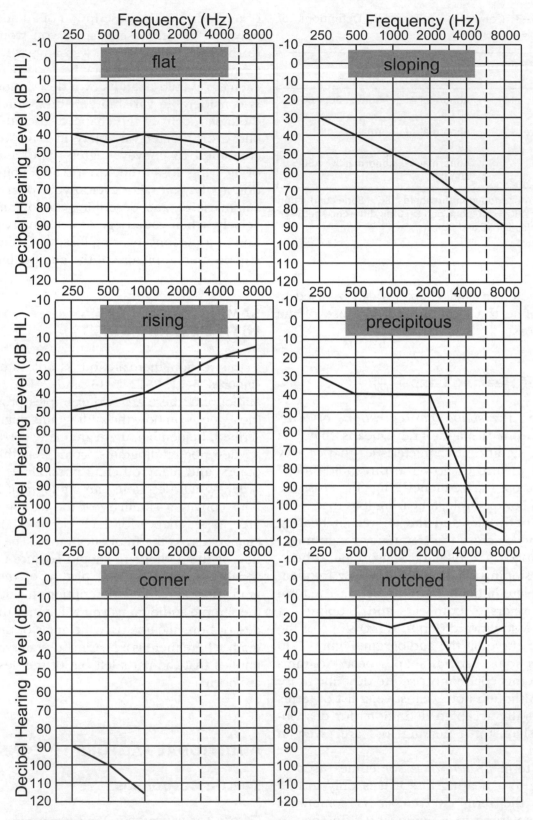

FIGURE 7–10. Common terms to describe different audiogram shapes (configurations). See text and Table 7-4 for definitions of the terms.

TABLE 7–4. Commonly Used Descriptions of Audiogram Shapes

Shape	Audiometric Threshold Characteristic
Bilateral	Similar in both ears
Relatively flat	Within 20 dB across the audiogram
Sloping	>20 dB per octave change toward high frequencies
Precipitous	Steeply sloping (e.g., >40 dB/octave) toward high frequencies
Rising	Improving >20 dB from low toward high frequencies
Notched	Worse in a narrow frequency region (typically 3000–6000 Hz)
Saucer/ cookie bite	Worse in mid frequencies; shallow concave appearance
Corner	Residual hearing ability only in the low frequencies

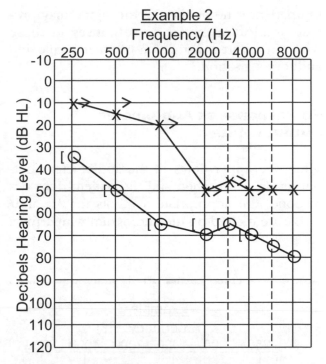

FIGURE 7–12. Audiogram example 2. Two possible descriptions of the audiogram are: (1) Pure-tone threshold testing for the left ear indicated hearing within the normal range through 1000 Hz, sloping to a moderate sensorineural hearing loss in the higher frequencies. The right ear showed a sloping, mild-to-severe, sensorineural hearing loss. (2) The left ear has a moderate sensorineural hearing loss from 2000 to 8000 Hz, with normal hearing in the lower frequencies. The right ear has a mild to moderate sensorineural hearing loss 250 to 500 Hz, with a moderately severe to severe sensorineural hearing loss 1000 to 8000 Hz. See the audiogram key in Figure 7–1 for definitions of the audiometric symbols.

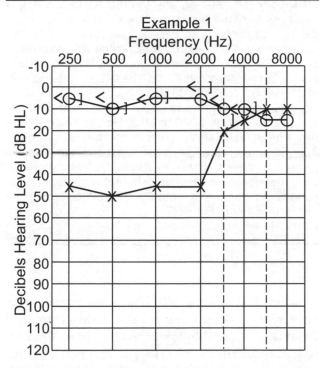

FIGURE 7–11. Audiogram example 1. Two possible descriptions of the audiogram are: (1) Pure-tone threshold testing for the left ear indicated a moderate conductive hearing loss through 2000 Hz, rising to normal in the higher frequencies. Hearing was within normal limits for the right ear. (2) Left ear showed a moderate conductive hearing loss through 2000 Hz. See the audiogram key in Figure 7–1 for definitions of the audiometric symbols.

hearing them (Boothroyd & Cawkwell, 1970; Nober, 1970). Clinically, tactile responses occur mostly by BC for the low frequencies. Tactile thresholds to BC have been shown to range from about 25 to 40 dB at 250 Hz, and 55 to 70 dB at 500 Hz. As illustrated in Figure 7–15, tactile responses will appear as an erroneous air–bone gap that may falsely imply a low frequency conductive component to the hearing loss. You should always be suspect of tactile responses when testing BC in the low frequencies, especially when there is an apparent air–bone gap, and make note of it on the audiogram. Asking the patient if he or she felt the signal may provide verification of tactile responses in those who can report a distinction between tactile and auditory sensation.

No Response at Audiometer Output Limits

When the upper limits of the audiometer's output levels are reached and the patient does not respond, the appropriate symbols for AC and/or BC are plotted on the audiogram with arrows

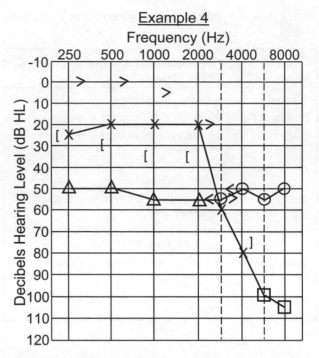

FIGURE 7–14. Audiogram sample 4. Two possible descriptions of the audiogram are: (1) Pure-tone threshold testing in the right ear indicated a relatively flat, moderately severe hearing loss, which was mixed (20 to 25 dB air–bone gaps) through 2000 Hz and sensorineural from 3000 to 8000 Hz. The left ear showed normal hearing through 2000 Hz with a sensorineural hearing loss that precipitously slopes to severe at 4000 Hz and profound from 6000 to 8000 Hz. (2) The right ear has a moderately severe, mixed hearing loss through 2000 Hz (20 to 25 dB air–bone gaps) and a moderately severe sensorineural hearing loss in the higher frequencies. The left ear has a moderate to profound sloping sensorineural hearing loss from 2000 to 8000 Hz. See the audiogram key in Figure 7–1 for definitions of the audiometric symbols.

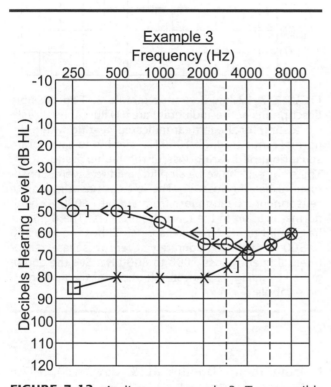

FIGURE 7–13. Audiogram example 3. Two possible descriptions of the audiogram are: (1) Pure-tone threshold testing in the right ear indicated a moderate to moderately severe sensorineural hearing loss. The left ear showed a severe, relatively flat, mixed hearing loss through 2000 Hz (with air–bone gaps ranging from 40 dB at 250 Hz to 20 dB at 2000 Hz), rising to a moderately severe sensorineural hearing loss in the higher frequencies. (2) The right ear has a sloping sensorineural hearing loss that ranges from mild at 250 Hz to moderately severe in the mid to high frequencies. The left ear has a severe, flat hearing loss with a conductive (air–bone gap) component from 250 to 2000 Hz. See the audiogram key in Figure 7–1 for definitions of the audiometric symbols.

attached to the symbols. The output limits may vary slightly depending on the audiometer, and BC has considerably lower output limits than AC (e.g., 80 dB HL vs. 120 dB HL, respectively). An example of how a patient's lack of responses (no responses at limits) would appear on an audiogram is shown in Figure 7–16. This patient has normal hearing in the right ear, but for the left ear most of the masked AC and BC thresholds are beyond the output limits of the equipment. It is common practice not to connect the AC symbols in regions where there are no responses (e.g., above 500 Hz in Figure 7–16). The purpose of the "no response" symbols on an audiogram is to show that testing was attempted at the limits of the audiometer, but the patient actually has worse thresholds than those indicated by the "no response" symbols. As you can see in Figure 7–16, there is the appearance of an air–bone gap; however, it is important not to describe this as an air–bone gap because it is simply due to the difference in output limits for BC and AC. For the example in Figure 7–16, based on the audiogram alone, you cannot be sure if there is any involvement of the conductive portions of the ear (cannot determine if it is a mixed hearing loss) because you were not able to test masked BC thresholds high enough to find the patient's true BC thresholds. Information from other tests in your battery (e.g., tympanometry) would be needed to help determine if there was a conductive component. For Figure 7–16, can you predict where the unmasked BC and unmasked AC responses would have been?

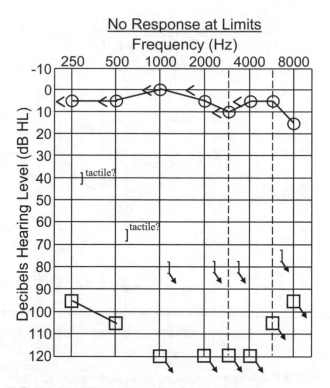

FIGURE 7–16. An example of an audiogram showing no responses (patient did not hear the tones) at the upper output limits of the equipment for the left ear bone conduction and air conduction thresholds. The threshold differences between the AC and BC symbols for the left ear do not imply any air–bone gaps because the actual thresholds for the left ear cannot be determined due to output limits of the transducers. The patient has a hearing loss in the left ear that is greater than that which could be tested. See the audiogram key in Figure 7–1 for definitions of the audiometric symbols.

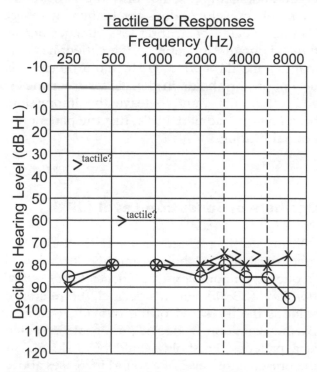

FIGURE 7–15. An example of an audiogram showing how to indicate the possibility that the low frequency bone conduction thresholds may be due to tactile sensations rather than auditory sensations. See the audiogram key in Figure 7–1 for definitions of the audiometric symbols.

Collapsed Canals

Collapsed canals can occur in some individuals with reduced elasticity in the cartilaginous portion of the external ear canal when supra-aural earphones are used for testing. The collapsed canals are only an artifact of the testing situation, whereby the force of the supra-aural earphone is enough to temporarily close off the ear canal. When the ear canal is collapsed by the supra-aural earphone, it will reduce the intensity of the AC pure tones, but not the BC pure tones, and can result in an erroneous air–bone gap. Figure 7–17 shows an example of an audiogram that would suggest collapsed canals. The effects

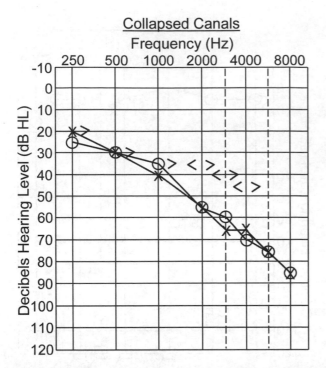

FIGURE 7–17. An example of an audiogram suggesting false air–bone gaps in the mid to high frequencies due to temporary collapsing (closing) of ear canals that may occur in some patients due to the pressure of supra-aural earphones. Retesting with insert earphones should eliminate the erroneous air–bone gaps. See the audiogram key in Figure 7–1 for definitions of the audiometric symbols.

of a collapsed ear canal are usually seen in the mid to high frequencies, showing up as a high frequency air–bone gap, whereas a true conductive component would include the low frequencies. Whenever there is a mid or high frequency air–bone gap using supra-aural earphones, the audiologist should be suspicious of a collapsed canal and use other means of AC testing, such as the use of insert earphones, hand-holding the supra-aural earphone loosely on the ear, or sound-field testing while masking the non-test ear.

Pure-Tone Average

Calculating a *pure-tone average* (PTA) for each ear is often done to provide a summary of the pure-tone thresholds over a particular frequency range. The PTA is calculated from the AC thresholds because the AC route includes all portions of the auditory system. The traditional PTA is the average of the thresholds at 500, 1000, and 2000 Hz. Other calculations of PTA may be done in certain situations, including a four-frequency PTA (500, 1000, 2000, 3000 Hz) or a high frequency PTA (1000, 2000, 3000, 4000 Hz), especially when calculating percent of hearing handicap for compensation cases. A two-frequency PTA (e.g., 1000 and 2000 Hz) is sometimes used when there is a steep slope to the audiogram. Clark (1981) recommends calculating the PTA from the three poorest thresholds between 500 and 4000 Hz. Whenever the PTA is not the standard (500, 1000, 2000 Hz), the frequencies used in calculating the average should be noted with the audiogram.

The PTA is sometimes used as an average value for describing the degree of hearing loss; however, the authors recommend describing the degrees of hearing loss as they change across the entire audiogram, and not only the PTA. A single number (average) does not adequately reflect how the degree of hearing loss changes across the audiogram. For example, if a patient has normal hearing through 2000 Hz and a precipitous decline in thresholds in the higher frequencies, you would not want to leave the impression, based on the traditional PTA, that the patient has normal hearing.

Decibels of Sensation Level (dB SL)

"Oh my gosh," you are probably thinking, "another decibel!" Yes, there is another decibel used frequently in audiology, called *decibel of sensation level* (dB SL). For this decibel, the reference value is the threshold of the individual patient: By the definition of decibel, a signal presented at a patient's threshold would be 0 dB SL. As the presentation level of a sound increases above a patient's threshold, so does the amount of dB SL. In other words, when using dB SL, you must always know the patient's threshold. Let's say that a patient has a threshold of 20 dB HL at a

SYNOPSIS 7–2

- A descriptions of an audiogram should provide a concise summary of the type of loss, degree of loss, and shape of loss as a function of frequency, without repeating all the threshold data that are on the audiogram.
- The following terms are in common use to describe the degree of hearing loss:
  - −10 to 15 dB HL   Normal
  - 16 to 25 dB HL   Normal for adults; slight or minimal in children
  - 26 to 40 dB HL   Mild
  - 41 to 55 dB HL   Moderate
  - 56 to 70 dB HL   Moderately severe
  - 71 to 90 dB HL   Severe
  - 91+ dB HL   Profound
- The following characteristics are used to describe the types of hearing loss:
  - Sensorineural   Air–bone gap ≤ 10 dB; AC and BC abnormal
  - Conductive   Air–bone gap >10 dB; AC abnormal, BC normal
  - Mixed hearing loss   Air–bone gap > 10 dB; AC abnormal, BC abnormal
- The following terms are in common use to describe the shape of the hearing loss:
  - Bilateral   Similar in both ears
  - Flat   Within 20 dB across audiogram
  - Sloping   >20 dB per octave toward high frequencies
  - Precipitous   Steeply sloping (e.g., >40 dB/octave)
  - Rising   Improving from low to high frequencies
  - Notched   Worse in a narrow region (typically 3 to 6 kHz)
  - Saucer/cookie-bite   Worse in mid frequencies; shallow concave appearance
  - Corner   Residual hearing only in the lower frequencies
- Tactile responses, in which the patient can feel the vibration during BC testing rather than hear it, can occur around 25 to 40 dB HL at 250 Hz, and around 55 to 70 dB HL at 500 Hz. For patients with more than a moderate hearing loss, these tactile BC thresholds may appear as false air–bone gaps.
- Some patients with severe to profound hearing loss may not respond at the output (level) limits of the audiometer. Because BC output limits are less than AC output limits, it may appear as an erroneous air–bone gap, and the extent of any conductive involvement cannot be determined from the audiogram and would need other information to make that determination.
- Collapsed canals can temporarily occur in some patients with highly compliant ear canals during testing with supra-aural earphones. Collapsed canals are characterized by air–bone gaps that occur in the mid to higher frequencies, but not in the lower frequencies. Collapsed canals can be avoided by using insert earphones.
- A pure-tone average (PTA) is often calculated from the thresholds at 500, 1000, and 2000 Hz. With a steeply sloping hearing loss, the PTA can be calculated using only 500 and 1000 Hz. Other variations of PTA can be used; however, this should be noted on the audiogram.
- Decibel sensation level (dB SL) is another way of referencing the level of sounds that are presented to patients. The reference value for dB SL is the patient's own threshold at each frequency. By definition, 0 dB SL = patient's threshold.

particular frequency; if a tone at that frequency is presented at 60 dB HL, this would be 40 dB SL (40 dB above the threshold). For a patient with a threshold of 40 dB HL, a sound presented at 60 dB HL would be 20 dB SL. As you will see in later chapters, there are some audiologic tests that are done at a specific dB SL, which would require a different dB HL for different patients, depending on their thresholds. For example, let's say a test is designed to be presented at 20 dB SL: For a patient with a threshold of 30 dB HL, the presentation level of the test would be set on the audiometer intensity dial to 50 dB HL; for a patient with a threshold of 60 dB HL, the presentation level of the test would be set on the audiometer intensity dial to 80 dB HL. Keeping track of dB HL and dB SL may sound a bit confusing at first, but keep in mind that dB HL is the level you set with the intensity dial on the audiometer (referenced to ANSI standards) and dB SL is the amount that a particular sound is relative to the patient's threshold (suprathreshold).

REFERENCES

American National Standards Institute [ANSI]. (2004). Methods for manual pure-tone threshold audiometry, *ANSI S3.21-2004*. New York, NY: Author.

American National Standards Institute [ANSI]. (2010). Specifications for audiometers, *ANSI S3.6-2010*. New York, NY: Author.

American Speech-Language-Hearing Association [ASHA]. (2005). Guidelines for manual pure-tone threshold audiometry. Retrieved from http://www.asha.org/policy

Boothroyd, A., & Cawkwell, S. (1970). Vibrotactile thresholds in pure-tone audiometry. *Acta Otolaryngologica, 69*, 381–387.

Clark, J. G. (1981). Uses and abuses of hearing loss classification. *ASHA, 23*(7), 493–500.

Goodman, A. (1965). Reference zero levels for pure-tone audiometer. *ASHA, 7*, 262–263.

Haggard, R. S., & Primus, M. A. (1999). Parental perceptions of hearing loss classification in children. *American Journal of Audiology, 8*(2), 83–92.

Jerger, J. (2013). Why the audiogram is upside-down. *International Journal of Audiology, Early Online*, 1–5.

Nober, E. H. (1970). Cutile air and bone conduction thresholds of the deaf. *Exceptional Children, 36*(8), 571–579.

Studebaker, G. A. (1967). Intertest variability and the air–bone gap. *Journal of Speech and Hearing Disorders, 32*, 82–86.

8 Speech Audiometry

After reading this chapter, you should be able to:

1. Describe how to calibrate the speech materials using the audiometer's VU meter and discuss why this must be done each time testing is performed.

2. Describe how to perform and interpret speech recognition threshold (SRT) tests.

3. Define what is meant by the speech banana and explain the general distribution of speech sounds as to frequency and intensity characteristics.

4. Describe how different degrees of hearing loss would affect understanding of speech.

5. Explain what is meant by the Speech Intelligibility Index (SII).

6. Understand how to use a count-the-dots audiogram to help a patient understand his or her hearing loss and how it might be applicable to different degrees of hearing loss.

7. Describe how to perform a suprathreshold test for word recognition score (WRS) and discuss issues related to selecting the presentation level for WRS testing.

8. Graph a performance intensity (PI) function for PB words (PI–PB) for cochlear versus 8th cranial nerve disorders and calculate the respective rollover ratios.

9. Calculate WRS using whole word and phoneme scoring, and determine whether two WRS values are significantly different from each other based on critical differences from the binomial distribution.

10. Use WRS to differentiate between a cochlear or 8th cranial nerve disorder with similar pure-tone averages.

11. Demonstrate familiarity with some speech in noise tests, such as the Hearing in Noise Test (HINT) and Quick Sentence in Noise Test (QuickSin).

12. Discuss variations that are used for speech testing of children.

Speech audiometry is a method used by audiologists to evaluate how well a patient can hear and understand specific types of speech stimuli. As mentioned in the previous chapter, knowing the lowest levels (thresholds) that we can hear pure tones is not very representative of what we listen to in our real-world environments. Most patients do not begin to notice their hearing loss until they are having trouble understanding speech, or when a family member notices that the person is having trouble communicating. Speech tests provide a formal way to determine the patient's ability to recognize speech, albeit in a controlled environment. Speech audiometry can also contribute to the diagnosis of different hearing disorders. For example, a problem in the cochlea can have a fairly predictable relation between the shape of the audiogram and understanding of speech, whereas a problem in the 8th cranial nerve often results in significantly poorer speech recognition than would be suggested by the audiogram. It is not unusual for two persons with identical audiograms to have different degrees of difficulty recognizing or processing speech.

Results of speech tests are used to compare and validate pure-tone thresholds, compare speech recognition ability between the two ears, and/or monitor changes across time. Speech audiometry can also help determine whether a patient is an appropriate candidate for a hearing aid or cochlear implant, or to compare a patient's performance with different amplification devices and settings. Speech audiometry includes two basic types of speech tests: (a) the establishment of a speech threshold and (b) a measure of speech recognition ability performed at a level above their threshold (suprathreshold). This chapter describes some of the basic speech tests routinely performed during an audiometric evaluation, and discusses ways to interpret these measures.

SPEECH TESTING EQUIPMENT AND CALIBRATION

Speech audiometry can be performed using the same comprehensive diagnostic audiometer that is used for pure-tone testing. The speech materials are presented to the patient through the speech channel of the audiometer. Figure 8–1 shows the main components of an audiometer that are used for speech testing. The speech channel has options for the tester to present the speech materials by talking into a microphone, referred to as *monitored live voice* testing, presenting *recorded speech materials* through an externally connected device such as a compact disk (CD) player, or by using speech materials stored in the audiometer or on a computer. The use of recorded or digitized speech materials is gener-

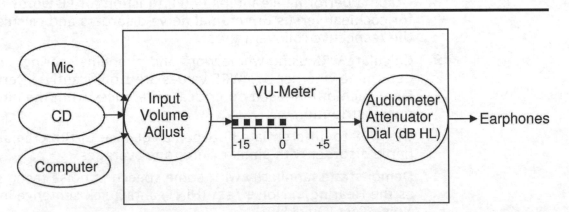

FIGURE 8–1. Block diagram showing the major components of a clinical audiometer that are used for speech testing. Speech materials can be delivered by microphone (Mic), compact disk (CD), or computer. The input volume must be adjusted until the volume unit (VU) meter peaks at zero so that the audiometer attenuator dial reading (dB HL) is presenting the proper level to the patient.

ally recommended because of their consistency and ability to be standardized, which improves comparisons across testing sessions or different patients. Speech testing with monitored live voice is acceptable in situations where flexibility is needed in presenting the speech materials to patients who may need some modifications; for example, those with limited vocabularies or those who are being assessed for auditory-visual speech perception abilities.

As with pure tones, the audiometer's output level (dB HL) for speech is calibrated based on the standards for audiometric speech levels set by the American National Standards Institute [ANSI] (2010), much like calibrating for pure tones. However, because words and sentences vary in intensity, it is difficult to set a precise level for words, per se. Instead, the reference sound pressure level for the speech channel is based on a 1000 Hz pure tone presented through the speech channel, so that the measured output is 12.5 dB SPL higher than the reference sound pressure level for a 1000 Hz pure tone for the appropriate transducer (see Table 8–1).

Whether presenting the speech by monitored live voice or recorded/digitized material, it is very important to adjust the input level of the speech materials before testing so that the level presented to the patient is at the appropriate dB HL. In other words, variations in the level of the tester's voice or the distance from the microphone can alter the level of the signal when using monitored live voice. In addition, since externally connected devices have their own variable output levels, the tester needs to adjust the incoming level to the audiometer's speech channel so that the values set by the audiometer's attenuator dial are accurate representations of the dB HL being presented to the patient. To ensure appropriate calibration levels, the input to the audiometer's speech channel can be adjusted by changing the input volume (see Input Volume Adjust in Figure 8–1) and monitoring the level through the use of the audiometer's volume unit (VU) meter, a meter that is readily visible on the audiometer (see Figure 8–1). As the materials are being presented, the VU meter has an indicator that fluctuates with the level of the incoming signal. The VU meter has a midpoint labeled 0 dB that represents the point where the speech channel is in calibration per ANSI (2010) and, therefore, the presentation level of the speech material to the patient is equal to the value on the audiometer attenuator dial (in dB HL). The typical VU meter has a range that goes from –20 dB to +10 dB relative to the calibration point at 0 dB. For example, when the VU meter is at –5 dB, the presentation level of the speech material is 5 dB lower than it should be, thus a presentation level of 40 dB HL is actually only presented at 35 dB HL to the patient. To compensate, the tester must increase the input volume by 5 dB so that the VU meter reads 0 dB. This is often referred to as peaking the VU meter.

The VU meter must be adjusted each time a new patient is tested or a different set of recorded speech materials is used. For monitored live voice testing, the tester must adjust the input level, before testing the patient, by saying a few words until the VU meter "peaks" at 0 dB when

TABLE 8–1. Air Conduction Reference Values for Speech Channel Corresponding to 0 dB HL (Audiometric Zero) Based on ANSI S3.6 (2010). Air Conduction Reference Values Are in dB SPL re: 20 μPa. Expected Calibration Levels Are 12.5 dB Above the Reference Value for a 1000 Hz Calibration Tone for the Respective Transducer.

Transducer	Model	1000 Hz	Speech Correction	Calibration dB SPL
Supra-aural phones[a]	TDH-50P	7.5	12.5	20.0
Insert phones[b]	ER-3A	5.5	12.5	18.0

[a]Calibrated with 6-cc coupler.

[b]Calibrated with occluded ear simulator. Values are different for HA-1 or HA-2 couplers (ANSI, 2010).

the words are presented. The tester must continuously monitor the VU meter throughout the test to ensure that the level remains stable. For recorded or computer-generated materials, there is a 1000 Hz calibration tone included with the materials that the tester uses to adjust the input level until the VU meter is at 0 dB.

SPEECH THRESHOLD MEASURES

One of the goals of speech audiometry is to find the lowest level a patient is able to produce a response to speech stimuli, which is called the speech threshold. Speech stimuli are generally more familiar to a patient than pure tones, and in cases where pure tones are not successful or contaminated by false positives or false negatives, speech thresholds may provide the only information about the patient's degree of hearing loss. Some audiologists prefer to start the hearing evaluation with speech threshold measures to get an idea of where to expect the pure-tone thresholds. The speech threshold is measured using the same dB HL scale as the pure-tone thresholds, and the degree of hearing loss for speech can be described by the same categories used for degree of hearing loss for pure-tone audiometry. The frequency distribution of speech generally falls within the 300 to 6000 Hz region of the audiogram; therefore, measures of speech thresholds provide estimates of the pure-tone thresholds most important for speech. Keep in mind, however, that the speech threshold is primarily representative of those frequencies where the patient has the best hearing; thus, the speech threshold is not able to predict the shape of the audiogram.

Another important use of the speech threshold is as a cross-check with the pure-tone thresholds. The speech threshold is usually equal to or slightly better than the pure-tone average (PTA), and should be within 10 dB HL of the PTA. If there is more than a 10 dB difference between the speech threshold and the PTA, then a determination of why there is a difference should be explored. When the speech threshold and the PTA do not agree, the possibilities to explore include the following:

- Could the discrepancy be due to the shape of the audiogram? For steeply sloping audiograms, are there one or two frequencies that could be providing the cues for the speech threshold (Fletcher, 1950; Silman & Silverman, 1991)?
- Could the discrepancy be related to limited proficiency in the language being used for the test or is there a foreign dialect?
- Were the speech materials properly calibrated with the VU meter?
- Were the pure-tone thresholds purposely exaggerated or contaminated in some way by the patient's response bias? See Chapter 12 for more information on the exaggerated (functional) hearing loss.

Speech Recognition Threshold (SRT)

The speech procedure most often used to determine the speech threshold is called the *speech recognition (reception) threshold* (SRT). The SRT procedure typically uses two-syllable compound words, called *spondee words*, that can be presented with nearly equal intensity and/or stress on each syllable, such as "baseball" and "railroad." With monitored live voice, the level of the words are adjusted so that the VU meter "peaks" at 0 dB for each syllable, and the tester should not put any excessive voice inflection on either syllable. The spondee word lists most commonly used today for SRT measurement (American Speech-Language-Hearing Association [ASHA], 1988) are modifications of materials (CID W-1 and W-2 Words Tests) developed at the Central Institute of the Deaf (CID) (Hirsh et al., 1952). Recorded lists of spondee words have been produced by Auditec Inc. and by the Department of Veteran Affairs. For adults, ASHA (1988) recommends a list of 15 spondees (see Table 8–2). Although basic SRT measures are usually performed with spondee words, sentence materials are also available for speech threshold testing, especially in noise (see Speech-in-Noise Tests later in this chapter).

The spondee SRT test requires the patient to correctly recognize the presented spondee words.

TABLE 8–2. Spondee Words in the ASHA (1988) Guidelines

Baseball	Inkwell	Railroad
Doormat	Mousetrap	Sidewalk
Drawbridge	Northwest	Toothbrush
Eardrum	Padlock	Woodwork
Grandson	Playground	Workshop

The SRT usually begins with a familiarization of the list of words at a comfortable listening level so that the words that are not correctly identified are omitted from the test list (Tillman & Jerger, 1959). The tester varies the presentation level of the spondees to find the lowest level that the patient can recognize at least 50% of the words. Recorded materials or monitored live voice are acceptable for SRT testing, and there are no appreciable differences in threshold between the two (ASHA, 1988). The patient is given instructions such as, "I am now going to find the softest level that you can recognize some common words. Please repeat the words that you hear, even if you have to guess."

There have been several different procedures in use for establishing the SRT. The "up-5-down-10" bracketing method, like the one used for pure-tone threshold testing, is used by many audiologists and has been described by Martin and Dowdy (1986); however, this bracketing procedure has not been incorporated into any professional standard or guideline as a method for obtaining an SRT. Other SRT procedures use blocks of words (4 to 5 words per block) at each level, with specific rules as to when to increase or decrease the presentation level. Most SRT procedures have an initial phase that quickly searches for an approximation of the patient's threshold in order to save time presenting too many words at levels that are too far below or too far above the patient's actual threshold. Some SRT procedures use a descending threshold search, *whereby* the blocks of words are first presented above a patient's estimated threshold and then at descending levels (American Speech-Language-Hearing Association [ASHA],

1988; Chaiklin & Ventry, 1964); other procedures use an *ascending threshold search*, whereby the blocks of words are first presented below the estimated threshold and then at ascending levels (Chaiklin, Font, & Dixon, 1967; Downs & Minard, 1996). In the following paragraphs, the Downs and Minard (1996) ascending SRT procedure will be described in more detail.

The Downs and Minard Method for Obtaining the SRT

The Downs and Minard (1996) method for obtaining an SRT is a relatively fast and easy procedure to perform using blocks of words, and produces results similar to those of other SRT procedures. The steps for the Downs and Minard SRT procedure are as follows (see also Figure 8–2):

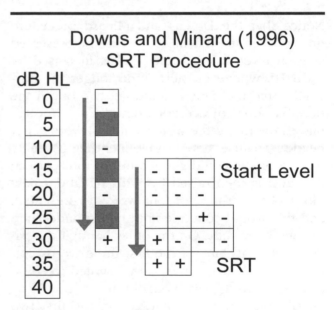

FIGURE 8–2. Illustration of how speech recognition threshold (SRT) is obtained using the Downs and Minard (1996) ascending procedure. The minus signs represent words not correctly identified and the plus signs represent words correctly identified. There is a pretest phase to establish the start level (15 dB HL) shown by the series of boxes immediately to the right of the dB HL column. For the threshold search phase (on the far right of the figure), two, three, or four spondees are presented in 5 dB ascending steps until two spondees are correctly identified. In this example, the SRT = 35 dB HL.

1. Familiarize the patient with the spondee words at a comfortable listening level. Remove any that the patient has difficulty understanding.
2. Instruct the patient that the words may be very faint and he or she is to repeat the words back to you.
3. Begin by presenting one spondee at the lowest audiometer setting or at least 30 dB below the estimated or known PTA (or at 0 dB HL if unable to estimate); continue presenting one spondee in 10 dB ascending steps until the patient repeats one spondee correctly.
4. Decrease the level by 15 dB (to get below threshold again): This is the starting level for the ascending threshold search phase.
5. At the starting level and at each 5 dB HL ascending step, present blocks of either two, three, or four spondees as needed until patient repeats two spondees correctly: This level is the patient's SRT.

Notice that the Downs and Minard procedure does not require that all four words be presented at each level: Instead, the level is increased by 5 dB HL whenever there is no longer the possibility that the patient could get two out of the possible four correct. For example, if he or she misses the first three words, a fourth word is not needed because there is no longer the possibility that he or she could get two out of four correct; the level is then raised by 5 dB HL and a new block of two, three, or four words is presented, and this would continue until two spondees are repeated correctly. On the other hand, if the patient gets only one of the first three words correct, a fourth word must be presented to see if he or she could get two out of four correct (50%). Of course, should the patient get the first two words of a block correct, that level would be the patient's SRT. On the rare occasion when the patient gets two correct at the original starting level, the starting level is lowered by 10 dB HL and the procedure begins at the new starting level.

Speech Detection Threshold

A *speech detection threshold* (SDT), sometimes referred to as a *speech awareness threshold* (SAT),

is a speech threshold measure that determines the lowest level a patient can simply detect speech rather than correctly recognize the speech. The SDT is usually 5 to 10 dB HL lower than the SRT because the SDT only depends on the patient reacting to the most audible frequency of the word (Cambron, Wilson, & Shanks, 1991). The SDT is only used when an SRT cannot be obtained, such as with adults with severe to profound hearing loss, young children, patients with speech or language impairments, or physically/mentally challenged patients. The choice of speech materials for obtaining an SDT is not that critical; they can be familiar two syllable words, such as "hello," familiar phrases such as "Can you hear me?," nonsense syllables such as "ba ba ba," continuous discourse such as reading a passage, and/or spondee words. Familiarizing the patient to the speech is also not required when obtaining an SDT. Generally, the intensity of the speech is adjusted in an ascending direction from below threshold until the patient responds in some instructed manner (raises hand) or by using a head-turn visual reinforcement audiometry (VRA) procedure. The SDT can also be established with some bracketing procedure, such as the up-5-down-10 method used for pure-tone thresholds (American Speech-Language-Hearing Association [ASHA], 1988). When using the SDT as a cross-check with the PTA, you must consider whether there is good agreement with the best pure-tone threshold between 250 and 4000 Hz. If the SDT is more than 20 dB lower than the average of the best two-frequency average, then either measure should be suspect and the discrepancy should be resolved (Brandy, 2002). When the SDT is obtained instead of the SRT, it should be clearly indicated on the audiogram report, and the type of speech stimuli used should also be specified. The SDT is a poor indication of the shape of a person's hearing loss, as it only reflects the best hearing frequency.

SUPRATHRESHOLD SPEECH RECOGNITION

Although the SRT is useful for cross-checking with the PTA or to give some limited estimate of a

SYNOPSIS 8–1

- Speech audiometry is part of the basic audiologic evaluation. Speech tests are used to validate pure-tone results, provide some information when pure-tone results are not able to be obtained, compare speech abilities between the ears, monitor changes over time, and as a measure of hearing aid suitability and/or performance.
- Speech materials are delivered through the speech channel of an audiometer and can be presented by monitored live voice (MLV), recorded materials through a compact disk (CD), or digitally generated by computer. Recorded or computer-generated materials should be used whenever possible.
- The ANSI standard for 0 dB HL of the speech channel is 12.5 dB SPL higher than the ANSI standard for a 1000 Hz pure tone for the respective AC transducer.
- To compensate for input level variations, the tester must always make adjustments to the input level of the audiometer by peaking the VU meter at 0 dB, so that a calibrated dB HL is presented to the patient.
- Speech recognition threshold (SRT) is usually tested with two-syllable words, called spondees. The patient is first familiarized with the words at a comfortable listening level and those words incorrectly identified are omitted from the threshold testing.
  - A commonly used ascending SRT method (but not advocated in any guideline) is the up-5-down-10 bracketing procedure (similar to that used for pure-tone, but with spondee words).
  - Another SRT ascending procedure that uses blocks of words at each level is the Downs and Minard (1996) procedure: Begin below the estimated threshold or the lowest level on the audiometer and give one spondee at each 10 dB increment until the patient gets one spondee correct; decrease the level by 15 dB (which sets the starting level); give two, three, or four spondees at each 5 dB increment until the patient gets two spondees correct; this level is the SRT.
- For patients who have difficulty with the SRT test, a speech detection threshold (SDT) can be obtained. The SDT is only a test of the lowest level at which the patient detects speech and does not require recognition, and is about 5 to 10 dB better than the SRT. The SDT reflects the patient's best pure-tone threshold and does not provide much information about the shape of the audiogram or the ability to recognize speech.
- The SRT should be within 10 dB of the patient's PTA. If the difference between SRT and PTA is more than 10 dB, it could indicate that the patient is exaggerating his pure-tone hearing loss; however, be sure to rule out the possibility of it being related to the steep slope of the audiogram (compare with a two-frequency PTA), language or dialect issues, or improper peaking of the VU meter.

patient's hearing ability, it is not representative of the levels that people listen to speech in their real environments. People generally listen to speech at a comfortable conversational level or at other suprathreshold levels. In addition, daily listening activities involve listening to speech in a variety of noisy situations.

The different speech sounds have different intensities and frequencies. For example, most vowels are higher in intensity and lower in frequency than most consonants. The average conversational level for speech is about 45 to 50 dB HL (Killion & Mueller, 2010; Thibodeau, 2007), which is related primarily to the intensity of the vowels; however, the range between the loudest vowels (e.g., 50 dB HL) and the softest consonants, especially the fricatives, e.g., /f/, /s/ (e.g., 20 dB HL), is about 30 dB. Figure 8–3 illustrates how the different speech sounds are distributed on an audiogram when spoken at a normal conversational level. The shaded region in Figure 8–3 represents an outline of the range of the speech sounds associated with conversational-level speech. This shaded region is often referred to as the *speech banana* due to its general shape. The normal distribution of the different speech sounds shown in Figure 8–3A is often included on an audiogram as a simple and easily understood way to explain to a patient what parts of the speech he or she can or cannot hear. Figure 8–3B is a more representative illustration of the ranges of the acoustic properties of the different speech sounds. Additionally, it is important to keep in mind that the recognition of speech depends on more than just detecting a specific frequency, such as: (a) recognition of vowels depends on the first and second formants, (b) recognition of some consonants (e.g., /b/ vs. /g/ vs. /d/) depends on the first and second formants of their associated vowels, (c) many voiced consonants and nasals have two or three energy bands, (d) consonant frequencies can vary depending on the preceding and following sounds (coarticulation), and (e) differences occur across talkers, especially across gender. Figure 8–4 shows how two different hearing losses could affect the audibility of the different speech sounds within the speech banana for speech presented at a relatively normal conversational level of 50 dB HL. Even with a mild high frequency hearing loss, you can see that many of the higher frequency components of consonant sounds (e.g., /f/, /s/, /th/, /t/, /z/, /v/) would be inaudible (below the patient's thresholds) and might cause some word confusion, such as in *fight* or *sight*. Of course, different degrees and shapes of hearing losses will result in different acoustic features being more or less audible to the patient.

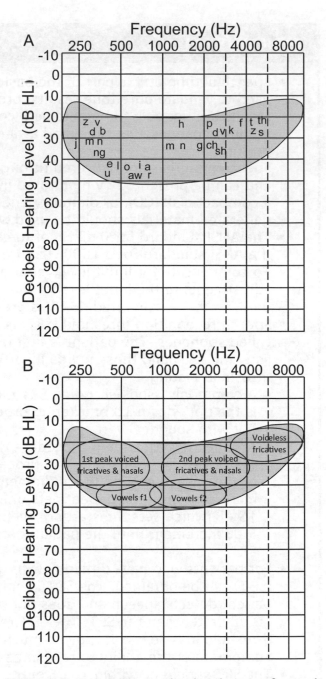

FIGURE 8–3. A AND B. The distribution of speech sounds superimposed on an audiogram, known as the speech banana during average conversational level (45 to 50 dB HL). **A.** Common speech sounds. **B.** Illustration of the ranges of different types of speech sounds within the speech banana.

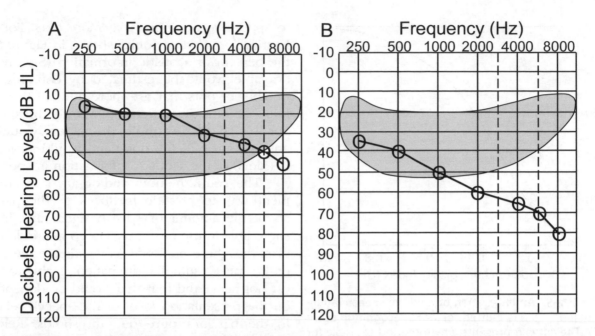

FIGURE 8–4. A AND B. Two hearing losses displayed on an audiogram along with the speech banana for average conversational level (45 to 50 dB HL). **A.** Mild high frequency hearing loss. This patient would do fairly well listening to people talking, but may have difficulty understanding some words because the high-frequency speech sounds (e.g., fricatives) would be inaudible. **B.** Mild to severe sloping hearing loss. This patient may be aware of people talking from the lower frequency, higher intensity vowels, but would have considerable difficulty understanding because much of the speech is inaudible.

Count-the-Dots Audiogram

As discussed above, it is often helpful to describe to a patient how a hearing loss might be expected to affect his or her hearing of speech in the real world by using the speech banana on the audiogram. Obviously, this is a very general approach and does not give any quantifiable information. Finding a systematic way to predict speech understanding based only on the speech spectrum has been the subject of research for quite some time. The earliest attempts to predict overall speech intelligibility was done by French and Steinberg (1947) and Fletcher (1950), known as the *articulation* or *audibility index* (AI); the earlier versions of the AI were later revised and renamed the *speech intelligibility index* (SII) (American National Standards Institute [ANSI], 1997). The basic principle of the SII lies in the fact that as less of the speech spectrum becomes audible (by external filtering or by the presence of

a hearing loss), speech intelligibility gets poorer. In addition, some frequency regions contribute more to intelligibility than others. The different frequencies within the speech stimuli are divided into a number of bands that are given weightings based on their importance to the overall recognition of the speech stimuli. The SII results in a number that ranges from 0.0 (none of the speech acoustic information is available) to 1.0 (all of the speech acoustic information is available). Actual calculations of the SII consider a variety of listening conditions and speech parameters, which are put into a complicated mathematical formula to derive a number that represents the amount of speech information that is usable to the listener. Figure 8–5 shows a hypothetical plot of the percent of correct word recognition as a function of the SII value to illustrate how a normal hearing listener might respond to single-syllable words as the amount of acoustic information is increased or decreased. As you

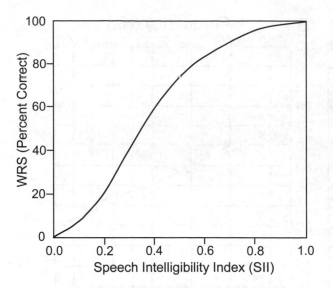

FIGURE 8–5. An illustration of how the speech intelligibility index (SII) is plotted for word recognition score (WRS). The curve represents a hypothetical example for normal hearing listeners. As the SII decreases, due to a reduction in usable acoustic information, there is a corresponding decrease in the WRS.

to speech recognition have more dots. For the hearing loss (left ear only) shown in Figure 8–6, the percent of acoustic information (SII) that is available would be estimated by counting the number of dots that are more audible than the line that joins the patient's pure-tone thresholds. For this specific example, the patient would be able to hear 66% (66 dots) and would miss 34% (34 dots) of the acoustic information in speech.

The count-the-dots audiogram is a convenient way to provide feedback to the patient about the amount of speech signal that he or she is able to use or not use. Keep in mind, however, that these methods only estimate the parts of the speech stimulus the patient is able to hear (or not hear) and that this would be dependent on the presentation level of the speech relative to the patient's pure-tone thresholds. Relying only on the pure-tone audiogram to predict a patient's speech recognition ability has not been

would expect, as the amount of available acoustic speech information increases, the better the speech recognition. The exact shape of the curve will depend on the type of speech stimuli used and the parameters included in the calculation of the SII.

For clinical purposes, the calculations of the SII in their original forms are much too burdensome. However, clinical versions of the SII concept have evolved that are much simpler and easier to use clinically (Humes, 1991; Killion & Mueller, 2010; Mueller & Killion, 1990; Pavlovic, 1988). One handy procedure is called the *count-the-dots audiogram*, an example of which is shown in Figure 8–6. The original count-the-dots audiogram was introduced by Mueller and Killion (1990) and in 2010 was updated by these authors (Killion & Mueller, 2010). As seen in Figure 8–6, the Killion and Mueller (2010) count-the-dots audiogram distributes 100 dots (each dot represents 1%) across the audiogram in a way that weights frequencies by the relative number of dots based on their contribution to the overall importance of speech recognition: Those frequencies with a greater contribution

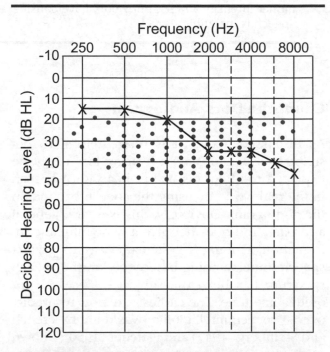

FIGURE 8–6. Count-the-dots audiogram to represent the SII in a simpler, clinically useable manner based on Killion and Mueller (2010). The acoustic speech information is divided, in a weighted fashion, across the audiogram by 100 dots. Each dot contributes 1% to the intelligibility. For the hearing loss shown in this example, there are 66 dots above the patient's threshold, which would result in 66% of the acoustic information being audible and 34% inaudible.

adopted as a routine procedure in the clinical setting; however, this approach may become more widely used in the future as more validation studies are done. For the present, there are other clinical procedures to measure speech recognition ability that are typically included as part of the basic audiometric evaluation and are discussed later in this chapter.

MOST COMFORTABLE AND UNCOMFORTABLE LOUDNESS LEVELS

Most of us prefer to listen to sounds at comfortable levels and we tend to avoid listening to sounds at uncomfortable levels. Audiometrically, the level (dB HL) at which a patient prefers to listen to speech is called the *most comfortable loudness level* (MCL) and the level (in dB HL) at which a patient finds speech to be too loud is called the *uncomfortable loudness level* (UCL) or *loudness discomfort level* (LDL). Information about a patient's MCL and UCL may be helpful in selecting the appropriate level at which to do speech testing. The most common way to determine a patient's MCL and UCL for speech is to use categorical ratings where the patient is asked to judge the loudness for increasing levels of words or sentences according to the following categories (a list of these categories is given to the patient) (Punch, Rakerd, & Joseph, 2004):

7. Uncomfortably loud
6. Loud, but OK
5. Comfortable, but slightly loud
4. Comfortable
3. Comfortable, but slightly soft
2. Soft
1. Very soft

As you will see later in this chapter, and in the chapter on hearing aids, information about a patient's MCL and UCL are useful to assess his or her ability to understand speech, and to evaluate how much range he or she has before speech becomes uncomfortably loud. The UCL represents the upper end of the range for a patient's hearing. Measures of UCL are important for hearing aid fittings so that the hearing aid output does not exceed the patient's UCL. Although MCL and UCL may be reported for a range of hearing levels (Dirks & Kamm, 1976), the normal hearing person's MCL for speech is generally between 40 and 55 dB HL, whereas the UCL for speech is approximately 100 dB HL. The amount of useable hearing for a patient, called the *dynamic range*, is the difference between the SRT and the UCL. In cochlear hearing losses, it is typical for the patient to have a UCL for speech that would be the same or slightly lower than someone with normal hearing; however, since the patient has an elevated SRT, the resulting dynamic range is greatly reduced (Kamm, Dirks, & Mickey, 1978).

PROCEDURES FOR SUPRATHRESHOLD SPEECH RECOGNITION

Suprathreshold speech testing is a routine part of the audiologic evaluation, and is used to evaluate how well a patient can recognize speech, using single-words or sentences, at one or more levels above his or her SRT or PTA. Typically, suprathreshold speech recognition is performed using single-syllable words, which are phonetically or phonemically balanced lists of single-syllable words (consonant-vowel-consonant), called *PB words*. The PB word lists were constructed to approximate the frequency of occurrence for different speech sounds or phonemes based on their occurrence in the English language. The two most popular sets of PB word lists in use today are the CID W-22 (phonetically balanced) developed by Central Institute for the Deaf (Hirsh et al., 1952), and the NU-6 (phonemically balanced) developed at Northwestern University (Tillman & Carhart, 1966).

The goal of a word recognition test is to obtain a *word recognition score* (WRS), which is the percent of items that the patient correctly identifies. The patient is given instructions such as "I am now going to measure your recognition of words that will be presented at an audible level. You will hear an initial phrase, 'Say the word, followed by the word that you are to repeat. Please repeat the words that you hear, even if you need to guess.'" For the commonly used WRS, the PB words are presented in an *open-set* format, meaning that the patient is not aware of what words are to be presented (no familiarization). In some situations, the PB words can be presented with and without the patient looking at the tester in order to assess his or her ability to recognize words with and without visual cues.

There are two ways to score the results for word recognition tests: One way is to count the number of words that are correctly identified and convert to the percentage of the number of words presented, called *whole word score*. The other way is to count the number of phonemes that are correctly identified, called *phoneme score*, where each phoneme (initial consonant, vowel, or final consonant) in each word is scored as an item, and converted to the percentage of the number of phonemes presented. The number of items used to obtain the WRS is not standardized. Each PB word list is comprised of 50 words, called a full-list; however, most audiologists divide the list in half (25 words), called a half-list. It is important to keep in mind that as the number of test items decreases, the variability increases; and as the variability increases, larger differences between scores must occur to be statistically significant (see Critical Differences in WRS Based on Binomial Distribution later in this chapter). Although many audiologists use lists of 25 words to save time, the larger variability, as well as the loss of phonemic balance associated with a half-list, makes the use of whole word scoring with 25 words less meaningful. On the other hand, a list with 50 words decreases the variability, but takes longer to administer. Using phoneme scoring, however, may provide a better trade-off between variability and the time to administer the test. With phoneme scoring, a half-list (25 words) would have 75 items that are scored. This larger number of items reduces the variability and saves time compared to presenting a list of 50 words. Phoneme scoring may also give a better representation of the patient's overall ability to understand speech because you can see the type of phoneme errors being made. Regardless of the chosen method, it is important to indicate on the audiometric worksheet the number of words used and whether the WRS is based on whole word or phoneme scoring so that any changes in the patient's ability over time are calculated using the same scoring format.

There are other open-set single-syllable materials available for speech recognition testing, including the High Frequency Word List, CUNY Nonsense Syllable Test, Edgerton–Danhauer Nonsense Syllable Test, and the Computer-Assisted Speech Perception Assessment Test (CASPA). Also available are *closed-set* tests such as the California Consonant Test and the Modified Rhyme Test, as well as sentence tests such as the AzBio Sentence Lists, CID Everyday Sentences, and the Connected Speech Test.

Selection of the Presentation Level for WRS Testing

The selection of the presentation level is an important consideration for WRS testing. There is no agreed-upon approach for selection of WRS test level, and this is still an area of debate. Often times, WRS is obtained at a single level for each ear; however, a more complete assessment of speech recognition ability can be done by testing WRS at more than one intensity level. One thing to keep in mind is the question you are trying to answer. For example, obtaining WRS at 50 dB HL (normal conversational level) might be done in order to demonstrate to the patient how his or her hearing loss affects his or her ability to understand normal levels of conversational speech, and how amplification or other rehabilitation strategy might provide an improvement in his or her ability to communicate. On the other hand, testing at a higher level, or even more than one level, might be done to find out the patient's best WRS.

Historically, WRS testing was done at a single level of 30 to 40 dB above the patient's SRT (30 to 40 dB SL). This level was based on data showing that normal-hearing listeners achieve maximum word recognition when words are presented at or above 30 dB SL, and those with relatively flat cochlear hearing losses achieve maximum word recognition at or above 40 dB SL (Maroonroge & Diefendorf, 1984). Today, a single level at 30 to 40 dB SL is still used by many audiologists to obtain a WRS; however, this approach must be interpreted with caution because it may not be the optimal level for a patient to demonstrate

Historical Vignette

Raymond Carhart, in the 1940s, made it his mission to rehabilitate soldiers returning from World War II who had sustained hearing loss. Carhart's task was to devise a set of procedures upon which to base a rational decision about which of several possible hearing aids to dispense to the service personnel. To accomplish this, he virtually invented, from scratch, what we now know as speech audiometry. He adapted the earlier work at the Harvard Psychoacoustic Laboratory on spondee and phonemically balanced (PB) word lists into the concepts of the speech reception threshold (SRT) and the maximum PB score (PB_{max}). Also during this time, John Gaeth, at Northwestern University, studied word recognition in the elderly, and concluded that one could not fully explain all of the word recognition difficulty from the audiogram alone. Something else seemed to be reducing PB_{max} scores in some elderly individuals, which he named "phonemic regression." Five decades later, many still find this concept difficult to accept, but we now know that, in addition to the undeniably important audibility factor, there are age-related changes in frequency resolution, temporal resolution, cognition, and central auditory processing.

his or her best (maximum) WRS performance, called *PB_{max}*.

If WRS is only obtained at 40 dB SL, you may underestimate the patient's ability to understand speech, especially when wearing a hearing aid. Brandy (2002) suggested that for sloping hearing losses, the WRS could be presented 40 dB above the patient's PTA of 500, 1000, 2000, 3000, and 4000 Hz, rather than 40 dB above the SRT. In many patients who have moderate to severe hearing loss, you may not even be able to pre-

sent words at 40 dB SL because this level would be above the patient's UCL (Kamm et al., 1978).

Another strategy, if you are interested in finding the patient's PB_{max}, is to perform WRS at the highest level possible without being uncomfortable, such as 5 dB less than his or her UCL (UCL −5 dB) or at a set level of 85 or 90 dB HL. As Figure 8–7 shows, more acoustic information would be audible to the patient if WRS testing was performed at UCL −5 dB, which in this case would be at 90 dB HL (65 dB SL relative to the SRT) rather than at 65 dB HL (40 dB SL relative to the SRT). The higher test level not only results in more of the speech frequencies to be above the patient's threshold, it also makes all the acoustic information much more audible.

Guthrie and Mackersie (2009) found that PB_{max} could best be determined by testing WRS at either UCL −5 dB (which requires finding/estimating UCL) or more quickly by setting the presentation level based on the patient's threshold at 2000 Hz depending on the degree of hearing loss as follows:

- If the 2000 Hz threshold is <50 dB HL, present words at 25 dB SL
- If the 2000 Hz threshold is 50 to 55 dB HL, present words at 20 dB SL
- If the 2000 Hz threshold is 60 to 65 dB HL, present words at 15 dB SL
- If the 2000 Hz threshold is 70 to 75 dB HL, present words at 10 dB SL

Testing for WRS at a single high intensity level may create its own problems, especially when evaluating a patient with a possible 8th cranial nerve disorder. For example, a patient with an 8th cranial nerve disorder characteristically shows poorer speech recognition performance at high intensities than for somewhat lower levels, called rollover. For these patients, if WRS is only tested at one presentation level, the WRS may give a misleading account of the patient's word recognition ability because the WRS may actually be better at a slightly lower level. One solution to this issue is to perform WRS at more than one level to get a complete picture of how the patient performs and to get a better estimate

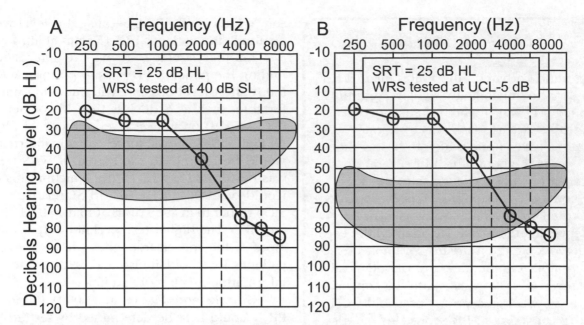

FIGURE 8–7. A AND B. Illustration of how an increase in word recognition test level can provide more acoustic information available to the patient. In these examples, the patient has an SRT = 25 dB HL and a sloping hearing loss. **A.** WRS presentation level at 40 dB SL (65 dB HL). **B.** WRS presentation level at UCL –5 dB (90 dB HL). SRT, speech recognition threshold. WRS, word recognition score. UCL, uncomfortable listening level.

of their maximum WRS, as discussed in the following section.

Performance-Intensity Function for WRS (PI-PB Function)

The optimal way to determine the patient's PB_{max} is to perform the WRS test at multiple presentation levels, called a *performance-intensity function for PB words* (PI–PB function). By graphing how the patient's WRS changes as a function of presentation level, you can better estimate the patient's PB_{max}. Figure 8–8 shows examples of documenting WRS scores using a PI–PB function. Figure 8–8A compares the PI-PB functions for a normal hearing listener to a patient who has a cochlear hearing loss (SRT = 30 dB HL), both of whom show that as the presentation level is increased, there is a rise in the WRS. At some point, the WRS reaches a maximum score whereby further increases do not improve the word recognition scores (reaches a plateau). The first point of the function where the curve reaches the highest score is the PB_{max}. Notice also, in this particu-

lar example, that the patient with the cochlear hearing loss would not have demonstrated his or her true PB_{max} (seen at 80 dB HL) had testing only been done at a single test level of 40 dB SL (70 dB HL). Figure 8–8B illustrates how a PI-PB function is also useful for differential diagnosis of a cochlear hearing loss from an 8th cranial nerve hearing loss. For normal hearing listeners and those with cochlear hearing losses, once PB_{max} has been reached the WRS remains close to that score for higher presentation levels (plateaus). However, patients with 8th cranial nerve disorders, such as acoustic tumors or neural loss due to aging, seem to have an inability to sustain neural activity when the auditory nerve is "stressed" at high intensity levels. Patients with an 8th cranial nerve disorder may show rollover at presentation levels above the level where he or she achieved his or her PB_{max} (Jerger & Jerger, 1971). The poorer WRS score seen at the highest test level is often referred to as PB_{min}. Remember, PB_{min} refers to the WRS obtained at a level higher than the level associated with the patient's PB_{max}. As you can see in Figure 8–8B, for example, the patient with the 8th cranial nerve disorder shows

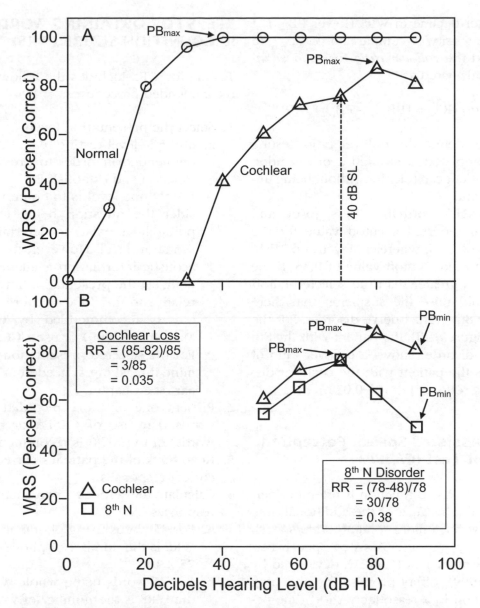

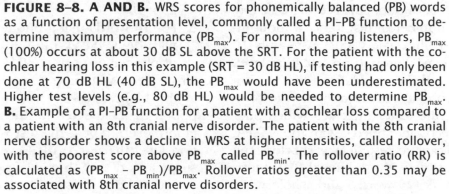

FIGURE 8–8. A AND B. WRS scores for phonemically balanced (PB) words as a function of presentation level, commonly called a PI–PB function to determine maximum performance (PB$_{max}$). For normal hearing listeners, PB$_{max}$ (100%) occurs at about 30 dB SL above the SRT. For the patient with the cochlear hearing loss in this example (SRT = 30 dB HL), if testing had only been done at 70 dB HL (40 dB SL), the PB$_{max}$ would have been underestimated. Higher test levels (e.g., 80 dB HL) would be needed to determine PB$_{max}$. **B.** Example of a PI–PB function for a patient with a cochlear loss compared to a patient with an 8th cranial nerve disorder. The patient with the 8th cranial nerve disorder shows a decline in WRS at higher intensities, called rollover, with the poorest score above PB$_{max}$ called PB$_{min}$. The rollover ratio (RR) is calculated as (PB$_{max}$ − PB$_{min}$)/PB$_{max}$. Rollover ratios greater than 0.35 may be associated with 8th cranial nerve disorders.

a much greater decline in WRS (lower PB_{min}) at the highest intensity. A comparison of PB_{max} to PB_{min} is called the *rollover ratio* (or *rollover index*), and is calculated as:

$$\text{Rollover ratio (RR)} = (PB_{max} - PB_{min}) / PB_{max}$$

To completely define the rollover ratio, testing should be completed at as high a presentation level as the patient can tolerate without being uncomfortably loud.

For the NU-6 word lists, Bess, Josey, and Humes (1979) reported a cutoff value for the rollover ratio of 0.25, whereas Meyer and Mishler (1985) reported a cutoff value of 0.35. If the rollover ratio is greater than the selected cutoff value, it should raise the suspicion that there may be some 8th cranial nerve disorder. For the example in Figure 8–8B, the patient with the 8th cranial nerve disorder shows a rollover ratio of 0.38, whereas the patient with the cochlear disorder shows a rollover ratio of 0.035.

Computer-Assisted Speech Perception Assessment Test (CASPA)

Unfortunately, a PI–PB function is often not performed clinically because of the additional time required. However, a more contemporary speech recognition test, Computer-Assisted Speech Perception Assessment Test (CASPA), developed by Boothroyd (1999), offers promise for obtaining a PI–PB function in a reasonably short time period. The CASPA uses phoneme scoring as a way to increase the number of test items without increasing the test time. The CASPA uses only 10 words (30 phonemes) at each presentation level. The word lists and the calculations of the phoneme and/or word scores are done by the computer software (the tester indicates which phonemes are correctly identified). With the CASPA, multiple levels can be tested in a shorter time period than possible with traditional PI–PB testing using half-lists (25 words) and whole word scoring. The CASPA has 16 different word lists balanced for phonemes and inter-list equivalency (Mackersie, Boothroyd, & Minniear, 2001), and also has 20 Spanish lists (Haro, 2005).

STEPS FOR OBTAINING WORD RECOGNITION SCORE (WRS)

Testing for WRS includes the following authors' recommended procedures:

1. Select the presentation level:
   a. Multiple-level testing (e.g., CASPA) is recommended in order to provide a PI–PB function and establish PB_{max}.
   b. If only one level is to be performed, consider the question being asked (many possibilities exist) to determine the presentation level. However, for maximizing acoustic information available to the patient, set the presentation level (in dB SL) relative to the 2000 Hz pure-tone threshold as recommended by Guthrie and Mackersie (2009) or use UCL –5 dB.
   c. For the selected presentation level, determine if masking is needed in the non-test ear (see Chapter 9).
2. Present one or more recorded lists of PB words. The use of CASPA or half-lists (25 words) of the NU-6 is recommended.
3. Keep track of the patient's correct and/or incorrect responses.
4. Calculate the WRS as a percentage of correct responses.
   a. For 25 words using phoneme scoring, the WRS is the number of phonemes correct/ 75 × 100.
   b. For 25 words using whole word scoring, the WRS is the number of words correct/ 25 × 100.
   c. For 10 words using phoneme scoring (as with the CASPA), the WRS is the number of phonemes correct/30 × 100.
5. (If needed) Assuming that testing was done at the highest level possible (or if WRS is poorer than expected for the chosen presentation level), repeat the test with a presentation level that is 20 dB lower (especially if suspicious of an 8th cranial nerve disorder).
   a. If the WRS is the same or worse at the 20 dB lower level, then use the score obtained at the higher level as the WRS (PB_{max}).
   b. If the WRS is better by more than 8% at the 20 dB lower level, additional testing

SYNOPSIS 8–2

- The distribution of speech sounds at a normal conversational level ranges from 20 to 50 dB HL: Consonants are generally lower in intensity and higher in frequency; vowels are generally higher in intensity and lower in frequency.
- The speech intelligibility index (SII) weights the acoustic properties of speech and attempts to predict how these properties affect recognition of speech. The SII derives a number from 0.0 (none of the acoustic speech components available) to 1.0 (all of the acoustic speech components available).
- A clinical version of the SII is called the count-the-dots audiogram (Killion & Mueller, 2010), whereby the frequency/intensity components are represented as 100 dots distributed across the audiogram with frequency weightings based on relative importance to speech recognition. When a patient's hearing loss is superimposed with the dots, it can be a useful counseling or planning tool.
- Word recognition score (WRS) is obtained as a routine part of the audiologic evaluation to estimate how a patient's hearing loss affects speech understanding at one or more selected presentation levels depending on the question to be answered.
- WRS testing involves presenting single-syllable phonemically balanced (PB) words, such as the NU-6 word list, and obtaining a percent correct score.
  - Although the NU-6 has several lists of 50 words (full-lists), most audiologists use lists of 25 words (half-lists) to save time.
  - WRS can be calculated as whole word scores or phoneme scores (three phonemes per word). Phoneme scoring has the advantage of more items to score for a limited number of words, and this can reduce the variability of the test.
- The selection of WRS presentation level will depend on the question you are trying to answer. Speech testing levels should always be lower than the patient's UCL. There are many options for selecting the presentation level for WRS including (where relevant):
  - Multiple levels (PI–PB function/CASPA)
  - X dB SL above 2000 Hz threshold based on Guthrie and Mackersie (2009)
  - UCL –5 dB or 85 dB HL
  - 30 to 40 dB above the SRT or the three- or four-frequency PTA
  - MCL
  - 50 dB HL (normal conversational level)
- A PI-PB function is used to assess WRS at multiple levels in order to identify a patient's true PB_{max} or to determine if there is rollover, a sign of an 8th cranial nerve disorder.
  - The authors suggest using the CASPA to efficiently define the PI–PB function.
  - Alternatively, it is suggested that testing be performed first at UCL –5 dB and then at a level that is 20 dB lower. If the lower level produces a better WRS, then additional levels should be tested to determine the PB_{max} and PB_{min}.
  - Rollover ratio is calculated as $(PB_{max} - PB_{min})/PB_{max}$. A rollover ratio for NU-6 word lists > 0.35 suggests the possibility of 8th cranial nerve involvement and should be evaluated in context with the other information or results.

at even lower levels is required to define the PB_{max} and to determine if there may be significant rollover.

INTERPRETING WORD RECOGNITION SCORES

Obtaining the WRS is a routine part of the audiologic evaluation and can be used to: (a) estimate how a patient's hearing loss affects speech understanding at normal conversational level (45 to 50 dB HL) or at a comfortable listening level, (b) compare performance between the two ears, (c) compare performance across time, and (d) provide a more relevant stimulus to assess how a patient performs with a hearing aid.

Audiologists typically report the WRS on the audiogram with some type of limited interpretation, such as, "Speech recognition ability appears to be good (or fair, or poor)." Table 8–3 gives some common categories for generally describing speech abilities based on WRS. For normal hearing listeners and those with conductive hearing losses, the WRS is usually above 90%. For cochlear hearing losses, the WRS will vary considerably depending on the degree and shape of the hearing loss. For an 8th cranial nerve disorder, such as an acoustic tumor, the WRS can be poorer than one would expect based on the audiometric configuration, called *phonemic regression*. Although the categorical descriptors might be useful in providing some simple feedback to the patient, they do not provide much useful information regarding the significance of the scores relative to what is expected for the de-

TABLE 8–3. Commonly Used Categories to Generally Describe Results of Word Recognition Score (WRS) Testing

WRS (% Correct)	Degree of Impairment	Word Recognition Ability
100–90	None	Excellent/normal
89–75	Slight	Good
74–60	Moderate	Fair
59–50	Poor	Poor
<50	Very poor	Very poor

gree of hearing loss, the significance of any differences between the two ears, or changes that occur over time. To be more meaningful, WRS interpretation must be based on available data in the literature, which leads to better decisions about the significance of the WRS appropriate for good evidence-based practice. In the following sections, you will learn how to answer some clinical questions regarding interpretation of WRS based on available data.

Critical Differences in WRS Based on the Binomial Distribution

Is there a significant difference in WRS between the two ears?

Has there been a significant change in WRS since the previous test?

Is the patient better off with a hearing aid than without one?

Is the WRS significantly better with one hearing aid or another?

The questions listed above involve making decisions about whether two word recognition scores are significantly different from each other, taking into account the inherent variability of the scores for selected test parameters. The appropriate answers to these questions can be found by referring to established data based on a *binomial distribution*, which was made popular by Thornton and Raffin (1978). The binomial distribution is a statistically derived table of probabilities to describe WRS variability (standard deviation) as a function of test items and test scores (Gelfand, 2015). The variability of the WRS test decreases as the number of test items increases, and at the extremes of the word recognition scores the variability is lower for a 50-item word list than for a 25-item word list, and is lower at the upper and lower ends of the WRS percent correct continuum. This means that a greater difference in scores is required for a 25-item word list compared to a 50-item word list in order to be significantly different, and a greater difference in scores is required for scores in the middle of the percent correct continuum, compared with the upper and lower extremes, in order to be significantly different.

The application of the binomial distribution to WRS data can be used to produce a *critical differences table* that can be used to compare any two word recognition scores. In other words, how different do two scores have to be from each other in order for the difference to be significantly different at the 95% confidence interval? The application of the binomial distribution can be used to determine critical difference values for whole word scores or for phoneme scores when properly adjusted (Boothroyd, 2008; Carney & Schlauch, 2007). Table 8–4 provides the critical differences (95% confidence intervals) based on the binomial distribution from Boothroyd (2008) that can be used to compare two WRS scores (whole-word or phoneme) for a specified numbers of test items. To use Table 8–4, find the row that represents the lower of the two scores being compared, then move horizontally to find where that row intersects the column that represents the number of words being scored; the number in the intersecting cell is the upper end of the confidence interval (critical value). To be significantly different from the patient's lower score, the patient's higher score must be greater than the intersecting column number. If the second score is less than or equal to the intersecting column number, the two scores cannot be considered significantly different (may occur due to some level of chance). For example, suppose you obtain word recognition scores of 68% and 88% for the right and left ears, respectively, based on whole word scoring for lists of 25 words. To determine if there is a significant difference in WRS between the two ears, find the row that corresponds to a score of 68%, and then find where that row intersects the column associated with 25 words; the critical value found in the intersecting cell is 91. That means that scores between 68% and 91% are not significantly different from each other. For this example, you should report that the word recognition scores between the two ears are not significantly different based on critical differences from the binomial distribution. The critical differences in Table 8–4 can also be used with phoneme scoring by multiplying the number of whole words by 2.5 phonemes per

word (rather than 3).[1] In other words, if phoneme scoring is used for a list with 25 words, you would use the column labeled 63 number of items. For example, suppose two phoneme scores being compared are 74% and 92%. The intersecting cell for 74% (row) and 63 items (column) shows a critical value of 88%; this means that the second phoneme score of 92%, which is higher than the critical value, is significantly different from 74%. Using these critical differences, based on the binomial 95% confidence intervals, you can assess if a patient performance is significantly different between the two ears, has changed over time, or shows better performance with one hearing aid over another hearing aid.

Differential Diagnoses of Cochlear versus 8th Cranial Nerve Disorders

The use of speech audiometry for differential diagnosis of cochlear related hearing loss versus 8th cranial nerve related hearing loss is not as important as it was 20 years ago. Since that time, audiologists have relied on physiologic tests, like acoustic reflexes and auditory brainstem responses, and there have also been tremendous advances in medical imaging techniques that are quite sensitive to 8th cranial nerve tumor diagnoses. However, since WRS is obtained as a routine part of the audiologic evaluation, its proper interpretation may signal the need for further evaluation if suspicions of an 8th cranial nerve disorder are raised. As described in an earlier section, a patient with an 8th cranial nerve disorder may have phonemic regression such that the WRS is disproportionately poorer than predicted based on the audiometric configuration and/or expectations for cochlear hearing losses. The calculation of a significant rollover ratio should raise your suspicion of an 8th cranial nerve disorder.

It would be nice to know, with confidence, how poor a WRS must be to suggest an 8th cranial nerve disorder. Unfortunately, there are very

---

[1]Because of the interdependence among the 3 phonemes, a multiplier of 2.5 is used instead of 3 (Boothroyd, personal communication, September 20, 2007).

TABLE 8–4. Critical Difference Values for PB Words Based on the Binomial Distribution

95% Confidence		Number of Items (phoneme scoring = 2.5 number of words)						Number of Items			
		10	25	50	63			10	25	50	63
The lower of the two scores being compared (in %)	0	33	15	8	6	The lower of the two scores being compared (in %)	50	91	77	70	68
	1	36	17	10	9		51	91	78	71	68
	2	38	20	12	11		52	92	79	71	69
	3	40	22	14	13		53	93	80	72	70
	4	41	23	16	14		54	93	81	73	71
	5	43	25	18	16		55	94	81	74	72
	6	45	27	19	17		56	95	82	75	73
	7	47	29	21	19		57	95	83	76	74
	8	48	30	22	20		58	96	84	77	75
	9	50	32	24	22		59	96	84	78	76
	10	51	33	25	23		60	97	85	78	77
	11	53	35	27	25		61	97	86	79	77
	12	54	36	28	26		62	98	87	80	78
	13	55	38	29	27		63	98	87	81	79
	14	57	39	31	29		64	99	88	82	80
	15	58	40	32	30		65	99	89	83	81
	16	59	42	33	31		66	100	90	83	82
	17	61	43	34	32		67	100	90	84	82
	18	62	44	36	34		68	100	91	85	83
	19	63	45	37	35		69	100	92	86	84
	20	64	47	38	36		70	100	92	87	85
	21	65	48	39	37		71	100	93	87	86
	22	66	49	41	38		72	100	93	88	86
	23	68	50	42	40		73	100	94	89	87
	24	69	51	43	41		74	100	95	89	88
	25	70	53	44	42		75	100	95	90	89
	26	71	54	45	43		76	100	96	91	89
	27	72	55	46	44		77	100	96	92	90
	28	73	56	47	45		78	100	97	92	91
	29	74	57	48	46		79	100	97	93	92
	30	75	58	50	47		80	100	98	94	92
	31	76	59	51	48		81	100	98	94	93
	32	77	60	52	50		82	100	99	95	94
	33	77	61	53	51		83	100	99	95	94
	34	78	62	54	52		84	100	100	96	95
	35	79	63	55	53		85	100	100	97	96
	36	80	64	56	54		86	100	100	97	96
	37	81	65	57	55		87	100	100	98	97
	38	82	66	58	56		88	100	100	98	97
	39	83	67	59	57		89	100	100	99	98
	40	83	68	60	58		90	100	100	99	98
	41	84	69	61	59		91	100	100	100	99
	42	85	70	62	60		92	100	100	100	99
	43	86	71	63	61		93	100	100	100	100
	44	87	72	64	62		94	100	100	100	100
	45	87	73	65	63		95	100	100	100	100
	46	88	74	66	64		96	100	100	100	100
	47	89	75	67	65		97	100	100	100	100
	48	89	75	68	66		98	100	100	100	100
	49	90	76	69	67		99	100	100	100	100

Note. Courtesy of Arthur Boothroyd and Carol Mackersie. Modified with permission. Find where lower score (*row*) intersects number of items scored (*column*).

little published data to make that determination. Dubno, Lee, Klein, Matthews, and Lam (1995) provided lower 95% confidence limits for PB$_{max}$ as a function of pure-tone average (PTA) for patients with confirmed sloping high frequency cochlear hearing losses. Table 8–5 shows the data from Dubno et al. as a function of PTA for 25-item word lists (whole-word scoring). Based on these data, if the PB$_{max}$ is below the lower 95% confidence limit for cochlear ears shown in Table 8–5, the score would be considered disproportionately low and further evaluation for a possible 8th cranial nerve disorder may be warranted. If the WRS is poorer than the lower 95% confidence limit, a PI–PB function should be obtained to determine if there is significant rollover before deciding that the WRS is suggestive of an 8th cranial nerve disorder. Validation of these values with a population of patients with confirmed 8th cranial nerve disorders has not been conducted; therefore, audiologists must use this method of interpretation with some caution based on a single study with cochlear hearing losses.

SPEECH-IN-NOISE TESTS

The speech measures described above are usually presented in quiet. However, there are many other speech measures that are designed to assess how well a patient can recognize speech in the presence of different levels of background noise, thus obtaining measures of speech recognition that may be more representative of real-world listening situations. A primary complaint for many people with hearing loss is that even though they may hear people talking, they have difficulty understanding what is being said, especially when there is background noise. These tests typically present speech materials for different levels of noise, called a speech-to-noise ratio (SNR). For example, if the speech material is presented at 50 dB HL and the noise is presented in the same ear at 45 dB HL, this would be considered a +5 SNR (also designated +5 S/N). Some commonly used speech-in-noise tests include the NU-6 with speech spectrum noise or multitalker babble, the Speech Perception in Noise (SPIN) test, the Synthetic Sentence Identification (SSI)

TABLE 8–5. Lower 95% Confidence Limits for WRS as a Function of PTA (500, 1000, 2000 Hz) in Ears with Cochlear Hearing Loss

PTA (dB HL)	Lower 95% Confidence Limit For WRS (percent) based on 25-item NU-6 word lists	PTA (dB HL)	Lower 95% Confidence Limit For WRS (percent) based on 25-item NU-6 word lists
–3.3	100	36.7	68
0.0	100	38.3	64
1.7	100	40.0	64
3.3	96	41.7	60
5.0	96	43.3	56
6.7	96	45.0	56
8.3	96	46.7	52
10.0	96	48.3	52
11.7	92	50.0	48
13.3	92	51.7	48
15.0	92	53.3	44
16.7	88	55.0	44
18.3	88	56.7	40
20.0	88	58.3	40
21.7	84	60.0	36
23.3	84	61.7	36
25.0	80	63.3	32
26.7	80	65.0	32
38.3	76	66.6	32
30.0	76	68.3	28
31.7	72	70.0	28
33.3	72	71.7	34
35.0	68		

Note: Data shown are for 25-item NU-6 word lists.

See Dubno et al. for results using a 50-item word lists.

Source: Confidence-limits for maximum word-recognition scores, by J. R. Dubno, F. S. Lee, A. J. Klein, L. J. Mathews, & C. F. Lam, 1995, *Journal of Speech and Hearing Research, 38.* Copyright 1995 by American Speech-Language-Hearing Association. Adapted with permission.

test with a competing story, the Quick Sentence in Noise (QuickSIN) test, Bamford-Kowal-Bench Speech in Noise (BKB-SIN) and the Hearing in Noise Test (HINT).

The QuickSIN test was developed by Etymotic Research (Niquette, Gudmundsen, & Killion, 2001) as a clinically useful method of quickly measuring speech identification in noise to evaluate a patient's performance with and without hearing aids. The QuickSIN test embeds key words in unpredictable sentences. The test sentences are presented in background noise that is made up of four people speaking different sentences (four-talker babble) with varying signal-to-noise ratios (SNRs). Each sentence has five key words that must be correctly identified. The test is given at 70 dB HL for those with a PTA less than 45 dB HL or at MCL for those with a PTA greater than 50 dB HL. The test presents one sentence at each SNR, beginning at +25 SNR (easiest) and decreasing in 5 dB steps to 0 SNR (most difficult). The patient's SNR is compared with the SNR expected for normal hearing listeners to get a final score, called SNR loss.

The HINT measures how well a person is able to correctly identify sentences as a function of different speech-to-noise ratios. The HINT has been standardized on a relatively large population (Nilsson, Soli, & Sullivan, 1994). The HINT is available as a computer-based software CD that can work with the audiometer or as a stand-alone unit in which everything is done through the computer. In either situation, the computer presents the sentence material, adjusts the level of the sentences following rules based on how the patient responds (i.e., the level is decreased for each correct response and increased for each incorrect response), and then calculates how the patient performs relative to the standardized database. The typical HINT has the background noise set at 65 dBA,[2] then the sentences are presented at varying levels until a speech-to-noise ratio is obtained that represents the point where 50% correct sentence identification occurs, called the reception threshold for sentences (RTS). The HINT can be used to test the ears binaurally (with sentences and noise presented to both ears at the same time) or with the sentences in one ear and the noise in the other ear. The HINT can be performed under earphones for diagnostic applications or in a sound field for hearing aid applications. The RTS can be used to compare the patient's performance with mean data from normal hearing listeners, or it can be used to determine how much the patient's hearing-in-noise ability is improved with different hearing aids.

VARIATIONS WITH YOUNG CHILDREN OR DIFFICULT-TO-TEST POPULATIONS

As with pure-tone audiometry, modifications are needed with speech audiometry when testing young children or other difficult-to-test populations. These modifications are usually necessary for children younger than 6 years of age or any patient who is difficult to test using the adult procedures. As a test stimulus, speech is more familiar to children than the more abstract pure-tone stimuli and has an inherently higher reinforcement value. In many cases, audiologists prefer to begin testing young children with speech audiometry in order to make the child more comfortable with the testing situation, and to obtain some information about their hearing abilities in case pure-tone testing cannot be completed. As with pure-tone audiometry, the tester must be enthusiastic, offer a lot of positive reinforcement, and be flexible. Earphones should always be attempted first to get ear-specific information; however, sound-field testing can be performed when needed. Typically, monitored live voice is used with young children due to the need for flexibility, but recorded materials are available. The primary goal is to obtain a speech recognition threshold and a measure of word recognition ability. The different strategies and speech materials for testing young children are described in the following sections.

Speech Recognition Threshold (SRT)

As with adults, the SRT requires that the child indicate somehow that he or she understands the word and/or is able to repeat the word correctly. When this is not possible, then an SDT should be obtained using VRA or conditioned-play techniques if necessary (see earlier section on SDT for interpretation). Obtaining an SRT for a young child is very important because it may be the

---

[2]dBA is a representation of a noise level as measured with a sound level meter with an A-weighted filter network designed to better match the human audibility curve. The A-weighting attenuates frequencies below 700 Hz and above 9000 Hz.

best indicator of his or her degree of hearing loss in the speech frequencies and can be a good validation of the pure-tone thresholds.

It is usually better to use words that are familiar to the child, so often the audiologist will use selected items from the adult spondee word list or ask the caregiver which words are in the child's vocabulary. There is also a list of children's spondee words available that is composed of words more likely to be in the child's vocabulary. For those children with a limited expressive vocabulary or reluctance to provide verbal responses, the SRT can be obtained by having the child point to spondee picture cards or objects (lay out four to six cards or objects). With advances in computer-based audiometry, these pictures may be displayed on the computer screen, and when the child touches the correct picture he or she receives some type of visual reward on the screen. Another commonly used strategy is to have the child point to different body parts ("Show me your nose."). This can also be done by having the child point to the body parts on an inanimate character, like a doll or clown. This differs from testing adults in that the words may not be spondees and there is a *carrier phrase*, but these variations are not problematic.

The procedure for finding the lowest level at which the child can respond to the speech stimuli is also less formalized than for adults. Since time is critical when testing children, many audiologists use an up-10-down-20 bracketing procedure, where one word is given at each level and the level adjusted up 10 dB if they do not respond correctly and down 20 dB if they do respond correctly. With a cooperative child, the up-5-down-10 bracketing could be used. Another approach is to present four to six words at each presentation level beginning 20 to 30 dB above threshold and decreasing in 5 dB (or 10 dB) steps until he or she misses half of the words. Whatever procedure is used, the goal is to estimate the SRT as the lowest level where the child responds to about half of the words.

Suprathreshold Speech Recognition Scores

Information about a child's ability to recognize speech is performed using procedures similar to those recommended for adults; however, the materials must be within the child's vocabulary. As with adults, the WRS is a percentage of words correctly identified. For children 5 to 6 years old, there is a PBK-50 word list (composed of words appropriate for children of kindergarten age) that is commonly used and presented in the same

---

SYNOPSIS 8–3

- The WRS is often categorized in descriptive terms, such as excellent, good, fair, or poor. Patients with normal hearing or conductive hearing losses are expected to have excellent WRS (WRS > 90%); those with cochlear hearing losses may vary across all categories in a generally predictable way based on the degree and shape of their hearing loss; those with 8th nerve involvement may have disproportionately poorer WRS than would be predicted from their audiogram.
- It is often useful to evaluate whether the WRS from one ear is different from the other, if there has been a change over time, or if performance is better with one hearing aid than another. To determine whether two scores are significantly different from each other, a table of critical difference values based on a binomial distribution table is required (e.g., see Table 8–4) that provides 95% confidence limits when comparing two scores (with similar methods). If the two scores are within the 95% confidence values provided by the binomial distribution, they cannot be considered statistically different from each other.

SYNOPSIS 8–3 (continued)

- Data showing lower 95% confidence intervals for the NU-6 word lists for cochlear hearing losses as a function of PTA are available (Dubno et al., 1995) (see Table 8–5). A WRS that is poorer than the lower 95% confidence interval for cochlear hearing losses suggests an 8th nerve disorder, and you should determine if the results are consistent with the other diagnostic information to suggest an 8th nerve problem or whether the patient has poor word recognition for other reasons.
- Speech recognition testing in the presence of background noise is sometimes included in the evaluation to obtain information about how a patient might be performing in more real-world situations. Commonly used speech-in-noise tests include the BKB-SIN, QuickSIN, and the HINT.
- For testing children between 3 and 6 years of age, there are special tests available to obtain a measure of suprathreshold speech recognition, most of which include pointing to the correct word from a group of four to six pictures of familiar objects. For SRT, pointing to pictures or to familiar body parts is often used.

way as the adult PB word lists. When interpreting speech recognition scores for children, it is important to use materials that are standardized for the age being tested and to interpret the findings according to the test's manual. Most of the standardized speech recognition tests for young children involve pointing to the requested picture from a group of four to six items. Examples of tests appropriate for children in the 3- to 6-year-old range include the Word Identification by Picture Identification (WIPI), Northwestern University Children's Perception of Speech (NU-CHIPS), and the Pediatric Speech Intelligibility (PSI). The WIPI and PSI can be tested with or without background noise. A special version of the HINT (HINT-C) is also available for children 6 to 12 years of age.

REFERENCES

American National Standards Institute [ANSI]. (1997). Method for the calculation of the speech intelligibility index, *ANSI S3.5-1997*. New York, NY: Author.

American National Standards Institute [ANSI]. (2010). Specifications for audiometers, *ANSI S3.6-2010*. New York, NY: Author.

American Speech-Language-Hearing Association [ASHA]. (1988). Guidelines for determining the threshold level for speech. *ASHA, 30*, 85–89.

Bess, F. H., Josey, A. F., & Humes, L. E. (1979). Performance intensity functions in cochlear and eighth nerve disorders. *The American Journal of Otology, 1*(1), 27–31.

Boothroyd, A. (1999). *Computer-Assisted Speech Perception Assessment (CASPA) (Version 3)*. Computer software available from Dr Boothroyd upon request.

Boothroyd, A. (2008). Table of critical differences based on the binomial distribution. Personal communication.

Brandy, W. T. (Ed.) (2002). *Speech Audiometry* (5th ed.). Baltimore, MD: Lippincott Williams & Wilkins.

Cambron, N. K., Wilson, R. H., & Shanks, J. E. (1991). Spondaic word detection and recognition functions for female and male speakers. *Ear and Hearing, 12*, 64–70.

Carney, E., & Schlauch, R. S. (2007). Critical difference table for word recognition testing derived using computer simulation. *Journal Speech Language Hearing Research, 50*, 1203–1209.

Chaiklin, J. B., Font, J., & Dixon, R. F. (1967). Spondaic thresholds measured in ascending 5 dB steps. *Journal Speech and Hearing Research, 10*, 141–145.

Chaiklin, J. B., & Ventry, I. M. (1964). Spondee threshold measurement: A comparison of 2 and 5-dB methods. *Journal of Speech and Hearing Disorders,* *29,* 47–59.

Dirks, D. D., & Kamm, C. (1976). Psychometric functions for loudness discomfort and most comfortable loudness levels. *Journal of Speech and Hearing Research, 19,* 613–627.

Downs, D., & Minard, P. (1996). A fast valid method to measure speech-recognition threshold. *Hearing Journal, 49,* 39–44.

Dubno, J. R., Lee, F. S., Klein, A. J., Matthews, L. J., & Lam, C. F. (1995). Confidence limits for maximum word-recognition scores. *Journal of Speech and Hearing Research, 38*(2), 490–502.

Fletcher, H. (1950). A method of calculating hearing loss for speech from an audiogram. *Acta Otolaryngologica Suppl,* 26–37.

French, N. R., & Steinberg, J. C. (1947). Factors governing the intelligibility of speech sounds. *Journal of the Acoustical Society of America, 19,* 90–119.

Gelfand, S. A. (2015). *Essentials of Audiology* (4th ed.). New York, NY: Thieme.

Guthrie, L., & Mackersie, C. L. (2009). A comparison of presentation levels to maximize word recognition scores. *Journal of the American Academy of Audiology, 20,* 381–390.

Haro, N. (2005). *Spanish Word Lists for Speech Audiometry* (AuD Doctoral Research Project). San Diego State University.

Hirsh, I. J., Davis, H., Silverman, S. R., Reynolds, E. G., Eldert, E., & Benson, R. W. (1952). Development of materials for speech audiometry. *Journal of Speech and Hearing Disorders, 17,* 321–337.

Humes, L. E. (1991). Understanding the speech-understanding problems of the hearing impaired. *Journal of the American Academy of Audiology, 2*(2), 59–69.

Jerger, J., & Jerger, S. (1971). Diagnostic significance of PB word functions. *Archives of Otolaryngology, 93,* 573–580.

Kamm, C., Dirks, D. D., & Mickey, M. R. (1978). Effect of sensorineural hearing loss on loudness discomfort level and most comfortable loudness judgments. *Journal of Speech and Hearing Research, 21*(4), 668–681.

Killion, M. C., & Mueller, H. G. (2010). Twenty years later: A new count-the-dots method. *The Hearing Journal, 63,* 10–17.

Mackersie, C. L., Boothroyd, A., & Minniear, D. (2001). Evaluation of the Computer-assisted Speech Perception Assessment Test (CASPA). *Journal of the American Academy of Audiology, 12*(8), 390–396.

Maroonroge, S., & Diefendorf, A. O. (1984). Comparing normal hearing and hearing-impaired subjects' performance on the Northwestern Auditory Test Number 6, California Consonant Test, and Pascoe's High-Frequency Word Test. *Ear and Hearing, 5*(6), 356–360.

Martin, F. N., & Dowdy, L. K. (1986). A modified spondee threshold procedure. *Journal of Auditory Research, 26,* 115–119.

Meyer, D. H., & Mishler, E. T. (1985). Rollover measurements with Auditec NU-6 word lists. *Journal of Speech and Hearing Disorders, 50,* 356–360.

Mueller, H. G., & Killion, M. C. (1990). An easy method for calculating the articulation index. *Hearing Journal, 43* 14–17.

Nilsson, M., Soli, S. D., & Sullivan, J. A. (1994). Development of the hearing in noise test for the measurement of speech reception thresholds in quiet and noise. *Journal of the Acoustical Society of America, 95,* 1085–1099.

Niquette, P., Gudmundsen, G., & Killion, M. C. (2001). *QuickSIN Documentation.* Elk Grove, IL: Etymotic Research.

Pavlovic, C. V. (1988). Articulation index predictions of speech intelligibility in hearing aid selection. *ASHA Leader, 30*(6–7), 63–65.

Punch, J., Rakerd, B., & Joseph, A. (2004). Effects of test order on most comfortable and uncomfortable loudness levels for speech. *American Journal of Audiology, 13,* 158–163.

Silman, S., & Silverman, C. (1991). *Auditory Diagnosis: Principles and Applications.* San Diego, CA: Academic Press.

Thibodeau, L. (2007). Speech audiometry. In M. Roeser, M. Valente, & H. Hosford-Dunn (Eds.), *Audiology Diagnosis* (2nd ed.). New York, NY: Thieme.

Thornton, A. R., & Raffin, M. J. (1978). Speech-discrimination scores modeled as a binomial variable. *Journal of Speech and Hearing Research, 21*(3), 507–518.

Tillman, T. W., & Carhart, R. (1966). An expanded test for speech discrimination utilizing CNC monosyllabic words, Northwestern University Auditory Test No. 6. *Technical Report SAM-TR-66-55.* Brooks AFB, TX: USAF School of Aerospace Medicine.

Tillman, T. W., & Jerger, J. F. (1959). Some factors affecting the spondee threshold in normal hearing subjects. *Journal of Speech and Hearing Research 2,* 141–146.

9

Masking for Pure-Tone and Speech Audiometry

After reading this chapter, you should be able to:

1. Understand why the non-test ear (NTE) needs to be masked in some cases in order to obtain true thresholds in the test ear (TE).

2. Know what is meant by interaural attenuation (IA) and the minimum IA values used for each transducer when making decisions about the need to obtain masked thresholds.

3. Recognize, from the unmasked thresholds, when masked thresholds must be obtained; apply the decision-making rules for masking when testing by air conduction (AC) using supra-aural earphones or insert earphones and by bone conduction (BC).

4. Describe the types of maskers used for pure-tone and speech testing.

5. Define effective masking (EM) and how the maskers are calibrated and used with the audiometer.

6. Describe the occlusion effect (OE) and why this needs to be considered when masking for BC.

7. Describe two advantages of insert earphones over supra-aural earphones as they relate to masking.

8. Define what is meant by a masking plateau and how much of a plateau is appropriate. Discuss why the width of the plateau is smaller when there is a potential bilateral moderate conductive loss.

9. Define overmasking and masking dilemma, and recognize situations in which these may occur.

10. Apply the specific steps for AC and BC masking using the plateau method for a variety of unmasked audiograms.

11. Apply the rules for determining if masking is needed for speech testing, and select adequate amounts of maskers for speech testing.

The process of putting noise, called a *masker*, into the non-test ear (NTE), while measuring responses from the test ear (TE), is called *masking* (or *clinical masking*). The threshold obtained in the TE is called the *masked* threshold, and implies that the masker was delivered to the NTE. In order to be able to deliver a masker into the NTE, a two-channel audiometer is needed so that the test sound (tones or speech) can be routed to the TE through one channel, and the masker can be routed to the NTE through the second channel. Most clinical audiometers automatically route the masker to the NTE when masking is selected.

In Chapter 7, some basic principles of masking were presented so that you would understand why unmasked or masked symbols are used on an audiogram to represent a patient's pure-tone thresholds. To be clinically useful, audiometric measures are expected to be true representations of the TE and not a reflection of hearing by the NTE. In Chapter 7, the principles of masking were presented as they pertained to thresholds for pure tones; however, as you will see in a later section of this chapter, when doing speech testing you must also be cognizant of the possible need for masking to prevent the speech signals from being heard in the NTE. This chapter provides details on when masking is needed and how to perform masking. The first part of the chapter will focus on masking for pure-tone thresholds and the second part of the chapter will focus on masking for speech tests.

There are many testing situations in which the sound presented to the TE can set up vibrations in the skull that potentially could be picked up by the NTE: When testing by bone conduction (BC) at any intensity level or when testing by air conduction (AC) at moderate and higher intensity levels, the sound vibrations can occur in the bones of the skull and, therefore, are able to be received by both cochleae through bone conduction. This becomes especially problematic when the NTE has better hearing than the TE, since the patient's response to the sound delivered to the TE could actually be a result of the patient hearing the sound through bone conduction in the NTE. When the signal delivered to the patient's TE is audible in the NTE, it is referred to as *cross-hearing*. Keep in mind that cross-hearing to the NTE (during AC or BC testing) always occurs by bone conduction (Studebaker, 1962; Zwislocki, 1953). Whenever cross-hearing could occur, masking of the NTE will be needed. To prevent the patient from hearing the sound that may be heard through cross-hearing in the NTE, a masker (noise) is delivered to the NTE. The patient is instructed to respond only to the pure tones or speech signals in the ear being tested, and to ignore the noise that he or she will hear in the other ear.

INTERAURAL ATTENUATION

It is fairly easy to understand that when the bone vibrator is on the mastoid of one ear, the other cochlea is also being stimulated because it is also imbedded in the skull. However, are both ears receiving the sound at the same intensity? In other words, is there some attenuation of the sound in the NTE compared to the TE? *Interaural attenuation (IA)* is a term that is used to quantify the difference in the level of the signal presented in the TE (by AC or BC) to the level of the signal that occurs in the NTE (by BC). Another way of thinking about this is to ask how much does the level of the signal in the TE have to be before it is capable of being heard in the NTE (by BC)? Furthermore, if the NTE is capable of hearing the sound presented to the TE (i.e., cross-hearing occurs), masking the NTE would be needed in order to establish the true thresholds in the TE.

Ranges of IA values have been determined for different transducers by several studies (e.g., Chaiklin, 1967; Coles, 1970; Sanders & Rintleman, 1964; Sklare & Denenberg, 1987; Studebaker, 1967). For BC testing, the IA is considered to be 0 dB, that is, the BC sound is the same level in both ears. For AC testing, the level of the pure tone presented to the TE that can cause vibrations of the skull are different for supra-aural earphones and insert earphones; insert earphones have a higher IA. The difference is primarily dependent on the relative surface area of the skull that is exposed to the sound from the different AC transducers; supra-aural earphones have a larger area of exposure to the skull than insert earphones. Figure 9–1 shows a comparison of the averages and ranges of IA values for supra-aural earphones and insert earphones. The IA varies somewhat across frequency, and will also vary across patients; however, for clinical purposes, minimum IA values are adopted instead of mean IA values to ensure that you do not miss masking someone with an IA below the average. The minimum IA for supra-aural earphones has been widely accepted as 40 dB. This means that, when testing with supra-aural earphones, vibrations of the skull can occur at levels greater than or equal to ($\geq$) 40 dB HL. For insert earphones, a single minimum IA value has not yet been universally accepted or described in any standards. As you can see in Figure 9–1, the IA values for insert earphones are greater in the lower frequencies than in the higher frequencies. The IA values for insert earphones can also vary depending on depth of the earphone insertion; if not inserted deep enough, the IA may be less. Some audiologists choose to use a different minimum IA depending on the frequency when using insert earphones. However, the authors of this textbook have adopted a minimum IA for insert earphones of 55 dB for all frequencies. This is a conservative, yet reasonable value, and simplifies the concept of masking with insert earphones by adopting one minimum IA value for all frequencies.[1] The following are the minimum IA values adopted for this textbook for the different transducers:

IA for bone vibrator = 0 dB

IA for supra-aural earphones = 40 dB

IA for insert earphones = 55 dB

The reliance on minimum IA values allows you to decide if masking is necessary, but does not necessarily mean that the patient's actual IA is at the minimum level. In fact, most patients

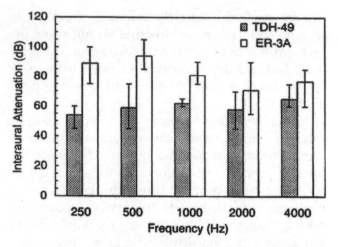

FIGURE 9–1. Comparison of interaural attenuation values for supra-aural earphones and insert earphones. *Source*: From Sklare and Denneberg, 1987, p. 298. Copyright 1987 by Lippincott Williams & Wilkins.

will have an IA higher than the minimum, but you do not know, nor have the time to measure the IA for each patient. However, in many cases, you can see from the unmasked thresholds on an audiogram that the patient's IA is higher than the minimum when you compare the unmasked AC threshold in the TE to the BC threshold in the NTE. For example, if a patient has an unmasked AC threshold in the TE of 65 dB HL and a BC threshold in the NTE of 5 dB HL, that patient's IA is at least 60 dB (and may even be more than 60 dB). However, you would still make the decision to use masking because 60 dB is greater than the minimum IA for either of the AC transducers.

MASKERS

It is important to remember that the masker is always delivered by an AC transducer. If the masker was to be delivered by a BC transducer, then the masker would always be heard in both ears, making it impossible to get a true response from the TE. But by presenting the masking noise with an earphone, there is a range of masker levels (at least 40 dB HL with supra-aural earphones and at least 55 dB HL with insert earphones) that

---

[1]This conservative minimum is based on the lowest IA, which occurs at 2000 to 4000 Hz. For lower frequencies, the minimum IA is at least 65 dB. Some audiologists may use IAs higher than the 55 dB minimum IA adopted for this textbook.

can be applied before the cochlea of the TE is stimulated by the noise. In other words, using insert earphones to present the masker to the NTE would allow at least 55 dB HL of noise to be used before there is any possibility of crossing over to the TE.

The masking noises used in pure-tone threshold audiometry are called *narrowband maskers* (or narrowband noises). For each of the audiometric test frequencies there is a corresponding band of noise (one-third octave wide) centered around the test frequency. Depending on the frequency being tested, you would select the appropriate narrowband masker. For example, if a 1000 Hz pure tone is being presented to the TE, a 1000 Hz narrowband masker would be presented in the NTE. When masking is used for speech testing, a *speech masker* is used instead of a narrowband masker. The speech masker is a broader spectrum noise that encompasses a range of frequencies important for speech recognition. Most audiometers automatically set the masker to the selected test stimulus.

The maskers are calibrated in terms of their *effective masking levels*. Effective masking is a calibrated amount of noise that will provide a threshold shift to a corresponding dB HL for the stimulus centered within the noise (Sanders & Rintleman, 1964; Yacullo, 1996, 2009). For example, 30 dB HL of effective masking for a pure tone will elevate the AC threshold of the corresponding pure tone to 30 dB HL. In practice, effective masking makes the signal no longer audible. The required amounts of noise that correspond to 0 dB HL of effective masking for each audiometric test frequency and speech are specified by the American National Standards Institute (American National Standards Institute [ANSI], 1996, 2010) The ANSI effective masker levels are built into the audiometer (just as for 0 dB HL for the pure tones). In this way, the attenuator dial of the audiometer channel used to deliver the maskers corresponds to the number on the dB HL dial for each needed level of effective masking that is presented to the NTE. To illustrate, if the attenuator dial for the masker is set to 40 dB HL, it means that the masker can effectively elevate/mask the AC threshold for the test signal (pure tone or speech) to 40 dB HL when presented in the same ear. The actual amount of the threshold change that occurs with the masker will depend on the patient's threshold. For example, if the patient's AC threshold is 30 dB HL, then putting in a 40 dB HL effective masker will elevate the patient's threshold *to* 40 dB HL, but the threshold change is only increased *by* 10 dB (40 dB HL effective masking minus 30 dB HL threshold). As you will come to see, it is very important to keep in mind that when you increase (elevate) the AC threshold in the NTE with masking, you also increase the BC threshold by the same amount, but not necessarily to the same dB HL. For instance, in cases where there is an air–bone gap in the NTE, the air–bone gap will remain. As an example, suppose the AC pure-tone threshold in the NTE is 50 dB HL and the BC threshold in the NTE is 30 dB HL (20 dB air–bone gap). When a masker is presented to the NTE by AC with an effective masking level of 60 dB HL, the AC threshold (in the presence of the masker) in the NTE will be elevated to 60 dB HL (a 10 dB increase in threshold) and, therefore, the BC threshold in the NTE will also increase by 10 dB to 40 dB HL (still a 20 dB air–bone gap).

As mentioned earlier, the masker is always presented to the NTE by an AC transducer. When testing for AC thresholds with insert earphones or supra-aural earphones, the sound is presented to the TE through one of the earphones and the masker is presented to the NTE by the other earphone. When testing for BC thresholds, the bone vibrator is placed on the mastoid of the TE and the masker is presented to the NTE by an insert earphone or a supra-aural earphone. If the masker is presented using a supra-aural earphone during BC testing, the other earphone on the headset is placed on the temple next to the eye on the side of the TE.

CENTRAL MASKING

Central masking refers to a small elevation in the threshold of a signal in the TE that occurs when masking noise is presented to the NTE. Central masking may occur even though the level of the noise, either narrowband noise or speech noise, is considerably less than any IA and, therefore, not audible in the TE. The source of this small masking effect is unknown, but is assumed to be due

SYNOPSIS 9–1

- The process of putting noise into the non-test ear (NTE), while measuring responses from the test ear (TE), is called masking. The threshold obtained in the TE is called the masked threshold.
- In order to deliver a masker into the NTE, a two-channel audiometer is needed so that the test tones or speech can be routed to the TE through one channel, and the masker routed to the NTE through the second channel.
- Testing anytime by bone conduction (BC), and testing at moderate to high levels by air conduction (AC) produces vibrations in the skull that can stimulate, through BC, both cochleae.
- Interaural attenuation (IA) is the difference in the level of the signal (by AC or BC) presented to the TE, compared to the level of the signal that occurs in the NTE (by BC).
- The recommended minimum IA values for the different transducers are:
  - BC IA (with bone conduction vibrator) = 0 dB
  - AC IA (with supra-aural earphone) = 40 dB
  - AC IA (with insert earphone) = 55 dB
- Cross-hearing can occur when the difference between the presentation level of the sound in the TE (by AC or BC) and the BC threshold of the NTE is equal to or greater than the minimum IA.
- A noise masker is a sound that is delivered to the NTE that covers/obscures a sound that may cross over to the NTE, thus making it inaudible (masked).
- Maskers used in audiometry are either narrowband noises when masking for pure-tone thresholds or speech spectrum noises when masking for speech tests.
- Central masking is a small (5 dB) threshold shift in the pure-tone or speech threshold that can occur in the TE when masking is presented to the NTE. Central masking is due to some (unknown) effects within the central auditory system. The small threshold shift is not of any real clinical significance.

to some central nervous system reaction to the masker (Konkle & Berry, 1983; Liden, Nilsson, & Anderson, 1959; Yacullo, 2009). The amount of threshold elevation in the TE due to central masking is only about 5 dB HL for pure tones or speech testing. The small effect of central masking can be expected during the masking process, but is generally not of any significance.

WHEN TO MASK FOR AIR CONDUCTION PURE-TONE THRESHOLDS

For AC pure-tone threshold testing, cross-hearing will occur when the IA is exceeded and the pure tone reaching the NTE is greater than the BC threshold of the NTE. The decision on whether to obtain masked thresholds can be determined by comparing the AC presentation level in the TE to the unmasked BC threshold in the NTE; if the difference is greater than the minimum IA for the specific transducer, then masking would be needed. In clinical practice, however, masking for AC is often done before obtaining the BC thresholds because it is more efficient to complete the testing of both ears while the earphones are in place, instead of switching back and forth between AC and BC for each ear. In that case, you can often make your decision to mask for AC testing based on an "assumed" BC threshold of the NTE. In many cases, your assumed BC thresholds of the NTE can be based on other information/test results (e.g., immittance measures). In cases where the difference between the AC thresholds between the two ears is greater than or equal to the minimum IA, you can assume that the BC threshold of the NTE would be at the same or better level than the AC threshold of the NTE, and the decision to mask would still hold. However, it is important to keep in mind that your assumed BC threshold in the NTE may turn out to be incorrect, and you may need to go back and find the masked AC thresholds after the BC thresholds are obtained: For example, if the difference between the AC thresholds of the two ears (AC TE compared to AC NTE) is less than the minimum IA you may decide that masking is not needed; however, after testing by BC, you may find that there is enough of an air–bone gap in the NTE so that the AC threshold in the TE compared to the measured BC threshold in the NTE exceeds the minimum IA, and retesting the AC threshold with masking would be needed. Decisions to mask based on comparing AC to AC of the two ears is only appropriate if the difference is equal to or greater than the minimum IA; if the difference is less than the minimum IA, the decision to mask may need to be delayed until the actual BC thresholds of the NTE are known. Figure 9–2 shows some situations to illustrate when AC masking thresholds would be needed or not (see figure legend for explanation). The general rule for deciding that masking is needed for AC testing is:

> Whenever the difference between the unmasked AC threshold of the TE and the assumed or measured BC threshold of the NTE is $\geq$ 55 dB for insert earphones (or 40 dB for supra-aural earphones), masking is needed to rule out the possibility that the AC threshold is coming from the NTE (by BC).

WHEN TO MASK FOR BONE CONDUCTION PURE-TONE THRESHOLDS

For BC pure-tone threshold testing, cross-hearing to the NTE is a frequent problem, and can occur in the following two conditions: (1) The AC threshold in one ear is $\geq$15 compared to the AC threshold in the other ear; and (2) there is the appearance of a potential air–bone gap for both ears. As discussed earlier, a 10 dB air–bone gap is typically not considered clinically significant, so masking would not be needed. In both of the above conditions, since the IA for BC is 0 dB, you will not know which ear is represented by the unmasked BC threshold. In fact, the unmasked BC symbol only represents the side on which the bone conduction vibrator was placed. Figure 9–3 shows some situations that illustrate when BC masked thresholds would be needed or not (see figure legend for explanation). The general rule for deciding that masking is needed for BC testing is:

> Whenever there is >10 dB difference between the unmasked BC threshold and the AC threshold of the TE (an apparent air–bone gap), masking is needed to rule out the possibility that the BC threshold is coming from the NTE.

APPLYING THE RULES FOR PURE-TONE MASKING

Figure 9–4 shows three examples of audiograms with unmasked thresholds. Each example has a table that indicates (+) where masked thresholds would be needed. In these examples, you should be able to see where the above rules were applied to decide which thresholds for AC or BC would have to be reestablished using masking (masked thresholds). Try covering up the tables and see if you come up with the same answers.

In Figure 9–4A, you do not know if the true right ear AC thresholds are the same as those shown by the unmasked AC thresholds or whether they are worse as a result of cross-hearing to the BC of the NTE. Of course, the answers depend on which transducer: For example, from 2000 to 8000 Hz, masking would be needed for supra-aurals but not for inserts because of the different IA values. Applying the rule for BC masking in Figure 9–4A, you can see that the differences between the right ear unmasked AC thresholds and the unmasked BC thresholds are each >10 dB.

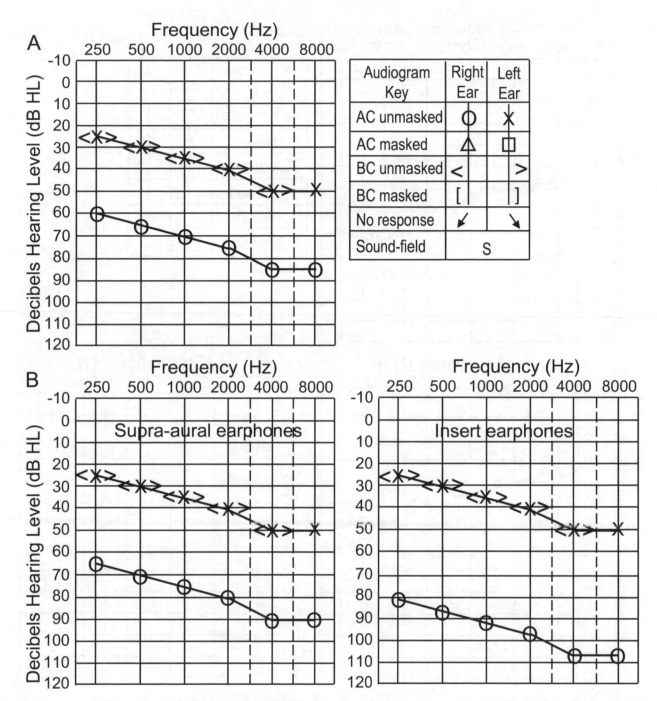

FIGURE 9–2. A–C. Examples of audiograms demonstrating situations where masking would be needed or not in order to establish true air conduction thresholds. In **A**, masking is not needed because the difference between the unmasked right ear air conduction thresholds compared to the unmasked left ear bone conduction thresholds equals 35 dB for each of the frequencies, which is less than the minimum interaural attenuation for supra-aural earphones (40 dB) and for insert earphones (55 dB). In **B**, masking is needed to obtain the true right ear air conduction thresholds because the differences between the right ear unmasked air conduction thresholds compared to the left ear unmasked bone conduction thresholds are equal to the minimum interaural attenuation for supra-aural earphones. In **C**, masking is needed to obtain the true right ear air conduction thresholds because the differences between the right ear unmasked air conduction thresholds compared to the left ear unmasked bone conduction thresholds are equal to the minimum interaural attenuation for insert earphones.

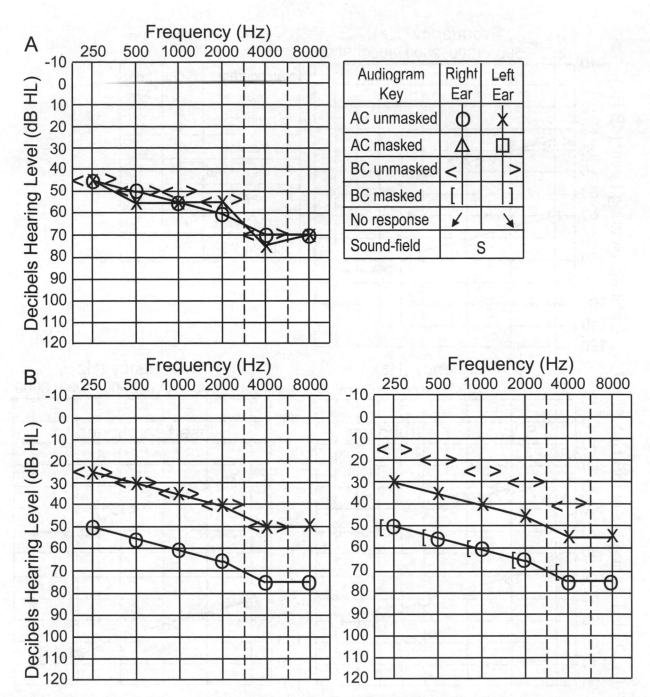

FIGURE 9–3. A–C. Examples of audiograms demonstrating situations where masking would be needed or not to establish true bone conduction thresholds. In **A**, masking is not needed because neither ear shows any air–bone gaps, that is, the bone conduction thresholds would not be any better than the unmasked thresholds nor would they be worse than the air-conduction thresholds. In **B**, masking is needed in order to obtain the true right ear bone conduction thresholds because of the air–bone gaps of more than 10 dB. The true right ear bone conduction thresholds could be anywhere from the right ear unmasked bone conduction thresholds to the right ear air conduction thresholds. In **C**, masking is potentially needed to obtain the true bone conduction thresholds of both ears. In this situation, the right ear masked results are also shown that show a shift from the unmasked thresholds. In this case, even though there are air–bone gaps in the left ear, the unmasked BC thresholds must be from the left ear; therefore, the masked BC thresholds for the left ear need not be obtained.

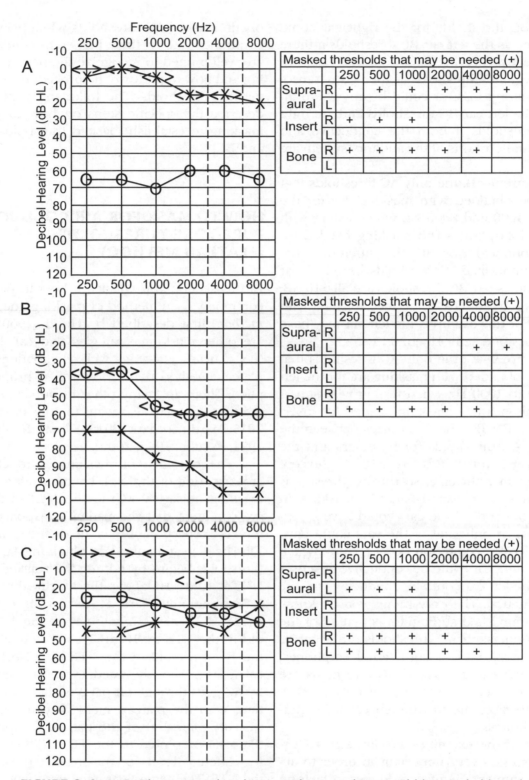

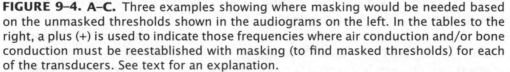

FIGURE 9–4. A–C. Three examples showing where masking would be needed based on the unmasked thresholds shown in the audiograms on the left. In the tables to the right, a plus (+) is used to indicate those frequencies where air conduction and/or bone conduction must be reestablished with masking (to find masked thresholds) for each of the transducers. See text for an explanation.

The true BC thresholds for the right ear could be the same as the left ear BC thresholds if there is a conductive hearing loss; could be equal to the right ear AC thresholds if there is a sensorineural hearing loss; or could be anywhere in-between the left ear BC thresholds and the right ear AC thresholds if both the conductive and sensorineural portions of the auditory system are involved.

In Figure 9–4B, the only AC thresholds that need to be obtained with masking are for the left ear at 4000 and 8000 Hz when testing with supra-aural earphones (no masking needed for insert earphones). For BC, the differences between the unmasked AC thresholds for the left ear and the unmasked BC thresholds are all >10 dB, so these would all have to be reestablished with masking. For this example, the left ear may have a mixed loss or a sensorineural loss.

In Figure 9–4C, the only AC thresholds that need to be obtained with masking are for the left ear at 250 to 1000 Hz when testing with supra-aural earphones (no masking needed for insert earphones). For BC, the differences between the unmasked AC thresholds for both ears and the unmasked BC thresholds are >10 dB (except at 4000 Hz in right ear), so the BC thresholds would have to be reestablished with masking. In this example, both of the ears could have a conductive loss or only one of the ears could have a conductive loss (and you do not know which one!). The right ear could be conductive or sensorineural; the left ear could be conductive, mixed, or sensorineural. The only things you do know from this unmasked audiogram is that all of the right ear unmasked AC thresholds are accurate for insert earphones or supra-aural earphones, all of the left ear unmasked AC thresholds are accurate for insert earphones, but only 2000 to 8000 Hz are accurate for the left ear for supra-aural earphones.

As all of the examples in Figure 9–4 illustrate, masking is very important in order to accurately document degrees and types of hearing loss. Failure to properly use masking may lead to improper descriptions of the type of hearing loss, misrepresentation of the severity of the hearing loss, and/or even which ear is responding. It should also be apparent that there is less need to obtain masked AC thresholds when using insert earphones due to their higher IA. Audiologists are well trained to recognize the need for masking and how to perform the procedures to obtain masked thresholds. The following sections will describe the specific steps on how to perform masking to establish masked thresholds for AC and BC.

HOW TO MASK FOR AIR CONDUCTION PURE-TONE THRESHOLDS (PLATEAU METHOD)

In this section you will learn how to perform a commonly used method of masking, the *plateau method*, first described by Hood (1960). There are other masking strategies that can be used (e.g., Turner, 2004), as well as variations of the plateau method that work well if properly applied. There are many other resources on masking that you may also want to consult (Gelfand, 2015; Martin & Clark, 2015; Silman & Silverman, 1991; Yacullo, 1996, 2009).

The objective of masking is to eliminate cross-hearing of the NTE by presenting enough masking noise (by AC) to the NTE so that you are confident that the patient's response to the tone is a reflection of what he or she hears in the TE. The plateau method for obtaining AC masked thresholds begins by putting the masker into the NTE at 10 dB HL above the AC threshold of the NTE, commonly referred to as the *initial masking level* (IML). This IML will elevate the AC threshold in the NTE by 10 dB HL and will also raise the BC threshold in the NTE by 10 dB HL because, as previously stated, everything presented by AC goes through all parts of the auditory system. With the plateau method, you keep track (usually mentally) of the patient's responses to the tone presented to the TE at different levels for different levels of the masker presented to the NTE. The general strategy is as follows:

- If the patient does not respond, raise the level of the tone.
- If the patient responds, raise the level of the masker.

- Repeat the above until a plateau is reached. This would be recognized when the patient responds at the same presentation level in the TE for increases in the masker level in the NTE.

This masking strategy would continue until you become confident that cross-hearing is no longer a factor and the patient's response represents a true threshold of the TE. You are confident when the presentation level of the sound in the TE, compared to the elevated (due to the masker) BC threshold in the NTE, is less than the IA. As you work through the following examples, they will seem very detailed and lengthy, but in actual practice the process goes fairly quickly. Audiologists usually keep mental track of the masking steps based on whether the patient responds or does not respond to the presented tone in the TE. The main thing to keep asking yourself is whether the patient's response could be due to hearing the sound in the NTE through cross-hearing (by BC). If this is still a possibility, you are not done masking; if it is no longer a possibility, then you have established the true threshold in the TE. As mentioned earlier, audiologists often decide to obtain masked AC thresholds based on where he or she *assumes* the TE BC thresholds are, rather than go back and forth between testing AC and BC to find the BC thresholds. However, for purposes of this textbook, NTE BC thresholds are provided in the examples to facilitate learning the steps for masking.

Examples of Masking for Air Conduction

Let's look at the details for the example in Figure 9–5, which shows an example of masking for the AC threshold at one frequency (500 Hz). The panel on the left shows the masking steps in an audiogram format. Each of the steps is indicated with a number to show how the AC threshold of the NTE (e.g., X1) and its corresponding change in BC threshold (>1) are elevated by the masker, as well as the corresponding AC response in the TE (O1). For the example in Figure 9–5, you can see that the difference between the right ear AC

unmasked threshold (60 dB HL) compared with the left ear BC unmasked threshold (10 dB HL) is equal to 50 dB, which exceeds the minimum IA for supra-aural earphones and, therefore, the right ear AC threshold needs to be established by putting the masker into the left ear. If the patient's IA was 40 dB, then the unmasked AC would have been at 50 dB HL.

The panel on the right side of Figure 9–5 shows a masking profile that plots each dB HL that the patient responded as a function of the different levels of the masker. The masking profiles are to illustrate what is occurring during masking from an academic perspective, and are not typically plotted for patients in a clinic setting. The orientation of the masking profile used in this text is similar to that used by Turner (2004) and the dB HL levels on the masking profile are matched to the audiogram format. The masking profile can show the undermasked stage (sometimes called the *chase*), as well as the plateau. The lowest level of masker that begins the plateau is called the *minimum masking level* (or change-over point). Although a 15 dB plateau would be considered adequate by the authors, some audiologists prefer to document a 20 or 30 dB plateau when possible by adding more masker increases after the tone threshold has stabilized. Although this wider plateau is not really necessary, it does illustrate the range of plateaus that you might see used by different audiologists. The highest level of masker used in defining the plateau is called the *final masking level (FML)* For the examples in this text, 20 dB plateaus will be demonstrated.

Of course, you do not want to put too much masking into the NTE and have it be uncomfortable for the patient. However, before you get too far and think you can just put in as much noise as the patient can tolerate, you must realize that the masker itself can cross back over to the TE if the IA is exceeded. When this occurs, it is called *overmasking*, and the masker will elevate (mask) the threshold to the tone in the TE and give a false threshold. As mentioned earlier, this would always be the case if you were to present the masker by BC. Instead, AC transducers are used to present the masker so there is a range of masker levels (e.g., 55 dB HL for insert

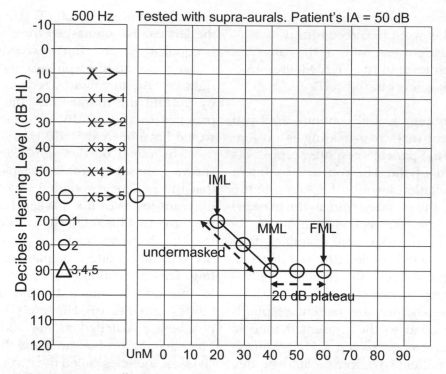

FIGURE 9–5. An illustration of the steps used for the plateau method for air conduction masking. On the left is a representation of the audiogram at 500 Hz and on the right is a masking profile showing how the corresponding air conduction threshold in the test ear (*y*-axis) shifts as a function of masker level (*x*-axis). In this example, the right ear unmasked air conduction threshold (O) must be reestablished with masking to obtain the true right ear threshold (Δ). The *numbered symbols* on the audiogram represent the thresholds for successive masking steps. In this example, the masker is presented to the left ear, so X1 represents the initial masking level; >1 is the elevation of the bone conduction threshold due to the X1 masker; and O1 is the air conduction response in the test ear in the presence of the X1 masker. The masking profile on the right shows the initial masking level (IML), the point where the plateau begins (MML), and the final masking level used (FML). The plateau is shown as a horizontal part of the masking profile where the test ear threshold does not change for increases in the masker presented to the non-test ear. On the audiogram portion, the corresponding plateau is indicated with the masked symbol with its corresponding series of masking steps where the threshold did not change (e.g., Δ3, 4, 5, 6). See text for explanation of the steps.

earphones; 40 dB HL for supra-aural earphones) that can be used before overmasking will occur. Again, the insert earphone has the advantage over supra-aural earphones because it has a wider range of masker levels possible before overmasking becomes a problem. In the examples given later in the chapter, you will see how overmasking can be a problem, called a *masking dilemma*, in some cases where there is an apparent air–bone gap in the unmasked thresholds for the NTE. Overmasking should not be a problem when there is normal hearing or a sensorineural loss in the NTE.

Let's go over the specific steps for the example shown in Figure 9–5. For this example, the IML is 20 dB HL (10 above the left ear AC threshold). This will elevate/mask the AC threshold in the left ear to 20 dB HL (X1) and will also raise the BC threshold to 20 dB HL (>1). For all the examples in this textbook, steps of 10 dB for the masker and 5 dB for the test tone will used.[2] The general (and relatively simple) procedure is to raise the level of the tone when the patient does not respond and raise the level of masker when the patient responds; continue these steps until sufficient masking has been applied: Masking is sufficient when the response in the TE compared with the elevated/masked BC threshold in the NTE is less than the patient's IA (in this case the patient's IA = 50 dB). You will know you have sufficient masking when the threshold to the tone does not change for additional increases of the masker level, which defines the plateau. To continue this example, the additional steps would be:

- Present AC tone at 60 dB HL in the right ear (the unmasked AC threshold); *patient does not respond*. Because the given audiogram already shows the true right ear AC (masked) threshold is at 80 dB HL, you can predict, in this case, that the patient would not respond to the tone because the difference between the tone being presented in the right ear (60 dB HL) and the elevated/masked BC threshold in the left ear (20 dB HL) is less than the patient's IA of 50 dB. So, at this point you still do not know the patient's true threshold because he or she no longer responds at 60 dB HL. Since the patient did not respond, you raise the level of the tone.
- Raise the AC tone to 65 dB HL (if going in 5 dB steps); *patient does not respond*.
- Raise the AC tone to 70 dB HL; *patient responds* (O1) because the difference between the level now being presented to the right ear (70 dB HL) and the elevated/

masked BC threshold in the left ear (20 dB HL) is again 50 dB and equal to patient's IA (50 dB). So, once again, you still do not know whether the response to the tone at 70 dB HL is from the right ear or the left ear (by BC); hence, you are still in the undermasking phase.

- Raise masker to 30 dB HL (X2, >2) and retest with the AC tone at 70 dB HL; *patient does not respond*.
- Raise AC tone to 75 dB HL; *patient does not respond*.
- Raise AC tone to 80 dB HL; *patient responds* (O2).
- Raise masker to 40 dB HL (X3, >3) and retest AC tone at 80 dB HL; *patient does not respond*.
- Raise AC tone to 85 dB HL; *patient does not respond*.
- Raise AC tone to 90 dB HL; *patient responds* (Δ3). Note: You have now reached the masked threshold as given in this example, so you know the *patient will respond*; however, with a real patient, you would not know this and would need to keep repeating the steps until you find the patient's true threshold.
- Raise masker to 50 dB HL (X4, >4) and retest AC tone at 90 dB HL; *patient responds* (Δ4). At this point, you are 10 dB less than the patient's 50 dB IA and have a 10 dB plateau.
- Raise masker to 60 dB HL (X5, >5) and retest AC tone at 90 dB HL; *patient responds* (Δ5). At this point you are 20 dB less than the patient's 50 dB IA and have a 20 dB plateau and are done masking for this frequency.
- It is good clinical practice to indicate on the audiogram the FML or range of masking levels used to define the plateau. For this example, you would indicate on the audiogram the masked AC symbol (Δ) at 90 db HL and a FML of 60 dB HL.

The main criticism of the plateau method is that you may go through a few unnecessary steps before arriving at the appropriate level of masking; however, it may be better to be cautious

---

[2]Alternately, you may (a) use 5 dB steps for tone and masker, (b) use 10 dB steps for tone and masker, (c) change from 10 dB steps to 5 dB steps when closer to threshold, and/or (d) finish masking after establishing the plateau by reducing the level by 5 dB to find the lowest response level.

with a few extra steps than to end up with the incorrect results, especially when learning how to mask. Once the masking concepts are mastered, you may choose to adopt other strategies to determine the proper amount of masking to put into the NTE.

To summarize, in order for you to know if the tone being presented to the TE by AC is actually being heard by the TE, you need to compare the level of the tone heard by AC in the TE to the BC threshold of the NTE (as elevated with the masker). If that difference is less than the IA, then the response to the tone must be coming from the TE because cross-hearing to the NTE can no longer be occurring. If the difference is greater than or equal to the IA, the response may still be due to hearing the tone in the NTE and more masking must be put into the NTE. Again, your goal is to put enough masking (by AC) in the NTE so that the NTE cannot hear (by BC) the tone being presented in the TE. And one final thing to keep in mind is to be sure that the level of the masker is not creating an over-masking situation, something to be concerned about only when the unmasked results show a bilateral moderate degree of hearing loss with an air–bone gap.

HOW TO MASK FOR BONE CONDUCTION THRESHOLDS (PLATEAU METHOD)

In general, the same masking procedures that are used for obtaining masked AC thresholds are used for obtaining masked BC thresholds, except that the minimum IA is 0 dB. In clinical practice, masking for BC thresholds is performed much more frequently than masking for AC thresholds because of the 0 dB IA. There is, however, an additional consideration that needs to be considered when masking for BC thresholds, and that is the occlusion effect (OE), which is not a factor during AC testing.

Occlusion Effect

When testing for BC thresholds without an earphone in place, the ears are said to be *unoc-cluded* (uncovered). However, in order to obtain masked thresholds, an earphone is placed on the NTE and the ears are said to be *occluded* (covered), which may create an *occlusion effect* (OE). The OE produces a noticeable increase in the intensity of low frequency tones presented by the bone vibrator, which translates into an improvement of the BC thresholds in the occluded condition compared to the unoccluded condition (Studebaker, 1967; Tonndorf, 1972; Yacullo, 2009). You can easily experience the OE by alternately closing off (occluding) and opening (unoccluding) your ear by cupping your hands over your ear or pushing in the tragus while sustaining the vowel "eeee." With the ear occluded, the perceived sound is louder than when the ear is unoccluded.

Figure 9–6 illustrates the concepts of the OE during BC testing. The primary source of the OE is the cartilaginous portion of the external ear canal, which can vibrate even during BC stimulation. When the ear is occluded with a supra-aural earphone (Figure 9–6A), the sound created by the vibrations of the cartilaginous portion of the ear canal cannot escape the ear to the same degree as they would in the unoccluded condition; therefore, the BC signal that the patient hears is actually increased in level because these vibrations within the ear canal send a small amount of energy into the ear by AC. This extra air-conducted energy combines with the energy created by the BC vibrator. The OE is primarily of concern when using supra-aural earphones to present the masker to the NTE. An insert earphone, when properly inserted (Figure 9–6B), has a reduced or nonexistent OE because the foam cuff occupies much of the cartilaginous portion of the external ear canal and, therefore, does not have the capability of vibrating to the BC sounds (Yacullo, 1996, 2009). A reduced OE is yet another advantage of insert earphones over supra-aural earphones when masking. However, the elimination/reduction of the OE with an insert earphone is dependent on its placement (Figure 9–6C).

The OE for supra-aural earphones only occurs at 250 to 1000 Hz, and the size of the OE increases as the frequency decreases. The mean OE for a supra-aural earphone varies slightly across studies. Roeser and Clark (2000) recommend 20 dB at 250 Hz, 15 dB at 500 Hz, and 5 dB

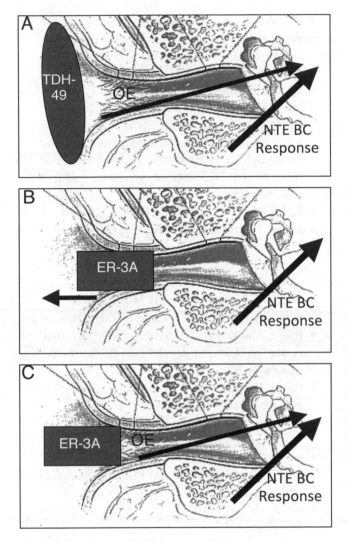

FIGURE 9–6. A–C. Illustration of the primary source of the occlusion effect (OE). During bone conduction testing, some vibrations can occur in the cartilaginous portion of the external ear canal that produce some air-conducted energy in the ear canal, which may or may not combine with the bone-conducted energy from the test tone depending on whether the ear is occluded (covered) or not. In **A**, a supra-aural earphone is placed over the non-test ear (NTE). In **B**, an insert earphone in the NTE is in place with proper depth of insertion. In **C**, an insert earphone in the NTE is in place with a shallow depth of insertion. See text for explanation.

at 1000 Hz. Yacullo (2009) recommends 30 at 250 Hz, 20 dB at 500 Hz, and 10 dB at 1000 Hz. For insert earphones, Yacullo (2009) recommends 10 dB at 250 Hz only. For the examples in this textbook, the following OE values will be used:

Supra-aural earphone:

250 Hz = 20 dB

500 Hz = 15 dB

1000 Hz = 5 dB

For insert earphones:

250 Hz = 10 dB

As an audiometric example of the OE, suppose the unoccluded (unmasked) BC threshold at 500 Hz is found to be 20 dB HL. When the BC threshold is retested with the NTE occluded with a supra-aural earphone, but before any masking noise is added, the BC threshold might be improved to 5 dB HL, indicating an OE of 15 dB for that tone. So how do you take into account the OE when obtaining masked BC thresholds? Because the occlusion effect causes the BC threshold to be better (lower), this creates an artificial air–bone gap that needs to be accounted for when selecting the IML. The IML would need to be increased by the amount of the OE in order to elevate/mask the BC threshold back to its original (unoccluded) starting point. Therefore, for BC testing, the IML to the NTE would be equal to the AC threshold in NTE + 10 dB + amount of any OE. After including the OE in the IML, the rest of the masking steps for BC are the same as those for AC. Another thing to keep in mind is that the OE is offset by any conductive loss because air–bone gaps of as little as 20 dB will preclude perceiving the increased intensity caused by the OE (Studebaker, 1967; Yacullo, 2009). So, in cases of a conductive loss in the NTE, the OE = 0 dB and will not be a factor in selecting the IML.

Some audiologists prefer to adopt specific amounts to use for the OE based on data from the literature; however, the actual size of the OE may be determined for each patient. This can be done by retesting the BC threshold in the occluded condition without the masking noise and comparing it to the unoccluded BC threshold. Once you have the amount of OE, this amount can be used in selecting the IML. Alternately, you can track the occluded BC threshold in the

NTE to decide when enough masking noise has been used to preclude the NTE from responding; both methods will require that the noise level be increased by the amount of OE, either at the beginning (IML) or at the end (FML), so that an adequate plateau is established.

Examples of Masking for Bone Conduction

Let's look at an example of masking for BC threshold for one frequency (500 Hz) as shown in Figure 9–7. See section on how to mask for AC for an explanation of the parts to the figure. The right ear masked BC threshold is shown in the figure, along with the right ear masked AC threshold. The goal is to describe all the steps that would get you to the masked BC threshold at 50 dB HL. The right ear will end up with a mixed hearing loss (as given by the masked threshold) which is not apparent from the unmasked BC threshold. The IML presented to the left ear is 35 dB HL (AC threshold of the left ear + 10 dB + 15 dB OE). This will elevate/mask the AC threshold in the left ear to 35 dB HL (X1) and will raise the BC threshold to 20 dB HL (>1). Note that the difference between the AC and BC elevated/masked levels will continue to be the amount of the OE (15 dB in this case). To continue this example, the additional steps would be:

- Present the BC tone at 10 dB HL (the unmasked BC threshold); *patient does not respond.* Because the given audiogram shows the true right ear BC (masked) threshold is at 50 dB HL, you can predict, in this case, that the patient does not respond to the tone because the difference between the tone being presented in the TE (10 dB HL) and the elevated/masked BC threshold (20 dB HL) is –10 dB, which is less than the patient's IA, but less than the patient's given masked threshold (which you would not know in a real patient). So, at this point you still do not know the patient's true threshold because he or she no longer responds at 0 dB HL.
- Raise the BC tone to 15 dB HL (if going in 5 dB steps); *patient does not respond.*

- Raise the BC tone to 20 dB HL; *patient responds* (<1) because the difference between the BC level now being presented to the TE (20 dB HL) and the elevated/masked BC threshold (20 dB HL) is again 0 dB and equal to the IA (0 dB). So, once again, you still do not know whether the response to the tone at 20 dB HL is from the right ear or the left ear (by BC); hence, you are still in the undermasked stage.
- Raise masker to 45 dB HL (X2, >2) and retest BC tone at 20 dB HL; *patient does not respond.*
- Raise BC tone to 25 dB HL; *patient does not respond.*
- Raise BC tone to 30 dB HL; *patient responds* (<2). Difference still 0 dB.
- Raise masker to 55 dB HL (X3, >3) and retest BC tone at 30 dB HL; *patient does not respond.*
- Raise BC tone to 35 dB HL; *patient does not respond.*
- Raise BC tone to 40 dB HL; *patient responds* (<3). Difference still 0 dB.
- Raise masker to 65 dB HL (X4, >4) and retest BC tone at 40 dB HL; *patient does not respond.*
- Raise BC tone to 45 dB HL; *patient does not respond.*
- Raise BC tone to 50 dB HL; *patient responds* ([4). You are now at the true threshold given to you in this case; however, you would not know this with a real patient. At this point you are at the MML, but still at 0 dB IA.
- Raise masker to 75 dB HL (X5, >5) and retest BC tone at 50 dB HL; *patient responds* ([5). At this point, you are 10 dB less than the patient's 0 dB IA (i.e., –10 dB) and have a 10 dB plateau.
- Raise masker to 85 dB HL (X6, >6) and retest BC tone at 50 dB HL; *patient responds* ([6). You are now 20 dB less than the patient's 0 dB IA (i.e., –20 dB) and have a 20 dB plateau.
- It is good clinical practice to indicate on the audiogram the FML or range of masking levels used to define the plateau. For this example, you would indicate on

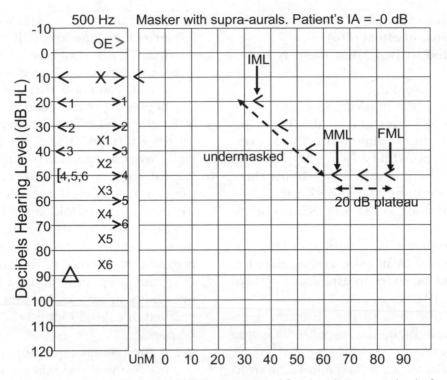

FIGURE 9–7. An illustration of the steps used for the plateau method of bone conduction masking. See Figure 9–5 for orientation to parts of the figure. In this example, the right ear bone conduction threshold (<) must be reestablished with masking to obtain the true right ear threshold ([). The *numbered symbols* on the audiogram represent the thresholds for successive masking steps. In this example, the masker is presented to the left ear, so X1 represents the initial masking level; >1 is the elevation of the bone conduction threshold due to the X1 masker; and <1 is the bone conduction in the test ear in the presence of the X1 masker. The masking profile on the right shows the initial masking level (IML), the point where the plateau begins (MML), and the final masking level used (FML). The plateau is shown as a horizontal part of the masking profile where the test ear threshold does not change for increases in the masker presented to the non-test ear (NTE). On the audiogram portion, the corresponding plateau is indicated with the masked symbol with its corresponding series of masking steps where the threshold did not change (e.g., [4, 5, 6). See text for explanation of the steps.

the audiogram the masked BC symbol (□) at 50 dB HL and a FML of 85 dB HL.

SUMMARY OF THE STEP-BY-STEP PROCEDURES FOR MASKING WITH THE PLATEAU METHOD

The plateau method of masking consists of a series of steps whose goal is to systematically elevate/mask the NTE until a stable TE response to the tone occurs as the masker is raised enough to establish a plateau. With sufficient masking in the NTE, cross-hearing cannot occur and the response to the tone is the true threshold of the TE. These plateau method steps can be adopted for AC or BC masking by appropriately adjusting for the IML and paying attention to the appropriate IA.

1. Present the appropriate IML to the NTE by AC: IML for AC testing = AC threshold of NTE + 10 dB;

IML for BC testing = AC threshold of NTE + 10 dB + occlusion effect (OE)
(No OE added to BC IML if there is a conductive loss).

2. Is the IML overmasking?
Compare the initial masking level (by AC in NTE) to the BC threshold in the TE to see if it exceeds the minimum IA; if so, overmasking is a possibility (will only occur in cases where the unmasked thresholds show a moderate air–bone gap in both ears).

2.1 If overmasking is not a possibility, go to step 3.

2.2 If overmasking is a possibility, the patient's actual IA may be greater than the minimum IA, so try to establish a plateau (5 to 15 dB). Go to step 7.

3. Present the test tone to the TE at the level where you last obtained a response. Does the patient respond?

3.1 If the patient does not respond (and overmasking is not a possibility), you know that the original unmasked response came from the NTE (by BC), so you are in the undermasking phase and still need to find the TE threshold; go to step 4.

3.2 If the patient responds, you know that the IML is the same as the minimum masking level and the beginning of the plateau; go to step 5.

4. Raise the tone in the TE in 5 or 10 dB steps until the patient responds; then compare the presentation level in the TE with the elevated (masked) BC threshold in the TE.

4.1 If the difference equals or exceeds the IA, the response could still be from the BC of the NTE, so you are in the under-masking stage and still need to find the true TE threshold; go to step 5.

4.2 If the difference does not equal or exceed the IA, you know that the masker is at the beginning of the plateau; go to step 5.

5. Raise the level of the masker in the NTE by 10 dB HL (could use 5 dB HL steps, especially when suspecting a small plateau).

6. Repeat steps 3 to 5 until at least a 15 dB plateau has been established: Record the TE masked threshold on the audiogram. It is also a good idea to record the maximum noise level (or range of noise levels) in the boxes at the bottom of the audiogram.

7. (Use this step only if overmasking was a possibility in step 1): Present tone at the unmasked threshold in the TE. Does the patient respond?

7.1 If the patient does not respond, you do not know if the masker is crossing over and elevating the threshold in the TE (a 5 dB increase could occur due to central masking, so you may need to try step 7.2); if patient does not respond, this is a masking dilemma: State on audiogram, "Could not mask because minimum amount of masking may be overmasking (masking dilemma)."

7.2 If the patient responds, he or she has an IA greater than the minimum IA and masking may be possible. Go to step 5, but keep in mind that the plateau may be narrow; for example, you may only be able to increase the masker by 5 or 10 dB before threshold starts increasing again

SYNOPSIS 9–2

- Masking of the NTE is needed in those conditions where there is the possibility that the tone presented to the TE may be heard through cross-hearing by BC in the NTE.
- The following is a general principle of when masking is needed:
  - Anytime the presentation level in the TE, whether by BC or AC, is equal to or greater than the minimum IA for the appropriate transducer, you must assume that the test signal can be heard by BC in the NTE and masking must be used.

SYNOPSIS 9–2 (*continued*)

- The rules for deciding if masking is needed are:
  - *BC masking*: Whenever there is >10 dB difference between the unmasked BC threshold and the AC threshold of the TE (i.e., an air–bone gap), masking is needed to rule out the possibility that the BC threshold is coming from the NTE.
  - *AC masking*: Whenever the difference between the AC threshold of the TE and the BC threshold of the NTE is greater than or equal to 55 dB (or 40 dB for supra-aural earphones), masking is needed to rule out the possibility that the AC threshold is coming from the NTE (by BC). In clinical settings, decisions on AC masking may be made before having the BC thresholds, and are based on assumed BC thresholds.
- A popular method of masking is called the plateau method. This method effectively eliminates the NTE when the patient's response to the TE does not change for a series of increases in the level of the masker in the NTE. When overmasking is not a problem, a plateau of 15–20 dB is recommended; however, some audiologists prefer larger plateaus (e.g., 20 to 30 dB).
- Overmasking is the situation in which the level of the masker in the NTE can result in cross-hearing in the TE, thus precluding accurate threshold measures. The same IA values for the AC transducers apply to overmasking.
- In cases of bilateral conductive hearing loss, only a small (5 to 10 dB) plateau may be possible before overmasking occurs.
- Insert earphones have an advantage over supra-aural earphones in that masking is not needed as often because of the greater IA for the insert earphones. The greater IA is related to a smaller surface area of the insert earphone that is in contact with the skull.
- When obtaining BC masked thresholds, be cognizant of increasing the level of the lower frequency BC sounds due to the occlusion effect (OE). The OE occurs when placing the AC transducer on the NTE. The source of the OE is vibration of the cartilaginous portion of the external ear canal. The OE is higher with supra-aural earphones than with insert earphones placed at appropriate depth.
- The basic steps for the plateau method of masking include:
  - Present the masker to the NTE at an initial masking level (IML):
    - IML for AC testing = AC threshold of NTE + 10 dB;
    - IML for BC testing = AC threshold of NTE + 10 dB + occlusion effect (OE)
  - Find the patient's threshold in the TE for each masker level.
    - If patient does not respond, then raise the level of the test tone.
    - If the patient responds, raise the level of the masker.
    - Continue process until patient's response to the test tone remains stable for a series of increases in the masker level (the plateau).
- A masking dilemma will occur when the initial masking level causes overmasking.
- Generally, it is better to obtain masked thresholds for the poorer ear first to reduce conditions that may be masking dilemmas.
- Insert earphones have the advantages when masking of having lower OE and higher IA.

(overmasking). Remember, there may be a narrower plateau in cases with bilateral air–bone gaps.

MASKING EXAMPLES

In this section, there are four different examples to illustrate the step-by-step procedures using the plateau method of masking. For each of the cases, there is a single-frequency audiogram (with both the unmasked and masked thresholds) and a corresponding masking profile, like the ones you already reviewed in detail in Figures 9–5 and 9–7. Also introduced in these examples is a masking tracking table (at the bottom of the figures) that the authors have found useful in helping students learn to apply the plateau method. The steps in the tracking table replace the steps shown in the earlier examples on the audiogram panel. Eventually, these steps will be tracked mentally, and with practice and precepted clinical training, masking will become easier. These examples are not exhaustive of the masking situations that may be encountered in clinical practice; however, they should illustrate concepts that will cover the majority of situations.

In the following examples, the masker is raised in 10 dB steps and the test tone raised in 5 dB steps. As mentioned earlier, some audiologists may prefer to increase both the masker and tone in either 5 or 10 dB steps. Keep in mind that 5 dB steps of the masker would be most appropriate when a small plateau is expected, such as when there is a bilateral air–bone gap. It may take some effort to track all the responses in these examples, but once the concepts are mastered, the steps flow faster when performing the masking on an actual patient, and the tracking form should no longer be needed.

Example 1: Air Conduction Masking Resulting in a Worse/Poorer Masked Threshold Than the Unmasked Threshold

As Figure 9–8 shows on the left, the unmasked right ear AC threshold (50 dB HL), when compared with the unmasked BC threshold (0 dB HL), is greater than the minimum IA for supraaural earphones (in this case, the patient's IA = 50 dB). The right ear masked AC threshold needs to be obtained (masking noise applied to left ear). In this example, you can see that the final masked AC threshold (Δ) has worsened when compared with the unmasked right ear threshold (O); therefore, you know that the unmasked right ear AC response was coming from the left ear (by BC). The following steps would have been used to establish the masked right ear AC threshold. The steps correspond to the information provided in the masking tracking table at the bottom of the figure, and the undermasking and plateau can be seen in the masking profile (on the right of the figure). Note that the masker is raised in 10 dB steps and the tone is raised in 5 dB steps; a 15 to 20 dB plateau is the goal. Also note in this example that the patient's IA is 50 dB (unmasked AC to unmasked BC). The specific steps can be seen in the tracking table shown at the bottom of Figure 9–8.

1. Put an initial masking level (IML) into the left ear by earphone of 10 dB HL (0 dB left ear AC threshold + 10 dB). This elevates the AC and BC threshold in the left ear to 10 dB HL.
2. Overmasking is not a possibility since masker level in left ear (10 dB HL) compared to unmasked BC threshold (0 dB HL) is less than the patient's IA (50 dB).
3. Present the AC tone to right ear at 50 dB HL (original unmasked AC threshold). *Patient does not respond.* This tells you that the right ear unmasked AC response had been from the left ear (by BC). You know this because the true threshold (80 dB HL) is given to you on the audiogram. However, when testing a real patient, you would not have this information, and would base your steps on whether the patient responds.
4. Increase the AC tone in the right ear to 55 dB HL (noise still at 10 dB HL). *Patient does not respond.*
5. Increase the AC tone in the right ear to 60 dB HL (noise still at 10 dB HL). *Patient responds.* Ask yourself: Could the patient's

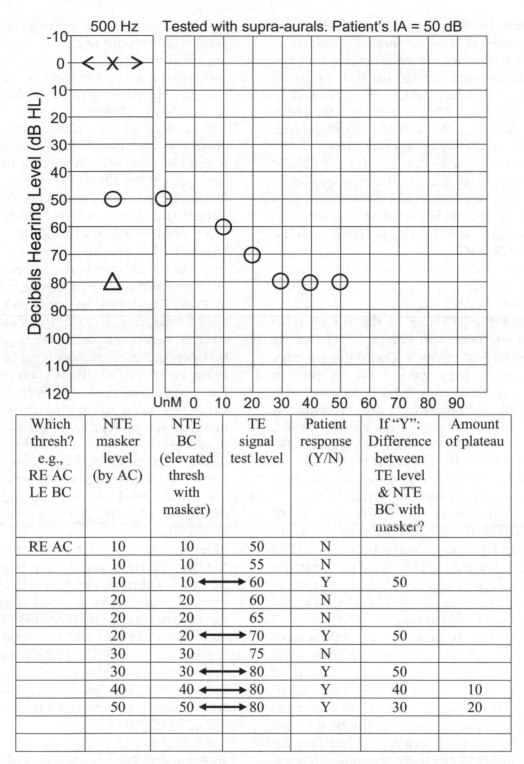

Which thresh? e.g., RE AC LE BC	NTE masker level (by AC)	NTE BC (elevated thresh with masker)	TE signal test level	Patient response (Y/N)	If "Y": Difference between TE level & NTE BC with masker?	Amount of plateau
RE AC	10	10	50	N		
	10	10	55	N		
	10	10 ⟷ 60	Y	50		
	20	20	60	N		
	20	20	65	N		
	20	20 ⟷ 70	Y	50		
	30	30	75	N		
	30	30 ⟷ 80	Y	50		
	40	40 ⟷ 80	Y	40	10	
	50	50 ⟷ 80	Y	30	20	

FIGURE 9–8. Example of air conduction masking resulting in a worse/poorer masked threshold than the unmasked threshold. See Figure 9–5 for orientation to parts of the figure. Also included at the bottom of this figure is a masking tracking table. See text for explanation of the masking steps. RE, right ear; LE, left ear; AC, air conduction; BC, bone conduction; IA, interaural attenuation; TE, test ear; NTE, non-test ear; Y, yes, patient responded; N, no, patient did not respond.

response be from the left ear? In this case, the answer is "yes" because the difference between the AC presentation level of the tone in the right ear (60 dB HL) compared with the elevated/masked BC threshold in the left ear (10 dB HL) is 50 dB HL, which is not less than the patient's IA (50 dB HL). You are in the undermasking phase.

6. Increase the masker in the left ear to 20 dB HL; present the tone to the right ear again at 60 dB HL. *Patient does not respond*. This tells you that the response the patient previously gave at 60 dB HL had been from the left ear (by BC).

7. Increase the AC tone in the right ear to 65 dB HL (noise still at 20 dB HL). *Patient does not respond*.

8. Increase the AC tone in the right ear to 70 dB HL (noise still at 20 dB HL). *Patient responds*. Ask yourself: Could the patient's response be from the left ear (by BC)? In this case, the answer is again "yes" because the difference between the presentation level of the tone in the right ear (70 dB HL) compared with the elevated/masked BC threshold in left ear (20 dB HL) is still not less than the patient's IA (50 dB). You are still in the undermasking phase.

9. Increase the masker in the left ear to 30 dB HL; present the tone to the right ear again at 70 dB HL. *Patient does not respond*. (Did you predict this?). This tells you that the previous response the patient gave at 70 dB HL had been from the left ear (by BC). (Are you seeing the pattern?)

10. Increase the AC tone in the right ear to 75 dB HL. *Patient does not respond*. (Did you predict this?)

11. Increase the AC tone in the right ear to 80 dB HL. *Patient responds*. Ask yourself: Could it be from the left ear (by BC)? In this case, the answer is again "yes" because the difference between the presentation level of the tone in the right ear (80 dB HL) compared with elevated/masked threshold in the left ear (30 dB HL) is still not less than the patient's IA. You are still in the undermasking phase. However, since the audiogram shows this to be the true threshold,

you know you are at the beginning of the plateau. You would not yet know this if testing a real patient.

12. Increase the masker in the left ear to 40 dB HL; present the tone to the right ear again at 80 dB HL. *Patient responds*. Ask yourself: Could it be from NTE? In this case, the answer is "no" because the difference between the presentation level of the tone in the right ear (80 dB HL) compared with the elevated/masked threshold in the left ear (40 dB HL) is now 40 dB, which is 10 dB less than the patient's IA (50 dB). You now have a 10 dB plateau.

13. Increase the masker in the left ear to 50 dB HL; present the tone to the right ear again at 80 dB HL. *Patient responds*. Ask yourself: Could it be from NTE? In this case, the answer is again "no" because the difference between the presentation level of the tone in the right ear (80 dB HL) compared with the elevated/masked threshold in the left ear is now only 30 dB HL, which is 20 dB less than the patient's IA (50 dB). You now have a 20 dB plateau. If a wider plateau is desirable, then increase the noise again and retest the tone (they should respond).

14. You would mark the masked right ear AC threshold at 80 dB HL and record a FML of 50 dB HL.

15. *Note*: If you had used 10 dB steps in the tone to the right ear, it may have gone a bit quicker (but probably not much); however, you may have jumped over the patient's true threshold by 5 dB. Therefore, you would need to end the series by presenting the tone to the right ear at 5 dB less than the value found. In this example, the patient would not have responded at 75 dB HL because you were given the true threshold of 80 dB HL.

In summary, this is a case in which the unmasked right ear AC threshold was not the true threshold, but instead was due to cross-hearing in the left ear (by BC). This became obvious when the original right ear threshold had to be raised when masking was introduced to the left ear at the IML. After that point, the process was a repeated series of steps in which the masker was increased, followed by the tone being increased until the right ear threshold remained stable for increases in the masker (plateau). Plateaus ranging from 15 to 45 dB could have been established in this example.

Example 2: Bone Conduction Masking Resulting in a Sensorineural Loss

In Figure 9–9, the unmasked thresholds indicate a potential air–bone gap greater than 10 dB in the left ear, which means that the left ear BC threshold must be reestablished with masking (noise in the right ear). In this example, the patient actually has a moderate sensorineural hearing loss in the left ear (shown by the]). Because the left ear BC threshold will shift to the left ear AC threshold, there will be several repeated steps (undermasking phase) until the plateau is established. The following steps are used to establish the 250 Hz masked BC threshold for the left ear. Be sure to recognize the use of the occlusion effect (OE) in setting the initial masking level (IML). Note that the masker is raised in 10 dB steps and the tone is raised in 5 dB steps; a 15 to 20 dB plateau is the goal. The patient's IA is assumed to be 0 dB. The specific steps can be observed in the tracking table shown in Figure 9–9.

1. Put an IML of 55 dB HL (35 dB HL right ear threshold + 10 dB + 10 dB OE) into the right ear by an insert earphone. This elevates the right ear AC threshold to 55 dB HL and the occluded BC threshold to 45 dB HL. Notice that the intent is to get the right ear BC elevated to 10 dB above the unmasked level similar to the strategy used for AC masking.

2. Overmasking is not a possibility (55 dB masker compared to 35 dB unmasked BC threshold is less than the 55 dB IA for an insert earphone).

3. Present the BC tone to the left ear at 35 dB HL (original unmasked BC threshold). *Patient does not respond.* You know this because the true masked threshold

(55 dB HL) is given to you. If testing a real patient, you would not know what to expect and subsequent steps are based on whether the patient responds.

4. Increase the BC tone in the left ear to 40 dB HL. *Patient does not respond.*

5. Increase the BC tone in the left ear to 45 dB HL. *Patient responds.* Ask yourself: Could the patient's response be from the right ear (by BC)? In this case, the answer is "yes" because the difference between the BC presentation level of the tone in the left ear (45 dB HL) compared with the elevated/masked BC threshold in the left ear (45 dB HL) is 0 dB, which is not less than the minimum IA (0 dB HL). You are in the undermasking phase.

6. Increase masker in the right ear to 65 dB HL; present tone again to the left ear at 45 dB HL. *Patient does not respond.*

7. Increase BC tone in the left ear to 50 dB HL. *Patient does not respond.*

8. Increase BC tone in the left ear to 55 dB HL. *Patient responds.* Ask yourself: Could the patient's response be from the right ear (by BC)? In this case, the answer is "yes" because the difference between the BC presentation level of the tone in the left ear (55 dB HL) compared with the elevated/masked BC threshold in the left ear (55 dB HL) is 0 dB, which is not less than the minimum IA (0 dB HL). You are still in the undermasking phase; however, since you know the true threshold is 55 dB HL from the audiogram, you are at the beginning of the plateau. Notice here, also, that the left ear masked BC threshold is the same as the left ear AC threshold, and since you know that the BC usually is not poorer than AC, you know that you are close to the true BC threshold for the left ear; however, it is good practice to establish a plateau to account for any variability.

9. Increase masker in the right ear to 75 dB HL; present tone again to the left ear at 55 dB HL. *Patient responds.* Ask yourself: Could the patient's response be from the right ear (by BC). In this case, the answer is "no" because the difference between the

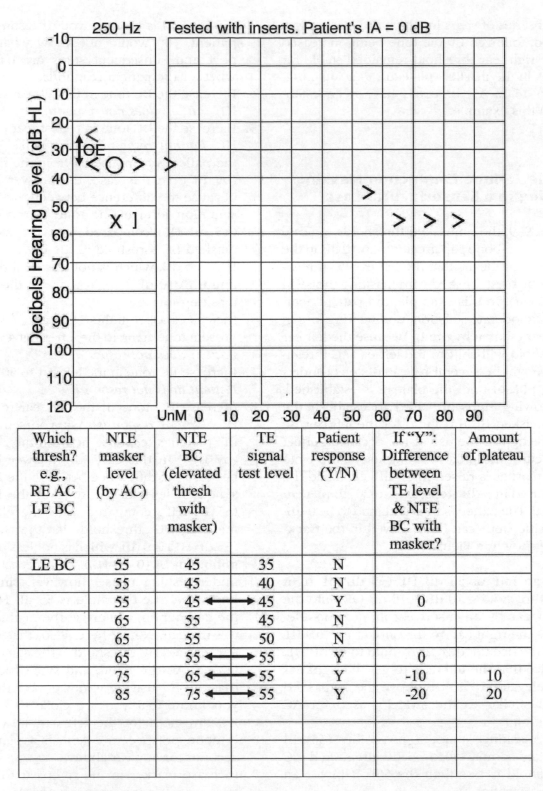

Which thresh? e.g., RE AC LE BC	NTE masker level (by AC)	NTE BC (elevated thresh with masker)	TE signal test level	Patient response (Y/N)	If "Y": Difference between TE level & NTE BC with masker?	Amount of plateau
LE BC	55	45	35	N		
	55	45	40	N		
	55	45 ⟷ 45	45	Y	0	
	65	55	45	N		
	65	55	50	N		
	65	55 ⟷ 55	55	Y	0	
	75	65 ⟷ 55	55	Y	-10	10
	85	75 ⟷ 55	55	Y	-20	20

FIGURE 9–9. Example of bone conduction masking resulting in a sensorineural loss for left ear. See Figure 9-8 for orientation to parts of the figure and abbreviations. The occlusion effect (OE) is also indicated on the audiogram. See text for explanation of the masking steps.

presentation level of the tone in the left ear (55 dB HL) compared with the elevated/masked BC threshold in the right ear (65 dB HL) is now −10 dB, which is less than the minimum IA (0 dB). You now have a 10 dB plateau.

10. Increase masker in the right ear to 85 dB HL; present tone again to the left ear at 55 dB HL. *Patient responds*. Ask yourself: Could it be from NTE? In this case, the answer is again "no" because the difference between the presentation level of the BC tone in the left ear compared with the elevated/masked BC threshold in the right ear is now −20 dB, which is less than the minimum IA (0 dB). You now have a 20 dB plateau.

11. Mark the masked left ear BC threshold at 55 dB HL and record a FML of 85 dB HL.

In summary, this is a case in which the unmasked BC threshold was not the true left ear BC threshold. This became obvious when the original BC threshold of the left ear had to be raised when masking was introduced to the right ear at the IML. From this point on, the process was a repeated series of steps of increasing the masker (10 dB step), then tone (5 dB step) until the left ear BC threshold remained stable for increases in the masker (plateau). A 20 dB plateau was obtained in this example, although a wider plateau could have been obtained by increasing the masker.

Example 3: Bone Conduction Masking Resulting in a Conductive Loss

In Figure 9–10, the unmasked thresholds indicate a potential air–bone gap greater than 10 dB in the left ear, which means that the left ear BC threshold must be re-established with masking. In this example, the patient actually has a conductive hearing loss in the left ear. Because the left ear masked BC threshold is the same as the unmasked BC threshold, there will not be any undermasking/chase phase and, therefore, fewer steps are needed to establish the masked thresholds than in the previous examples. The follow-

ing steps are used to establish the 250 Hz masked BC threshold for the left ear. These steps can be observed in the tracking table in Figure 9–10.

1. IML = 30 dB HL (10 dB HL right ear AC threshold +10 dB + 10 dB OE). This elevates/masks the BC threshold in the right ear to 20 dB HL.

2. Overmasking is not a possibility (30 dB HL masker compared to 10 dB HL unmasked BC is less than the minimal IA for insert earphones [55 dB]).

3. Present the BC tone to the left ear at 10 dB HL (original unmasked threshold). *Patient responds*. Ask yourself: Could the patient's response be from the right ear (by BC)? In this case, the answer is "no" because the difference between the presentation level of the BC tone in the left ear (10 dB HL) compared with the elevated/masked BC threshold in right ear (20 dB HL) is now −10 dB, which is less than the minimum IA (0 dB). You now have a 10 dB plateau. In this case, the IML already represents a 10 dB plateau since there was no shift in the original threshold with the masker 10 dB above the NTE threshold. The following additional steps are added to establish a wider plateau to account for any variability.

4. Increase the masker in the right ear to 40 dB HL; present the BC tone again to the left ear at 10 dB HL. *Patient responds again*. Ask yourself: Could the patient's response be from the right ear (by BC)? Again, the answer is "no" because the difference between the presentation level of the BC tone in the left ear (10 dB HL) compared with the elevated/masked BC threshold in the right ear (30 dB HL) is now −20 dB, which is less than the minimum IA (0 dB). You now have a 20 dB plateau.

5. Increase the masker in the right ear to 50 dB HL; present the BC tone again to the left ear at 10 dB HL. *Patient responds again*. Ask yourself: Could the patient's response be from the right ear (by BC)? Again, the answer is "no" because the difference between the presentation level of the BC tone in the left ear (10 dB HL) compared with the elevated/

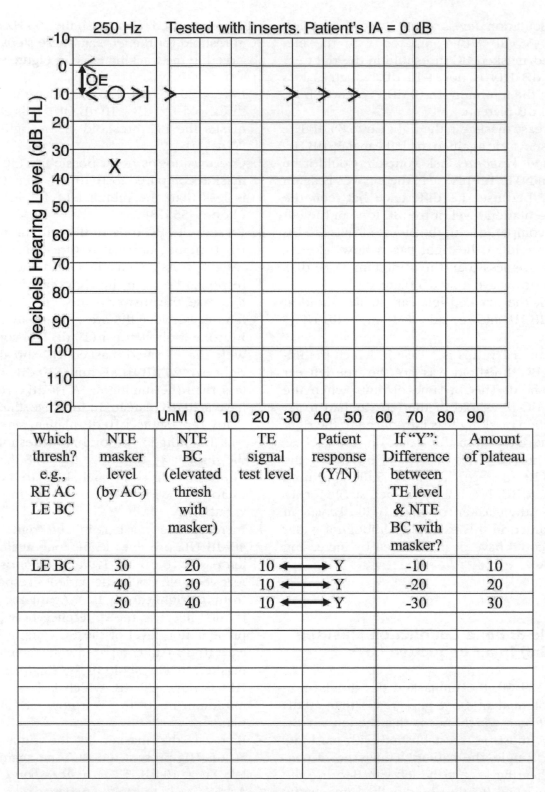

Which thresh? e.g., RE AC LE BC	NTE masker level (by AC)	NTE BC (elevated thresh with masker)	TE signal test level	Patient response (Y/N)	If "Y": Difference between TE level & NTE BC with masker?	Amount of plateau
LE BC	30	20	10 ⟷ Y		-10	10
	40	30	10 ⟷ Y		-20	20
	50	40	10 ⟷ Y		-30	30

FIGURE 9–10. Example of bone conduction masking resulting in a conductive hearing loss for left ear. See Figure 9-8 for orientation to parts of the figure and abbreviations. The occlusion effect (OE) is also indicated on the audiogram. See text for explanation of the masking steps.

masked BC threshold in the right ear (40 dB HL) is now –30 dB, which is less than the minimum IA (0 dB). You now have a 30 dB plateau.

6. Mark the masked left ear BC threshold at 10 dB HL and record a final masking level of 50 dB HL (if ending with a 30 dB plateau).

In summary, this is a case in which the original unmasked threshold was actually the true left ear BC threshold. This became obvious when the original BC threshold of the left ear did not shift when masking was introduced to the right ear at the IML. At that point, you already had a 10 dB plateau (some audiologists might not count this as part of the plateau). The process can continue by adding additional steps of noise to widen the plateau. In this case, a 30 dB plateau was established, although a 20 dB plateau would have been sufficient.

Example 4: Masking Dilemma

In Figure 9–11, the unmasked thresholds indicate the possibility of a moderate bilateral conductive hearing loss. In this example, you cannot be sure of which ear the AC or BC thresholds represent. You only know that at least one of the ears has the AC threshold at the unmasked level, but the other ear could be the same or worse. The unmasked BC thresholds also indicate that at least one ear has the threshold at the unmasked level, but the other ear could be the same or worse, and you do not know the type of hearing loss in the poorer ear. In fact, this patient could have a profound sensorineural hearing loss in the poorer ear, which from the unmasked results could be either ear! To be able to answer these questions, masked thresholds must be obtained; however, as we will see, masked AC or BC thresholds in this example cannot be obtained due to a masking dilemma. In this type of situation, before concluding that it is a masking dilemma, masking should be attempted, using 5 dB increases in masker and tone, in order to see if a small plateau can be obtained. The first set of steps attempts to establish the masked AC threshold for one of the ears. The second set of steps attempts

to establish the masked BC thresholds for one of the ears. In this example, the steps would be the same for each ear. Both sets of steps (for either ear) can be observed in Figure 9–11.

For AC masked thresholds (with supra-aural earphones):

1. IML = 60 dB HL (55 dB HL AC threshold + 5 dB) to the NTE (same for either ear). This elevates the BC threshold in the NTE to 15 dB HL. Notice that only 5 dB above the AC threshold was included in the IML because of the expectation of a small plateau, if any, before overmasking may occur. In addition, given the conductive loss in the NTE, no OE was added to the IML.

2. Overmasking is a possibility. The 60 dB HL of AC masker level compared to the 10 dB BC threshold = 50 dB, which is greater than the patient's potential IA of 45 dB (obtained by comparing the 55 dB unmasked AC threshold to the 10 dB unmasked BC threshold). When there is a possibility of overmasking, you should always mask because the patient may have a higher IA than appears from the unmasked thresholds, but remain suspicious of a possible masking dilemma.

3. Present the AC tone to TE at 55 dB HL (original unmasked threshold). *Patient does not respond.* Note that if the patient had responded at this level, you may have the beginning of a small plateau.

4. Increase AC tone in TE to 60 dB HL. *Patient responds.* Ask yourself: Could the patient's response be from NTE (by BC)? In this case, the answer is "yes" because the difference between the AC presentation level of the tone in the TE (60 dB HL) compared with the elevated/masked BC threshold in the left ear (15 dB HL) is 45 dB, which is not less than the patient's potential IA (45 dB HL). At this point, you are essentially in a masking dilemma; however, you could try a couple more steps to be sure a plateau cannot be established.

5. Increase masker to 65 dB HL, which elevates/masks the BC threshold in the NTE to 20 dB HL. Then present tone in the TE at

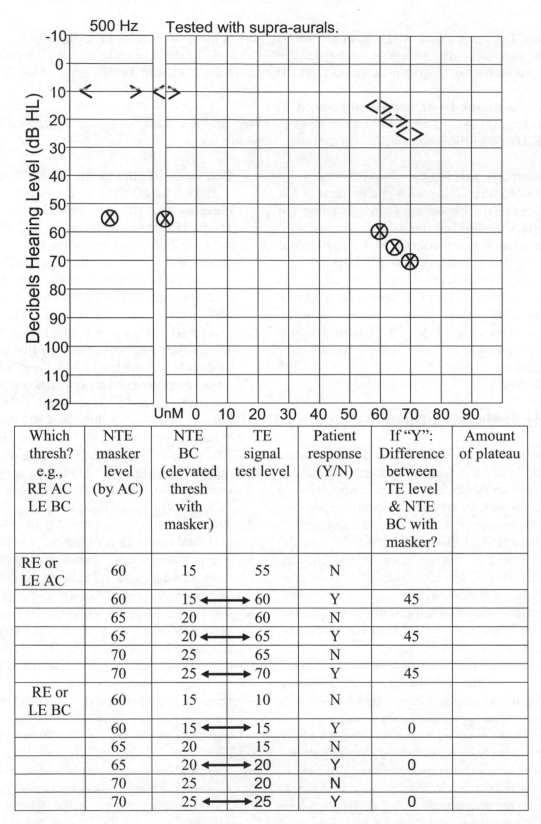

Which thresh? e.g., RE AC LE BC	NTE masker level (by AC)	NTE BC (elevated thresh with masker)	TE signal test level	Patient response (Y/N)	If "Y": Difference between TE level & NTE BC with masker?	Amount of plateau
RE or LE AC	60	15	55	N		
	60	15 ←→ 60		Y	45	
	65	20	60	N		
	65	20 ←→ 65		Y	45	
	70	25	65	N		
	70	25 ←→ 70		Y	45	
RE or LE BC	60	15	10	N		
	60	15 ←→ 15		Y	0	
	65	20	15	N		
	65	20 ←→ 20		Y	0	
	70	25	20	N		
	70	25 ←→ 25		Y	0	

FIGURE 9–11. Example of masking that results in masking dilemmas for both ears by air conduction and bone conduction. See Figure 9–8 for orientation to parts of the figure and abbreviations. See text for explanation of the masking steps.

60 dB HL (where patient last responded). *Patient does not respond.*

6. Increase tone to 65 dB HL. *Patient responds.* Ask yourself: Could it be from NTE? In this case, again the answer is "yes" because the difference between the AC presentation level of the tone in the TE (65 dB HL) compared with the elevated/masked BC threshold in the left ear (20 dB HL) is 45 dB, which is still not less than the patient's potential IA (45 dB HL).

7. Increase masker to 70 dB HL, which elevates BC threshold in NTE to 25 dB HL. Then present tone in TE at 65 dB HL. *Patient does not respond.*

8. Increase tone to 70 dB HL. *Patient responds.* Ask yourself: Could it be from NTE? In this case, again the answer is "yes" because the difference between the AC presentation level of the tone in the TE (70 dB HL) compared with the elevated/masked BC threshold in the left ear (25 dB HL) is 45 dB, which is still not less than the patient's potential IA (45 dB HL).

9. *Note:* The same pattern would continue and you will never establish a plateau.

10. Indicate on the audiogram, "The initial masking may be overmasking (masking dilemma)." In this case, you cannot determine the true AC threshold for either ear. You can state that at least one ear has that degree of hearing loss, but you do not know which ear, and you do not know the degree of hearing loss in the other ear.

For BC masked thresholds (masker presented by supra-aural earphone):

1. IML = 60 dB HL (55 dB HL AC threshold + 5 dB + 0 dB OE). This elevates the BC threshold in NTE to 15 dB HL. Notice that only 5 dB was included in the IML because of the expectation of a small plateau, if any, before overmasking may occur. Notice also that there is no additional masker added for the OE because of the potential air–bone gap in the NTE.

2. Overmasking is a possibility (same as for AC masking). The 60 dB HL of AC masker level compared to the 10 dB BC threshold = 50 dB, which is greater than the patient's potential IA of 45 dB (obtained by comparing the 55 dB unmasked AC threshold to the 10 dB unmasked BC threshold). When there is a possibility of overmasking, you should always mask because the patient may have a higher IA than appears from the unmasked thresholds, but remain suspicious of a possible masking dilemma.

3. Present the BC tone to the TE at 10 dB HL (original unmasked threshold). *Patient does not respond.* Note that if the patient had responded at this level, you may have the beginning of a small plateau.

4. Increase BC tone to the TE at 15 dB HL. *Patient responds.* Ask yourself: Could it still be from the NTE? In this case, the answer is "yes" because the difference between the BC presentation level of the tone in the TE (15 dB HL) compared with the elevated/masked BC threshold in the left ear (15 dB HL) is 0 dB, which is still not less than the patient's potential IA (0 dB HL). At this point, you are essentially in a masking dilemma; however, you could try a couple more steps to be sure a plateau cannot be established.

5. Increase masker in NTE to 65 dB HL; present BC tone to TE at 15 dB HL. *Patient does not respond.*

6. Increase BC tone in TE to 20 dB HL. *Patient responds.* Ask yourself: Could it still be from the NTE? In this case, the answer is again "yes" because the elevated (masked) BC threshold in NTE is also at 20 dB HL.

7. Increase masker in NTE to 70 dB HL; present tone to TE at 20 dB HL. *Patient does not respond.*

8. Increase tone to 25 dB HL. *Patient responds.* Ask yourself: Could it still be from the NTE? In this case the answer is again "yes" because the elevated (masked) BC threshold in NTE is also at 25 dB HL.

9. The same pattern would continue and you will never establish a plateau.

10. Indicate on the audiogram, "The initial masking may be overmasking (masking dilemma)." In this case, you cannot determine the true BC thresholds for either ear. You

can state that at least one ear has a conductive loss, but you do not know which ear.

In summary, for situations in which there is a potential bilateral air–bone gap, you should suspect a possible masking dilemma. As you can surmise from Figure 9–11, each time a "yes" was obtained, the difference between the BC presentation level in the TE, when compared with the elevated/masked BC threshold in the NTE, still equaled the patient's IA (0 dB) and you could not conclude that it was from the TE. With additional increases of masker and subsequent increases of the tone in the TE (AC or BC), not even a small plateau could be established. However, when faced with the potential for a masking dilemma, masking should always be attempted because the actual patient's IA may be higher than the minimum based on the unmasked thresholds. In some cases, a small (e.g., 10 dB) plateau may be established and provide some evidence of the true thresholds. If that occurs, it should be noted on the audiogram and/or clinical report. The use of an insert earphone may allow a small plateau. As indicated earlier, in cases where there is an asymmetric hearing loss, it is best to try to obtain masked responses from the poorer ear first because the IML would be lower in the better ear, and if the masked BC thresholds of the poorer ear reveal a shift (e.g., sensorineural loss), then the original unmasked BC would represent the other ear and masking would not be needed, thus avoiding a masking dilemma. If you attempt to obtain masked thresholds first for the better hearing ear, the IML would be more likely to show a masking dilemma. Ultimately, however, you may need to attempt masking in both ears.

MASKING FOR SPEECH TESTING

The principles of masking for speech testing are the same as for pure-tone threshold testing, and in fact apply to any clinical tests in which the NTE may be contributing to the signals presented to the TE. Recall that clinical masking is necessary whenever the IA is exceeded and the signal being presented to the TE can be heard in the NTE by bone conduction (BC). For speech testing, masking would be needed whenever the presentation level of the speech materials in the TE exceeds the IA and cross-hearing to the NTE (by BC) can occur. Since the speech materials have a relatively broad spectrum, any of the bone conduction thresholds in the NTE may provide enough information for the patient to correctly respond; therefore, when making decisions about masking for the speech tests you must compare the presentation level of the speech (by AC) in the TE to the *best* BC threshold in the NTE. As mentioned in an earlier section on pure-tone masking, often the decision for AC masking is made while the earphones are on, but before the BC thresholds are obtained; in that case, the masking is based on assumed BC thresholds. For speech testing, many audiologists make decisions to mask for the speech measures while the earphones are still on and, therefore, also would need to make assumptions about the BC thresholds. For the examples in this textbook, the actual BC thresholds are provided. However, the following should serve as a guiding principle in masking for speech tests:

> Sufficient speech spectrum noise must be presented to the NTE by AC to elevate the actual or assumed best BC threshold in the NTE so that the speech being presented to the TE would not be heard in the NTE.

Of course, the IA for speech will depend on the type of transducer; insert earphones have a greater IA value than supra-aural earphones, just as for pure-tone testing. Establishing an IA for speech materials is complicated by the variations in the intensity among speech sounds that occur naturally and may be different for different types of materials. Estimates of the IA for spondee words range from 48 to 76 dB for supra-aural earphones, and for speech detection may be as low as 35 dB (Yacullo, 2009). For insert earphones, Sklare and Denenberg (1987) reported a range of 68 to 84 dB. However, to make things easier to remember it seems reasonable to use the same minimum IAs used for pure-tones, that is, 40 dB and 55 dB for supra-aural earphones and insert earphones, which are the IA values used in the following examples.

Masking for Speech Recognition Threshold (SRT)

For speech recognition threshold (SRT) testing, decisions about the need for masking follow the same principles as for pure-tone threshold testing. If masking for SRT is needed, then the goal is to deliver enough speech masking noise to the NTE so that you are confident the words presented to the TE are not heard in the NTE (by BC). Keep in mind, however, that if you masked for pure tones and found that the masked AC pure-tone thresholds were the same as the unmasked thresholds (i.e., no shift in thresholds occurred), then masking would not be required for SRT testing.

Unlike masking for pure-tone thresholds, masking for speech does not use the plateau method of masking; instead a single level of noise is selected based on the expected level of the speech. Therefore, when masking is needed for SRT you would select a single speech masker level that is sufficient to elevate/mask the *best* BC threshold in the NTE to a level whereby the BC of the NTE cannot contribute to the recognition of the speech materials presented in TE. In other words, the level of the masker is chosen so that the difference between the estimated/expected SRT in the TE minus the elevated/masked *best* BC threshold in the NTE is less than the IA for the AC transducer being used. If you have the pure-tone masked thresholds, then you can estimate the SRT based on the corresponding AC threshold of the best BC threshold or use the PTA. As discussed earlier, the minimum IAs for speech will be the same as for pure-tones, 40 dB for supra-aurals and 55 dB for inserts. Generally, the goal is to select the level of the masker so that it elevates/masks the best BC threshold so the difference between the level of the speech and the best BC is 5 dB less than the minimum IAs (35 dB for supra-aurals and 50 dB for inserts).

Figure 9–12 shows a typical example of masking for SRT testing using supra-aural earphones for a selected level of the speech masker. From the PTA (63 dB HL) of the right ear, you can anticipate that the right ear SRT would be within 10 dB of this level, and most likely will be about 60 dB HL. In addition, you can see (or assume) that the best BC threshold in the left ear is 0 dB

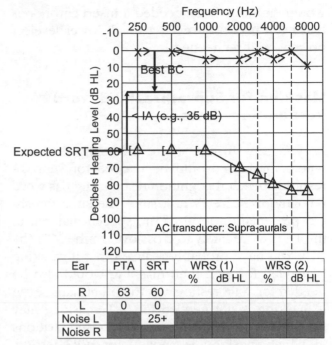

Ear	PTA	SRT	WRS (1)		WRS (2)	
			%	dB HL	%	dB HL
R	63	60				
L	0	0				
Noise L		25+				
Noise R						

FIGURE 9–12. Example of masking for speech recognition threshold (SRT). A single speech masker level is selected based on the expected SRT or PTA of the right ear, which when compared to the elevated/masked best bone conduction threshold in the left ear is sufficient to eliminate the possibility of cross hearing. For this example, the minimum speech masking level is 25 dB HL; however, higher levels of noise could have been selected to achieve the same goal of eliminating cross-hearing to the left ear. See text for explanation. AC, air conduction; BC, bone conduction; IA, interaural attenuation; R, right ear; L, left ear.

HL; thus there is more than a 40 dB difference between the AC threshold in the right ear and the best BC threshold in the left ear. Subtracting 35 dB from the expected level of the words indicates that the best BC threshold would have to be elevated to at least 25 dB HL; therefore, in this example, the minimum level of the masker would need to be 25 dB HL in order to elevate/mask the left ear BC threshold to 25 dB. The selected level is a minimum, and higher levels of the masker would accomplish the same goal as long as overmasking does not occur. The SRT for the right ear would be recorded in the appropriate box on the audiometric worksheet, along with the level of masking noise that was used in the left ear. Notice that in this example, masking would have also been needed if insert earphones had been used; however, a much lower level of noise would be needed.

Masking for Suprathreshold Word Recognition Tests

As you can surmise, there are many instances where masking would be needed for suprathreshold speech recognition testing, such as word recognition score (WRS), since the suprathreshold presentation level of the speech material in the TE is more likely to cross over to the NTE (by BC). You have probably realized that if masking is needed for SRT, then masking would also be needed for WRS testing. On the other hand, even if masking is not needed for SRT, masking may be needed for WRS testing. For those situations in which masking is needed for WRS testing, a single level of speech masker would also be selected for each level that the words are presented. The selected level of the speech masker would also be dependent on the selected WRS presentation level. As with masking for SRT, the level of the speech masker is selected so that it effectively elevates the best BC threshold in the NTE so that it cannot contribute to the recognition of the speech being presented to the TE.

Figure 9–13 is a continuation of the previous audiogram and shows how to select the level of masking for a specific presentation level of the words, in this case 85 dB HL using supra-aural earphones. The difference between the presentation level of the words in the right ear (85 dB HL) compared to the best BC threshold in the left ear (0 dB HL) is equal to 85 dB, thus exceeding the minimum IA for either supra-aural earphones or inserts. In this example, the level of masker selected in the left ear would be at least 50 dB HL, which elevates/masks the left ear AC and BC thresholds to 50 dB HL. With this masker level, the difference between the right ear presentation level (85 dB HL) and the left ear BC threshold with masking (50 dB HL) is equal to 35 dB, which less the target of at least 5 dB is less than the minimum IA for speech with supra-aural earphones. Notice also that higher levels of the speech masker (e.g., 65 dB HL) could also

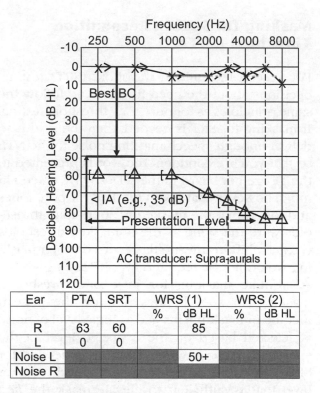

FIGURE 9–13. Example of masking for word recognition score (WRS). A single speech masker level is selected based on the presentation level of the words in the right ear, which when compared to the elevated/masked best bone conduction threshold in the left ear eliminates the possibility of cross hearing. For this example, the minimum speech masking level is 50 dB HL; however, higher levels of noise could have been selected to achieve the same goal of eliminating cross-hearing to the left ear. See text for explanation. AC, air conduction; BC, bone conduction; IA, interaural attenuation; R, right ear; L, left ear.

be used. The WRS scores are recorded on the audiogram worksheet along with the WRS presentation level (dB HL) and the masking level.

A rule of thumb used by many audiologists is to select the level of the speech masker in the NTE that 20 dB less than the level of words being presented in the TE. This practice would be appropriate in most situations; however, you must be cautious of overmasking, especially if there is an air–bone gap in the TE. As with pure-tone masking, a masking dilemma may occur when there is a moderate potentially bilateral air–bone gap (conductive component), because the minimum level of masking could be overmasking.

SYNOPSIS 9–3

- Masking is needed for speech testing whenever there is the possibility of cross-hearing, as for pure-tone testing.
- The authors' recommended minimum IA for speech is 40 dB HL and 55 dB for supra-aural and insert earphones, respectively.
- Masking for SRT is needed if the pure-tone thresholds were obtained with masking.
- Masking for WRS is needed more often than SRT because it is performed at a suprathreshold level. Masking for WRS may be needed even if masking for SRT is not needed.
- For speech masking, a single level of speech masker is selected for each level of speech testing, so that the difference between the presentation level of the speech compared with the best BC threshold of the NTE is less than the IA.
- There is often a range of speech masker levels that would satisfy the criteria of minimum masking and not overmasking.
- Presentation levels and masker levels are typically included on the audiogram worksheet.

REFERENCES

American National Standards Institute [ANSI]. (1996). Specifications for audiometers, *ANSI S3.6-1996*. New York, NY.

American National Standards Institute [ANSI]. (2010). Specifications for audiometers. *ANSI S3.6-2010*. New York, NY: Author.

Chaiklin, J. B. (1967). Interaural attenuation and cross-hearing in air-conduction audiometry. *Journal of Auditory Research*, 7, 413–424.

Coles, R. R. A., & Priede, V. M. (1970). On the misdiagnosis resulting from incorrect use of masking. *Journal of Laryngology and Otolaryngology*, 84, 41–63.

Gelfand, S. A. (2015). *Essentials of Audiology* (4th ed.). New York, NY: Thieme.

Hood, J. D. (1960). The principles and practice of bone-conduction audiometry. *Laryngoscope*, 70, 1211–1228.

Konkle, D. F., & Berry, G. A. (1983). Masking in speech audiometry. In D. F. Konkle & W. F. Rintelmann (Eds.), *Principles of Speech Audiometry* (pp. 285–319). Baltimore, MD: University Park Press.

Liden, G., Nilsson, G., & Anderson, H. (1959). Masking in clinical audiometry. *Acta Otolaryngologica*, 50, 125–136.

Martin, F. N., & Clark, J. G. (2015). *Introduction to Audiology* (12th ed.). Boston, MA: Pearson Education, Inc.

Roeser, R. J., & Clark, J. G. (2000). Clinical masking. In R. J. Roeser, M. Valente, & H. Hossford-Dunn (Eds.), *Audiology Diagnosis* (pp. 253–279). New York, NY: Thieme.

Sanders, J. W., & Rintleman, W. F. (1964). Masking in audiometry. *Archives of Otolaryngology*, 80, 541–556.

Silman, S., & Silverman, C. (1991). *Auditory Diagnosis: Principles and Applications*. San Diego, CA: Academic Press.

Sklare, D. A., & Denenberg, L. J. (1987). Interaural attenuation for tubephone insert earphones. *Ear and Hearing*, 8(5), 298–300.

Studebaker, G. A. (1962). On masking in bone-conduction testing. *Journal of Speech and Hearing Research*, 5, 215–227.

Studebaker, G. A. (1967). Clinical masking of the non-test ear. *Journal of Speech and Hearing Disorders*, 32, 360–367.

Tonndorf, J. (1972). Bone conduction. In J. V. Tobias (Ed.), *Foundations of Modern Auditory Theory* (pp. 84–99). New York, NY: Academic Press.

Turner, R. G. (2004). Masking redux ii. A recommended masking protocol. *Journal of the American Academy of Audiology*, 15, 29–46.

Yacullo, W. S. (1996). *Clinical Masking Procedures*. Boston, MA: Allyn and Bacon.

Yacullo, W. S. (2009). Clinical masking. In J. Katz, L. Medwetsky, R. Burkard, & L. Hood (Eds.), *Handbook of Clinical Audiology* (6th ed., pp. 80–115). Philadelphia, PA: Wolters Kluwer Lippincott Williams & Wilkins.

Zwislocki, J. (1953). Acoustic attenuation between the ears. *Journal of the Acoustical Society of America*, 25, 752–759.

10 Outer and Middle Ear Assessment

After reading this chapter, you should be able to:

1. Define admittance and describe how the admittance of the middle ear is measured using tympanometry and acoustic reflex threshold tests.

2. Recognize and describe tympanogram shapes (types) and their clinical interpretations.

3. Understand how and when to use high frequency probe-tone tympanometry and acoustic reflex measures.

4. Describe and interpret measures of wideband acoustic immittance (reflectance and absorbance).

5. Interpret acoustic reflex threshold patterns (ipsilateral and contralateral) and acoustic reflex decay measures.

6. Use acoustic reflex threshold criteria for cochlear ears (based on data by Gelfand et al.) to differentiate cochlear, 8th cranial nerve, and functional hearing loss.

Behavioral hearing tests evaluate the auditory system from the point where the sound wave hits the auricle to where the auditory cortex associates it with the sound that started the vibration. However, more information is available from each portion of the auditory system that cannot be obtained from behavioral tests. As audiologists, we need to assess each section of the system and compare a variety of test results to make a diagnosis as to the type and degree of hearing loss. There are several audiologic tests, not done with an audiometer, that are used to assess function from specific parts of the auditory system, and are referred to as objective tests because they usually do not require participation from the patient. These objective tests are used in conjunction with the behavioral tests, not in replacement of them, and when available are combined with audiometric results to create a more complete picture of the patient's overall hearing problem. These objective tests require specific instrumentation beyond the audiometer. The following sections provide an introductory look at the instrumentation, procedures, and interpretations of the objective tests that are commonly used in clinical audiology to assess the outer ear and middle ear, as well as the assessment of neural pathways associated with the acoustic reflex involving the stapedius muscle. *Otoscopy* is a method to visually inspect the ear canal and auricle; this procedure is usually accomplished before any test or hearing aid fitting, especially when you need to place anything into the ear. Tympanometry, wideband acoustic immittance, and acoustic reflexes are included in the *immittance test battery*, and are of such importance that they are routinely included in the basic audiological evaluation, along with pure-tone and speech audiometry. Immittance tests provide a look at how well sound energy can be transmitted through the outer ear and middle ear.

OTOSCOPY

The ability to peer into an ear canal to determine the status of the outer and middle ear has been available for more than 650 years since the first description of the *otoscope* (Feldmann,

1996). This tool is routinely used by otologists to help diagnose ear disorders; however, it is also used by audiologists to examine the ear canal and tympanic membrane to determine the color, shape, and general appearance of the structures to determine if they appear normal. Today's standard otoscopes are designed to illuminate and magnify the view down the ear canal. In addition, there are video otoscopes that allow for visualization, projection on a screen, and capture of the images for recordkeeping or showing to the patient.

Figure 10–1 shows photos of a standard otoscope and a video otoscope. The standard otoscope includes a head, handle, and a speculum (plural, *specula)*. The speculum is a plastic, funnel-shaped piece that attaches to the head of the otoscope and is the part that is placed into the ear canal of the patient. The specula are either sterilized or disposed of between patients so cross-contamination does not occur. The head of the otoscope contains a light source and magnification lens. There are a variety of heads for otoscopes, but the one most often used by audiologists consists of an LED light and enclosed lens. An LED light provides a bright white light that

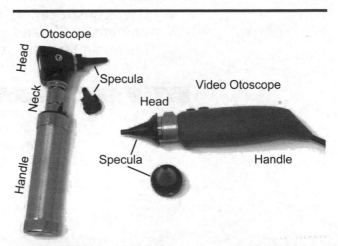

FIGURE 10–1. Otoscopes used in visualizing the ear canal and tympanic membrane. The otoscope on the left is a hand-held unit with a rechargeable battery pack in the handle and uses disposable specula to place in the ear canal. On the right, is a video otoscope with a disposable speculum. There is a small camera in the unit that displays the image on a monitor and can record the video feed for off-line viewing or printing.

lasts a long time and is cool to the touch. Otoscopes can have different levels of magnification from 2 to 4 times to allow you to better see the features of the external canal and tympanic membrane. The handle is used to hold onto the otoscope and houses the battery and power switch. Clinics can choose between non-reusable batteries, rechargeable batteries, or electrical corded handles according to their preference. The otoscopes with the non-reusable batteries are thinner and lighter because they use AA batteries. Otoscopes with rechargeable batteries are designed to place the handle onto a desktop charger or plug into the wall. The corded otoscopes are usually wall mounted and mobility is limited to the length of the cord. The video otoscope comes in either a standard otoscope configuration with a handle, head, and specula or as an in-line configuration as shown is Figure 10–1. Most video otoscopes require a connection to a computer to display, capture, and record the image. The specula for the video otoscopes are similar to those used with the standard otoscopes. The head of the video otoscope also has a button or wheel for adjusting the focus and a button (or floor switch) for capturing the picture or video.

When using an otoscope, proper technique is required to protect the patient. Unlike some medical professionals, the audiologist usually holds the otoscope with a pencil grip, as demonstrated in Figure 10–2, to allow bracing of the hand against the patient's head. Bracing is done to protect the patient from accidental injury as the speculum is inserted, and in case the patient suddenly moves when the otoscope is in her or his ear canal, the brace will allow the otoscope to move with the patient instead of causing damage to her or his ear canal. Holding the otoscope in the recommended position may seem awkward at first, but is generally easiest if held pencil-style between the thumb and next three fingers close to the head of the instrument, with the "pinky" finger extended to make contact with the head. The external ear is grasped by the tester's hand and pulled up and back to straighten out the ear canal. The otoscope speculum is inserted into the canal, and the otoscope is rotated to allow inspection of all landmarks of the ear canal and tympanic membrane. Otoscopy should be com-

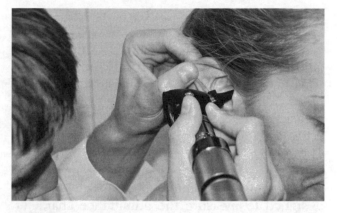

FIGURE 10–2. When viewing the tympanic membrane through an otoscope it is important to use a proper bracing technique where one hand pulls up and back on the auricle and the fingers of the other hand are placed against the head so as to not allow the speculum to be pushed further into the canal if the patient moves during visualization.

pleted on every patient before any test instrument is placed in the ear canal to verify that there is no foreign object that could damage the structures if hit, or other condition that may negate placing anything into the ear canal. When performing otoscopy for removing cerumen, which may contain bodily fluids, or whenever there is some discharge in the ear canal, personal protective gear (typically nitrile gloves) must be worn and properly disposed.

IMMITTANCE

Immittance audiometry infers the extent to which sound energy is transferred through the outer and middle ear systems. If we apply a known sound source to the ear, the acoustic and mechanical properties of the outer and middle ears provide a certain amount of opposition to the flow of energy. The opposition to the flow of energy is called *impedance*, such that a high impedance system has a greater opposition to the flow of energy. The reciprocal of impedance is called *admittance*, which is a measure of how much of the applied energy flows through the system, such that a high admittance system has a greater flow of energy. A high admittance system has a low impedance, and vice versa. If either impedance or admittance is known, the other can be determined by a relatively simple calculation, since they are reciprocals. Impedance is usually designated as Z and measured in units of *ohms*; admittance is usually designated as Y and measured in units of *millimhos*. These two properties are related such that Y = 1/Z or Z = 1/Y. The term *immittance* is used to encompass the concepts of both admittance and impedance. However, today's immittance instruments are designed to measure the admittance characteristics of the auditory system and the results are reported in terms of the admittance values (Y).

The instrument used in immittance audiometry goes by a variety of names, such as an "immittance instrument," "admittance instrument," or "middle ear analyzer." As shown in Figure 10–3, a variety of immittance instruments are commercially available from different manufacturers. Figure 10–4 shows the basic components of an admittance instrument. To obtain a measure of admittance, an 85 dB SPL pure tone (usually 226 Hz), called the *probe tone*, is presented to the ear through a probe assembly placed at the entrance to the ear canal. A microphone, which is also part of the probe assembly, is used to monitor the level of the probe tone in the ear canal. For infants younger than 6 months, conventional tympanometry with a 226 Hz probe tone is not a valid measure, and other probe-tone frequencies are recommended (as described later in this chapter).

For a normal outer and middle ear system, there is an expected admittance associated with a given probe tone. Modern instruments use an *automatic gain control* (AGC) circuit to automatically adjust the output level of the probe tone to maintain it at 85 dB SPL in the ear canal. Any change in dB SPL performed by the AGC circuit is a reflection of how much energy is admitted by the system, and is used to calculate the admittance. The measured admittance is compared with the admittance characteristics of known cavity sizes to which the equipment is calibrated. For example, for a 226 Hz probe tone, 1.0 mmho is approximately equal to the admittance associated with a 1.0 cubic centimeter (cm^3) or 1.0 milliliter (ml) volume of air at sea level. Although the mmho is the preferable unit, some instruments plot the admittance in units of cm^3 or ml (which are all essentially equivalent). This simple relationship of admittance to volume is one of the reasons why 226 Hz is used as the probe tone. Figure 10–5 shows that, as cavity size increases,[1] the admittance of an acoustic system increases and, therefore, the AGC circuit must increase the SPL to maintain the 226 Hz probe tone at 85 dB SPL. Because of the relation of admittance to cavity size, the clinical measures of admittance are calibrated to be equivalent to different cavity sizes that approximate the range of

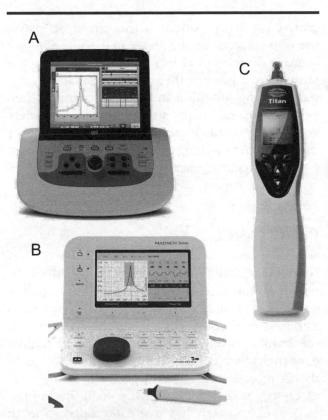

FIGURE 10–3. Some examples of middle ear analyzers for clinical assessment of the middle ear. **A.** Grason-Stadler Model TympStar Pro. **B.** Interacoustics Model Titan. **C.** Madsen Model Zodiac. *Source*: Photos courtesy of Grason-Stadler Inc. (A), Interacoustics (B), Otometrics/Audiology Systems (C).

---

[1]Acoustic immittance (Y_a) is equal to volume velocity (U) divided by the pressure (P). As cavity size increases (larger U), the admittance increases for a constant pressure. Likewise, as admittance increases, the cavity size increases for a constant pressure.

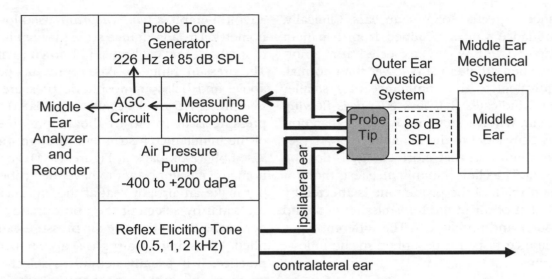

FIGURE 10–4. Block diagram showing the key components of an admittance instrument or middle ear analyzer. The air pressure pump is used to apply air pressure during tympanometry. The reflex eliciting tones (ipsilateral and contralateral) are used for acoustic reflex testing. See text for an explanation on how the probe tone is used to measure the admittance of the outer and middle ear. *AGC*, automatic gain circuit.

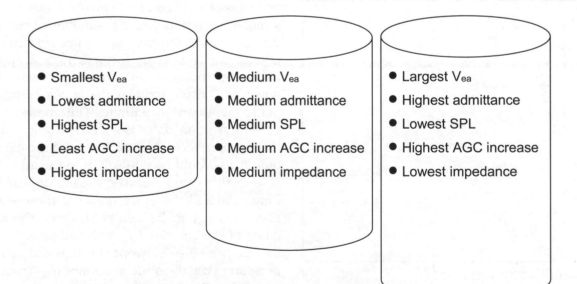

FIGURE 10–5. Illustration of the relationship between the volume of a cavity and measures of admittance or impedance. As cavity size increases, the admittance increases due to a reduced sound pressure level (*SPL*) of the probe tone, and more gain is required by the automatic gain circuit (*AGC*) to maintain the 85 dB SPL probe-tone level in the ear canal. Clinically, admittance measures are related to the admittance of cavities of known volumes and compared with the expected admittance for normal ears.

admittance expected for human ears. Clinically, the admittance values obtained from a patient are compared with what is expected from a normal ear. When admittance is lower than normal, it is equivalent to the admittance of a smaller cavity and indicates that less energy is flowing into the ear. When admittance is higher than normal, it is equivalent to the admittance of a larger cavity and indicates that more energy is flowing into the ear. The clinical immittance tests monitor how the dB SPL of the probe tone is affected by changes that occur in the transmission of sound in the outer and middle ear. The different types of immittance tests are described in the following sections.

TYMPANOMETRY

Tympanometry measures how the admittance changes as a function of applied air pressure and how this function is affected by different conditions of the middle ear. Figure 10–6 shows

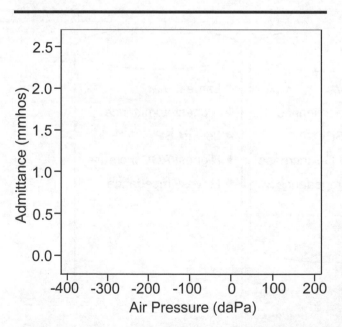

FIGURE 10–6. A typical graph that is used to display tympanograms. The admittance instrument is used to measure the admittance in millimhos (mmhos) along the *y*-axis, as a function of applied air pressure in decaPascals (daPa) along the *x*-axis. The 0 daPa value represents the atmospheric pressure, and the other daPa values are above (+) or below (–) atmospheric pressure.

a typical graph, a *tympanogram*, used for tympanometry. The admittance scale (*y*-axis) is in units of mmhos or ml calibrated to known cavity sizes. The pressure range (*x*-axis) represents pressures above and below atmospheric pressure, which is represented by 0 decaPascals (daPa). The air pressure is delivered by the air pressure pump of the immittance instrument through the probe assembly (look back at Figure 10–4). For tympanometry, it is important to have the probe assembly make an airtight seal at the entrance to the ear canal by selecting the appropriate-size rubber probe tip so that the air pressure can be applied. Obtaining an airtight seal may take some practice; it is usually helpful to select a probe tip that is slightly larger than the ear canal and to pull up and back on the auricle to straighten the cartilaginous portion of the ear canal as the probe is inserted, then let the ear canal close around the probe tip. It is important not to conduct tympanometry on ears with active middle ear disease (i.e., ear canal drainage) as this fluid can enter the probe during testing.

Figure 10–7 illustrates the principles of recording a tympanogram at three different amounts of air pressure. Tympanometry provides a means of separating the admittance related to the ear canal from the admittance related to the middle ear. This is performed by first applying maximum positive air pressure (+200 daPa), which effectively reduces the ability of the tympanic membrane to vibrate: The admittance recorded at +200 daPa is a relatively low admittance that reflects the admittance of the ear canal only. This would be equivalent to the admittance of a smaller cavity because the middle ear is not functional and, therefore, does not allow as much sound energy to be admitted. Once the admittance of the ear canal is obtained at +200 daPa, the air pressure is swept through the range of pressures (usually done automatically) from +200 to −400 daPa. For a normal functioning middle ear, there should be a maximum admittance at 0 daPa (atmospheric pressure) because that is where the air pressure in the external ear canal is equal to the air pressure in the middle ear, and is where the tympanic membrane vibrates most effectively. The maximum admittance measured at 0 daPa is equivalent to the volume of a larger cavity than at +200 daPa and reflects the

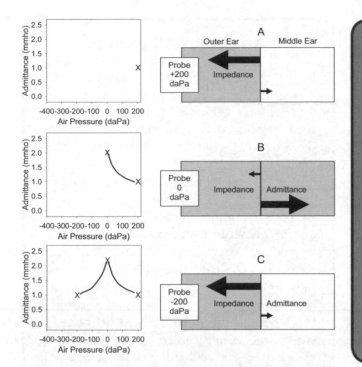

FIGURE 10–7. A–C. Illustration of how a normal tympanogram is generated. In **A**, the applied air pressure is at +200 daPa above atmospheric pressure and results in a minimum admittance that is equivalent to a relatively small cavity. This small admittance represents the admittance of only the outer ear because the tympanic membrane is not able to vibrate normally. In **B**, when the applied air pressure is lowered to 0 daPa (atmospheric pressure), the admittance reaches a maximum because the tympanic membrane can now vibrate most effectively. In this case, the admittance is equivalent to a larger cavity that represents the admittance of the outer and middle ear. In **C**, when the applied air pressure is at –200 daPa, the tympanic membrane does not vibrate effectively and the admittance is again equivalent to a small cavity that represents the admittance of only the outer ear. The actual admittance of the middle ear itself is represented by the difference between the maximum admittance and the admittance at +200 daPa.

admittance of both the outer ear and middle ear in the transmission of the probe tone. As the applied air pressure becomes negative, the admittance again decreases (equivalent to the volume of a smaller cavity) because the tympanic membrane does not vibrate as efficiently and reflects the admittance of the ear canal only. The actual admittance of the middle ear is represented by the difference between the admittance obtained

at +200 daPa and the admittance obtained at 0 daPa (or the point of maximum admittance).

Figure 10–8 shows a normal tympanogram, conventionally called a *Type A tympanogram*. The shape of the normal (Type A) tympanogram has the peak admittance occurring at 0 daPa and a systematic reduction in admittance at the higher and lower pressures. The pressure where the tympanogram peak occurs is called the *tympanometric peak pressure* (TPP). The admittance obtained at +200 daPa is related to the *acoustic equivalent volume of the ear canal* (V_{ea}), which is described in more detail in the next section. The overall peak of the tympanogram (Peak Y) includes the admittance of both the outer ear and the middle ear; therefore, the actual *admittance of the middle ear* (Y_{tm}), as calculated at the tympanic membrane, is the difference in admittance between Peak Y and V_{ea}. The way the tympanogram is displayed in Figure 10–8 is called a *non-compensated tympanogram*, which means that the graph displays the admittance value for the ear canal (V_{ea} at +200 daPa) and the additional admittance that is related to the middle ear (Y_{tm} at 0 daPa). Today's immittance instruments can also display the tympanogram as a *compensated tympanogram*, which is shown in Figure 10–9.

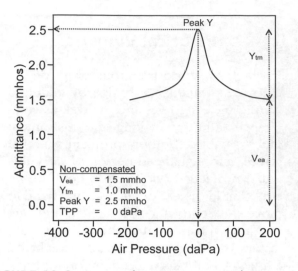

FIGURE 10–8. A normal *non-compensated* tympanogram. The admittance of the outer ear (V_{ea}) is first obtained at +200 daPa and is then subtracted from the overall admittance (Peak Y) to obtain the admittance of the middle ear (Y_{tm}). The air pressure where the peak of the tympanogram occurs is called the tympanometric peak pressure (TPP).

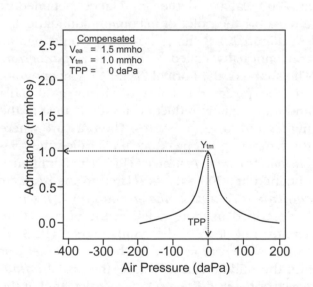

FIGURE 10–9. A normal *compensated* tympanogram. The admittance of the outer ear (V_{ea}) is first obtained at +200 daPa but is not displayed on the graph; instead the tympanogram is automatically displaced downward by the amount of the V_{ea} so that the peak admittance is a direct reflection of the admittance of the middle ear (Y_{tm}). The V_{ea} is only displayed as a numerical value. The air pressure where the peak of the tympanogram occurs is called the tympanometric peak pressure (TPP).

A compensated tympanogram automatically removes the admittance due to the ear canal (V_{ea} at +200 daPa) in the graph, and the tympanogram displays only the admittance of the middle ear. The compensated tympanogram begins at +200 daPa with an admittance of 0 mmhos. With a compensated tympanogram, the admittance of the ear canal (V_{ea}) is provided on the printout in numerical format. Compensated tympanograms are popular because the admittance on the y-axis is a direct measure of the middle ear admittance (Y_{tm}). Most of the tympanograms in this text will be displayed in the compensated format.

The ranges of normative values for the different tympanometric measures vary across studies and are dependent on a variety of parameters, including age, gender, pump speed, and direction of pressure change. Some normative values for the different tympanometric measures are shown in Table 10–1. As you can see, the normal admittance values have a relatively wide

TABLE 10–1. Normative Tympanometric Measures of Acoustic Equivalent Volume of Ear Canal (V_{ea}), Static Acoustic Admittance of the Middle Ear (Y_{tm}), Tympanometric Peak Pressure (TPP), and Tympanometric Width (TW)

Age Group	V_{ea} (ml or cc)	Y_{tm} (mmhos)	TPP (daPa)	TW (daPa)
Adults (>10 yr)	0.80 to 2.20	0.30 to 1.70	–105 to +5	<125
Children (>18 mo to 10 yr)	0.60 to 1.20	0.30 to 1.05	–75 to +25	<200
Children (6 mo to 18 mo)	0.50 to 1.00	0.20 to 0.70	–75 to +25	<250
Infants[a] (<6 mo)	0.20 to 0.80	0.40 to 2.10	NA	<150
AAA child screening fails	Not used	<0.20	<-200	>250

[a]1000 Hz probe tone; +200 compensation.
Data compiled from the following sources:
Roush et al. (1995)
American Academy of Audiology [AAA] (2011)
Margolis and Hunter (2000)
Hunter (2013)

range; however, when a measure is outside these norms, there is a good correlation with an abnormal middle ear condition.

Acoustic Equivalent Volume of the Ear Canal

The acoustic equivalent volume (V_{ea}) of the ear canal, as estimated from the admittance obtained at +200 daPa, can provide some diagnostic information about the condition of the tympanic membrane or ear canal. For a normal ear canal and tympanic membrane, the admittance at +200 should be within the normal range of ear canal volumes (see Table 10–1). Figure 10–10 illustrates how the V_{ea} can be used to determine the status of the tympanic membrane or the ear canal for different conditions. In Figure 10–10A, the tympanic membrane is intact and the V_{ea} (a reflection of the volume of the ear canal) is within the normal range. In Figure 10–10B, the tympanic membrane has a perforation or a pressure equalization (PE) tube surgically inserted for the treatment of a chronic ear infection, resulting in a V_{ea} that is larger than the normal range because it is now equivalent to a larger cavity that includes the outer ear and middle ear. Alternately, as shown in Figure 10–10C, if the V_{ea} is lower than the expected normal range it may be an indication that the exter-

nal ear canal is obstructed by a foreign object or has impacted cerumen. For either of these abnormal V_{ea} conditions, the tympanogram will not show any changes in admittance as the applied air pressure is varied and appears as a flat line. As cautionary notes, a small V_{ea} may also be caused by a plugged probe assembly, or the probe assembly is pushed up against the ear canal wall. It is also possible that an ear with a perforation could show a normal V_{ea} if there is thick fluid or other tissue mass that is filling the middle ear space. Therefore, it is imperative that you complete an otoscopic examination prior to making any measurement in the ear canal. In some patients, you may not be able to obtain an adequate seal of the probe tip because the applied positive air pressure or a swallow by the patient may open the eustachian tube and release the air pressure. In those cases, it is useful to set the tympanogram to measure V_{ea} at –200 daPa (which can hold the eustachian tube in its naturally closed position) and ask the patient not to breathe while performing the tympanogram, which sweeps through the air pressure range from negative to positive.

Tympanometric Width

Another way to quantify a tympanogram's shape is to measure the width of the tympanogram,

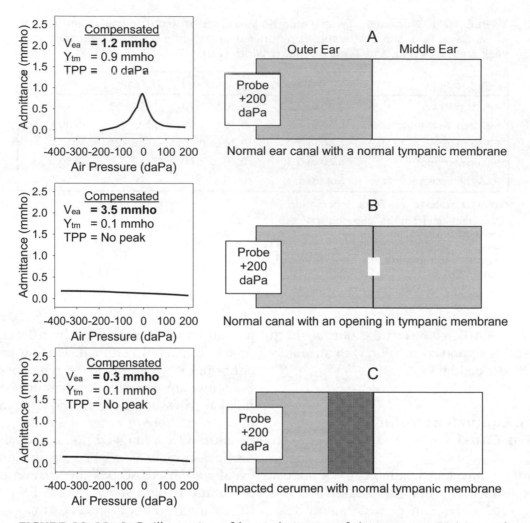

FIGURE 10–10. A–C. Illustration of how admittance of the outer ear (V_{ea}) is used clinically. In **A**, the tympanic membrane is intact, as evidenced by a normal-shaped tympanogram and a normal V_{ea}. In **B**, the tympanic membrane has a perforation, as evidenced by the flat tympanogram and larger than normal V_{ea}. In **C**, the ear canal is impacted with earwax (cerumen), as evidenced by a flat tympanogram and a smaller than normal V_{ea}. Y_{tm}, admittance of the middle ear; TPP, tympanometric peak pressure.

tympanometric width (TW), at a defined point. Tympanometric width is defined as the absolute value of the pressure range, in daPa, that corresponds to the width of the tympanogram at half the height of the peak of the tympanogram. Figure 10–11 illustrates how TW is calculated. First establish the point that is half of the height of the compensated Y_{tm}; then draw a horizontal line at this half-height point to intersect the positive and negative sides of the tympanogram. At each of the two intersection points, drop a vertical line down to the two corresponding pressure points along the x-axis: The TW is the difference between these two pressure points and is expressed in daPa. Most modern instruments automatically calculate and display the value of TW. Figure 10–12 shows examples of abnormally wide tympanograms. An abnormal TW is usually associated with middle ear fluid that is either accumulating or resolving; and as the condition of

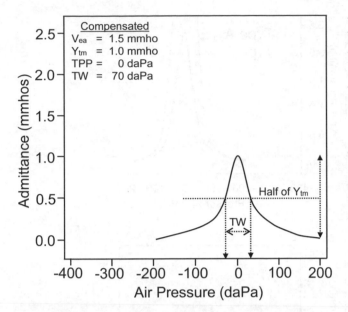

FIGURE 10–11. Illustration of how to calculate tympanometric width (TW). First, find the value on the y-axis that represents half the height of the admittance of the middle ear (Y_{tm}) and draw a horizontal line so that it intersects the tympanogram on both sides. Then draw vertical lines down from the two intersecting points to the air pressure scale. The TW is the absolute value of the difference between the two pressure points. Most admittance instruments can automatically calculate the TW. V_{ea} admittance of the outer ear; TPP, tympanometric peak pressure.

the middle ear changes, the tympanogram may become a flat line or may become normal. Refer to Table 10–1 for normal ranges of TW based on several studies. For example, a TW > 200 daPa would be abnormal for children 1.5 to 12 years old based on the consolidated data in this table.

Types of Tympanograms

A commonly used scheme to describe tympanograms is based on the types described by Jerger (1970). As already described, the normal tympanogram is referred to as a Type A tympanogram (see Figure 10–9). Abnormal tympanograms, as illustrated in Figure 10–13, are labeled *Type A_s*, *Type A_d*, *Type B*, and *Type C* tympanograms. While Jerger's classification scheme is widely used, not everyone reading an audiology report will know what the types mean. A more useful approach is to describe the actual characteristics of the tympanogram, for example, "a flat tympanogram" or "a normal-shaped tympanogram with the peak admittance occurring at −300 daPa." The different types of tympanograms and their descriptions are briefly described below.

Normal admittance (Type A) tympanogram has a characteristic peak shape with the Y_{tm} and

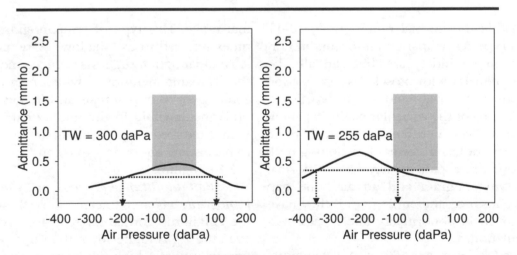

FIGURE 10–12. Two examples in which the tympanic width (TW) is abnormally wide. The normal range for TW is indicated by the *shaded box*. Calculation of TW is independent of the tympanic peak pressure (TPP).

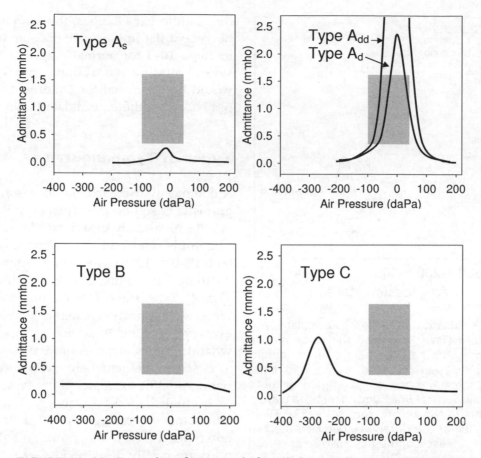

FIGURE 10–13. Examples of commonly found abnormal tympanograms and their labels based on the Jerger (1970) classification scheme. See text for descriptions of these tympanogram types and their associated pathologies.

the TPP within the normal range (Table 10–1). A normal (Type A) tympanogram occurs in normal functioning middle ears, but can also be found in some ears with otosclerosis (a fixation of the stapes in the oval window) or disarticulation (disruption) of the ossicular chain. A patient with a normal (Type A) will not have an air–bone gap if the patient has a normal functioning middle ear; however, a patient may have a normal (Type A) tympanogram and an air–bone gap (conductive loss) on the audiogram if they have an ossicular chain abnormality like otosclerosis or disarticulation.

Reduced admittance (Type A_s) tympanogram has a characteristic peak shape with the TPP in the normal range as for Type A; however, the Y_{tm} is lower than the lower end of the nor-

mal range. This type of tympanogram is sometimes referred to as "shallow." A reduced (Type A_s) tympanogram suggests reduced movement of the tympanic membrane, which may be seen in some cases of otosclerosis and in some cases of otitis media (fluid in the middle ear). A patient with a reduced (Type A_s) tympanogram is likely to have some air–bone gaps (conductive loss) on the audiogram.

High admittance (Type A_d or Type A_dd) tympanogram has a characteristic peak shape with the TPP in the normal range as for Type A; however, the Y_{tm} is higher than the upper end of the normal range. A high admittance (Type A_d) tympanogram suggests a highly mobile tympanic membrane, which may be seen in some cases of disarticulation of the ossicular chain or cases of thinned tympanic membranes resulting from previous middle ear infections. A high admittance (Type A_{dd}) tympanogram has an extremely high-value Y_{tm}; in fact, the admittance may go off the chart. These high admittance types (Type A_d or Type A_{dd}) are highly suggestive of a disarticulation of the ossicular chain and will usually have an air–bone gap (conductive loss) on their audiogram.

Flat (Type B) tympanogram does not have the characteristic peak shape seen for Type A, but instead appears as a relatively flat tracing across the pressure range. A flat (Type B) tympanogram is quite common in cases of otitis media with effusion (fluid in the middle ear). A flat (Type B) tympanogram will also occur when there is a perforation in the tympanic membrane or if a pressure equalization (PE) tube has been put into the tympanic membrane as a treatment for otitis media; however, perforations or PE tubes can be differentiated from otitis media by a larger than normal V_{ea}. A flat (Type B) tympanogram can also occur with impacted cerumen, a clogged probe assembly, or with the probe pushed against the ear canal wall; however, these conditions will be accompanied by a lower than normal V_{ea}. The audiologist must be sure that a flat (Type B) tympanogram is not due to poor placement or poor operation of the probe assembly. Patients with a flat (Type B) tympanogram may or may not have an audiogram with air–bone gaps depending on the reason for the flat tracing: A flat (Type B) tympanogram with a normal V_{ea} is expected to have air–bone gaps on the audiogram; a flat (Type B) tympanogram with a large V_{ea}, due to a small perforation or PE tube, most likely will not have air–bone gaps on the audiogram; a flat (Type B) tympanogram with a low V_{ea}, due to a foreign object or impacted cerumen, may have small air–bone gaps on the audiogram.

Negative pressure (Type C) tympanogram has a characteristic peak shape as seen with Type A; however, the TPP is shifted to a more negative pressure point. A negative pressure (Type C) tympanogram indicates that the pressure in the middle ear space is not equalized to the atmospheric pressure. Some negative pressure is common in ears as a temporary condition due to sniffling or after a recent airplane flight. These situations are generally not of much clinical significance, and in many cases chewing or swallowing opens the eustachian tube equalizing the pressure and causes the ears to "pop." This causes the negative pressure (Type C) tympanogram to change to a normal (Type A) tympanogram. However, when the TPP is outside the normal ranges and a negative pressure (Type C) tympanogram persists for an extended period of time, it may suggest poor eustachian tube function due to an allergy or cold. Poor eustachian tube function can lead to fluid in the ear, at which point the tympanogram will change to flat (Type B). A patient with a negative pressure (Type C) tympanogram will usually not have air–bone gaps on the audiogram unless the Type C tympanogram is also accompanied by a reduced Y_{tm} or an abnormal TW.

In summary, an abnormal tympanogram is a good indication of some middle ear involvement that affects the admittance characteristics of the middle ear. However, the tympanogram is not a predictor of the amount (if any) of conductive hearing loss and is most useful when used in conjunction with the pure-tone audiogram or other information about the patient. It is important to keep in mind also that the shape of the tympanogram does not always define the precise pathology, since some of the shapes can occur for different middle ear conditions. For example, when a normal, Type A, tympanogram is obtained you should not assume that the middle ear is normal because this can be found in some cases of otosclerosis or disarticulations; however, patients with these disorders should have air–bone gaps on their audiograms (see Chapter 12). A normal (Type A) tympanogram without any air–bone gaps on the audiogram rules out middle ear involvement, however, if there is an air–bone gap on the audiogram a normal Type A (or A_s) suggests some involvement of the ossicular chain, but rules out fluid in the middle ear (which should have a flat Type B tympanogram). In addition, a normal (Type A) tympanogram rules out a perforation in the tympanic membrane, obstruction of the ear canal, and fluid in the middle ear. Tympanometry is a valuable tool and is routinely included as part of the basic audiological test battery. In some cases, especially with children or other difficult-to-test populations

SYNOPSIS 10–1

- Physiological tests such as tympanometry and acoustic reflex thresholds are routinely included in the basic hearing evaluation. When used in conjunction with the history, pure-tone audiometry, and/or speech audiometry, these physiological measures can help differentiate or confirm different types of hearing disorders.
- Immittance is a term that refers to measures of impedance or admittance. Admittance is the ease with which the energy flows through a system. Impedance is the opposition to the flow of energy through a system.
- Most clinical instruments measure the admittance using a probe assembly sealed at the entrance to the ear canal. The probe assembly has a miniature speaker to deliver a probe tone (usually 226 Hz at 85 dB SPL) and a microphone to monitor the dB SPL of the probe tone.
- In tympanometry, air pressure is applied over a range of +200 to –400 daPa relative to atmospheric pressure (0 daPa) and the change in admittance as a function of air pressure is graphed on a tympanogram. At the extreme positive and negative applied pressures, the admittance is reduced due to the immobility of the tympanic membrane caused by the applied air pressure. The positive pressure point allows for the estimation of the ear canal volume (V_{ea}) that is subtracted from the overall admittance to provide a measure of the middle ear admittance (Y_{tm}). A larger than normal V_{ea} can indicate a tympanic membrane perforation or pressure equalization tube. A smaller than normal V_{ea} can indicate a cerumen-impacted ear canal or blocked probe. Other tympanogram measures include the pressure where peak admittance occurs (TPP) or the width of the tympanogram at half its maximum height (TW). Tympanograms have conventional types and descriptions as follows:
  - Normal (Type A) tympanogram: Peak shape with a normal Y_{tm} occurring with a TPP around 0 daPa. Suggestive of normal functioning middle ears and some cases with otosclerosis or ossicular disarticulation.
  - Reduced admittance (Type A_s) tympanogram: Peak shape with a reduced (shallow) Y_{tm} occurring with a TPP around 0 daPa. Suggestive of otosclerosis or otitis media.
  - High admittance (Type A_d or A_{dd}) tympanogram: Peak shape with a higher than normal Y_{tm} occurring with a TPP around 0 daPa. Suggestive of ossicular disarticulation or highly mobile/flaccid tympanic membrane.
  - Flat (Type B) tympanogram: Low admittance and flat tracings (no change in Y_{tm} across the pressure range). Suggestive of otitis media with effusion. Also occurs with a tympanic membrane perforation or pressure equalization tube; however, these can be identified by the V_{ea}.
  - Negative pressure (Type C) tympanogram: Peak shape with a normal or reduced Y_{tm} occurring with a TPP in the negative pressure range. Suggestive of temporary eustachian tube dysfunction and/or resolving or developing stages of otitis media with effusion.
- See Table 10–1 for normative tympanometric values.

in which the pure-tone audiogram is not obtainable or is incomplete, tympanometric data can be helpful if you keep in mind the limitations of interpretation and use the information with other relevant patient information.

PROBE TONE FREQUENCY

In the previous section, the tympanometric measures were described for recordings made with a conventional low frequency (226 Hz) probe tone. The use of the low frequency probe tone may be justified when evaluating middle ear pathologies that predominantly affect the stiffness component of the middle ear system. However, there are some middle ear pathologies that are dominated by the mass component of the middle ear system, and these are better assessed using higher frequency probe tones (e.g., 678 or 1000 Hz). Mass dominant pathologies might include those that add mass to the system, such as scar tissue on the tympanic membrane or adhesions on the middle ear ossicles, or a break in the ossicular chain (disarticulation) that becomes mass dominant due to the reduction of the stiffness component. In addition, research has shown that infants younger than 4 months of age are better assessed with higher frequency (1000 Hz) probe tones due to developmental differences in outer and/or middle ear systems, and residual mesenchyme in the middle ear for a short period after birth (Hall & Swanepoel, 2010; Shanks & Shohet, 2009). Tympanometry using higher frequency probe tones can more readily differentiate between stiffness and mass dominant pathologies. For example, knowledge about the relative contributions of the stiffness and mass components provides differential diagnosis of pathologies due to fixation of the ossicular chain (otosclerosis) or disarticulation, both of which show up as a conductive hearing loss on the audiogram, and may even have relatively normal appearing tympanograms to low frequency probe tones.

Multifrequency tympanometry, in which the probe tone is automatically swept across a wide frequency range, has also been used to define the resonant frequency of the middle ear, which is much higher than normal for a stiffening pa-

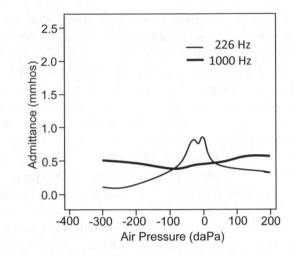

FIGURE 10–14. Tympanograms 226 and 1000 Hz in a 2-month-old infant.

thology like otosclerosis, and much lower than normal for a mass dominant pathology like disarticulation. The interested reader is referred to Hunter and Shahnaz (2013) for further information. The use of multifrequency tympanometry is not in widespread use today as a standard clinical test. With the development of wideband acoustic immittance measures, it is unlikely that the earlier method of using multifrequency tympanometry with pure tones will be adopted. However, one outcome that has emerged from the study of probe tone frequencies is the use of 1000 Hz probe tone for assessing newborns. Tympanometry conducted with 226 Hz probe tones often led to double-peaked tympanograms and conflicting interpretations of those results. Figure 10–14 shows both a 226 Hz and a 1000 Hz tympanogram from a 2-month-old infant; notice the difference in the shape of the tympanograms. It is possible for infants with middle ear fluid in their ear to have a normal 226 Hz tympanogram, but have an abnormal 1000 Hz tympanogram leading to an incorrect determination of type and degree of loss (Hunter & Margolis, 1992; Hunter, Tubaugh, Jackson, & Prospes, 2008; Shahnaz, Miranda, & Polka, 2008). Middle ear status can be detected with better sensitivity and specificity using 1000 Hz than 226 Hz probe tones in the newborn population (Zhiqi, Kun, & Zhiwu, 2010). With the development of newborn hearing screening, there was the impetus to accurately determine ears with normal middle ear function from those ears with fluid or other abnormalities. Therefore, the Joint Committee on Infant Hearing (JCIH) recommends the use of 1000 Hz tympanometry on infants less than 6 months of age (JCIH, 2007). Tympanometry with higher frequency probe tones has become a standard procedure when evaluating the hearing of infants. Tympanometry (1000 Hz) can be compared to normative data as shown in Table 10–1 to determine if the result is within the expected range. This assessment can be used as the cross-check to provide further evidence of the type of hearing loss.

WIDEBAND ACOUSTIC IMMITTANCE

Another, relatively new, method for measurement of middle ear properties is called *wideband acoustic immittance* (WAI) (Feeney et al., 2013).

The WAI is the overall set of measurements that includes both power-based and impedance-based measures, including the wideband power-based response functions of acoustic impedance, admittance, and reflectance. Previously, names such as wideband middle ear power, wideband reflectance, middle ear reflectometry, and wideband reflectance tympanometry, were utilized but they did not cover the entire spectrum of measurements (Feeney, Grant, & Marryott, 2003; Hall & Swanepoel, 2010; Hunter et al., 2008); therefore, WAI is the preferred term. The two most common ways to measure WAI are power reflectance and power absorbance.

If sound energy is presented down the ear canal, the amount of power reflected at the tympanic membrane is the power reflectance and the amount of sound transmitted through to the middle ear is the power absorption. Power reflectance is similar to multifrequency tympanometry, in that it measures the stimulus power that is reflected from the tympanic membrane (not

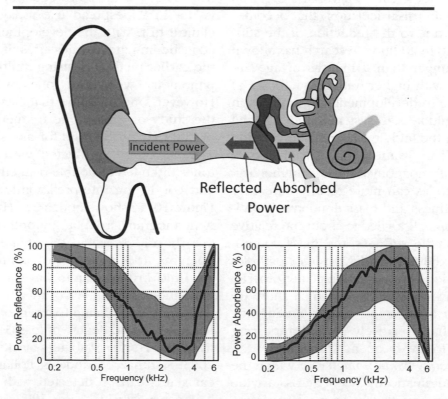

FIGURE 10–15. In WAI, the sound is sent down the ear canal and the power reflected back is shown (as a percentage) on the left and the power absorbed is shown (as a percentage) on the right.

admitted into the middle ear) for a variety of applied frequencies. Figure 10–15 shows the incidence wave traveling down the ear canal toward the eardrum; the reflected sound energy is the power reflected from the ear drum and the absorbance is the energy that is transmitted through the system. In most systems, some of the energy is reflected back, some is absorbed. Power reflectance is the ratio of the reflected sound energy to the incident sound energy, and equals the square of the magnitude of the pressure reflectance or $|R(f)|^2$. The power reflectance is constant along the tube and is determined by the acoustic impedance and the cross-sectional area at the terminating end. The result is displayed as a simple ratio from 0 to 1 (or as a percentage), where 0 indicates that all the sound is absorbed and 1 means that all the sound is reflected. The absorbance is equal to $1 - |R(f)|^2$ and is the sound power that is absorbed by the tympanic membrane expressed in percent. In other words, there is a relationship between the two measures as shown in Figure 10–15.

$$\text{Power Reflectance} = \frac{\text{Reflected Power}}{\text{Incident Power}}$$

and

$$\text{Power Absorbance} = \frac{\text{Absorbed Power}}{\text{Incident Power}}$$

When wideband stimuli, such as *chirps*, are used as the incident stimulus, the reflected energy can be analyzed by frequency. Measurements may be taken at ambient pressure, or at a range of ear canal air pressures, as employed in traditional tympanometry. Currently there are two FDA approved units which measure WAI; one unit measures at ambient pressure and reports power reflectance (Figure 10–16A) and the other unit measures absorbance at multiple

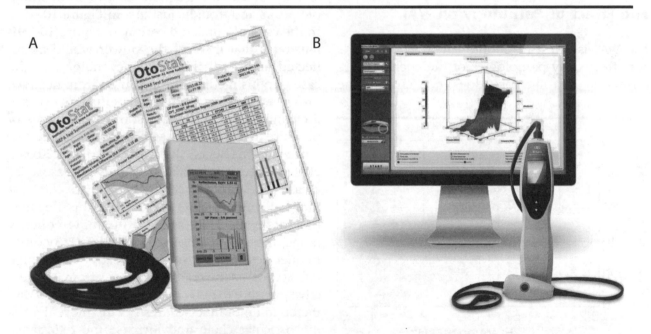

FIGURE 10–16. Wideband acoustic immittance (WAI) devices. **A.** Mimosa Acoustics Model OtoStat is a device that measures WAI at ambient pressure and reports in reflectance or absorbance at frequencies from 256 to 6000 Hz. **B.** Interacoustics Model Titan is a wideband tympanometer that measures the acoustic energy absorbed into the middle ear as a function of both frequency (from 226 to 8000 Hz) and pressure. As shown on the monitor, it uses those measurements to create a 3D graph of the absorbance where the audiologist can compare results from absorbance measurements to various pathologies. *Source*: Photos courtesy of Mimosa Acoustics (A) and Interacoustics (B).

frequencies and displays them in a 3D plot that shows absorbance, frequency, and pressure (Figure 10–16B).

Ambient pressure devices show the amount of power reflected (*y*-axis) as a function of frequency (*x*-axis). An ambient response for a normal ear is shown in Figure 10–17; there is a dip (less energy reflected) representing the least amount of reflected energy around the ear's resonance frequency, and there is a systematic increase in the amount of reflected energy in the frequency ranges above and below the most sensitive region. Figure 10–18 shows the 3D plot that comes from measuring the absorbance while manipulating the air pressure in the ear canal across a range of frequencies from 200 to 8000 Hz. From this, you can review either the absorbance at a single pressure or the absorbance across the frequency range depending on the axis you are viewing. Figure 10–18 (inset) shows the absorbance across pressures in a single slice at 1000 Hz that shows a measure similar to tympanometry.

The Effect of Pathology on WAI

The WAI is a test of middle ear function and is not affected by pathologies of the cochlea. Sensorineural hearing loss does not change the

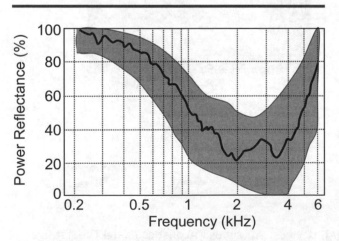

FIGURE 10–17. Example of an ambient wideband acoustic immittance (WAI) measure, showing how the reflected energy changes as a function of stimulus frequency. The normal range is represented by the *shaded portion*, which is characterized by a dip (less energy reflected) in the region where the ear is most sensitive (resonance).

results and ears with hearing loss do not have power reflectance curves that are different than those without (Feeney et al., 2003). The WAI response in Figure 10–17 is an example of a power reflectance across 256 frequencies from a normal hearing adult overlaid on a normative adult population. The results reveal that in the low frequencies (<1.0 kHz) reflectance is typically above 80%, then decreases below 30% due to improved middle ear efficiency from 1 to 5 kHz. Reflectance begins to increase above 4 kHz due to poorer efficiency of the middle ear in the high frequencies (Allen, Jeng, & Levitt, 2005). The average power reflectance curve shows a single trough near 1.5 to 2 kHz, but individual curves often show multiple troughs (as does the example shown in Figure 10–17). Theoretically, changes in the middle ear status will lead to changes in the WAI response. For example, Figure 10–19 illustrates different reflectance responses for various outer and middle ear conditions. If the stiffness of the middle ear changes, from a perforation, for example, reflectance would be hypothesized to drop in the low frequencies and show multiple peaks and troughs just like in Figure 10–19A. In the case of impacted cerumen, Figure 10–19B illustrates that most of the power would be reflected across all the frequency ranges. In the case of otitis media, where you go from negative pressure to otitis media with effusion, we see a change in the mass and stiffness. Changes of pressure in the middle ear will change the reflectance pattern (Beers, Shahnaz, Westrick, & Kozak, 2010; Hunter et al., 2008). Negative pressure increases the reflectance in the 600 to 2000 Hz range. Figure 10–19C shows that this negative pressure will affect the low to mid-frequency range, most noticeable around 1000 Hz because frequencies lower than that already have a high reflectance. As the condition moves from just negative pressure to otitis media with effusion (OME), the build-up of fluid will restrict the movement of the ossicular chain and increase the reflectance (Figure 10–19D) across a broad frequency range (Feeney et al., 2003).

Otosclerosis, a fixation of the stapes, will increase the stiffness of the middle ear system. This results in an increase in the reflectance in the frequency range below 1000 Hz (Allen et al., 2005; Shahnaz et al., 2009). Ossicular discontinuity

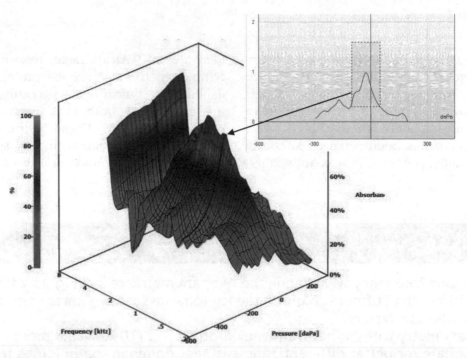

FIGURE 10–18. Example of pressurized wideband acoustic immittance (WAI) measure, showing a 3D image of the absorbance across pressure and frequency. Note the peak in the mid-frequencies close to 0 daPa. The absorbance measure (slice) at 1000 Hz is shown in the box on the right, indicating the absorbance at that frequency as the pressure is changed from positive to negative.

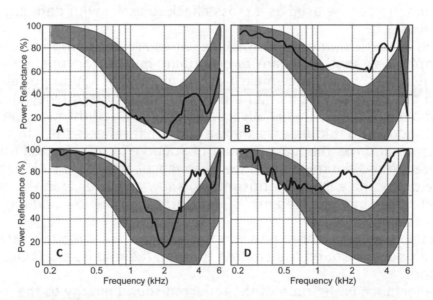

FIGURE 10–19. Examples of reflectance responses to various outer and middle ear conditions. (**A**) TM perforation causes a decrease in the reflectance in the low frequencies. (**B**) Impacted cerumen results in more reflectance across the frequency range. (**C**) Negative middle ear pressure increases the reflectance in the 500 to 1500 Hz range. (**D**) Otitis media with effusion causes an increase in the reflectance in the high frequencies.

also shows a change in the frequencies below 1000 Hz; however, this condition causes a decrease in the reflectance between 375 and 800 Hz. This notch shows a significant decrease in the reflectance at approximately 600 to 800 Hz which disappears after it has been repaired surgically (Feeney et al., 2003; Feeney, Grant, & Mills, 2009).

Measures of WAI are faster than multifrequency tympanometry and are becoming more established as a clinical test, especially now that the instruments are both FDA approved and commercially available. These instruments are also combined with otoacoustic emission and other testing equipment, making it more versatile.

SYNOPSIS 10–2

- Probe tone frequency will change the tympanometric recording; low frequency tones affect the stiffness, high frequency tones assess the mass component of the middle ear system.
- Tympanometry with higher frequency probe tones (1000 Hz) is more appropriate for better differentiating stiffness dominant pathologies from mass dominant pathologies than tympanometry with the more conventional low frequency probe tone (226 Hz).
- Measuring tympanometry in newborns (<6 months) should be done with a 1000 Hz probe tone. Infants with middle ear fluid may have a normal 226 Hz tympanogram but an abnormal 1000 Hz tympanogram, which could lead to an incorrect determination of the type of loss.
- Tympanometry can be used as a cross-check to assist with defining the type of hearing loss.
- Wideband acoustic immittance (WAI) measures are becoming more commonplace as another means of describing middle ear function.
- In WAI measures, reflectance measures the amount of sound power that is reflected off the tympanic membrane as a function of frequency and absorbance is the amount of power that is absorbed or transmitted through the TM. Normal functioning middle ears show a trace that reflects the ear's sensitivity to frequency and has the least amount of sound energy reflected (or most absorbed) around the most sensitive (resonance) area. Ears with negative pressure or middle ear fluid (otitis media) show an increase in the amount of sound energy being reflected (or least absorbed) in the low and high frequency ranges, respectively.
- Reflectance is the amount of power reflected from the tympanic membrane and the amount of sound transmitted through the middle ear is the power absorbance.
- Power reflectance is the ratio of the reflected sound energy to the incident sound energy, and equals the square of the magnitude of the pressure reflectance or $|R(f)|^2$ whereas power absorbance is the ratio of the absorbed sound energy to the incident sound energy and is equal to $1 - |R(f)|^2$.
- WAI can be measured at ambient pressure or while sweeping across pressure as in tympanometry.
- Various pathologies will result in different patterns in the reflectance/absorbance.

ACOUSTIC REFLEX THRESHOLD MEASUREMENT

Another part of the immittance evaluation is the *acoustic reflex threshold* (ART) test. The ART is done with the same immittance instrument, and is usually performed right after obtaining a tympanogram. As you recall from Chapter 5, the ear has an involuntary middle ear reflex in response to loud sounds that causes a contraction of the stapedius muscles. The acoustic reflex pathway is shown again in Figure 10–20 so that you can refer to it when interpreting results from ART testing. It is important to remember that the acoustic reflex is a bilateral response. A loud tone delivered to one ear will result in contraction of the stapedius muscle in both ears. The contraction of the stapedius muscle alters the transmission of sound through the ossicular chain, hence decreases the admittance of the probe tone. The clinical utility of measuring ARTs extends beyond just the assessment of outer and middle ear pathologies. As you can see from Figure 10–20, abnormalities of the cochlea, 8th cranial nerve, lower brainstem,

and/or the 7th cranial nerve may also influence the ability to record an acoustic reflex.

Recording Principles

Acoustic reflex testing monitors any change in admittance of the probe tone (226 Hz, 85 dB SPL) that should occur when the middle ear muscle (stapedius) contracts in response to a loud tone, the *reflex eliciting tone*, that is presented to the ear. Referring to Figure 10–4, you can see that the immittance instrument has a second tone generator that has the capability of delivering reflex eliciting tones to either ear. Typically, 500, 1000, and 2000 Hz tones are used as reflex eliciting tones when testing for ARTs. The reflex eliciting tone used for ART testing is usually about 1 s in duration. The contraction of the stapedius muscle is measured with the immittance instrument as an abrupt reduction in admittance of the probe tone due to the stiffening of the ossicular chain that is in response to the reflex eliciting tone (e.g., 1000 Hz). The acoustic reflex measures are performed at a single pressure, usually at the point of tympanometric peak pressure (TPP). When the reflex eliciting tone is presented to the same ear where the admittance is being measured, it is called an *ipsilateral acoustic reflex* ("ipsi"). When the reflex eliciting tone is presented to the opposite ear from where the admittance is being measured, it is called a *contralateral acoustic reflex* ("contra").

For most reflex eliciting tones, the tone level must be at least 70 dB HL to produce a measurable reflex. Some normative ART data are shown in Table 10–2 (Wiley, Oviatt, & Block, 1987). The normal range for ART is generally considered to be 75–95 dB HL. The ART for broadband noise is about 20 dB lower than for tones.

Figure 10–21 illustrates a series of acoustic reflex measures for different levels of a reflex eliciting tone. The ART is established by changing the level of the reflex eliciting tone until the minimum dB HL is found that produces a criterion change in admittance. The ART is commonly defined as the lowest dB HL of the reflex eliciting tone that produces a repeatable admittance

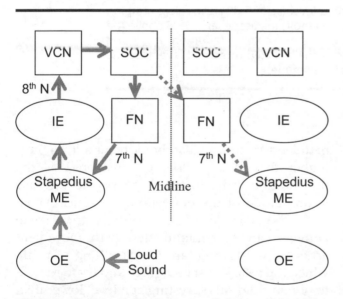

FIGURE 10–20. Block diagram of the acoustic reflex pathway for stimulation of one ear. Notice that there is an ipsilateral and contralateral pathway that results in bilateral contraction of the stapedius muscles. See Chapter 5 for more details. SOC, superior olivary complex; VCN, ventral cochlear nucleus; FN, facial nerve; IE, inner ear.

TABLE 10–2. Mean Acoustic Reflex Thresholds (in dB HL) with Standard Deviation (in parentheses) for Normal Hearing Ears in Young Adults.

	500 Hz	1000 HZ	2000 Hz	BB Noise
Ipsilateral Stimulus 5th–95th %ile	79.9 (5.0) 72–90	82.0 (5.2) 75–90	86.2 (5.9) 77–95	64.6 (6.9) 55–75
Contralateral Stimulus 5th–95th %ile	84.6 (6.3) 75–95	85.9 (5.2) 75–95	84.4 (5.7) 75–93.25	66.3 (8.8) 55–80

Based on Wiley et al. (1987).

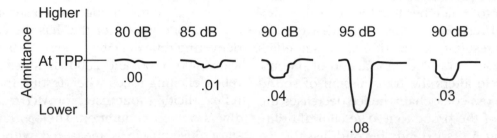

FIGURE 10–21. Illustration of acoustic reflex measures for different levels of the reflex eliciting tone. The acoustic reflex threshold is defined as the lowest level of the reflex eliciting tone that produces a downward deflection (reduced admittance) ≥ 0.02 mmhos. In this example, the acoustic reflex threshold is 90 dB HL. However, to help differentiate the acoustic reflex from possible artifact (see text), it is good practice to demonstrate that there is no deflection at the level 5 dB below the selected threshold level (see 85 dB HL in this example), and that the deflection should get larger in amplitude at the level 5 dB above the selected threshold level (see 95 dB HL in this example). In addition, it is good practice to show a repeatable deflection at the selected threshold level (see the two similar deflections at 90 dB HL in this example).

change of at least 0.02 mmhos (or 0.02 ml) (Schairer, Feeney, & Sanford, 2013). When the dB HL of the reflex eliciting tone is below the stapedius reflex threshold, there is no measurable change in admittance; however, when the dB HL of the reflex eliciting tone is high enough to cause the stapedius to contract, the admittance decreases during the presentation of the short duration reflex eliciting tone. As the dB HL of the reflex eliciting tone increases above the ART, there is a range in which the stapedius contraction strengthens and the size (amplitude) of the downward deflection of the acoustic reflex increases with increasing dB HL. To have more confidence in establishing the ART, it is recommended that testing also be done at a level 5 dB higher than what is being considered as the threshold in order to see the expected increase in amplitude of the deflection. In clinical situations, the acoustic reflex recordings from some patients can be contaminated with movement artifacts, swallowing, and/or clenching of teeth, which the tester must recognize and try to resolve to obtain valid ARTs. Testing at a level lower than 70 dB HL is a good strategy to determine if any deflections are present due to artifacts.

The equipment's maximum level for the reflex eliciting tones is typically 110 to 115 dB HL. Although relatively rare, it has been reported that some patients have experienced some tinnitus or additional hearing loss because of testing acoustic reflexes above 105 dB HL (Hunter, Ries, Schlauch, Levine, & Ward, 1999), and it is important to exercise caution when testing at levels higher than 105 dB HL.

The ARTs are typically recorded for both ipsilateral and contralateral conditions for each ear. It is conventional to describe contralateral ART testing as it relates to the ear receiving the reflex eliciting tone. For example, a right contralateral ART means that the reflex eliciting tone was presented to the right ear and the probe assembly was in the left ear. To be unambiguous, it is recommended that the contralateral ARTs be recorded in a manner that clearly indicates which ear the reflex eliciting tone in ("stim ear") and which ear the probe was in ("probe ear"); for example, "Stim R/Probe L". The ART for each frequency and recording condition is usually recorded on the audiometric data sheet along with the audiogram, tympanogram, and speech test results.

INTERPRETATIONS OF ACOUSTIC REFLEX THRESHOLDS

The clinical interpretations of ARTs involve looking at the patterns of results for both ipsilateral and contralateral recording conditions for each ear. The pattern of results will depend on the location of the problem in the acoustic reflex pathway, including the outer ear, middle ear, cochlea, 8th cranial nerve, lower brainstem nuclei, and 7th cranial nerve. While certain characteristic patterns for ARTs can be established, they are much more useful when used in conjunction with the tympanogram, audiogram, and/or patient complaints/history. A summary of the expectations for ARTs in different types of pathologic conditions is presented in Table 10–3. However, learning how to interpret ARTs can be facilitated by considering the following three general conditions, all of which are necessary to elicit an acoustic reflex:

1. **The ear with the probe assembly must not have any outer or middle ear pathology.**

If there is evidence of a conductive hearing problem with any degree of an air–bone gap on the audiogram and/or an abnormal tympanogram, the immittance instrument will not be able to record a change in admittance (even though the stapedius is activated). In this situation, the acoustic reflex is usually reported as no response or absent. Acoustic reflexes will also show no response when the ear with the probe assembly has a perforation or a pressure equalization tube in the tympanic membrane, even though there may not be an air–bone gap on the audiogram. Acoustic reflexes will also show no response when the ear canal is impacted with cerumen.

2. **The ear with the reflex eliciting tone must receive a tone that is loud enough.** If condition 1 (see above) is met, this second condition can be affected in different ways depending on the type of hearing loss. For a conductive hearing loss in the ear receiving the reflex eliciting tone, using contralateral test condition, an air–bone gap acts to reduce (attenuate) the level of the reflex eliciting tone reaching the cochlea. To offset this, the tester would increase the dB HL of the reflex eliciting tone to see if a reflex can be obtained before the upper limit of the equipment (usually 115 dB HL) is reached. If one assumes an average ART of 85 dB HL, then the level of the reflex eliciting tone can only be increased by 30 dB HL before the equipment limit is reached. Therefore, if the amount of air–bone gap in the stimulus ear is greater than 30 dB HL, the acoustic reflex will usually show no response because the reflex eliciting tone cannot be increased enough before the equipment limit is reached to offset the amount of conductive hearing loss. On the other hand, if the air–bone gap is less than or equal to 30 dB HL the acoustic reflex should be observed, but the level of the reflex eliciting tone needed to produce the ART will be outside the normal expected range, that is, the ART would be expected between 100 and 115 dB HL.

For a cochlear hearing loss, there is an entirely different expectation. It is well

TABLE 10-3. Summary of the Most Expected Acoustic Reflex Thresholds Results (italics) for the Different Types of Pathologies and Degrees of Hearing Loss

Pathology	Contra (probe in affected ear)	Contra (stim in affected ear)	Contra (probe & stim in affected ear)	Corollary
Conductive	If any ABG: (*No response*) If perforation, PE tube, or impacted cerumen: (*No response*)	If ABG ≤ 30 dB: (*100–115*) If ABG > 30 dB (*No response*)	If any ABG (*No response*) If perforation, PE tube, or impacted cerumen: (*No response*)	If reflex is in normal range, there should not be any OE/ME path in the probe ear.
Cochlear	Not relevant (dependent on stimulus in the affected ear)	If loss ≤ 45 dB (*≤95*) If loss 50–70 dB (*≤Gelfand et al. 90th %iles*) If loss > 70 dB (*No response*)	If loss ≤ 45 dB HL: (*≤95*) If loss 50–70 dB (*≤Gelfand et al. 90th %iles*) If loss > 70 dB (*No response*)	Expect acoustic reflex for most cochlear losses Normal reflex does not rule out cochlear hearing loss, nor does it define the degree of cochlear loss
8th nerve	Not relevant (dependent on stimulus in the affected ear)	If any loss (*No response or >Gelfand et al. 90th %iles*) If reflex ≤ 105 (*Abnormal reflex decay*)	If any loss (*No response or >Gelfand et al. 90th %iles*) If reflex ≤ 105 (*Abnormal reflex decay*)	If no reflex and hearing loss ≤ 70 dB = "red flag" for 8th N pathology If reflex is >Gelfand et al. 90th %iles = "red flag" for 8th N pathology
7th nerve	If distal to stapedial branch (*≤95*) If proximal to stapedial banch: (*No response or 100–115*)	Not relevant (dependent on probe in the affected ear)	If distal to stapedial branch: (*≤95*) If proximal to stapedial branch: (*No response or 100–115*)	
Functional	Not relevant (dependent on stimulus in the affected ear)	<Gelfand et al. 10th %iles	<Gelfand et al. 10th %iles	If reflex is not consistent with type or degree of hearing loss, then suspect functional

Based on using a 1000 Hz reflex eliciting tone with 115 dB HL upper limit. Gelfand et al. (1990). Data are based on contralateral recordings; however, those data are also used in this table to represent ipsilateral recordings. ABG, air-bone gap; Contra, contralateral; Ipsi, ipsilateral; PE, pressure-equalization; OE/ME, outer/middle ear.

established that loudness is not affected in the same way in cochlear hearing losses as for conductive hearing losses. Instead of the loudness of the reflex eliciting tone being attenuated, as occurs for a conductive hearing loss, the loudness of the reflex eliciting tone for a sensorineural hearing loss of cochlear origin is similar to that of a normal ear at these higher stimulus levels. This is related to a process called *recruitment*, in which there is an abnormal growth of loudness in an ear with a cochlear hearing loss. In an ear with recruitment, as the intensity of a tone is increased above the behavioral threshold, the perceived loudness increases at a faster rate than for normal hearing ears; and when the tone reaches moderately high intensity levels, the perceived loudness level is similar to that perceived by a normal ear. This loudness recruitment phenomenon is seen in the ARTs for cochlear hearing losses as well. In fact, a cochlear hearing loss up to about 70 dB

HL can be expected to have a measurable acoustic reflex.

Interpretation of ART as a function of degree of cochlear hearing loss is based on data by Gelfand, Schwander, and Silman (1990). Figure 10–22 shows an example of the Gelfand et al. data for contralateral ARTs obtained at 1000 Hz for different degrees of known cochlear hearing loss (Gelfand, 2015). The data show the 90th, 50th, and 10th percentiles of ARTs for those with normal hearing and for those with different degrees of cochlear hearing loss. For clinical interpretation, it is generally recommended that the upper (90th percentile) end of the range be used as the upper cutoff for the expected ARTs as a function of degree of cochlear hearing loss. For example, one would expect 90% of ears to have an ART less than or equal to 95 dB HL for a cochlear hearing loss up to 45 dB HL (same as expected for a normal hearing ear). For a cochlear hearing loss between 50 and 70 dB HL, the 90th percentile expected value increases from 100 to 115 dB HL. As you can also see in Figure 10–22, even 50% of persons with cochlear hearing losses would be expected to have an acoustic reflex with hearing loss as great as 80 dB HL. A useful way to describe ARTs for those with cochlear hearing loss is to say something such as "The ARTs are within the expected range for cochlear hearing losses based on the 90th percentile data of Gelfand et al. (1990)." The benefit of using this description will be apparent after describing, in the next section, the expectations for ARTs when the sensorineural hearing loss is due to a problem in the 8th cranial nerve.

Table 10–4 lists the 90th percentile values for normal hearing listeners and those with cochlear hearing loss from Gelfand et al. (1990) that should be considered when interpreting ARTs from patients with sensorineural hearing loss. The Gelfand et al. (1990) data are for contralateral ART testing, but similar patterns are found for ipsilateral ART testing (Cohen & Prasher, 1992) if the probe ear is free of any middle or outer ear pathology. The Gelfand et al. (1990) data are for 226 Hz probe tones

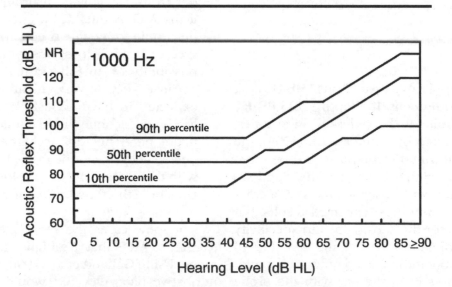

FIGURE 10–22. Data from Gelfand et al. (1990) showing the 90th, 50th, and 10th percentiles for acoustic reflex thresholds in ears with cochlear losses. Acoustic reflex thresholds above the 90th percentile curve should raise suspicion of possible 8th nerve disorder. See also Table 11–3 for 90th percentile values for 500, 1000, and 2000 Hz. *Source*: From Gelfand et al., 1990, p. 245. Copyright 1990 by American Speech-Language-Hearing Association.

TABLE 10–4. 90th Percentile Values for Acoustic Reflex Thresholds (ART) for Contralateral Recordings

Hearing Threshold (dB HL)	ART at 500 Hz (dB HL)	ART at 1000 Hz (dB HL)	ART at 2000 Hz (dB HL)
0	95	95	95
5	95	95	95
10	95	95	95
15	95	95	95
20	95	95	95
25	95	95	95
30	95	95	100
35	95	95	100
40	95	95	100
45	95	95	105
50	100	100	105
55	105	105	110
60	105	110	115
65	110	110	115
70	115	115	120
75	120	120	125
80	120	125	NR
85	NR	NR	NR
>90	NR	NR	NR

Source: Based on data from Gelfand et al. (1990).

and can be applicable up to the 115 dB HL limit of today's equipment. If adopting 105 dB HL as a safer limit for the reflex eliciting tones, as recommended by Hunter et al. (1999), the use of Gelfand's 90% criteria would be more limited at the higher degrees of hearing loss. However, one could use Gelfand's 50% criterion values as the most expected results, but this would alter the sensitivity and specificity of ARTs. Remember, the Gelfand et al. (1990) data only apply if there is no outer ear or middle ear pathology in the ear with the probe assembly and there is no air–bone gap in the ear with the reflex eliciting tone.

3. **The neural pathway must be adequate to activate the contraction of the stapedius**. The acoustic reflex pathway includes both the 8th (sensory) and 7th (motor) cranial

nerves; therefore, one would expect different patterns depending on the type and extent of neural dysfunction. For 8th cranial nerve disorders (e.g., acoustic neuroma), there is a compromise in the neural impulses from the stimulus ear that affects the activation of the ipsilateral and contralateral acoustic reflex pathways. It does not take very much of a disruption in neural activity to eliminate the acoustic reflex when the stimulus is presented to the ear with the 8th cranial nerve disorder. Therefore, the most expected result for an ear with an 8th cranial nerve disorder is that the ipsilateral and contralateral ARTs will show no response most of the time when the reflex eliciting stimulus is in the affected ear, even with a mild degree of hearing loss. Since 8th cranial nerve disorders usually affect only one ear, the ARTs for stimulation of the non-involved ear will be normal unless some other pathology is also present. There are, however, some patients with an 8th cranial nerve disorder in which an acoustic reflex can be obtained. In these cases, the same data from Gelfand et al. (1990) can be used to differentiate an 8th cranial nerve disorder from a cochlear disorder. For example, if the ART is outside (higher than) the 90th percentile for cochlear ears for a specific degree of hearing loss, this would suggest the possibility of an 8th cranial nerve disorder because very few cochlear ears would be expected to have acoustic reflexes at those levels. A recommended clinical description might be, "The ART is higher than the expected 90th percentile range for cochlear ears with that degree of hearing loss and suggests possible 8th cranial nerve involvement."

In some cases the term "elevated" is used to refer to ARTs that are higher than the normal range. Using Gelfand et al. (1990) 90th percentile normative data, elevated would be considered ARTs in the range of 100 to 115 dB HL, recognizing that a small number of those with normal hearing could have thresholds as high as 100 dB HL; however, as you can see, this would not be very useful to differentiate types of hearing loss, since ARTs in this range can occur with some cochlear, 8th cranial nerve, and conductive losses with air–bone gaps less than or equal to 30 dB HL in the stimulus ear.

For 7th cranial nerve involvement (e.g., Bell palsy), the acoustic reflex test is useful to differentiate whether the problem in the 7th cranial nerve is located *proximal* (more central) or *distal* (more peripheral) to the stapedial branch of the nerve (see the diagram of the 7th cranial nerve shown in Chapter 5, Figure 5–2). A hearing loss must also be ruled out prior to interpreting the acoustic reflex thresholds relative to 7th cranial nerve function. When the immittance probe is in the ear on the same side as the 7th cranial nerve problem, the ARTs will show no response if the problem is proximal to the stapedial branch and present when the problem is distal to the stapedial branch. Stated differently, if the ARTs are normal with the probe assembly in the ear on the affected side, the 7th cranial nerve problem is distal to the stapedial branch; and if the ARTs show no response, the problem is proximal to the stapedial branch. For 7th cranial nerve problems that are proximal to the stapedial branch, monitoring of the ARTs over time may be useful to determine recovery of function.

The ART can also be affected by pontine level brainstem disorders, although these cases are quite rare. For example, when there is a problem in the pathways that cross from one side of the brainstem to the other at the level of the superior olivary complex (SOC), referred to as an intra-axial lesion, the ARTs may be present for ipsilateral testing from each ear and show no response for contralateral testing from each ear. In this case, the 7th and 8th cranial nerve pathways are intact on each ipsilateral side; however, the neural information is not carried across the brainstem to the 7th cranial nerve on the other side due to some lesion in the midline of the pontine region of the brainstem.

EXAMPLES OF ART INTERPRETATIONS

Figure 10–23 is a decision-tree to help interpret pathological conditions related to ART outcomes. You should use this decision-tree as you work through the hypothetical cases shown in Table 10–5. For the decision tree and the following examples, it was assumed that the normal range for ARTs is less than or equal to ($\leq$) 95 dB HL and that testing could be performed up to 115 dB HL. For each of the cases in Table 10–5, ask yourself if each of the three previously described conditions for eliciting a reflex have been met, for ipsilateral and contralateral recordings. All conditions must be met to be able to record an acoustic reflex. It is a good idea to look first for any outer or middle ear pathology in either ear. If outer or middle ear pathology is ruled out, then look at the stimulus ear for interpretation. The following explanations are for the examples shown in Table 10–5.

Example 1: Reflexes show no response when the probe is in the right ear (R Ipsi and Stim L/Probe R) because the right ear has a pathology in the conductive pathway. When the reflex eliciting tone is in the right ear (Stim R/Probe L), the reflex is elevated because the degree of conductive loss is less than 30 dB and the level of the reflex eliciting tone can be increased (up to 115 dB limit) to overcome the attenuation. The reflex is normal when the probe and the reflex eliciting tone are in the left ear (L Ipsi).

Example 2: Reflexes show no response for all recording conditions because both ears have a conductive pathology. Note that any pathology or degree of conductive loss in the ear with the probe assembly will override the ability to increase the level of the reflex eliciting tone to offset the degree of conductive loss in that ear during ipsilateral recording.

Example 3: The interpretation of reflexes should focus on the ear with the reflex eliciting tone because the ear with the probe does not have any outer or middle ear pathology. Reflexes are expected to be present for all conditions because both ears have cochlear hearing losses and, therefore, recruitment of loudness is expected. The ARTs would be expected to be less than or equal to the 90th percentile data from Gelfand et al. (1990) (see Table 10–4). In this case, the ART is less than or equal to 95 dB HL for the

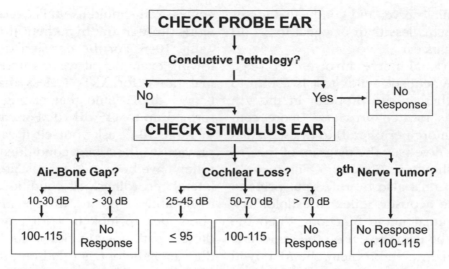

FIGURE 10–23. A decision-matrix to help interpret pathological conditions related to ART outcomes. The upper end of the normal range is considered to be 95 dB HL, based on Gelfand et al. (1990).

TABLE 10–5. Hypothetical Examples of Expected Acoustic Reflex Threshold (ART) Patterns

		Expected ART in dB HL			
Ex	Hypothetical Conditions	R Ipsi	L Ipsi	Stim R Probe L	Stim L Probe R
1	R: 20 dB conductive loss L: normal hearing and function	NR	≤95	100–115	NR
2	R: 20 dB conductive loss L: 20 dB conductive loss	NR	NR	NR	NR
3	R: 45 dB cochlear loss L: 65 dB cochlear loss	≤95	≤110	≤95	≤110
4	R: normal hearing with perforation L: normal hearing and function	NR	≤95	≤95	NR
5	R: 8th N tumor, mild SN loss L: normal hearing and function	NR or 100–115	≤95	NR or 100–115	≤95
6	R: 20 dB conductive loss L: 7th N lesion distal to stapedius	NR	≤95	100–115	NR

R, right ear; L, left ear; Ipsi, ipsilateral; Stim, stimulus; ART, acoustic reflex threshold; NR, no response.

Cochlear losses based on data from Gelfand et al. (1990).

45 dB cochlear loss (R Ipsi and Stim R/Probe L), and the ART is less than or equal to 110 dB HL for the 65 dB cochlear loss (L Ipsi and Stim L/Probe R).

Example 4: Reflexes show no response when the probe is in the right ear (R Ipsi and Stim L/Probe R) because the right ear has a pathology in the conductive pathway. In this case,

there is no conductive hearing loss; however, there is a perforation in the tympanic membrane that precludes the measurement of a reflex. The R Ipsi reflex is normal when the probe is in the left ear because the left ear has normal hearing and no outer or middle ear pathology. For the right contralateral condition (Stim R/Probe L), the reflex is normal because the right ear does not have any hearing loss, so the level of the reflex eliciting tone in the right ear should be normal; the reflex should be measurable in the left ear because the left ear does not have any outer or middle ear pathology.

Example 5: Reflexes are most likely to show no response when the reflex eliciting tone is presented to the right ear (R Ipsi and Stim R/Probe L) because the 8th nerve tumor does not allow adequate neural activity to activate the reflex even with the mild sensorineural hearing loss. Reflexes are normal when the reflex eliciting tone is presented to the left ear (L Ipsi and Stim L/Probe R) because there is no hearing loss in the left ear and neither ear has any outer or middle ear pathology. In some cases, reflexes can be present, but should be higher than the 90th percentile values from Gelfand et al. (1990).

Example 6: Reflexes show no response when the probe is in the right ear (R Ipsi and Stim L/Probe R) because the right ear has a pathology in the conductive components. The reflex is expected to be present when the probe is on the left ear (L Ipsi) because the left-sided 7th cranial nerve lesion is distal (more peripheral) to the stapedial branch of the 7th cranial nerve; however, because there is also a 20 dB conductive hearing loss in the right ear, the reflex is elevated for Stim R/Probe L.

It is also important to keep in mind the following caveats regarding interpretations of ARTs:

- Normal ARTs do not mean normal hearing.
- Abnormal reflexes can result from different pathologies.
- When differentiating cochlear versus 8th cranial nerve pathology, be sure to rule out any outer or middle ear pathology.
- Ears may have multiple pathologies; failure of any rule can cause abnormal ARTs.

ACOUSTIC REFLEX DECAY

Acoustic reflex decay is an additional measure of the acoustic reflex activity to provide evidence of possible 8th cranial nerve pathology. The acoustic reflex decay is measured using a reflex eliciting tone that is presented for 10 s at a level that is 10 dB above the acoustic reflex threshold. Figure 10–24 shows what happens during stimulation and recording of acoustic reflex decay. For a normal functioning ear, the response to the reflex eliciting tone is displayed as a well-defined deflection (reduced admittance) at the initiation of the reflex eliciting tone that continues at generally the same amplitude for the entire 10 s. However, if the amplitude of the deflection decreases (drifts back toward baseline) by more than 50% within 5 s, it is considered a positive acoustic reflex decay and is a positive sign for abnormal 8th cranial nerve involvement (e.g., an acoustic neuroma). The abnormal acoustic reflex decay is related to the inability of the 8th cranial nerve fibers to sustain adequate neural information, also called abnormal *adaptation*, which is not sufficient to maintain the acoustic reflex during prolonged stimulation by the reflex eliciting tone.

It is recommended that acoustic reflex decay testing be done with 500 and/or 1000 Hz reflex eliciting tone using a contralateral recording condition. Higher frequency tones are not useful because many normal hearing ears show positive acoustic reflex decay above 1000 Hz. Testing for acoustic reflex decay requires that the acoustic reflex threshold be established first and that the acoustic reflex thresholds occur within a range that allows an additional 10 dB to be added. Assuming equipment limits of 115 dB HL, the acoustic reflex threshold must be less than or equal to 105 dB HL to be able to test for acoustic reflex decay. If one adopts the recommended safe level of 105 dB HL, the acoustic reflex threshold must be less than or equal to 95 dB HL to test for acoustic reflex decay and may limit the cases in which acoustic reflex decay testing can be used to differentiate cochlear from 8th cranial nerve disorders. Keeping in mind that most patients with 8th cranial nerve disorders will not have acoustic reflexes, therefore, acoustic reflex decay testing cannot be performed. In some cases, a patient may have normal hearing thresholds and normal acoustic reflex thresholds, but show an abnormal acoustic reflex decay, and this may be the only suspicious sign of a possible 8th cranial nerve tumor. The acoustic reflex decay test is often routinely included in the immittance test

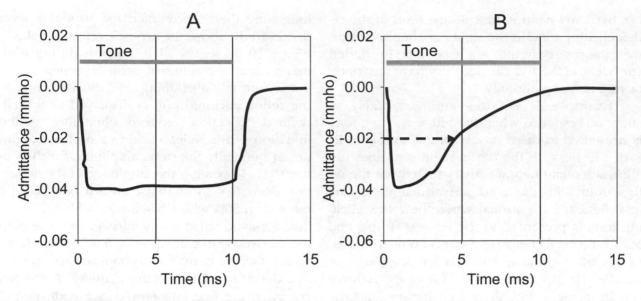

FIGURE 10–24. A AND B. Illustration of acoustic reflex decay measures. For acoustic reflex decay testing, a reflex eliciting tone is presented at a level of 10 dB above the acoustic reflex threshold, and is presented for 10 ms (illustrated by the *tone bar*). During stimulation, there is an expected decrease in admittance (downward deflection) due to the contraction of the stapedius muscle, which should be sustained for the duration of the tone. In **A**, the amplitude of the deflection remained fairly constant for the duration of the 10 s tone; however, in **B**, the amplitude of the deflection returned toward baseline (referred to as decay) by 50% within the first 5 s of stimulation. Clinically, if there is acoustic reflex decay of more than 50%, it is considered positive acoustic reflex decay and suggestive of an 8th nerve disorder; otherwise, it is considered negative acoustic reflex decay.

SYNOPSIS 10–3

- The immittance instrument can be used to monitor the contraction of the stapedius muscle by briefly stimulating the ear with a loud reflex eliciting tone (500, 1000, and/or 2000 Hz) and measuring any changes in the admittance of the 226 Hz probe tone. A reduction in admittance (≥0.02 mmhos) during stimulation indicates that the stapedius muscle contracted, assuming artifacts have been ruled out.
- The acoustic reflex is a bilateral response to tones; therefore, recordings can be made for stimulation of one ear while recording the admittance with the probe in the other ear (contralateral reflex) or in the same ear as the stimulation (ipsilateral reflex).
- The normal range for the acoustic reflex threshold to tones is 75–95 dB HL. Acoustic reflex thresholds are reported as no response (absent) if not measurable at the upper range of testing.
- Clinical interpretation of acoustic reflex threshold testing is guided by the following:
  - Any outer or middle ear pathology (with or without air–bone gaps) in the ear with the probe (probe ear) will result in no response.

SYNOPSIS 10–3 (continued)

○ An air–bone gap greater than 30 dB in the ear with the reflex eliciting tone (stim ear) will result in no response because the tone cannot be made loud enough before reaching equipment limits. For air–bone gaps less than or equal to 30 dB HL in the ear with the reflex eliciting tone, the acoustic reflex threshold should be measurable between 105 and 115 dB HL.

○ For cochlear hearing losses, loudness recruitment causes acoustic reflexes to be measurable for hearing losses as high as 70 to 80 dB HL in the ear receiving the reflex eliciting tone. Gelfand et al. (1990) data should be consulted to determine the 90% criterion for acoustic reflex thresholds for different degrees of cochlear hearing loss. For example, at 1000 Hz, the acoustic reflex threshold is expected to be less than or equal to 95 dB HL in 90% of ears with cochlear hearing losses up to 45 dB HL and 100 to 115 in 90% of ears with hearing losses from 50 to 70 dB, respectively. See Table 10–3.

○ For 8th cranial nerve pathologies, the neural activity of the 8th cranial nerve from the ear receiving the reflex eliciting tone (stim ear) is usually not adequate to produce a measurable acoustic reflex. The acoustic reflex threshold data can be used to differentiate cochlear versus 8th cranial nerve pathologies by referring to the Gelfand et al. (1990) data. For example, an 8th cranial nerve disorder is suspected if the acoustic reflex threshold is greater than 90% criterion value for a specific degree of sensorineural hearing loss. For most 8th cranial nerve pathologies, the acoustic reflex shows no response even with relatively good pure-tone audiometric thresholds. Positive acoustic reflex decay is also an 8th cranial nerve sign.

○ For 7th cranial nerve pathologies, the activation of the stapedius can be assessed relative to the probe ear. The acoustic reflex threshold will show no response if the 7th cranial nerve pathology is proximal to the stapedial branch of the 7th cranial nerve and present if the pathology is distal to the stapedial branch.

battery because it does not take much more additional time and it is important not to miss a patient that may have an 8th cranial nerve tumor. It is recommended that acoustic reflex decay testing be included in the test battery whenever you are suspicious of an 8th cranial nerve problem, especially when there is an asymmetric high frequency hearing loss.

REFERENCES

Allen, J. B., Jeng, P. S., & Levitt, H. (2005). Evaluation of human middle ear function via an acoustic power assessment. *Journal of Rehabilitation Research & Development*, *42*, 63–78.

Beers, A., Shahnaz, N., Westrick, B., & Kozak, F. (2010). Wideband reflectance (WBR) in normal school-aged children and in children with otitis media with effusion (OME). *Ear and Hearing*, *31*, 221–233.

Cohen, M., & Prasher, D. (1992). Defining the relationship between cochlear hearing loss and acoustic reflex thresholds. *Scandinavian Audiology*, *21*(4), 225–238.

Feeney, M. P., Grant, I. L., & Marryott, L. P. (2003). Wideband energy reflectance measurements in adults with middle-ear disorders. *Journal of Speech, Language, and Hearing Research*, *46*(4), 901–911.

Feeney, M. P., Grant, I. L., & Mills, D. M. (2009). Wideband energy reflectance measurements of ossicular chain discontinuity and repair in human temporal bone. *Ear and Hearing, 30*, 391–400.

Feeney, M. P., Hunter, L. L., Kei, J., Lilly, D. J., Margolis, R. H., Nakajima, H. H., Neely, S. T., Prieve, B. A., Rosowski, J. J., Sanford, C. A., Schairer, K. S., Schahnaz, N., Stenfelt, S., & Voss, S. E. (2013). Consensus statement: Eriksholm workshop on wideband absorbance measures of the middle ear. *Ear and Hearing, 34*(Supplement 1), 78–79.

Feldmann, H. (1996). History of the ear speculum. Images from the history of otorhinolarygology, hilighted by instruments from the collection of the German Medical History Museum in Ingolstadt. *Laryyngorhinootologie, 75*(5), 311–318.

Gelfand, S. A. (2015). *Essentials of Audiology* (4th ed.). New York, NY: Thieme.

Gelfand, S. A., Schwander, T., & Silman, S. (1990). Acoustic reflex thresholds in normal and cochlear-impaired ears: effects of no-response rates on 90th percentiles in a large sample. *The Journal of Speech and Hearing Disorders, 55*(2), 198–205.

Golding, M., Doyle, K., Sindhusake, D., Mitchell, P., Newall, P., & Hartley, D. (2007). Tympanometric and acoustic stapedius reflex measures in older adults. *Journal of the American Academy Audiology, 18*, 391–403.

Hall, J. W. I., & Swanepoel, D. W. (2010). *Objective Assessment of Hearing.* San Diego, CA: Plural.

Hunter, L. L., & Margolis, R. H. (1992). Multifrequency tympanometry of the eardrum impedance of human ears. *American Journal of Audiology, 1*, 33–43.

Hunter, L. L., Ries, D. T., Schlauch, R. S., Levine, S. C., & Ward, W. D. (1999). Safety and clinical performance of acoustic reflex tests. *Ear and Hearing, 20*(6), 506–514.

Hunter, L. L., & Shahnaz, N. (2013). *Acoustic Immittance Measures: Basic and Advanced Practice.* San Diego, CA: Plural.

Hunter, L. L., Tubaugh, L., Jackson, A., & Prospes, S. (2008). Wideband middle ear power measurements in infants and children. *Journal of the American Academy of Audiology, 19*, 309–324.

Jerger, J. (1970). Clinical experience with impedance audiometry. *Archives of Otolaryngology, 92*, 311–324.

Shahnaz, N., Bork, K., Polka, L., Longridge, N., Bell, D., & Westrick, B. (2009). ER and tympanometry in normal and otosclerotic ears. *Ear and Hearing, 30*, 219–233.

Shahnaz, N., Miranda, T., & Polka, L. (2008). Multifrequency tympanometry in neonatal intensive care units and well babies. *Journal American Academy Audiology, 19*, 392–418.

Shanks, J. E., & Shohet, J. (Eds.) (2009). *Tympanometry in Clinical Practice* (Vol. 6). Baltimore, MD: Lippincott Williams & Wilkins.

Schairer, K. S., Feeney, M. P., & Sanford, C. A. (2013). Acoustic reflex measurement. *Ear and Hearing, 34* Supplement 1, 43S–47S.

Wiley, T. L., Oviatt, D. L., & Block, M. G. (1987). Acoustic-immittance measures in normal ears. *Journal of Speech and Hearing Research, 30*(2), 161–170.

Zhiqi, L., Kun, Y., & Zhiwu, H. (2010). Tympanometry in infants with middle ear effusion having been identified using spiral computerized tomography. *American Journal of Otolaryngology, 31*, 96–103.

11 Evoked Physiologic Responses

After reading this chapter, you should be able to:

1. Describe the measurement of transient evoked otoacoustic emissions (TEOAEs) and distortion product otoacoustic emissions (DPOAEs).

2. Relate the presence and absence of otoacoustic emission (OAE) measures to the degree of hearing loss and differentiation of cochlear and neural disorders.

3. Describe the normal expected auditory brainstem response (ABR) waveform and how it changes with intensity, frequency, and rate.

4. Interpret ABR results as they relate to hearing thresholds and 8th cranial nerve disorders.

5. Give a general description of the auditory steady state response (ASSR) and their clinical application.

We turn our attention in this chapter to other measures of auditory function that do not require the patient to understand the task or to make any subjective responses. Given the limitations of behavioral tests, like pure-tone and speech audiometry, to differentiate cochlear from neural types of hearing losses, and for testing young infants and other difficult-to-test populations, there has been a long history in the field of audiology directed toward developing reliable physiological measures of the auditory system. In Chapter 10, you learned about the immittance test battery, primarily for obtaining objective measures from the outer ear and middle ear. In this chapter, other physiological tests, specifically *otoacoustic emissions (OAEs)* and *auditory brainstem responses (ABRs)*, are described. As with immittance, these physiological tests require instrumentation that is usually separate from the audiometer. Although these physiological tests are considered objective in nature, they require the patient to be relatively cooperative or sedated to obtain valid responses. It is also important to keep in mind that the monitoring and interpretation of the physiological tests rely, to a certain extent, on the skill and subjective interpretation of the audiologist. Although not an actual measure of hearing per se, physiological measures often provide the only information about the function of specific parts of the auditory system. In addition, physiological measures can often provide a crosscheck with other results, and/or can provide information that may suggest a particular course of follow-up or treatment. When physiological measures are combined with case history information, audiometric results and/or medical imaging, a more complete picture of the patient's problem can be determined.

The OAE and ABR tests are part of what is called *auditory evoked responses*, and are widely used as part of newborn "hearing" screening programs (see Chapter 13) and/or when behavioral tests are inappropriate or unsuccessful. Auditory evoked responses may also be useful for providing helpful information relative to the diagnosis of possible 8th cranial nerve or central auditory system disorders that cannot be ascertained from the basic audiometric test battery. The OAE test measures electroacoustic "echoes" within the ear canal that are emitted as part of the normal physiological activity of the cochlea, thought to be primarily related to outer hair cell (OHC) activity. The ABR test measures the underlying neural activity (*neuroelectric potentials*) of the 8th cranial nerve and brainstem using electrodes taped on the surface of the scalp. In addition to information about the integrity of the underlying neural pathways, the ABR test can be used to evaluate different types and degrees of peripheral auditory disorders by monitoring how the neural activity emanating from the cochlea is affected by conductive and cochlear types of hearing losses. The following sections provide an introductory look at the instrumentation, procedures, and interpretations of these physiological tests as they are commonly used in clinical audiology.

OTOACOUSTIC EMISSIONS (OAES)

Otoacoustic emissions (OAEs) are low-intensity acoustic vibrations measured in the ear canal with a sensitive microphone. As discussed in Chapter 5, the discovery of OAEs by Kemp (1978) went hand in hand with new discoveries about the active processes in the cochlea, especially the motility of the OHCs (Brownell, 1983). The emissions originate in a normally functioning cochlea, predominantly because of the movement of the OHCs that enhance the vibrations on the basilar membrane. The emissions travel outward along the basilar membrane, through the middle ear ossicles, and vibrate the tympanic membrane to produce OAEs in the ear canal. The OAEs are on the order of -10 to 20 dB SPL (Glattke & Robinette, 2007; Lonsbury-Martin, Martin, & Whitehead, 2007; Probst & Harris, 1993). The OAEs can be recorded with a sensitive microphone in the ear canal when coupled to a specialized computer that enhances the low-level OAEs and reduces the unwanted signals, such as background noise, in a process called *signal averaging*. Because the active process of the OHCs is operational only at low to moderate intensity levels, a mild cochlear hearing loss due to a loss of OHC function is sufficient to eliminate OAEs.

Historical Vignette

The successful recording of evoked and spontaneous emissions from the inner ear by David Kemp (1978) set off a flurry of activity around the world. It seemed that here, at last, a truly objective method for measuring degree of hearing sensitivity without the need for active cooperation from the person being evaluated had been discovered. As luck would have it, otoacoustic emissions (OAEs) turned out to be too sensitive: They are so sensitive to the status of the outer hair cells that they drop out altogether when degree of loss exceeds 40 to 50 dB HL. However, this did set the stage for their use in newborn hearing screening. Also, as so often happens in our field, other applications of the OAEs have turned out to be even more interesting and valuable. One such application, the efferent suppression of OAEs, first described by Lionel Collet and his colleagues in France, continues to show great promise in the evaluation of central auditory processing, especially at the low brainstem level. Ever at the forefront of innovation, Charles Berlin and his colleagues at the Louisiana State University Medical Center pioneered the clinical applications of efferent suppression.

Measurements of OAEs can be done in a couple of minutes for each ear, which has made them very popular for clinical use. In just a few minutes of testing, the function of the OHCs can be determined. During the 1990s, measurement of OAEs became widely adopted as an efficient and effective audiological procedure. Over the next decade, there was widespread implementation of mass newborn hearing screening programs, primarily because of OAEs, and today all 50 states have some form of a newborn hearing screening program (see Chapter 13 for more on newborn hearing screening with OAE and/or ABR).

Many audiologists include OAE testing as part of the basic audiologic evaluation of all patients, especially children, because they can be quickly administered and can provide a good cross-check with audiometric information. Because OAEs reflect preneural events, they can also be used to determine if a sensorineural hearing loss is due to a problem in the cochlea or in the neural pathway. For example, if a patient has a sensorineural hearing loss identified with behavioral audiometry, but has normal OAEs, this would suggest that the cochlea is functioning normally and the problem lies in the 8th cranial nerve or central auditory pathway. It is important to keep in mind that OAEs can only determine whether the OHCs are functioning normally or not; they do not provide a measure of how much hearing loss a patient may have since OAEs will be absent for even a mild to moderate degree of hearing loss, as well as for a profound hearing loss. The presence of robust OAEs can provide strong evidence of normal cochlear (OHC) function.

When evaluating OAE results, it is also important to determine if there is any problem with the outer or middle ear, which can interfere with both the inward and outward transmission of the cochlear-generated OAEs. Inward transmission of the stimuli through an abnormal middle ear reduces the sound energy reaching the cochlea, and the reduced energy creates a smaller output from the OHC. The energy will also be reduced as it transmits back out through the middle ear because of the conductive loss. The energy as it transmits back out through the middle ear. Most middle ear problems will result in absent OAEs; however, they can usually be recorded in ears with negative middle ear pressure when done at the tympanometric peak pressure (Hof, Anteunis, Chenault, & van Dijk, 2005). In addition, many ears with functioning pressure equalization tubes show OAEs (Dhar & Hall, 2012). If OAEs are present, then you can conclude that the outer hair cells are functioning. However, if OAEs are absent, the conclusion is not as simple. The clinical utility of OAE testing lies in its integration with other audiological tests. However, the presence of OAEs argues for normal auditory function in the outer ear, middle ear, and cochlea (OHCs) of the auditory system.

There are two main types of evoked[1] OAEs that are commonly used in clinical settings, those evoked by transients, called *transient evoked otoacoustic emissions (TEOAEs)*, and those evoked by two closely spaced pure tones that create additional tones in the cochlea, called *distortion product otoacoustic emissions (DPOAEs)*. Only a brief description of each of these OAEs is provided in this introductory text. For further information on the instrumentation and recording parameters, see other resources (Dhar & Hall, 2012; Gorga, Neely, Johnson, Dierking, & Garner, 2007; Hall & Swanepoel, 2010; Robinette & Glattke, 2007).

Transient Evoked Otoacoustic Emissions (TEOAEs)

Transient evoked otoacoustic emissions (TEOAEs) are evoked by the presentation of a series of brief transients (clicks). Because of the brief duration, the clicks have a broad frequency spectrum and, therefore, stimulate a wide portion of the basilar membrane. With TEOAEs, the emissions are recorded during the short silent intervals between the successive clicks and occur with a characteristic time delay after each click, called *latency*. Figure 11–1 illustrates the basic stimulation and recording of TEOAEs in a normal ear. The TEOAE is dependent on the stimulus used to stimulate the cochlea. Before making a recording of the TEOAE, you should review the stimulus (labeled A in Figure 11–1) to verify that it is appropriate in both time and frequency. The click stimulus should have an instantaneous rise/fall time and end (die out) quickly. The stimulus must

also have a spectrum measured in the ear canal ranging from about 100 to 4000 Hz (labeled B in Figure 11–1), allowing it to generate a response across that range if the OHCs are functioning. Due to recording constraints, the TEOAEs can only be measured between 1000 and 4000 Hz. This limitation is partly due to the requirement that the forward-directed traveling wave from the click needs to end (die out) before the recording of the backward-directed (OAE portion) can begin. A 5 ms delay is removed from the recording so that the response can be recorded without being contaminated by the click. However, since the high frequencies are returned to the ear canal first, they also get removed because of the recording delay; therefore, the TEOAEs are only able to be recorded as high as 4000 to 5000 Hz.

The actual time-domain waveform of the TEOAEs recorded in the ear canal is also displayed in a TEOAE recording (labeled D in Figure 11–1). The response is recorded and displayed as two separate files (A and B). The instrument stores the OAE responses to half of the stimuli into one memory file and the other half into the other memory file. The two memory files are displayed on top of each other to provide a visual look at the *reproducibility*. The resulting TEOAE is generated by adding waveforms A and B, whereas any random background or physiologic noise, called the *noise floor* is determined by subtracting A and B. A simple subtraction of the emission (A + B) from the noise floor (A – B) yields a signal-to-noise ratio (SNR). From the recorded TEOAE waveform, the OAE instrument performs a fast Fourier transform (FFT) analysis to calculate and display the spectrum of the TEOAE response, as well as the noise that is present in the recording (labeled E in Figure 11–1).

The expected latency period of the TEOAE components is between 5 and 15 ms, which relates to the frequencies of the response. In other words, if you look carefully at the waveform in Figure 11–1, you should be able to see that the peaks at the beginning part of the waveform have shorter periods (higher frequencies) than those at the later parts of the waveform (lower frequencies). The TEOAEs reflect the relatively broad frequency range along the basilar membrane activated by the clicks. Due to the tono-

---

[1]Evoked OAEs are produced by an externally applied stimulus and found in nearly all normal functioning cochleae. Spontaneous OAEs are another class of cochlear emissions that can also be recorded in the ear canal, but which occur in the absence of any externally applied stimulus. Spontaneous OAEs are only found in about half of normally functioning cochleae, and thus are not well suited for clinical use.

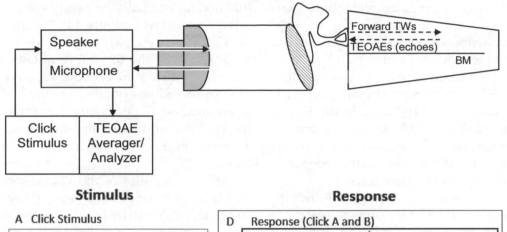

Stimulus   **Response**

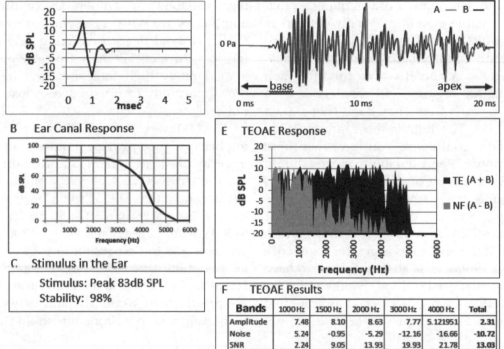

FIGURE 11–1. A block diagram of TEOAE stimulating and recording equipment. The top panel illustrates the principles of TEOAE generation and recording. The lower panels describe the TEOAE stimulus and response from a normal hearing ear. Panel A shows the click. Panel B shows the spectrum of the response to the click in the ear canal. Panel C indicates the level of the click stimulus and the stability of its presentation. Panel D shows the emission waveforms from two memory buffers (A and B) superimposed. The TEOAEs from the higher frequencies occur with shorter latencies and have shorter periods, while the TEOAEs from the lower frequencies occur with longer latencies and have longer periods. The amount of correlation between these two tracings at the different frequencies is called the reproducibility (REPRO) in some OAE equipment. Panel E shows the amplitude of the TEOAE and the background noise. Panel F provides the amplitude of the TEOAE relative to the noise, called signal-to-noise ratio (SNR), shown for the different frequency regions and the overall frequency range (Total).

topic organization of cochlea, high frequencies in the base and low frequencies in the apex, the TEOAEs are distributed over a latency range that reflects the time course of the traveling wave (forward and reverse) along the basilar membrane; the higher frequency (basal) portion of the basilar membrane is reflected in the shorter latency parts of the TEOAE waveform, and the lower frequency (apical) portion of the basilar membrane is reflected in the slightly longer latency parts of the TEOAE waveform.

The interpretation of the TEOAE test involves looking at the TEOAE results (labeled F in Figure 11–1) to determine those frequencies that show an acceptable emission, usually defined as an SNR of 6 dB (Dhar & Hall, 2012). Some instruments calculate a *reproducibility value* (correlation between the A and B waveforms) for each of the frequency regions and displays it as a percentage for each frequency band (not shown in Figure 11–1). The higher the reproducibility value, the more confidence you have that there is a true response. Reproducibility values should be at least 50% at each of the frequency regions (Kemp, Ryan, & Bray, 1990), and even a higher criterion (e.g., 75%) may be more appropriate for clinical applications. An emission is only considered present if the SNR ratio is greater than 6 dB, otherwise the emission is absent. Failure to have a TEOAE that is at least 6 dB above the noise for any of the frequency regions would indicate that the OHCs from those frequency regions are not

functioning normally or overly contaminated by a high noise level. Figure 11–2 shows examples of TEOAEs from two ears, one with present TEOAEs across the the full frequency range and the other with absent TEOAEs. Figure 11–3 shows TEOAE recordings obtained using a slightly different method of displaying the results, in which the emission and noise amplitudes are displayed as a bar graph showing results in half-octave bands.

The amplitudes of the TEOAEs vary considerably across people and ages (they are much larger in infants than in adults). Because of the high variability in amplitudes of the TEOAEs, amplitudes are not very useful for estimating an OAE threshold or for predicting degree of hearing loss. In fact, TEOAEs are only measured at a moderately high intensity level to maximize the opportunity to obtain a response above the noise.

TEOAEs are well suited for auditory screening because they provide a quick estimate of the integrity of the peripheral auditory function over the 1000 to 4000 Hz frequency range. It is generally accepted that TEOAEs will be absent if hearing loss is greater than 30 to 35 dB HL. According to Robinette, Cevette, and Probst (2007), TEOAEs are expected to be present in 99% of ears when all pure-tone thresholds are better than 20 dB HL, always absent when all pure-tone thresholds are greater than 40 dB HL, and may or may not be present with pure-tone thresholds between 25

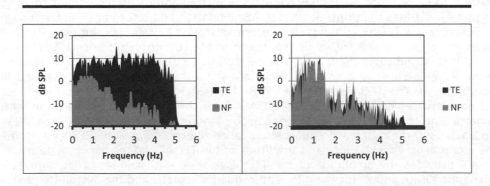

FIGURE 11–2. TEOAE responses. (**A**) Results from an ear with normal hearing; amplitudes of the TEOAEs are larger than the noise floor across the frequency range. (**B**) Results from an ear with hearing loss; amplitudes of both the response and noise floor are low indicating no emissions from the cochlea. Background noise is usually larger in the low frequencies.

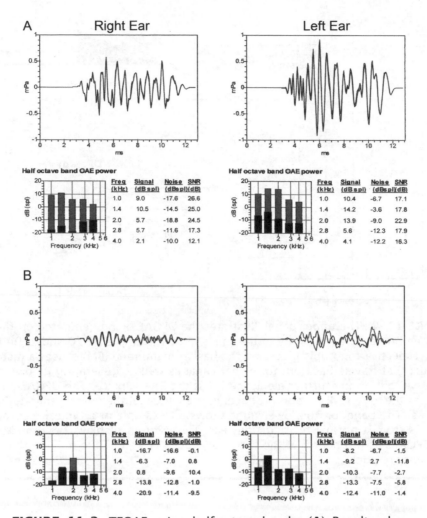

FIGURE 11-3. TEOAE using half-octave bands. (**A**) Results show normal TEOAEs in both ears as evidenced by the large emission amplitudes and large (>6 dB) SNR at all frequencies. (**B**) Results show abnormal (absent) TEOAEs for these ears as evidenced by very small emission amplitudes and small SNR (except at 2 kHz).

and 35 dB HL. TEOAEs effectively separate those with normal function from those who need further follow-up evaluations. Studies have shown that a fair number (10 to 15%) of newborns fail the initial TEOAE screening, most likely due to some transient middle/outer ear condition; however, upon rescreening the majority of those will pass (Prieve, 2007).

The presence of TEOAEs indicates cochlear function no worse than 35 dB HL, and that there is no significant outer and middle ear involvement. If a patient has normal TEOAEs and shows more than a mild sensorineural hearing loss, the hearing problem lies more central to the cochlea

(8th cranial nerve or central auditory system), or the pure-tone thresholds are not an accurate representation of the patient's hearing loss.

Distortion Product Otoacoustic Emissions (DPOAEs)

The cochlea is a non-linear system, which means that there are additional tones, called *distortion products*, generated in the cochlea that were not present in the externally applied stimulus. Figure 11-4 illustrates how DPOAEs are generated and recorded. When two pure tones (f_1 and f_2,

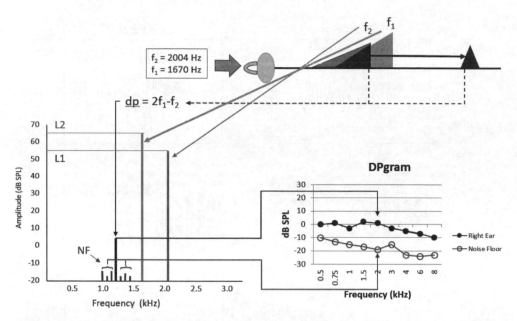

FIGURE 11–4. The upper panel illustrates the DPOAE being generated on the basilar membrane. The proximity of the tones in this example (1670 and 2004 Hz) in their respective tonotopic places on the basilar membrane (BM) causes a distortion product that travels back out to the ear canal as well as generating its own traveling wave that occurs further along the BM at the $2f_1 - f_2$ place. The DPOAE analyzer extracts the $2f_1 - f_2$ distortion products in the ear canal that were generated in the cochlea. The panel on the lower right shows an example of a typical recording of DPOAEs from a normal hearing right ear. The DPgram displays the amplitude of the DPOAEs as a function of the f_2 primary tone, as well as the noise within those frequency regions.

where f_1 is lower in frequency than f_2) are simultaneously presented to a human ear, the most prominent distortion product occurs at a frequency equal to $2f_1 - f_2$, the *cubic difference tone*. The externally presented pure tones are called the *primary tones*, and the $2f_1 - f_2$ is the distortion product tone that is generated in the cochlea. For example, if the primary tones are 1000 and 1200 Hz, the $2f_1 - f_2 = 800$ Hz. The $2f_1 - f_2$ distortion product occurs at least 50 dB lower than the level of f_1. The $2f_1 - f_2$ DPOAE is largest when the ratio of f_2/f_1 is equal to about 1.22. The level (dB SPL) of f_1 (L_1) is usually set to about 65 dB SPL and the level of f_2 (L_2) should be 10 to 15 lower than L_1 (e.g., 65 and 50 dB SPL) (Dhar & Hall, 2012; Gaskill & Brown, 1990; Whitehead, Stagner, Lonsbury-Martin, & Martin, 1995).

The DPOAE recording instrument filters out the frequencies of the two primary tones (f_1 and f_2) and focuses its measurement only on the distortion product frequency ($2f_1 - f_2$). Unlike TEOAEs, where the responses are recorded after each stimulus, the DPOAE method measures the responses during cochlear activation; however, it is not clear whether the different types of stimulation have any clinical significance. By changing the frequencies of the two primary tones (maintaining f_2/f_1 at 1.22), distortion products can be generated from different frequency regions in the cochlea. The DPOAEs are recorded for different pairs of primary tones, which are typically swept across the frequency range from 1000 to 6000 Hz. The frequency sweep is repeated and responses are recorded with signal averaging until the background noise is sufficiently reduced and the DPOAEs are enhanced. Generally, it takes about four or five sweeps across the frequency range to establish acceptable DPOAEs above the noise floor. The analysis of the DPOAE recording typically involves looking at the absolute amplitude of the DPOAE and/or the ratio of the DPOAE relative to the noise floor with the primaries at standard intensity levels (e.g., 65 and 50 dB SPL for f_1 and f_2, respectively). Generally, the DPOAE amplitude should be at least 6 dB above the noise floor (Kimberley, Brown, & Allen, 1997). DPOAEs can also be measured as a function of changing the stimulus level of the primary tones. In this procedure, an *input–output function* is generated by varying the level of f_1 or f_2 separately, or both f_1 and f_2 together, to obtain an input–output function to estimate the DPOAE threshold. The use of DPOAE input–output functions is not yet in widespread clinical use.

Although the instrument is measuring the amplitude of the $2f_1 – f_2$, it is the place along the basilar membrane where the two primary tones are interacting that must be functioning normally to generate the distortion product. The typical DPOAE results are plotted as a function of f_2 (Figure 11–4) because the OHC function within that region of the primary tones is primarily responsible for generating the distortion product for any given pair. The noise floor is an estimate of the noise in close proximity around the frequency of the emission. While the graphic display of the DPOAEs (DPgram) has the appearance of an audiogram, it not a representation of audiometric thresholds.

As with TEOAEs, it is generally accepted that DPOAEs are present in normal ears and absent in ears with cochlear hearing loss. The degree of cochlear hearing loss that is sufficient to eliminate DPOAEs is not firmly established. DPOAEs are expected to be present with pure-tone thresholds better than 25 dB HL and absent for hearing losses greater than 40 dB when using moderate level primary tones; however, they may also be present, with reduced amplitudes, for hearing losses as high as 50 to 60 dB HL, especially when higher level primary tones are used (Gorga et al., 2007). This could make the DPOAEs less attractive as a newborn screening tool than TEOAEs because some infants who have a mild cochlear hearing loss may pass the DPOAE screening. More research is needed to determine if decreased amplitudes (or smaller SNRs) of DPOAEs can provide any specific information regarding the degree of hearing loss.

As with TEOAEs, the DPOAEs are also affected by the presence of any involvement of the middle ear and, therefore, conductive loss must be considered/ruled out when DPOAEs are absent. The presence of normal DPOAEs is evidence of good peripheral auditory function (OHCs). As with TEOAEs, if DPOAEs are present in a patient with a moderate or worse sensorineural hearing loss, this would suggest that the hearing loss may be due to a problem in the neural portions of the auditory system.

AUDITORY BRAINSTEM RESPONSE (ABR)

The auditory brainstem response (ABR)[2] is one of a series of auditory evoked responses that can be measured from the neural pathways of the auditory system using small cup or disposable electrodes placed on the surface of the head. The electrodes are connected to a signal-averaging computer (as for OAEs) that averages the synchronous neural responses occurring within the 8th nerve and brainstem that generate neuroelectric (far-field) potentials that can be measured from the scalp, much like an electroencephalogram (EEG). Figure 11–5 shows a couple of examples of the equipment used for ABR recordings.

The ABR was first identified in the late 1960s and early 1970s (Jewett, Romano, & Williston, 1970; Sohmer & Feinmesser, 1967) and became a well-established special clinical test by the late 1970s, before the discovery of OAEs. The ABR occurs with a very short latency after the onset of the transient. The latency of the normal ABR is within 10 ms after stimulation by a click stimulus. Other transient evoked auditory responses, such as the *middle latency response* (*MLR*) that occurs 10–50 ms after stimulation, and the *late latency response* (*LLR*) that occurs 50–250 ms after stimulation, were discovered prior to the ABR. Although the MLR and LLR have some clinical utility, they are affected by subject state and aneasthesia, and are not used as routinely as ABR, especially for testing young children.

The ABR is not part of the basic audiometric test battery, but it is a very useful physiological

---

[2]Sometimes, the ABR is called the brainstem evoked response (BSER) or the brainstem auditory evoked response (BAER).

measure that is routinely performed by audiologists for special populations, including: (a) testing young children or other difficult-to-test patients whose behavioral thresholds are not able to be obtained or are questionable, (b) as a newborn hearing screening test, (c) as a follow-up for infants who fail a newborn hearing screening test, and (d) evaluation of patients suspected of 8th cranial nerve disorders. The interested reader is referred to other references for more detailed information on the ABR and other evoked electrical potentials (Burkard, Don, & Eggermont, 2007; Hall & Swanepoel, 2010; Hood, 1998; Small & Stapells, 2017).

The observation of an ABR is dependent on *neural synchrony*, which refers to the condition in which a relatively large number of auditory neurons discharge (fire) nearly simultaneously. To achieve neural synchrony, the ABR requires the use of brief acoustic signals with rapid onset times, *transients* (*clicks*) or *tone bursts*. A click has a broadband spectrum, whereas a tone burst has a more restricted spectrum around its center frequency. The computer measures the neuroelectric activity that occurs during a relatively short time period (10 to 20 ms) after each stimulus; in other words, the response is *time-locked* to the onset of each stimulus. A typical ABR requires about 2000 time-locked stimuli, presented at a rate of about 11 to 41/s. When the response is averaged over many stimuli, the synchronously responding activity from the auditory neural pathway (ABR response) is enhanced, while the background electrical activity (EEG) or other noise is reduced because it occurs randomly (non-time locked). The activity from the neural pathways of the ABR is quite small, especially when recorded relatively far from its sources; therefore, successful recording requires that the patient be very still or preferably asleep (natural or sedated). The clinical utility of the ABR is enhanced by the fact that the responses are unaffected by level of attention, sleep-state, or drugs, and can be reliably recorded across all ages, including premature infants.

The ABR is characterized by a series of six to seven waves (peaks) as shown in Figure 11–6. To improve interpretation, each recording condition is replicated (repeated) and typically the replications are plotted on top of each other. The earliest positive wave is called *wave I*, which is a reflection of the synchronous discharge of neurons in the distal (more peripheral) portion of the auditory portion of the 8th cranial nerve as it is leaving the cochlea. The subsequent waves are generated by the synchronous neural activity in the proximal part of the 8th cranial nerve (wave II), cochlear nucleus (wave III), superior olivary complex (wave IV), lateral lemniscus, and input to the inferior colliculus (wave V) (Møller, 1994). Although the neural generators for the different ABR waves are in the 8th cranial nerve and brainstem, the overall response latencies and thresholds are also characteristically affected by peripheral hearing disorders that can affect the output

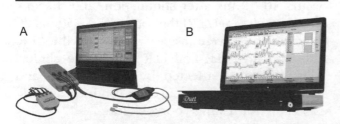

FIGURE 11–5. A AND B. Some examples of ABR units used to record neurodiagnostic and threshold ABRs. **A.** Vivosonic Integrity 500. **B.** Intelligent Hearing Systems Duet. *Source*: Photos courtesy of Vivosonic Inc. (A) and Intelligent Hearing Systems (B).

Historical Vignette

Few test procedures have had the same profound effect on audiological practice as the auditory brain stem response (ABR). It has truly revolutionized diagnostic evaluation. Gone today are the SISI, ABLB, and Békésy-type audiograms. They have been replaced by a single powerful tool that objectively differentiates cochlear loss from 8th cranial nerve disorders with high sensitivity and acceptable specificity. Donald Jewett stumbled upon this response almost by accident. He was looking at later evoked electroneural responses measured from the scalp when he noticed what appeared to be repeatable bumps in the first 10 ms after stimulus onset. Previous investigators missed them because it was the fashion at that time to band-pass filter the EEG rather narrowly around the frequency region of interest, which for the middle and late electroneural responses was well below 100 Hz; thus, activity in the 500 to 1000 Hz range, where the ABR response is maximal, was, in effect, discarded (filtered out). But no one told Jewett that you were supposed to filter so narrowly, and his much wider filter setting allowed the ABR peaks to be viewed.

to the 8th cranial nerve and brainstem. *Wave V* is the most prominent wave in the ABR waveform and is the wave most often used for clinical assessment of ABR threshold estimation because it is the only wave present near threshold.

Stimulus Related Principles of ABR

The ABR waveform acts according to a set of physiological principles tied to different parameters of the stimulus. The waveform changes in a predictable fashion according to changes in the stimulus intensity, frequency, and rate. It is im-

portant to understand these principles and how they are used in identifying peaks in the waveform and for proper interpretation of the overall results.

Stimulus Intensity

Figure 11–7 shows a series of ABR waveforms to click stimuli as a function of intensity for a normal hearing ear. Notice how wave V remains the most visible waveform as intensity decreases, and is characterized by a systematic increase in latency as intensity decreases. At low intensities, the ABR wave V latency to click stimuli reflects the synchronous neural activity from around the 2000 Hz region, which has better auditory sensitivity than other frequencies. For a normal ear, as intensity is increased, the wave V latencies shorten to reflect the activity from neurons in the higher frequency basal regions of the cochlea, which are stimulated earliest and where the faster traveling wave velocity produces greater neural synchrony. The ABR threshold recorded from clicks could be used as an estimate (within 10 to 15 dB) of the degree of hearing loss in the 2000 to 4000 Hz region (Bauch & Olsen, 1986).

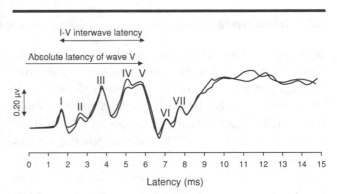

FIGURE 11–6. A normal auditory brainstem response (ABR) waveform to a click at a relatively high intensity level showing the waves (positive peaks) labeled I–VII. The latency (time) of each wave is called the absolute latency, which is relative to the onset of the brief stimulus (at 0 ms). An example of absolute latency is shown for wave V, which is usually the most prominent wave. The latency difference between any two waves is called the interpeak latency difference. The I–V interpeak latency difference is the one most often used clinically. Waves II, IV, VI, and VII are often difficult to discern and are not used clinically.

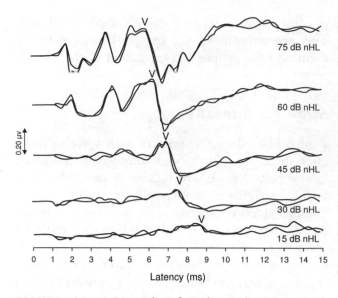

FIGURE 11–7. Example of auditory brainstem response (ABR) recordings as a function of stimulus (click) intensity level for a normal hearing ear. The click intensity levels are referenced to normal behavioral threshold to the clicks, and are labeled dB nHL to differentiate from dB HL used for audiometric stimuli. At lower intensities, wave V is the only wave that is observable, and it is usually present down to levels of 15 to 20 dB nHL in quiet recording conditions. Wave V latency systematically increases as intensity decreases.

Stimulus Rate

Stimulus rate refers to the number of clicks per second presented to the ear. The lower the rate, the better the morphology of the waveform: Rates of approximately 10 to 19 clicks yield robust waves I, III, and V (for moderate to high stimulus intensities). Figure 11–8 illustrates the effects of stimulus rate on the ABR, as the stimulus rate increases, the latency of wave V increases, but the latency of the earlier waves increase less than wave V, producing a greater interpeak latency difference between wave I and V (Hood, 1998) and/or waves I and III tend to disappear in the recording. Clinic protocols compare the latency of wave V at a slow rate (i.e., 11.1/s) to a fast rate (i.e., 80.5/s) as shown in Figure 11–8. While there is a normal increase in latency with rate for normal ears, there tends to be an abnormal increase in latency with rate in those with an 8th cranial nerve disorder.

Stimulus Frequency

The stimuli, as previously mentioned, can be either clicks or more frequency-specific tone bursts. As shown in Figure 11–9, as the frequency of the tone burst increases the latency of wave V decreases. The higher frequency tone bursts (i.e., 4000 Hz) stimulate more basal cochlear locations and have sharper peaks because of greater neural synchrony (traveling wave velocity is faster at the base); the lower frequency tone bursts (i.e., 500 Hz), especially at low intensities, stimulate more apical regions and have broader peaks because of less neural synchrony (traveling wave velocity is slower as it moves toward the apex). Notice that a recording time window of 15 to 24 ms would be needed to see the responses to the 500 Hz tone burst. Keep in mind, however, that lower frequency tone bursts, when delivered at a high intensity, are not very frequency specific because they cause stimulation nearer the base (remember, all traveling waves progress from base to apex) where the greater neural synchrony dominates the response.

The ABR and Types of Hearing Loss

The wave V latency is often plotted as a *latency-intensity (L-I) function* as shown in Figure 11–10. The shape of the L-I function is often helpful

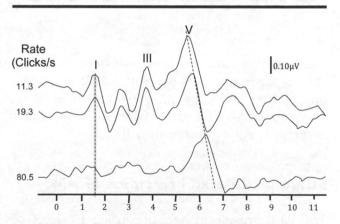

FIGURE 11–8. Examples of click-generated high-intensity ABRs to different stimulus rates. As the rate of stimulation increases, the latency of wave V increases, while the latency of wave I stays the same, thus the interpeak latency interval (I–V) increases.

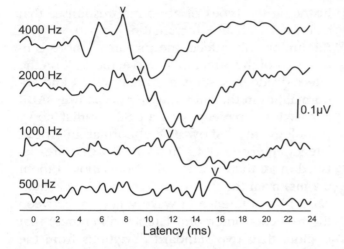

FIGURE 11–9. Examples of a series of tone-burst generated waveforms. Wave V is the only wave labeled on all tracings. As the frequency decreases, the latency of wave V increases.

in identifying the type of hearing loss. A patient with a flat conductive hearing loss will have an L-I function that parallels the normal L-I function due to the reduction in stimulus intensity at each recording level due to the conductive hearing loss. A patient with a sloping or relatively flat high frequency cochlear hearing loss will have an elevated threshold, but may also have a steeper than normal L-I function. The steeper L-I function begins with a delayed wave latency near threshold due to the hearing loss in the mid to high frequencies. As the stimulus intensity is increased, it crosses the thresholds in the higher frequencies where latency reflects the basal responding regions that occur with shorter latency and with greater synchrony, thus dominating the waveform. At the highest intensities, the cochlear hearing loss has wave V latency within the normal expected range, and the waveform is indistinguishable from a normal ear. In cases with a very steep or severe high frequency hearing loss, the L-I function may not end within the normal latency region at the higher intensities because there are not enough high frequency neurons to stimulate.

It is also important to realize that the ABR to clicks become problematic in identifying cases in which there is a low frequency hearing loss with better hearing in the high frequencies. In these

cases, the ABR will reflect only the more synchronously responding higher frequency regions once the stimulus is high enough to exceed their thresholds. Therefore, whenever there is good high frequency hearing, the ABR to clicks may not be effective and the L-I function could be entirely within the normal range due to the dominance by the more synchronously responding, normally functioning, basal (high frequency) region. In these situations, the ABR to clicks or tone bursts can provide frequency specific information by using different high-pass or band-pass maskers to eliminate the more synchronously responding high frequency regions (Don & Eggermont, 1978; Kramer & Teas, 1979; Stapells, Picton, Durieux-Smith, Edwards, & Moran, 1990).

NEURODIAGNOSTIC ABR

In the early use of ABR, clinicians often used ABR to identify possible 8th cranial nerve pathologies. The ABR was seen to be much less costly and invasive than a computerized tomography (CT) scan, and studies showed the ABR to be more sensitive to smaller tumors than CT scans. Any patient who had an asymmetric

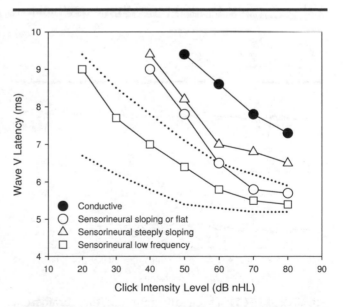

FIGURE 11–10. Examples of click-generated wave V latency-intensity (L-I) functions for different types of hearing losses. The dotted curves represent two standard deviations of the normal expected L-I function.

sensorineural hearing loss was routinely referred for a neurodiagnostic ABR. For neurodiagnostic assessment, the latency differences between the various waves, especially wave I–III, III–V, and/or wave I–V interpeak latency values are calculated and compared to normal expected values. An abnormal wave I–III (and I–V) interpeak latency difference suggests an abnormality in the 8th cranial nerve; an abnormal wave III–V (and I–V) interpeak latency difference suggests a problem in the brainstem. The presence or absence of a response, the overall shape of the waveform (*morphology*), the absolute latencies of the different waves, especially wave V, the interpeak latency differences between waves (I–III, III–V, I–V), wave V latency difference between ears (interaural latency difference), and effects of stimulus rate are the most often evaluated results of the ABR for neurodiagnostic purposes to assess neural transmission through the 8th cranial nerve and lower brainstem pathways.

When using the ABR to evaluate 8th cranial nerve or brainstem function, recordings are done at a relatively high stimulus level to maximize the likelihood of seeing all the waves. Results for a patient with an acoustic neuroma (tumor on the 8th cranial nerve) may show different types of abnormal recordings. Figure 11–11 shows the ABR recording from three different patients il-lustrating the types of abnormal responses that can occur with an 8th cranial nerve pathology. If the tumor only affects the proximal (more central) part of the 8th cranial nerve, the ABR on the affected side may show a normal wave I and abnormalities in the later waves. Alternatively, ABR results for a patient with an 8th cranial nerve pathology may show (a) abnormal interpeak latency intervals (I–III and/or I–V) that are delayed more than two standard deviations (about 0.4 ms) from the normal interpeak latency intervals; (b) a difference in wave V latency between the two ears (interaural latency difference) that is more than two standard deviations from the normal interaural latency difference; or (c) no discernible waves even though there is sufficient hearing to expect normal wave latencies.

THRESHOLD ABR

The use of ABR for threshold estimation utilizes a test protocol that determines the lowest level that a repeatable wave V response can be obtained and to diagnose the type of hearing loss (recall the L-I function). ABRs can be recorded using air and bone conduction, which is useful in determining if an air–bone gap exists. Figure 11–12 shows characteristic changes in the ABR waveform (wave V) for different frequencies presented at relatively low intensity levels within the range of normal hearing for neonates. Frequency specific ABRs can be obtained down to levels of 10 to 20 dB for frequencies as low as 500 Hz, with a quiet patient and proper recording parameters. The ABR cannot evaluate frequencies less than 500 Hz (and sometimes 500 Hz is difficult) because there is not enough neural synchrony in those lower frequency regions. For tone-bursts at 500 and 1000 Hz, the waveform morphology usually shows only a broadened wave V peak as seen in Figure 11–12, and the wave V latency is increased as one would predict because the neural response is originating at the more apical regions of the cochlea (longer traveling wave time). To assist with determining infant ABR thresholds, normative data for tone burst wave V latencies were recently published for 500, 1000, 2000, and 4000 Hz at thresholds from 10, 20, and 30 dB (Elsayed et al., 2015).

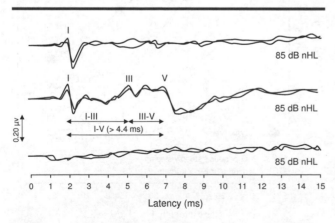

FIGURE 11–11. Three different auditory brainstem response (ABR) waveforms illustrating some of the different abnormal recordings that are associated with 8th nerve disorders. For neurological evaluations, it is best to make the recordings at a high intensity to try to obtain waves I, III, and V.

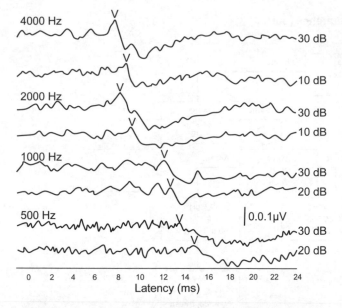

FIGURE 11–12. Tone-burst ABR waveforms recorded near threshold ("threshold ABR"). Results show wave V at each frequency from 500 to 4000 Hz at 30 dB and at either 10 or 20 dB; this would be considered normal thresholds for this neonate, indicating that this neonate has normal auditory function at least through the brainstem (and most likely has normal hearing).

the ABR only represents the neural function reflecting cochlear output and neural conduction along the lower brainstem pathway and, therefore, is not a measure of conscious hearing. Hearing loss can still be present even though ABR is normal when the hearing loss is from more central nervous system involvement or due to a functional component (feigning a hearing loss).

In many cases, the ABR is used as a screening test at a single preset intensity, say 30 or 40 dB, to determine a pass or fail. Those who fail the ABR screening are referred for follow up evaluations, that include threshold ABR and, if older than 6 months, a behavioral hearing test. Since newborns cannot be tested using behavioral techniques, as discussed in previous chapters, the audiologist must use ABR to provide an estimate of a baby's auditory thresholds. As with OAEs, the ABR is not a test of hearing, and only inferences can be made about any potential degree of hearing loss. Since ABR is a relatively quick, objective measure of hearing sensitivity, especially in newborns, young infants, or other difficult-to-test populations, ABR for threshold estimates has far surpassed the neurodiagnostic applications of ABR.

In a clinical evaluation of auditory sensitivity, a protocol should be developed that will sequence the test in a fast and efficient method to provide most clinical information before the infant wakes up from natural sleep. Using this type of protocol, results from at least three frequencies per ear can be obtained for most infants (>80%) in about 1 hour (Janssen, Usher, & Stapells, 2010). In many cases, the ABR is done under sedation with medical approval and monitoring. A test strategy proposed by Stapells (2002)

Table 11–1 gives guidelines (BCEHP, 2012; Small & Stapells, 2017) for the maximum threshold values for tone-burst ABRs (for air and bone conduction) that would be considered normal responses for infants, and the recommended correction amounts to apply to get an estimate of the behavioral threshold expectations (eHL). Although there is generally good agreement between ABR thresholds and pure-tone behavioral thresholds, it is important to keep in mind that

TABLE 11–1. Maximum Levels for ABR Thresholds for Normal Hearing and Estimated Hearing Levels (eHL)

	Air Conduction				Bone Conduction	
Frequency (Hz)	500	1000	2000	4000	500	2000
Maximum level for normal hearing (dB nHL)	30–35	30–35	20–30	20–25	20	30
Estimated threshold correction (eHL in dB)	10–15	5–10	0–5	–5–0	–5	5

Source: From BCEHP (2012) and Small & Stapells (2017).

Tone-ABR Test Sequence (partial)

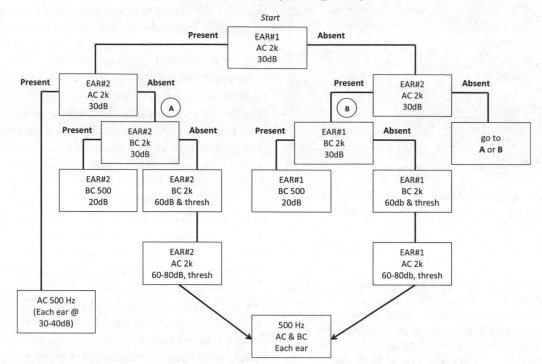

FIGURE 11–13. Flow chart to optimize the strategy in a time efficient manner for diagnostic tone-burst "threshold ABRs" in infants who did not pass the ABR or OAE screening. Start with the ear that did not pass the hearing screening, but switch between ears and transducers (air and bone). *Source*: From Stapells, 2002, p. 16. Copyright 2002 by Wolters Kluwer Health, Inc.

can be seen in Figure 11–13. The test sequence should be based on the response obtained from the preceding stimulus level and will change for each infant tested based on the outcome of the previous ABR waveform. A complete test with proper interpretation is important to provide appropriate information to the parent, proper referral, and overall management of the young child.

AUDITORY STEADY-STATE RESPONSE (ASSR)

Another physiologic test used clinically for estimating thresholds, especially in infants, is the *auditory steady state response* (ASSR) (Rance, Rickards, Cohen, De Vidi, & Clark, 1995). The ASSRs are periodic responses evoked by periodic (modulated) stimuli. The stimuli can be amplitude modulated or frequency modulated (or both) at different rates (modulation frequencies), either simultaneously or sequentially (Hall & Swanepoel, 2010; Rance, 2008; Stapells, 2008). The various modulation frequencies (e.g., 1000 Hz carrier tone amplitude modulation at 80 Hz) are processed at their appropriate tonotopic places along the basilar membrane. These modulations are carried up the auditory neural pathways to the brain, where they can be recorded with surface electrodes similar to other evoked potential measures. The ASSR is a reflection of how different levels of the brain react to the modulation frequencies of the stimuli. The carrier frequency determines where on the basilar membrane the stimulation is taking place, and the modulation rate determines the periodicity of the neural response in a normal hearing person. The ASSR as seen in Figure 11–14 is analyzed by measuring

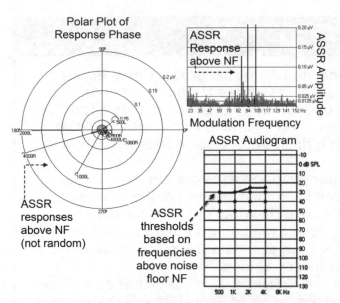

FIGURE 11–14. The use of an ASSR to determine an individual's threshold. The instrument analyzes the response signal-to-noise ratio, as well as the phases of the response components to assist in determining if a response is present. A correction factor is then subtracted from the lowest level detected and plotted in an audiogram format to show estimated thresholds at each frequency.

the carrier frequency. The filter settings of the recording instrument should be set to maximize the modulation frequencies and not the carrier frequencies, for example, 30 to 300 Hz. With today's clinical instruments, the spectra are automatically subjected to statistical rules to determine if a steady-state response is significantly above the noise floor. Modulation frequencies in the range 70 to 110 Hz produce steady-state responses that are not affected by levels of sleep or maturation, and most likely represent activity arising primarily at the level of the brainstem. To estimate air-conducted thresholds, a regression analysis based on normative ASSR data or a correction factor analysis is performed by the recording instrument (Hall & Swanepoel, 2010). This will result in an ASSR threshold and can be converted to an audiogram format by the addition of a correction factor. It is also possible, and clinically useful, to simultaneously present stimuli at different carrier frequencies (to one or both ears), each with a different modulation rate, to get a more rapid analysis of the patient's auditory function across a broader frequency range. ASSR responses are mostly used with air-conducted stimuli as bone-conducted stimuli can produce "spurious" responses in infants with hearing loss (Small & Stapells, 2017). For more details on ASSR, the interested reader should consult other sources (Hall & Swanepoel, 2010; Rance, 2008; Small & Stapells, 2017).

both the spectrum and phase of the neural response to determine if it is producing activity at the modulation rate and, hence, determine the extent to which the patient is able to process

Synopsis 11–1

- In response to sound, the normal cochlea produces additional mechanical energy due to the motility of the OHCs, and these vibrations are transmitted out of the ear where they are recorded as OAEs in the ear canal. OAEs are preneural events but can be affected by hearing loss in the cochlea, middle ear, or ear canal.
- Because OAEs are preneural, their presence would suggest normal cochlear function, and lead one to suspect that a sensorineural hearing loss was due to a neural (8th cranial nerve or central) disorder, or that they may be feigning a hearing loss.
- A normal TEOAE should be at least 6 dB above the noise floor at each of the measurable frequencies (1000, 2000, 3000, 4000 Hz) and show a reproducibility of more than 75%. TEOAEs are not reliable for frequencies below 1000 Hz or above 4000 Hz.

Synopsis 11–1 (*continued*)

- DPOAEs are recordings of cochlear generated distortion product frequencies, which occur for different pairs of primary tones, called f1 and f2 (where f2/f1 = 1.22, L1 = 65 dB SPL, and L2 = 50 dB SPL). DPOAEs are plotted as a function of f2 frequency, which is varied between 1000 and 6000 Hz. A normal DPOAE should show a response that is at least 6 dB above the noise floor at each f2 frequency.

- TEOAEs are typically absent with cochlear hearing losses greater than 30 dB HL, which makes them ideal for newborn hearing screening. Neither TEOAEs nor DPOAEs are able to quantify the degree of hearing loss because they would be absent for peripheral hearing losses ranging from mild to profound. Disorders of the middle ear and outer ear can eliminate OAEs and confound the interpretation of OAEs in newborn hearing screenings.

- The ABR is characterized by a series of wave peaks that occur within 2 to 10 ms following a brief click or tone burst and are recorded with electrodes taped to the head. The ABR is a reflection of the synchronous neural activity that occurs only with rapid onset stimuli (transients). Wave I originates from the peripheral portion of the 8th cranial nerve and the later waves from lower brainstem pathways. Each of these waves is affected by the peripheral auditory system, as well as the neural conduction through the 8th cranial nerve and low brainstem pathways. The most prominent peak is called wave V. Wave V is typically recordable in a normal ear to within 10 dB of behavioral threshold.

- A latency-intensity (L-I) function may be useful in characterizing possible hearing loss. A conductive hearing loss shows an elevated threshold and delayed wave V latency at each intensity level. A cochlear hearing loss shows an elevated threshold with a longer wave V latency near threshold, but at high intensities wave V latency occurs within the normal range when there are enough higher frequency neurons that are stimulated. A very steep high frequency cochlear hearing loss shows wave V latency flattens out before reaching the normal latency range. Noise masking (high-pass or band-reject) can be used to eliminate the higher frequency regions and improve frequency specificity, especially in cases where there is a mid frequency hearing loss with better high frequency sensitivity.

- For neural assessment, the absence or abnormal delay of the peaks after wave I is evaluated. For example, an 8th cranial nerve tumor could have a wave I, but the later waves may be absent or the latency interval between waves I and V could be prolonged.

- Auditory steady-state response (ASSR) produces responses that reflect the rates of modulation (e.g., 70 to 110 Hz) for different carrier frequencies, and show promise for estimating frequency specific auditory thresholds, including the lower frequencies. ASSRs are subjected to a spectral analysis to determine which frequency regions are producing/following the modulation rate for the applied frequencies. A statistical analysis is done to determine if a steady-state response is significantly above the noise floor.

REFERENCES

Bauch, C. D., & Olsen, W. O. (1986). The effect of 2000-4000 Hz hearing sensitivity on ABR results. *Ear and Hearing, 7*(5), 314–317.

Brownell, W. E. (1983). Observations on a motile response in isolated outer hair cells. In W. R. Webster & L. Aitken (Eds.), *Mechanisms of Hearing* (pp. 5–10). Clayten, Australia: Monash University Press.

Burkard, R. F., Don, M., & Eggermont, J. J. (2007). *Auditory Evoked Potentials*. Baltimore, MD: Kluwer Lippincott.

Dhar, S., & Hall, J. W. (2012). *Otoacoustic Emissions*. San Diego, CA: Plural.

Don, M., & Eggermont, J. J. (1978). Analysis of the click-evoked brainstem potentials in man using high-pass noise masking. *The Journal of the Acoustical Society of America, 63*(4), 1084–1092.

Elsayed, A., Hunter, L. L., Keefe, D. H., Feeney, M. P., Brown, D. K., Meinzen-Derr, J. K., Sullivan-Mahoney, M., Francis, K., & Schaid, L. G. (2015). Air and bone conduction tone-burst auditory brainstem thresholds using a Kalman filtering approach in non-sedated normal hearing newborns. *Ear and Hearing, 36*, 471–481.

Gaskill, S. A., & Brown, A. M. (1990). The behavior of the acoustic distortion product, 2f1-f2 from the human ear and its relation to auditory sensitivity. *Journal of the Acoustical Society of America, 88*, 821–839.

Glattke, T. J., & Robinette, M. S. (Eds.) (2007). *Transient Evoked Otoacoustic Emissions in Populations with Normal Hearing Sensitivity* (3rd ed.). New York, NY: Thieme.

Gorga, M. P., Neely, S. T., Johnson, T. A., Dierking, D. M., & Garner, C. A. (2007). *Distortion Product Otoacoustic Emissions in Relation to Hearing Loss. In M. S. Robinette & T. J. Glattke (Eds.). Otoacoustic Emissions: Clinical Applications* (3rd ed.). New York, NY: Thieme.

Hall, J. W. I., & Swanepoel, D. W. (2010). *Objective Assessment of Hearing*. San Diego, CA: Plural.

Hof, J. R., Anteunis, L. J. C., Chenault, M. N., & van Dijk, P. (2005). Otoacoustic emissions at compensated middle ear pressure in children. *International Journal of Audiology, 44*(6), 317–320.

Hood, L. J. (1998). *Clinical Applications of the Auditory Brainstem Response*. San Diego, CA: Plural.

Janssen, R. M., Usher, L., & Stapells, D. R. (2010). The British Columbia's Children's Hospital tone-evoked ABR protocol: How long do infants sleep, and how much information can be obtained in one appointment? *Ear and Hearing, 31*, 722–724.

Jewett, D. L., Romano, M. N., & Williston, J. S. (1970). Human auditory evoked potentials: possible brain stem components detected on the scalp. *Science, 167*, 1517–1518.

Kemp, D. T. (1978). Stimulated acoustic emissions from within the human auditory system. *The Journal of the Acoustical Society of America, 64*(5), 1386–1391.

Kemp, D. T., Ryan, S., & Bray, P. (1990). A guide to the effective use of otoacoustic emissions. *Ear and Hearing, 11*(2), 93–105.

Kimberley, B. P., Brown, D. K., & Allen, J. B. (1997). Distortion product emissions and sensorineural hearing loss. In M. S. Robinette & T. J. Glattke (Eds.), *Otoacoustic Emissions Clinical Applications*. New York, NY: Thieme.

Kramer, S. J., & Teas, D. C. (1979). BSR (wave V) and N1 latencies in response to acoustic stimuli with different bandwidths. *The Journal of the Acoustical Society of America, 66*(2), 446–455.

Lonsbury-Martin, B., Martin, G., & Whitehead, M. (2007). Distortion product otoacoustic emissions in populations with normal hearing sensitivity. In M. Robinette & T. Glattke (Eds.), *Otoacoustic Emissions: Clinical Applications* (3rd ed., pp. 107–130). New York, NY: Thieme.

Møller, A. R. (1994). Neural generators of auditory evoked potentials. In J. T. Jacobson (Ed.), *Principles and Applications in Auditory Evoked Potentials*. Boston, MA: Allyn and Bacon.

Prieve, B. A. (2007). Otoacoustic emissions in neonatal hearing screening. In M. S. Robinette & T. J. Glattke (Eds.), *Otoacoustic Emission: Clinical Applications* (pp. 365–402). New York, NY: Thieme.

Probst, R., & Harris, F. P. (1993). Transiently evoked and distortion-product otoacoustic emissions. Comparison of results from normally hearing and hearing-impaired human ears. *Archives of Otolaryngology—Head & Neck Surgery, 119*(8), 858–860.

Rance, G. (2008). *Auditory Steady-State Response: Generation, Recording, and Clinical Applications*. San Diego, CA: Plural.

Rance, G., Rickards, F. W., Cohen, L. T., De Vidi, S., & Clark, G. M. (1995). The automated prediction of hearing thresholds in sleeping subjects using auditory steady-state evoked potentials. *Ear and Hearing, 16*(5), 499–507.

Robinette, M. S., Cevette, M. J., & Probst, R. (Eds.). (2007). *Otoacoustic Emissions and Audiometric Outcomes Across Cochlear and Retrocochlear Pathology* (3rd ed.). New York, NY: Thieme.

Robinette, M. S., & Glattke, T. J. (2007). *Otoacoustic Emission: Clinical Applications* (3rd ed.). New York, NY: Thieme.

Small, S. A., & Stapells, D. R. (2017). Threshold assessment in infants using the frequency-specific ABR and

ASSR. In R. Seewald & A. M. Tharpe (Eds.), *Comprehensive Handbook of Pediatric Audiology*. San Diego, CA: Plural.

Sohmer, H., & Feinmesser, M. (1967). Cochlear action potentials recorded from the external ear in man. *The Annals of Otology, Rhinology, and Laryngology, 76*(2), 427–435.

Stapells, D. R. (2002). Tone-evoked ABR: Why it's the measure of choice for young infants. *The Hearing Journal, 55,* 14–18.

Stapells, D. R. (Ed.) (2008). *The 80 Hz Auditory Steady-State Response Compared with Other Auditory Evoked Potentials*. San Diego, CA: Plural.

Stapells, D. R., Picton, T. W., Durieux-Smith, A., Edwards, C. G., & Moran, L. M. (1990). Thresholds for short-latency auditory-evoked potentials to tones in notched noise in normal-hearing and hearing-impaired subjects. *Audiology: Official Organ of the International Society of Audiology, 29*(5), 262–274.

Whitehead, M. L., Stagner, B. B., Lonsbury-Martin, B. L., & Martin, G. K. (1995). Effects of ear-canal standing waves on measurements of distortion-product otoacoustic emissions. *The Journal of the Acoustical Society of America, 98*(6), 3200–3214.

12 Disorders of the Auditory System

After reading this chapter, you should be able to:

1. Define terminology used to describe the time of onset and duration of hearing disorders.

2. Define some medical terms used to describe auditory disorders.

3. Identify a variety of disorders of the outer ear and middle ear.

4. Identify a variety of disorders of the inner ear and 8th cranial nerve.

5. Describe the physical characteristics, patient complaints, audiologic results, and treatment options for a variety of auditory disorders.

6. Understand how audiometric results can help provide differential diagnoses of common auditory disorders.

7. Match hearing disorders to their type of hearing loss, for example, normal, conductive, or sensorineural.

8. Create representative audiograms for different pathologies.

9. See the relationship among a variety of audiologic test results characteristic of different auditory disorders.

10. Recognize the patient and audiometric characteristics of a functional hearing loss. Describe and interpret the Stenger test.

11. Understand the differences between subjective and objective tinnitus. Recognize when to make medical referrals for tinnitus. Describe three methods for treating subjective tinnitus.

This chapter provides general descriptions of some selected auditory disorders and their associated pathologies. The auditory disorders are separated into those that affect the different parts of the auditory system, the outer ear, middle ear, inner ear, 8th cranial nerve, and central pathways. Keep in mind, however, that some auditory disorders can affect more than one part of the ear, and a patient may have more than one type of auditory disorder from different causes at the same time, such as a sensorineural hearing loss from noise trauma and a conductive hearing loss from an ear infection. This chapter also briefly covers nonorganic (functional) hearing losses, where the patient may be exaggerating or feigning a hearing loss. At the end of the chapter, there is a discussion of *tinnitus* ("ringing" in the ears), which is a common symptom of many hearing disorders. As you will see, not all auditory disorders have associated hearing losses, and many types of hearing losses are not outwardly visible. Where appropriate, the disorders covered in this chapter are accompanied by a figure that highlights results from a variety audiologic tests that you learned about in earlier chapters, as well as a summary of underlying causes, symptoms, complaints, and treatments. Familiarity with auditory disorders/pathologies is useful for proper slection and interpretation of audiological tests, making decisions about follow-up management and for making appropriate referrals to medical practitioners.

DESCRIBING AUDITORY DISORDERS

Before getting into the specific disorders, some associated concepts and terminology will be addressed. One important component in describing auditory disorders is to define which part (or parts) of the ear is (are) affected, called *differential diagnosis*. One of the most important parts of an audiological assessment is getting some pre-assessment information about the patient, called a *case history*. From the case history, you can learn important information about the patient's primary complaints and symptoms, as well as answers to some directed questions about the extent of any hearing and communication problems, when the problem began, whether it has worsened, came on suddenly or gradually, is associated with dizziness and/or tinnitus (ringing in the ears). Additional information you may explore in the case history might include how family members perceive the patient's problem, any associated circumstances or activities that brought on the conditions, medications taken, family history, previous hearing tests and/or surgeries, and the use of hearing aids. Based on the patient's answers to these questions and/or information from other sources, additional questions may be appropriate.

Audiologic test results are also important to help differentially diagnose auditory pathologies by determining if there is any hearing loss and, if so, determine whether it is conductive, mixed, sensorineural, unilateral, or bilateral. Information from speech tests, immittance tests, otoacoustic emissions, and/or auditory evoked potentials may also be useful in reaching a proper diagnosis and course of treatment. For example, audiologic test results may help localize the disorder to a possible perforation of the tympanic membrane or suggest that there may be pathology of the 8th cranial nerve. It is important to keep in mind that a medical diagnosis can only be determined by a physician, who conducts a thorough medical examination and may order lab work, imaging studies, or other diagnostic tests. All medically related auditory disorders must be referred by hearing health care professionals to a physician for evaluation and ongoing care. In cases where an adult has a sensorineural hearing loss, with no apparent medical or neural involvement, the audiologist may provide appropriate services without the need for medical evaluation; however, any hearing loss in a child should be referred to a physician for evaluation, and if hearing aids are warranted, medical approval from the physician must be obtained or a waiver signed by the patient; however, keep in mind that these requirements may change with the addition of over-the-counter hearing aids.

There are many other terms that provide information about auditory disorders. A *genetic hearing loss* (also called hereditary hearing loss or familial hearing loss) is due to differences in the genes that are passed on through a hereditary source. The recent Human Genome Project (https://www.genome.gov/10001772/all-about-the-human-genome-project-hgp), which is attempting to identify and map all the genes in human DNA, has led to an abundance of new knowledge regarding genes that are associated with hearing loss and deafness. Hearing loss may be the only consequence of a genetic condition, such as that caused by a genetic protein mutation known as *connexin-26*, which is the most common genetic cause of hearing loss, and which may be expressed at birth or at a later prelinguistic stage (Nance & Dodson, 2007). Although most genetic hearing losses are not related to other syndromes, some genetic hearing losses are associated with known genetic and/or hereditary syndromes, including those that affect the outer and/or middle ear, such as Treacher Collins, DeGeorge, Goldenhar, Paget, and Apert; those that affect the cochlea, such as Usher, Jervell and Lange-Nielsen, Herrmann, Alport, Klippel–Feil, and Waardenburg; and those that can affect either or both the conductive and sensorineural portions, such as Down, CHARGE association, Crouzon, Hunter, and Möbius. According to Nance and Dodson (2007), there have been more than 150 genes identified that are associated with hearing loss. Genetic hearing losses do not always have a hereditary link, and can occur spontaneously during development. Some genetic hearing disorders do not manifest any problems until after birth, referred to as *early-onset genetic hearing loss* (during infant–toddler stage) or *late-onset genetic hearing loss* (during childhood or adult stages). A *congenital hearing loss* is one that is present at birth, resulting from *prenatal* (prior to birth) or *perinatal* (during birth) factors. A congenital hearing loss can be due to genetic factors or other pathologic causes. A list of factors known to have a high association with congenital or developmental hearing losses is known as the *high-risk register* (Joint Committee on Infant Hearing, 2007). The interested reader is referred to other textbooks (Shprintzen, 2001; Toriello & Smith, 2013) for additional information on genetic and other congenital hearing disorders.

A hearing loss that is not of genetic or congenital origin is called an *acquired hearing loss*, which is a hearing loss that occurs after birth and is usually caused by disease, trauma, drugs, or aging. Hearing losses can also be described in terms of their time course: An *acute disorder* is one that is in its initial phase and lasts a relatively short duration; a *chronic disorder* is a condition that is persistent over a relatively long period of time; an *intermittent disorder* is a condition that comes and goes or reoccurs often. Other terms or conditions that are associated with auditory disorders include *otorrhea*, which refers to fluid (usually infected) that is draining into the external auditory canal from the middle ear, *aural fullness*, which is a sense of pressure in the ear reported by patients and can be a sign of fluid in the middle ear or some types of sensorineural hearing loss, and *otalgia*, which means pain in the ear and often comes from different cranial nerves innervating the ear, face, teeth, temporomandibular joint, or throat (Jordan & Roland, 2000). In many cases, the cause of a hearing loss is of unknown cause, called *idiopathic*, especially when referring to a *sudden hearing loss*.

OUTER EAR DISORDERS

Disorders of the outer ear can occur in the auricle or external ear canal. Outer ear disorders are usually visible with the eye and/or with an otoscope. Outer ear disorders require medical evaluation, and in most cases, can be medically or surgically treated. Outer ear disorders can result from embryological developmental abnormalities causing anatomical defects, or can be acquired due to infections, cancer, trauma, tumors, or obstructions. Many outer ear disorders do not have any associated hearing loss related to the outer ear condition, but some outer ear abnormalities may suggest a hearing loss in other parts of the auditory system, especially those related to congenital disorders.

Disorders of the Auricle

Auricular (pertaining to the auricle) pathologies generally do not have any associated hearing loss. Congenital auricular abnormalities result from alterations of the embryologic developmental events at various stages or cell location. These events may lead to structural variations of the auricle that range from slight variations in the size, location, angle, or differences between the two ears, or to complete absence of one or both auricles, called *anotia*. An abnormally small and malformed auricle is called *microtia*. Even bilateral anotia and/or microtia do not result in any appreciable hearing loss or communication problems. In cases of anotia or microtia, it is important to determine if there are other abnormalities, especially of the outer ear canal or middle ear (Roland & Rohn, 1997). Other auricular developmental anomalies include a small dimple just anterior to the tragus, called *preauricular pit* or *sinus*, or a small skin growth, called *preauricular appendage* or *tag*. Treatments for congenital auricular abnormalities are usually done in later childhood for cosmetic reasons and involve surgical corrections or attachment of a realistic looking plastic ear. Surgical decisions must take into account problems in other parts of the auditory system, whether the problem is unilateral or bilateral, and an assessment of hearing abilities.

Acquired auricular disorders are usually due to some form of trauma that results in cosmetic damage. Sources of trauma include physical blows to the auricle, frostbite, burns, penetrating object, bites, abrasions, or pulling on an earring. Trauma due to blunt forces can produce *auricular hematoma*, which is internal bleeding within the auricle that may lead to damage to the cartilage (Kinney, Kinney, & Vidimos, 1997). In most cases, the acute damage to the auricle heals itself, but the cartilage may remain misshapen. Patients may elect to have cosmetic surgery to repair the damage or appearance. Acquired auricular disorders may also occur from disease, infections, or cancer. Infections may be bacterial, such as impetigo due to staphylococcus infection. Infections may also be viral, such as herpes zoster (Ramsay Hunt syndrome) or herpes simplex, and can cause severe pain, vesicles, and facial nerve problems. Antibiotics may be prescribed to treat infections that occur in auricular disorders. Neoplasms, which are abnormal tissue growth or tumors, can also invade the auricle. Some neoplasms are benign cysts; however, others may be cancerous, including squamous cell carcinoma, basal cell carcinoma, or melanoma, for which surgical treatment is typically required.

Disorders of the External Ear Canal

Disorders of the external canal may or may not have any associated hearing loss, depending on the extent and type of disorder. Congenital embryological abnormalities of the external ear canal can occur in isolation or with some concomitant auricular involvement, and/or involvement in other parts of the auditory system, including the middle ear or the cochlea.

Atresia (atretic ear) is the absence of an external auditory canal due to embryologic events, and may be unilateral or bilateral. The absence of the ear canal may be due to failure of the canal to form an opening in the temporal bone, or it may be due to the canal being filled with tissue. Atresia will cause a maximum conductive hearing loss of around 50 to 60 dB HL, due to the blockage of sound through the outer ear to the middle ear. If the atresia is bilateral, there most likely will be a masking dilemma (see Chapter 9) that makes it difficult to determine the extent of hearing loss in each ear or whether there is any sensorineural hearing loss in one of the ears. Figure 12–1 summarizes the background and audiologic profile for a young child with unilateral atresia. Unilateral atresia is usually not surgically corrected; the patient may do quite well as a unilateral listener. Treatment for bilateral atresia is often surgery in one of the ears, but this decision is dependent on the type and degree of hearing loss in each ear. An audiologic treatment option is to fit the patient with a bone–anchored implant (BAI) (see Chapter 15).

Impacted cerumen (ear wax) is an acquired disorder of the external auditory canal that occurs when there is an over-accumulation of cerumen that becomes impacted somewhere along the length of the canal. A normal amount of cerumen has important functions and has a natural migration out of the ear canal; however, it can occasionally become trapped, especially with the use of cotton-tipped cleaning swabs that tend to push the cerumen deeper into the ear

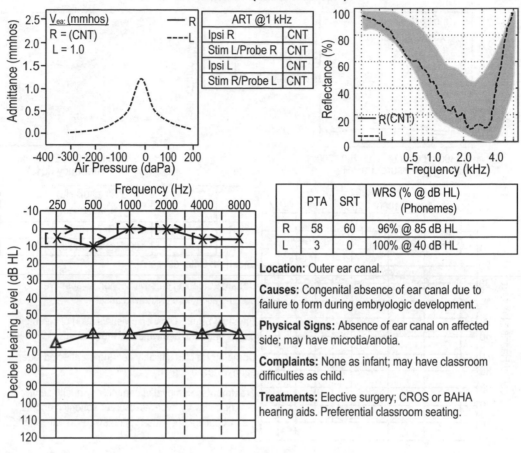

ATRESIA (UNILATERAL)

ART @1 kHz	
Ipsi R	CNT
Stim L/Probe R	CNT
Ipsi L	CNT
Stim R/Probe L	CNT

	PTA	SRT	WRS (% @ dB HL) (Phonemes)
R	58	60	96% @ 85 dB HL
L	3	0	100% @ 40 dB HL

Location: Outer ear canal.

Causes: Congenital absence of ear canal due to failure to form during embryologic development.

Physical Signs: Absence of ear canal on affected side; may have microtia/anotia.

Complaints: None as infant; may have classroom difficulties as child.

Treatments: Elective surgery; CROS or BAHA hearing aids. Preferential classroom seating.

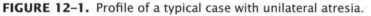

FIGURE 12–1. Profile of a typical case with unilateral atresia.

canal where it is more difficult to migrate out of the ear. Over time, this trapped cerumen can completely block off part of the ear canal and cause a mild conductive hearing loss. The hearing will return to normal following removal of the cerumen. Impacted cerumen is usually unilateral, but can occur in both ears if the patient continues the action that causes the cerumen accumulation and delays seeking medical treatment. Figure 12–2 summarizes the features and audiological profile for a case with unilateral impacted cerumen. Medical treatment for cerumen impaction is to have the cerumen removed by a trained health care provider (including audiologists) who use special instruments to remove it: curettes to physically pull it out, suction tube

to suction it out or by lavage/irrigation of the ear canal with a forced flow of water. Over-the-counter cerumen-softening agents are also available and may be an effective treatment in mild cases. An accumulation of cerumen that comes in contact with the tympanic membrane, even without being impacted, can affect the movement of the tympanic membrane due to a greater mass, and may produce a mild conductive hearing loss in the higher frequencies only.

Foreign objects can find their way into the ear canal, especially with young children. Some examples of foreign objects that find their way into the ear include cotton swabs, sand, insects, earrings, clay, food, beads, pen caps, small batteries, and pieces of glass. Hearing loss from foreign objects

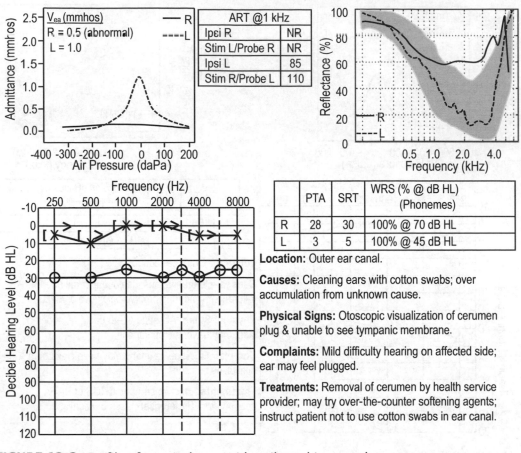

IMPACTED CERUMEN (UNILATERAL)

ART @1 kHz	
Ipsi R	NR
Stim L/Probe R	NR
Ipsi L	85
Stim R/Probe L	110

Vₑₐ (mmhos)
R = 0.5 (abnormal)
L = 1.0

	PTA	SRT	WRS (% @ dB HL) (Phonemes)
R	28	30	100% @ 70 dB HL
L	3	5	100% @ 45 dB HL

Location: Outer ear canal.

Causes: Cleaning ears with cotton swabs; over accumulation from unknown cause.

Physical Signs: Otoscopic visualization of cerumen plug & unable to see tympanic membrane.

Complaints: Mild difficulty hearing on affected side; ear may feel plugged.

Treatments: Removal of cerumen by health service provider; may try over-the-counter softening agents; instruct patient not to use cotton swabs in ear canal.

FIGURE 12–2. Profile of a typical case with unilateral impacted cerumen.

depends on if the object blocks off a part of the ear canal, in which case there may be a mild conductive hearing loss (similar to cerumen impaction). Objects in the ear canal may be uncomfortable, painful, or can cause lacerations, abrasions, cerumen impaction, or infections. Treatment for foreign objects is to have the object removed by a trained medical health care provider.

Stenosis (stenotic ear) is an abnormal narrowing of the external auditory canal, usually due to developmental anomalies. According to Roland and Rohn (1997), if an ear canal is less than 4 mm in diameter it should be considered a stenotic ear. Stenosis does not result in any conductive hearing loss, if there is some amount of opening that can allow sounds to strike the tympanic membrane; however, the patient may be more prone to ear infections or to hearing loss from impacted cerumen or foreign objects because of the narrower opening.

Exostosis (*exostoses*), often referred to as surfer's ear, is a condition of bony outgrowths, covered with skin, that occur in the external ear canal. These bony outgrowths result from irritation of the ear canal due to repeated and prolonged exposure to cold water, typical of surfers; however, the precise cause of these benign bony growths is not known. Exostosis is characterized by multiple bumps and is usually bilateral. Exostosis is painless and generally non-problematic, unless the bumps create enough of a narrowing of the ear canal to cause cerumen impaction

SYNOPSIS 12–1

- Audiologic results can help in the differential diagnosis of ear disorders by documenting any hearing loss and determining if it is related to the conductive or sensorineural parts of the auditory system.
- Audiologists must recognize medically related hearing disorders and make appropriate referrals for medical evaluation and treatment decisions.
- Hearing loss at birth is referred to as a congenital hearing loss. These may be due to hereditary links, genetic mutations during development, or infections or trauma during the prenatal and perinatal periods. Acquired hearing disorders are those that occur later in life from noncongenital factors.
- Hereditary (genetic) hearing losses can manifest as congenital hearing losses or can develop as early- or late-onset hearing losses that can occur during childhood or even in the adult years.
- Hearing disorders can be described relative to their time of onset and/or duration; acute = initial phase; chronic = persisting over a period of time; intermittent = resolves and reoccurs.
- Some common terms associated with ear disorders include otorrhea (ear drainage), otalgia (ear pain), aural fullness (pressure feeling in ear), and idiopathic (of unknown cause).
- Outer ear disorders are usually visible with the eye or otoscope, and many do not have any associated hearing loss.

or trap debris and moisture that lead to infections, or impinge on the tympanic membrane. In problem cases, the exostoses can be surgically removed, but will likely reoccur with continued exposure to cold water. Hearing loss does not occur from exostosis unless it leads to a secondary problem.

Osteoma is a rounded bony growth, typically pearl shaped, that can also occur in the ear canal. An osteoma is a benign tumor that occurs spontaneously and usually does not cause any problems; therefore, surgical treatment is generally not required. An osteoma may be confused with exostosis; however, an osteoma is usually a single bump and occurs unilaterally. Hearing loss does not occur from osteoma, unless it leads to a secondary problem.

Otitis externa is an infection of the tissues lining the external ear canal. These infections are usually caused by bacteria or fungus; however, the herpes zoster virus (Ramsay Hunt syndrome) can also produce lesions in the external ear canal. Otitis externa is sometimes called swimmer's ear when it is caused by bacterial infections from improperly maintained swimming pools. The most common bacteria causing otitis externa is pseudomonas, which is quite common in the environment. Pseudomonas is usually prevented from multiplying because of the acidity of cerumen; however, when the cerumen is washed out by swimming, the protection is gone and there is an increased risk of developing otitis externa, especially problematic in the summer months when swimming is popular (Jordan & Roland, 2000). Otitis externa is often painful and may be accompanied by swelling and/or a fluid discharge. Treatment for otitis externa is with topical or oral antibiotics, depending on the severity. Wearing earplugs when swimming may also help prevent otitis externa.

Table 12–1 summarizes the disorders of the outer ear covered in this chapter.

TABLE 12–1. Summary of Outer Ear Disorders

Disorder	Description	Type of Hearing Problem
Anotia/microtia	Absent or misshapen auricle; congenital pathology, genetic origin	None, unless accompanied by atresia
Atresia	Absence of external ear canal	Maximum (50 to 60 dB HL) conductive loss
Exostosis (Surfer's ear)	Mounds of bony growth in ear canal; acquired from repeated exposure to cold water	No hearing loss; may lead to secondary problems (impacted cerumen, infections)
Foreign object	Variety of objects that find their way into the ear	No hearing loss unless completely blocks off canal or causes blockage of cerumen; may be painful or lead to infection; needs to be removed by physician
Hematoma	Bleeding under skin of auricle; acquired pathology from trauma	No hearing loss; needs medical attention
Impacted cerumen	Accumulation of cerumen that blocks off ear canal; often from cleaning ears with cotton swabs	Mild conductive hearing loss
Osteoma	Benign pearl-shaped bony tumor in ear canal; spontaneous origin	No hearing loss; usually does not cause any medical problem
Otitis externa (Swimmer's ear)	Bacterial, fungal, or viral (Herpes zoster) infections of the ear canal	No hearing loss; can be painful; needs medical attention
Pits or tags	Indentations or skin tags anterior to auricle; congenital pathology, genetic origin	None, unless genetic disorder affects other parts of the ear
Stenosis	Small diameter ear canal; usually congenital disorder; genetic origin	No hearing loss; may lead to secondary problems (impacted cerumen, infections)

MIDDLE EAR DISORDERS

Disorders of the middle ear commonly cause conductive hearing loss due to changes in the tympanic membrane, ossicular chain, growths, or fluid accumulation resulting from poor eustachian tube dysfunction. Some middle ear disorders can be observed with an otoscope, including those of the tympanic membrane, as well as some that are visible through the semi-transparent tympanic membrane. Most middle ear disorders require medical evaluation, and in most cases, can be medically or surgically treated.

Otitis Media

Otitis media is an accumulation of fluid, called *effusion*, which occurs in the middle ear. When the fluid in the middle ear is clear and non-infected, it is called *serous otitis media*. When the fluid becomes thickened or puss-like (with or without active bacteria), it is called *mucoid otitis media*, purulent otitis media, or glue ear. While the fluid in the middle ear is infected, it is called *acute otitis media*. If fluid remains in the middle ear for an extended period of time, it is called *chronic otitis media*. Otitis media is a common cause of conductive hearing loss, especially in young children. It can be unilateral or bilateral. The degree of conductive hearing loss from otitis media can range from mild to moderate depending on the amount and consistency of the fluid in the ear.

Otitis media can occur in all ages; however, young children have the highest prevalence of otitis media due to the anatomical and functional differences in the eustachian tube (see Chapter 4). The general sequence underlying the occurrence of otitis media begins with *eustachian tube dysfunction*, in which the eustachian tube is unable to equalize the air pressure in the middle ear, creating a negative pressure in the middle ear as the remaining air becomes absorbed by the tissues of the middle ear. Eustachian tube dysfunction can be related to developmental differences or may be due to swelling of the nasopharynx that can occur with an upper respiratory infection, allergy, or enlarged adenoids.

Negative middle ear pressure may also result from a relatively sudden change in external air pressure, called *barotrauma*, as can occur during an airline flight or underwater diving. Prolonged negative middle ear pressure, in some cases, can lead to effusion from the mucous lining of the middle ear, leading to serous otitis media. If the fluid becomes invaded with bacteria, which may occur when the person with an upper respiratory infection coughs or sneezes, the condition advances to acute otitis media. The acute otitis media stage can be painful and accompanied by fever or pulling at the ears.

For acute otitis media, the treatment options include simply allowing the ear to resolve the condition on its own over a few weeks, and/or prescribing oral antibiotics. Persistent cases generally require antibiotic treatment and possibly removal of the fluid with a needle-type syringe, a procedure called *myringotomy*, which is performed by a physician. For patients with chronic or reoccurring otitis media, a physician may recommend the placement of a *pressure equalization* (PE) *tube*. A PE tube is a small grommet-like tube inserted into the tympanic membrane to allow the fluid to drain, and provides a mechanism to equalize air pressure in the middle ear. The PE tube remains in place for a few months and can be effective in reducing the chance of reoccurring ear infections. In most cases, as the tympanic membrane regrows over the incision, the PE tube is pushed out and the tympanic membrane is healed. Treatment decisions for otitis media are also guided by the extent and duration of hearing loss, as well as whether the age of the patient is an important learning period. In most cases, the conductive hearing loss will be resolved. It is important to realize that it is the fluid in the middle ear that causes the conductive hearing loss because it alters the transmission of vibrations across the ossicular chain. Antibiotics only kill the bacteria but do nothing about the fluid in the middle ear. A patient who does not have an active ear infection or who is being treated for an ear infection may continue to have the conductive hearing loss when fluid is present in the middle ear. Figure 12–3 summarizes the features and audiologic profile for a case with bilateral otitis media.

Tympanic Membrane Perforation

A *perforation* is a hole that occurs in the tympanic membrane. Perforations can occur from trauma, such as a slap to the ear, explosion, or a patient-induced puncture from a cotton-tipped applicator, paper clip, or hairpin. Your parents were right when they told you not to put anything smaller than your elbow in your ears! It is not uncommon for someone to be cleaning his or her ears with a cotton swab and another person bumps his or her arm when opening the medicine cabinet door. Trauma-induced perforations can be of different sizes and locations on the tympanic membrane. Tympanograms will be flat (Type B) with a large V_{ea}. With a relatively large perforation, there may be a mild conductive hearing loss; however, a smaller perforation may not result in any appreciable hearing loss.

A perforation can also occur from otitis media. In this case, there is considerable fluid buildup in the middle ear that erodes the tympanic membrane from the inside until it ruptures to relieve the fluid pressure. Most tympanic membrane perforations spontaneously heal themselves but may cause scar tissue or create an area in the tympanic membrane without the fibrous tissue layer, called a *monomere* (or monomeric tympanic membrane). The healed tympanic membrane does not usually have any associated hearing loss. The presence of a *patent* (open) PE tube in the tympanic membrane acts like a very small perforation, and usually does not cause any conductive hearing loss. Figure 12–4 summarizes the features and audiologic profile for a case with a mild unilateral perforation.

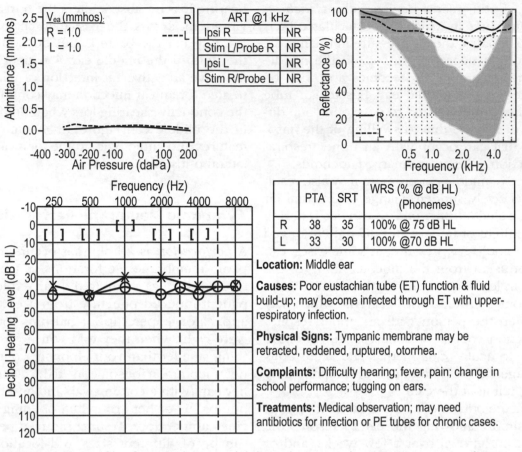

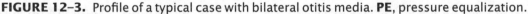

FIGURE 12–3. Profile of a typical case with bilateral otitis media. **PE,** pressure equalization.

Cholesteatoma

A *cholesteatoma* is a benign mass (pseudotumor) that develops in the middle ear space. It usually arises secondary to a perforation or otitis media. The mass consists of dead skin tissue and keratin that are normally sloughed off from healthy skin tissue but become trapped in a surrounding area of healthy skin. The tissue mass continually expands as more skin cells are sloughed off. This keratinizing, moist mass of tissue may lead to a foul-smelling otorrhea. The cellular makeup, growth pattern, and enzymes can destroy the middle ear structures and the bony shelf between the middle ear and the brain to invade the mastoid; therefore, this disorder is considered a medical condition that requires immediate attention and surgical removal. The most common origin

of an acquired cholesteatoma is from a *retraction pocket* in the pars flaccida region of the tympanic membrane, whereby the negative middle ear pressure pulls the pars flaccida partially into the middle ear space. The retraction pocket is lined with healthy skin cells that continually slough off and are trapped in the retraction pocket. A cholesteatoma may also occur from the tympanic membrane tissue around a perforation or PE tube as the tissue is healing itself but migrates into the middle ear (Myerhoff, Marple, & Roland, 1997). Cholesteatomas are usually unilateral. The hearing loss associated with a cholesteatoma can vary. In the early stages, there may not be any symptoms or hearing loss; however, as the mass enlarges, and depending on the direction of growth, it may erode the ossicles or affect their vibration. The cholesteatoma may also cause a perforation in

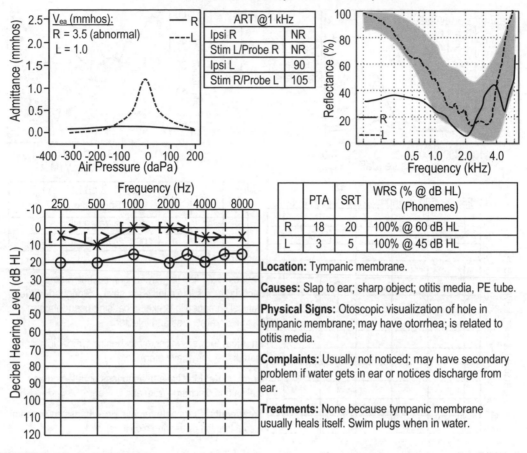

PERFORATION (UNILATERAL)

V$_{ea}$ (mmhos):	— R
R = 3.5 (abnormal)	---- L
L = 1.0	

ART @1 kHz	
Ipsi R	NR
Stim L/Probe R	NR
Ipsi L	90
Stim R/Probe L	105

	PTA	SRT	WRS (% @ dB HL) (Phonemes)
R	18	20	100% @ 60 dB HL
L	3	5	100% @ 45 dB HL

Location: Tympanic membrane.

Causes: Slap to ear; sharp object; otitis media, PE tube.

Physical Signs: Otoscopic visualization of hole in tympanic membrane; may have otorrhea; is related to otitis media.

Complaints: Usually not noticed; may have secondary problem if water gets in ear or notices discharge from ear.

Treatments: None because tympanic membrane usually heals itself. Swim plugs when in water.

FIGURE 12–4. Profile of a typical case with unilateral tympanic membrane perforation. **PE,** pressure equalization.

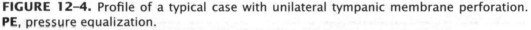

the tympanic membrane resulting in otorrhea, and in some cases the cholesteatoma may invade the round window and cause a sensorineural hearing loss or mixed hearing loss. Following surgery, the conductive or mixed hearing loss may persist depending on the damage caused by the cholesteatoma. Figure 12–5 summarizes the features and audiological profile for a case with unilateral cholesteatoma.

Otosclerosis

Otosclerosis is a disorder that is caused by an outgrowth of the bony wall of the inner ear, usually around the stapes footplate. The otosclerosis begins as a spongy bony growth (otospongiosis) that eventually becomes hardened or sclerotic. Otosclerosis is more prevalent in females and begins to show up between the ages of 20 and 40 years (House, 1997). The cause of otosclerosis is not completely understood; however, a popular theory is that in many cases it appears to be due to a late-onset genetic disorder. This embryologic origin may be related to the incomplete developmental process of bone formation around the oval window, which is the last area that bone formation occurs (Myerhoff et al., 1997). In young adulthood, the otosclerosis begins to reveal itself, often exacerbated by hormonal changes, especially in women. When the bony growth encapsulates the footplate of the stapes (*stapes fixation*) and causes a conductive

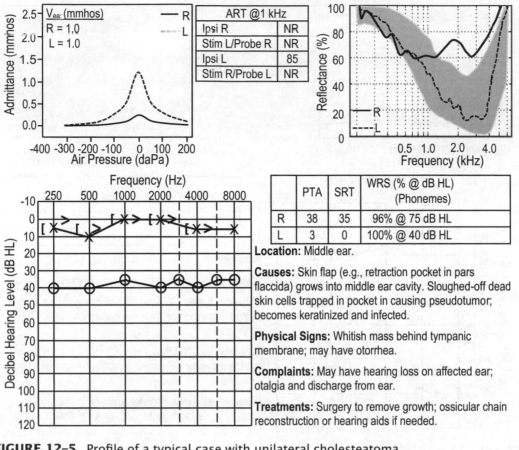

CHOLESTEATOMA (UNILATERAL)

ART @1 kHz	
Ipsi R	NR
Stim L/Probe R	NR
Ipsi L	85
Stim R/Probe L	NR

	PTA	SRT	WRS (% @ dB HL) (Phonemes)
R	38	35	96% @ 75 dB HL
L	3	0	100% @ 40 dB HL

Location: Middle ear.

Causes: Skin flap (e.g., retraction pocket in pars flaccida) grows into middle ear cavity. Sloughed-off dead skin cells trapped in pocket in causing pseudotumor; becomes keratinized and infected.

Physical Signs: Whitish mass behind tympanic membrane; may have otorrhea.

Complaints: May have hearing loss on affected ear; otalgia and discharge from ear.

Treatments: Surgery to remove growth; ossicular chain reconstruction or hearing aids if needed.

FIGURE 12–5. Profile of a typical case with unilateral cholesteatoma.

hearing loss, the otosclerosis becomes a clinical disorder.

Otosclerosis often shows up as a conductive hearing loss in one ear, but typically progresses to a bilateral conductive loss. There may be some asymmetry between the ears as well, but the conductive loss typically progresses from a mild to moderately severe degree in the low to mid frequencies. The audiometric pattern also shows a slight dip in the bone conduction threshold around 2000 Hz, known as *Carhart's notch*. This notch in the bone conduction threshold is not a reflection of any sensorineural loss but instead results from a loss of the normal middle ear resonance due to the fixation of the ossicular chain. The bone conduction threshold at 2000 Hz usually improves following surgical treatment of the otosclerosis. Immittance results often show

a characteristic pattern for otosclerosis; typically a normal-shaped tympanogram (Type A) or reduced admittance (Type A_s); however, acoustic reflex testing shows no responses. Reflectance measures show an increased reflectance (lower absorbance) due to the stiffening effects on the tympanic membrane.

Surgery is one treatment option for otosclerosis, which usually involves replacing part of the stapes with a prosthetic device that connects the incus to the oval window, called *stapedectomy*, or connecting the prosthesis through a hole drilled in the stapes footplate, called a *stapedotomy*. There are a variety of prostheses, including wires or pistons made from metal or synthetic material. Surgery for otosclerosis is quite successful in eliminating or significantly reducing the conductive hearing loss. However, pa-

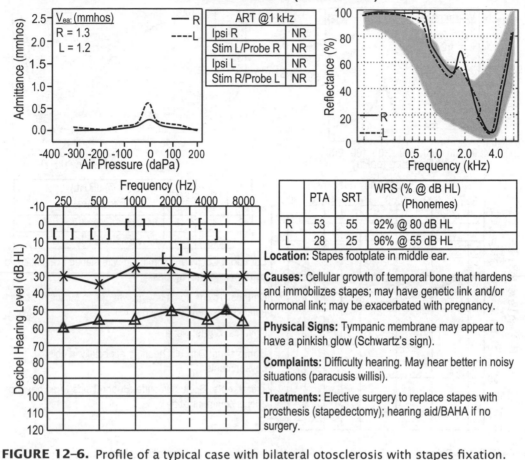

FIGURE 12–6. Profile of a typical case with bilateral otosclerosis with stapes fixation.

tients may also decide to be fit with a hearing aid or do nothing at all. Figure 12–6 summarizes the features and audiometric profile for a case with bilateral, *asymmetric* middle ear otosclerosis.

Otosclerosis can also invade the inner ear, which is called *cochlear otosclerosis*. In cochlear otosclerosis, the otospongiosis of the temporal bone around the oval window invades the inner ear and either produces toxins or alteration of the blood supply that destroys the hair cells (Myerhoff et al., 1997). Cochlear otosclerosis produces a slow, progressive, sensorineural hearing loss, usually stabilizing with a moderate degree of hearing loss in the middle frequency range (saucer/cookie bite configuration). Cochlear otosclerosis can be unilateral or bilateral. Treatment for cochlear otosclerosis may include sodium fluoride to slow or stabilize the process (Shambaugh,

1983) and/or hearing aids as needed for the sensorineural hearing loss. Figure 12–7 summarizes the features and audiometric profile for a case with bilateral, asymmetric cochlear otosclerosis.

Ossicular Disarticulation

Ossicular disarticulation (or ossicular discontinuity) refers to a separation of the ossicular chain or a break in one of the ossicles, typically a dislocation of the long process of the incus from the stapes (Jordan & Roland, 2000). A disarticulation may occur because of damage from a variety of causes, including a slap on the side of the head, head injury, waterskiing accident, or necrosis (cell destruction) from otitis media or cholesteatoma. Ossicular disarticulations are usually

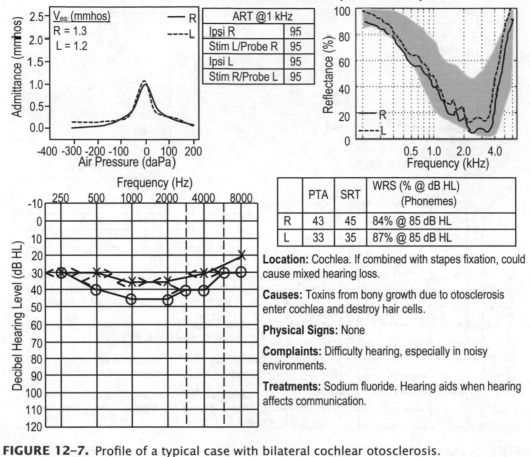

FIGURE 12–7. Profile of a typical case with bilateral cochlear otosclerosis.

unilateral and result in a moderate to moderately severe conductive hearing loss. The immittance results show a characteristic normal-shaped tympanogram with a high admittance (Type A$_d$) and acoustic reflexes are absent. The disarticulation reduces the stiffness of the ossicular chain and makes the ear more mass dominant. Reflectance measures shows a deep notch below 1000 Hz, a slight increase in the mid-frequencies, and within the normal range in the high frequencies (Feeney et al., 2003). Reflectance patterns are useful in differentiating disarticulation from otosclerosis, both of which have similar audiograms. Disarticulations may be repaired or replaced with a prosthetic device, in a surgical procedure called *ossiculoplasty*. Surgery for disarticulation may not completely eliminate the conductive hearing loss in many cases (Jordan & Roland, 2000).

Figure 12–8 summarizes the features and audiometric profile for a case with unilateral ossicular disarticulation.

Glomus Tumors

A *glomus tumor* is a benign, slow-growing tumor of the middle ear. It is a highly vascularized (composed of blood vessels) tumor stemming from glomus cells arising from neural tissues (paraganglia cells) in the middle ear. Glomus tumors arise from the jugular bulb that runs along the floor of the middle ear (called *glomus jugulare*) or other nerves running in the middle ear along the promontory (called *glomus tympanicum*). A

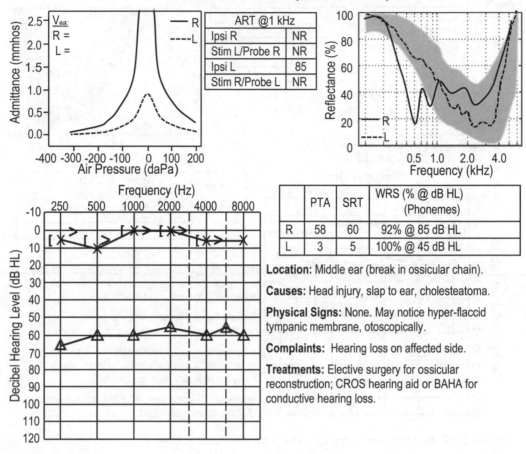

FIGURE 12–8. Profile of a typical case with unilateral ossicular disarticulation.

glomus tumor is usually visible with an otoscope and appears as a reddish-purple mass due to its vascularity. Glomus tumors occur more often in older female adults and may arise spontaneously or have a hereditary link (Lustig & Jackler, 1997). The effects of a glomus tumor depend on its size and location but may include aural fullness, a pulsing sound related to the blood flow, and a unilateral conductive hearing loss in about half of the patients (Woods, Strasnick, & Jackson, 1993). Immittance results typically show a normal tympanogram (Type A) and the acoustic reflex pattern depends on the extent of the conductive hearing loss. Treatment for a glomus tumor is surgery to completely remove the mass. Figure 12–9 summarizes the features and a possible audiometric profile for a case with a unilat-

eral glomus tumor affecting the movement of the ossicular chain.

ACQUIRED COCHLEAR DISORDERS

Acquired disorders of the cochlear portion of the inner ear usually show sensorineural hearing losses of varying degrees from a variety of causes. The disorders described here do not include congenital/hereditary sensorineural hearing loss. An acquired sensorineural hearing loss may occur during different stages of life and involve damage to hair cells from noise, aging, drugs, infections, autoimmune disease, or head trauma. Cochlear damage may occur also from an imbalance of the inner ear fluids or rupture of the oval or round

GLOMUS TUMOR (UNILATERAL)

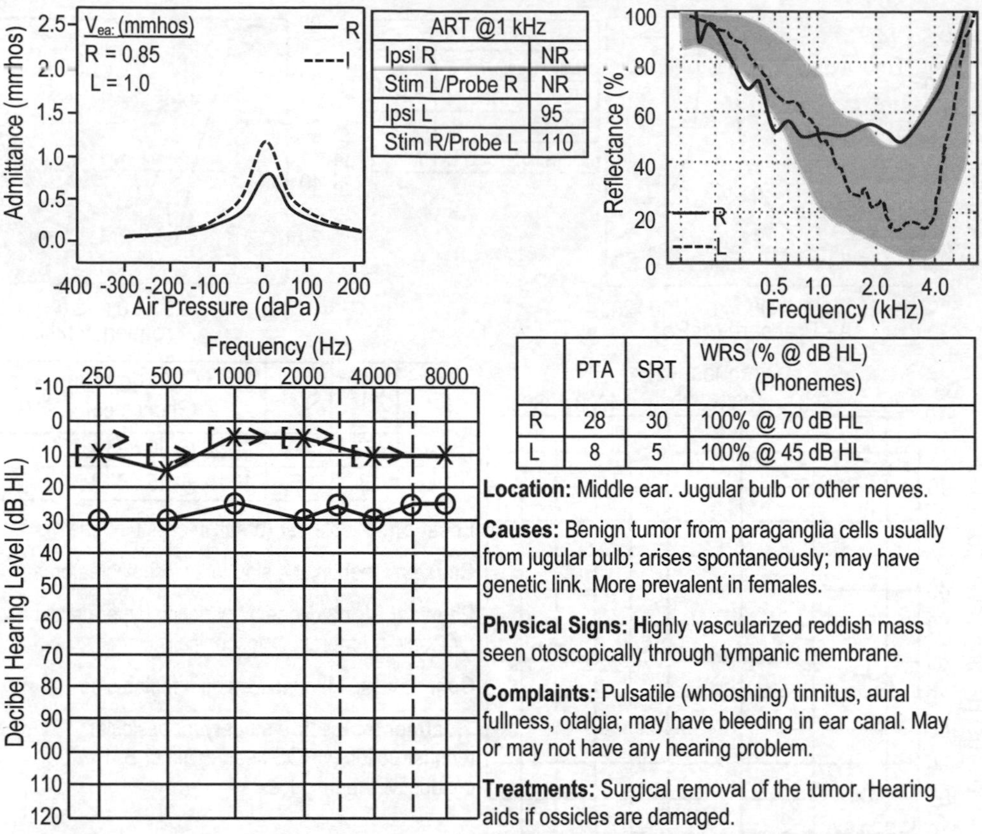

ART @1 kHz	
Ipsi R	NR
Stim L/Probe R	NR
Ipsi L	95
Stim R/Probe L	110

	PTA	SRT	WRS (% @ dB HL) (Phonemes)
R	28	30	100% @ 70 dB HL
L	8	5	100% @ 45 dB HL

Location: Middle ear. Jugular bulb or other nerves.

Causes: Benign tumor from paraganglia cells usually from jugular bulb; arises spontaneously; may have genetic link. More prevalent in females.

Physical Signs: Highly vascularized reddish mass seen otoscopically through tympanic membrane.

Complaints: Pulsatile (whooshing) tinnitus, aural fullness, otalgia; may have bleeding in ear canal. May or may not have any hearing problem.

Treatments: Surgical removal of the tumor. Hearing aids if ossicles are damaged.

FIGURE 12–9. Profile of a typical case with a unilateral glomus tumor.

SYNOPSIS 12–2

- Hearing disorders of the middle ear typically result in a conductive hearing loss. Most middle ear pathologies occur unilaterally; however, some (e.g., otitis media and otosclerosis) occur in or progress to both ears.
- Otitis media, an accumulation of fluid in the middle ear, is the most common cause of middle ear disorders. Otitis media begins with poor eustachian tube function leading to accumulation of fluid (effusion). If bacteria invade the middle ear, an acute infection may occur. Antibiotics treat the infection but do not eliminate the fluid. Otitis media often resolves on its own, but may require myringotomy or pressure equalization tubes.
- Trauma-induced middle ear disorders include tympanic membrane perforations and ossicular chain disarticulations. Tympanic membrane perforations usually heal spontaneously. Disarticulations can be managed with prosthetic reconstruction, called ossiculoplasty.
- Otosclerosis originates from a bony growth of the temporal bone around the oval window that may begin between 20 and 40 years of age. The bony growth

SYNOPSIS 12–2 (*continued*)

may fixate the stapes leading to a conductive hearing loss, or may invade the cochlea where its toxins may damage the hair cells leading to a sensorineural hearing loss. The cause of otosclerosis is not known, but is thought to have a hereditary link (late onset). Surgical replacement of the stapes with a prosthesis is called stapedectomy.

- Tumors can also arise in the middle ear; the most common are cholesteatoma (pseudotumor) and glomus tumors.
- Table 12–2 summarizes disorders of the middle ear covered in this chapter.

TABLE 12–2. Summary of Middle Ear Disorders

Disorder	Description	Type of Hearing Problem
Otitis media	Inflammation of the middle ear, usually accompanied by fluid (effusion); acquired from poor eustachian tube function; common in children	Conductive hearing loss due to the fluid; hearing loss improves when otitis media is resolved, spontaneously or with surgery (PE tubes); antibiotics may be prescribed if accompanied by bacterial infection
Perforation	Puncture or rupture of the tympanic membrane; can vary in size; PE tube may act like a small perforation	Normal hearing to mild conductive hearing loss; membrane usually heals itself
Cholesteatoma	Skin flap growing in the middle ear, usually from retraction pocket; sloughed-off skin builds up and becomes infected; continues to grow in middle ear and may rupture tympanic membrane producing smelly discharge	Hearing loss depends on where cholesteatoma grows and structures that it damages; usually erodes the ossicles and results in moderate conductive loss; needs medical referral for surgery
Otosclerosis	Spongy growth of temporal bone around oval window; can encapsulate stapes or invade cochlear (cochlear otosclerosis); begins in second to fourth decade; some hereditary link	Usually fixates stapes and causes moderate conductive hearing loss in affected ear; usually unilateral, but may progress to bilateral; cochlear otosclerosis causes sensorineural loss due to toxin damaging hair cells; stapedectomy to replace stapes with prosthesis
Disarticulation	Trauma-induced break in the ossicular chain or fracture in one of the ossicles	Moderate to moderately severe conductive hearing loss; elective surgical reconstruction (ossiculoplasty)
Glomus tumors	Benign vascularized tumors arising in the middle ear from paraganglia cells associated with jugular bulb or other nerves in middle ear; occur spontaneously	Hearing loss depends on location of tumor; about half present with a conductive loss; refer for surgical treatment

PE, pressure equalization.

windows. Cochlear disorders are not able to be visualized with an otoscope. Many cochlear disorders do not require medical treatment; however, some do require medical evaluation and treatment. Most hearing losses from cochlear disorders are treated with hearing aids.

Noise-Induced Hearing Loss

A *noise-induced hearing loss* (NIHL), also called acoustic trauma, is a hearing loss that occurs from exposure to extremely loud noise. Noise-induced hearing loss is one of the most common causes of acquired sensorineural hearing loss. Noise damage can occur from impulsive-type sounds, like an explosion or gunshot, or more commonly from longer-term exposures to high-level industrial, military, and/or recreational noises, such as jackhammers, airplanes, machinery, or music. The damage can involve the hair cell stereocilia, tectorial membrane, metabolic changes to the hair cell, rupture of Reissner's membrane, or a combination of those factors. Typically, the sensorineural hearing loss damages the outer hair cells of the cochlea, but with continued exposure can affect the inner hair cells as well.

A NIHL can be characterized by a *temporary threshold shift* (TTS) or a *permanent threshold shift* (PTS). The TTS may occur when exposed to loud noise levels for a few hours, as might occur from a music concert or loud stereo; and one may notice that sounds seem muffled and there is a high-pitched tinnitus (see section on tinnitus near end of this chapter). The TTS will, by definition, return to normal within a few hours. With continued exposure to loud sounds for several years, the hearing loss and tinnitus will become permanent and progressive, generally beginning with a loss of function in the outer hair cells, and then a loss in the inner hair cells with continued exposure. However, even a single occurrence to an impulsive, high-intensity sound can cause mechanical damage to the cochlea, and may also involve rupture of the tympanic membrane and disarticulation of the ossicles. An NIHL is usually bilateral, and begins with a mild to moderate hearing loss only in the 3000 to 6000 Hz region, often called a *noise notch*. With prolonged exposure, the notch may widen to other frequencies and the amount of hearing loss worsens. Figure 12–10 summarizes the features and audiometric profile for a case with noise-induced notched hearing loss. The sound pressure levels and durations of exposure that cause PTS are complicated and may vary depending on the type of noise, one's susceptibility, other health factors, or exposure to chemicals or drugs that may damage the ear. In general, there are standards (National Institute for Occupational Safety and Health [NIOSH], 1998; Occupational Safety & Health Administration [OSHA], 1983) that set acceptable limits for industrial noise exposures within a 24-hour period, called *damage risk criteria*. The most conservative standard (NIOSH) begins with a maximum allowable exposure of 85 dBA[1] for 8 hours (within a 24-hour period), and for every 3 dB increase in noise level above 85 dBA the exposure time is cut in half; for example, 88 dBA = 4 hours of exposure, 91 dBA = 2 hours of exposure. The OSHA standards use 90 dBA as the maximum allowable exposure to which one can be exposed for a period of 8 hours (within a 24-hour period), and for every 5 dB increase in noise level above the 90 dBA the exposure time is cut in half; for example, exposure to continuous noise level of 95 dBA would only be allowed for a maximum of 4 hours. Exposures less than the damage risk criteria are considered safe for most people. Continued exposure to levels exceeding the damage risk criteria can result in PTS. Workplaces with the potential for exposure to loud sounds should have in place a *hearing conservation program* to educate the employees about effects of noise, monitor their hearing, provide *hearing protection devices (HPDs)* such as noise reduction headsets or earplugs, and make changes in the work environment if possible.

Recreational music can also result in NIHL. For instance, music venues can often exceed 100 dBA; therefore, you should consider limiting the time of exposure depending on the level of the noise (unfortunately, the level is not usually known or provided). For example, using the NIOSH standard, if the music level is 103 dBA, you should limit exposure to about 7 minutes! Even with the OSHA standards, 105 dBA would be limited to about 30 minutes. Of course, hearing protection devices can help reduce the level of noise (by about 15 to 20 dB) and are highly recommended (and required by industry) when in situations where the sounds are too loud. Other treatment options are to reduce exposure to excessive noise and consider hearing aids when the degree of hearing loss is more advanced.

---

[1] dBA refers to the measurement of the level of a sound using an A weighted filtering that is closer to the threshold of audibility curve (e.g., non-audible frequencies are filtered out).

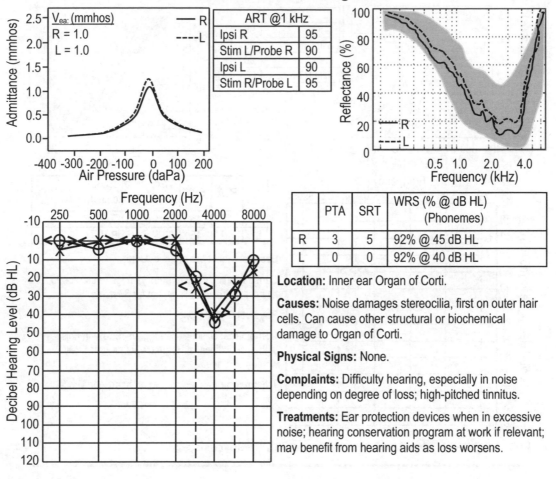

FIGURE 12–10. Profile of a typical case with permanent noise-induced hearing loss. OHC, outer hair cells; IHC, inner hair cells.

Hearing Loss Due to Aging (Presbycusis)

Presbycusis is the term used for hearing loss related to aging. Presbycusis is the most common form of adult-acquired sensorineural hearing loss. Close to half of persons 65 to 75 years of age have some degree of high frequency hearing loss. Presbycusis is characterized by a bilateral sloping high frequency sensorineural hearing loss that can begin around the sixth decade of life and may slowly progress with age. Patients often complain of difficulty understanding speech, especially in noisy situations (Committee on Hearing, 1988; Humes, 1996). The sensorineural hear-

ing loss associated with aging is typically a result of a loss of outer hair cell function followed by a loss of inner hair cell function; however, involvement of the central auditory pathways or the stria vascularis has also been shown. Figure 12–11 summarizes the features and audiologic profile for a patient with presbycusis. Although there is a high correlation between age and increasing sensorineural hearing loss, it is difficult to separate any concomitant effects of noise exposure, genetic predisposition, smoking, alcohol, diet, or other health factors (Roush, 1985). Treatment for presbycusis is primarily audiological with the fitting of hearing aids and aural rehabilitation programs as needed.

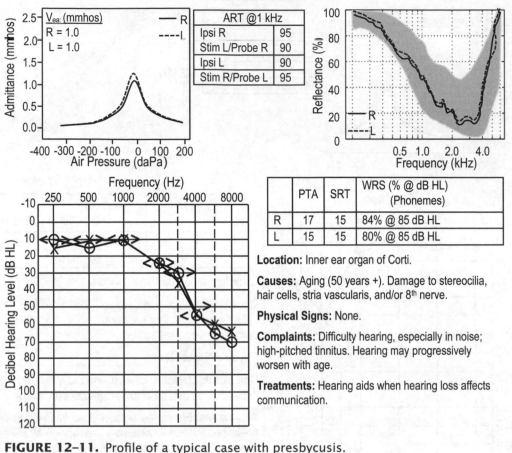

FIGURE 12–11. Profile of a typical case with presbycusis.

Ménière Disease

Ménière disease is a disorder that is characterized usually by four conditions; (a) episodes of vertigo, often severe with vomiting, (b) low frequency sensorineural hearing loss, which can fluctuate in early stages, (c) aural fullness, and (d) low pitched tinnitus ("ocean roar"). Ménière disease is related to a buildup of excessive endolymph in the scala media and vestibular labyrinths, called *endolymphatic hydrops*, the cause of which is not well understood, and may occur spontaneously, occur with a viral attack, or may have some genetic predisposition (Roland & Marple, 1997). Ménière disease occurs typically in the 30- to 60-year-old range. The severity, duration, and repeatability of the vertigo attacks vary across patients. The fluctuating nature of the disease has been shown to correspond to a buildup of endolymph, causing

the hearing loss, and then a rupture of Reissner's membrane, causing a vertiginous attack. The membrane fairly quickly repairs itself and the attack subsides and hearing may even improve; however, the process of endolymph buildup begins again. The patient may learn to predict the vertigo attacks by sensing the buildup of aural pressure, hearing loss, and tinnitus.

The hearing loss begins as a unilateral sensorineural loss, but may progress to bilateral in about 20% of patients (Jordan & Roland, 2000). The hearing loss usually begins in the low frequencies and may even fluctuate between moderate and normal hearing levels during the early stages, but then progresses to a relatively flat moderate hearing loss (often with the best hearing at 2000 Hz). Ménière disease requires medical evaluation, and most patients improve with treatment. Treatment may begin with elimination

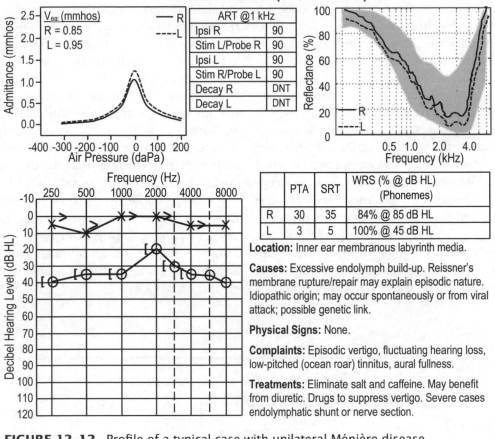

FIGURE 12–12. Profile of a typical case with unilateral Ménière disease.

of caffeine, nicotine, and salt in the diet, followed by a prescribed diuretic. In severe cases without resolution from other treatments, an *endolymphatic shunt* operation may be performed to provide for drainage of the endolymph into tissues, or a more invasive approach may be used to destroy the vestibular organs by infusing vestibulotoxic drugs into the inner ear through the middle ear, or by surgery (*labyrinthectomy* or *vestibular nerve section*). Figure 12–12 summarizes the features and audiologic profile of a case with unilateral Ménière disease.

Ototoxicity

Ototoxicity is the hearing loss that occurs from therapeutic drugs or other noxious chemicals. For the most part, the drugs are being used to treat some other disease and have associated side effects that can cause hearing loss. It is important for the audiologist to be involved as early as possible with patients being treated with ototoxic medications. Patients being treated with drugs that are ototoxic should have a baseline audiogram before treatment begins and regular audiograms during the treatment to monitor any changes in hearing. In some cases, if hearing loss begins to show up, the physician may alter the drug dose; however, most of the time the underlying illness is more important than the hearing. There may be the need for subsequent audiologic treatment with hearing aids and aural rehabilitation. There are five general categories of medications that are associated with hearing loss; (a) aminoglycosides, (b) chemotherapeutic agents, (c) loop diuretics, (d) salicylates (e.g., aspirin), and (e) antimalarial drugs (e.g., quinine). Aminoglycoside and chemotherapeutic agents can cause permanent bilateral sensorineural hearing loss, whereas the loop diuretics, salicylates, and antimalarial drugs usually cause temporary, bilateral sensorineural hearing loss that returns to normal soon after the drug therapy is stopped. *Aminoglycosides* (also referred to as the antibiotic "mycin" drugs) are the most damaging to the auditory and/or vestibular system. However, they are very important in treating infections which is why they are commonly used. Some common aminoglycosides that are primarily ototoxic are amakicin, tobramycin, dihydrostreptomycin, and neomycin. Other aminoglycosides, such as streptomycin and gentamycin, are more toxic to the vestibular system and may be used to preserve hearing during treatment. Damage to the cochlea from aminoglycosides is dose and duration dependent, but occurs first in the outer hair cells and can progress to the inner hair cells over lon-

ger treatment periods. If a hearing loss occurs, it is bilateral and begins first in the extended high frequencies (above 8000 Hz). Estimates of hearing loss caused by aminoglycosides range from 2 to 15% (Monsell, Teixido, Wilson, & Hughes, 1997). Evaluations of patients treated with aminoglycosides is one of the main clinical applications for performing extended high frequency audiometry. With time, the hearing loss may progress to the conventional frequency range. Although monitoring hearing during aminoglycoside treatment is a good idea, it may not always be possible because of the severity of the illness. In some cases, the hearing loss will continue to progress long after the treatment is terminated. Figure 12–13 summarizes the features and audiological profile of a case with aminoglycoside ototoxicity.

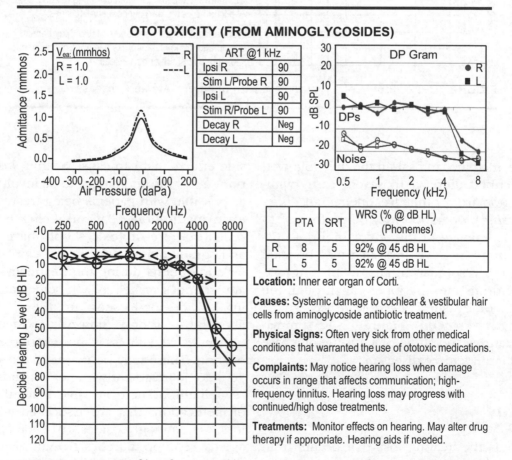

FIGURE 12–13. Profile of a typical case with ototoxicity from aminoglycoside antibiotics.

Chemotherapeutic (neoplastic) agents also pose a significant risk for cochlear damage. These drugs are used to treat some forms of cancer. The drugs most commonly associated with hearing loss are *cisplatin* and *carboplatin*. Cisplatin is used to treat tumors of the head and neck as well as ovarian or testicular cancer. Hearing loss with cisplatin occurs in about 17% of patients (Martini & Prosser, 2003), and is typically a permanent, bilateral, high-frequency sensorineural hearing loss, similar to that seen with aminoglycosides.

Loop diuretics are often used to treat patients with edema that is associated with congestive heart failure, lung disease, or renal disease. These types of diuretics act upon the loop of Henley in the kidney and cause high levels of diuresis. The most common loop diuretics associated with hearing loss are furosemide, bumetanide, and ethacrynic acid. The hearing loss from loop di-

uretics is related to effects on the stria vascularis and is usually temporary and characterized by a bilateral, moderate sensorineural hearing loss (Gallagher & Jones, 1979). The use of loop diuretics in conjunction with aminoglycosides or cisplatin may exacerbate their ototoxic effects and increase the risk for permanent sensorineural hearing loss (Brummett, Bendrick, & Himes, 1981). Figure 12–14 summarizes the features and audiological profile of a case of hearing loss from loop diuretics.

Salicylates are anti-inflammatory drugs, the most common being aspirin. Aspirin in high doses, as sometimes used in the treatment of rheumatoid arthritis, can cause tinnitus and a bilateral, flat, mild to moderate, temporary sensorineural hearing loss. The audiometric pattern for aspirin-induced ototoxicity is similar to that for loop diuretics (see Figure 12–14). The hearing

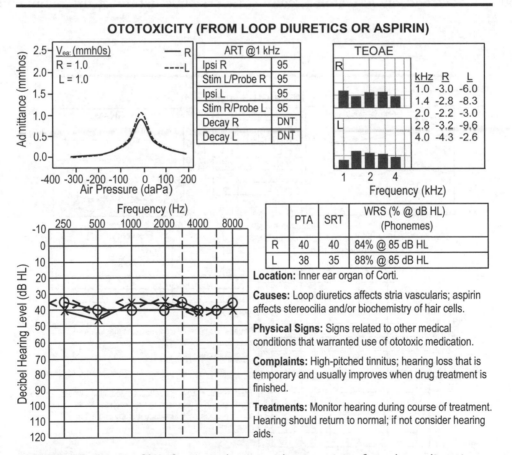

FIGURE 12–14. Profile of a typical case with ototoxicity from loop diuretics or aspirin.

loss and tinnitus disappear when the salicylate treatment is terminated. The amount of aspirin needed to produce tinnitus and hearing loss is about 6 to 8 g/day (Roland & Marple, 1997).

Antimalarial drugs, like quinine and chloroquine, are also capable of producing hearing loss and tinnitus. These drugs are usually used to prevent malaria or severe leg cramps. The hearing loss is generally a bilateral, high frequency sensorineural loss. As with salicylates, the hearing loss is usually temporary.

Infections

Bacterial infections that affect the inner ear are less common than those that affect the external and middle ear. Inner ear infections and associated hearing loss may be secondary to other infections like *meningitis*, gaining access through the cochlear aqueduct or internal auditory canal, or from otitis media and cholesteatoma, gaining access through the oval or round windows (Roland & Marple, 1997). Hearing loss from inner ear bacterial infections is usually severe and permanent. Treatment of bacterial infections is with antibiotics and corticosteroids. Viruses can also invade the inner ear and cause sudden sensorineural hearing loss of varying degrees, and in some cases, may even be temporary. *Cytomegalovirus (CMV)* is a common viral infection that generally does not cause hearing loss or much illness, other than a slight flu; however, if the mother contracts CMV during pregnancy, a small percentage of the time the baby will be born with a CMV infection that can lead to a progressive sensorineural hearing loss. CMV is a leading cause of sensorineural hearing loss in young children. Usually the hearing loss with CMV has a delayed onset and is progressive. Other childhood viruses, like rubella (German measles) or mumps, can also cause sensorineural hearing losses of varying degrees. Despite the systemic nature of the mumps virus, when

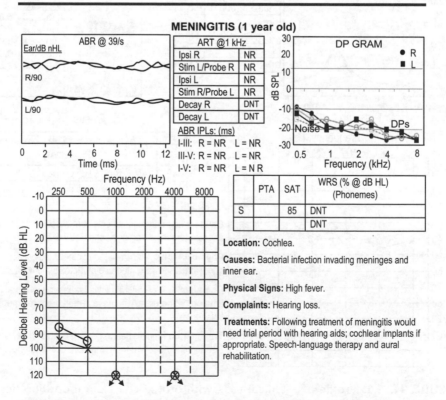

FIGURE 12–15. Profile of a typical case with bacterial infection resulting in meningitis.

there is a hearing loss it is most often unilateral and profound. The unilateral hearing loss may go unnoticed until later in life and may be traceable to early childhood mumps. Syphilis and herpes zoster can also cause severe bilateral sensorineural hearing loss, especially if exposed in utero. Systemic infections are relatively rare today in developed countries because of pediatric vaccinations. Hearing aids and aural rehabilitation are required to treat any concomitant hearing loss from bacterial or viral infections. Figure 12–15 summarizes the features and audiological profile for a case with inner ear infection due to meningitis.

Sudden Sensorineural Hearing Loss

Sudden sensorineural hearing loss is not a disease per se, but a term used to describe a sensorineural hearing loss that comes on rapidly, typically in a few hours or when one wakes up at night. The hearing loss usually begins as a moderate sensorineural loss accompanied by aural fullness and tinnitus. It usually is a unilateral hearing loss, but in some cases, depending on the causes, may affect the other ear later. The degree of hearing loss varies and in some cases, may spontaneously recover or can be restored with drug treatment if begun quickly; therefore, any sudden hearing loss should be treated as a medical emergency. There are many known causes of sudden sensorineural hearing loss, including viral attacks, vascular embolisms, autoimmune disorders, Ménière disease, acoustic neuroma, and closed-head trauma. A rupture in the oval or round window membrane, called a *perilymph fistula*, may also result in a sudden sensorineural hearing loss, along with dizziness. In many cases, a cause for the hearing loss cannot be identified, in which case it is referred to as an idiopathic sudden sensorineural hearing loss. In many cases, like with autoimmune or idiopathic sudden sensorineural hearing loss, immediate treatment with corticosteroids may be prescribed in the hope of stabilizing or improving the hearing loss. Figure 12–16

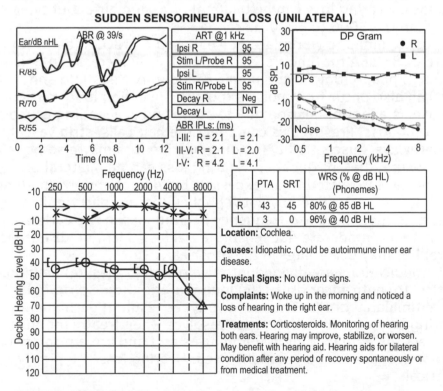

FIGURE 12–16. Profile of a typical case with unilateral sudden sensorineural hearing loss.

summarizes the features and audiological profile for a case with sudden sensorineural hearing loss.

Temporal Bone Fractures

A non-penetrating trauma to the skull (also called *closed-head injury*) from car accidents, sports, physical abuse, or falls can cause fractures to the temporal bone and lead to hearing loss and dizziness. Temporal bone fractures are identified through computerized tomography as part of the medical evaluation for those experiencing a blow to the head. In some closed-head injuries, including concussions, there may be some stretching of nerves in the brainstem or temporal lobe lesion, causing some subtle hearing problems. A *transverse fracture* of the temporal bone is one that is perpendicular to the petrous portion of the temporal bone and causes damage to the inner ear structures, leading to a sensorineural hearing loss (Bergemalm & Borg, 2001). If the fracture runs parallel along the edge of the petrous portion of the temporal bone it is called a *longitudinal fracture* and usually results only in middle ear involvement, including fluid/blood in the middle ear or a disarticulation of the ossicles. A longitudinal fracture is most often caused by a blow to the side of the head. Transverse fractures are less common and can occur from a blow to the front or back of the head. Often the damage is some combination of longitudinal and transverse (oblique fracture) and is better described as to whether or not the damage involves the otic capsule (inner ear) or spares the otic capsule. (Saraiya & Aygun, 2009), and the resulting

---

SYNOPSIS 12–3

- Aural pathologies that affect the cochlea result in sensorineural hearing losses. Noise-induced hearing loss (NIHL) is a leading cause of acquired sensorineural hearing loss. Hearing loss can be bilateral or asymmetric, but typically begins as a notch in the 3000 to 6000 Hz range.
- Safe exposure limits to workplace noise (based on NIOSH) allow for a maximum exposure of 85 dBA for 8 hours, and for each 3 dB increase in noise level the maximum exposure time is cut in half. Temporary threshold shifts (TTS) and tinnitus can also occur from noise exposure, including loud music.
- Presbycusis is a loss of hearing due to aging and is a leading cause of acquired adult hearing loss. Presbycusis can affect the hair cells, stria vascularis, or neural pathways. Susceptibility to aging hearing loss may also be related to noise exposure, diet, or genetics. Hearing loss can be bilateral or asymmetric.
- Ménière disease is related to an excessive buildup of endolymph (endolymphatic hydrops). It is characterized by a low pitched (ocean roar) tinnitus, vertigo, aural fullness, and fluctuating low frequency hearing loss in the early stages, followed by a permanent, moderate flat sensorineural loss. Ménière disease is usually unilateral but may occur later in the other ear.
- Ototoxic medications are divided into five general types: (a) aminoglycoside antibiotics, (b) anticancer drugs, (c) loop diuretics, (d) aspirin in high doses, and (e) antimalarial drugs. The first two types result in permanent hearing loss; the hearing loss with the other types resolves when treatment ends. Ototoxic drugs affect the extended high frequencies first and are a primary population where high frequency audiometry is used. Hearing loss is typically bilateral and symmetrical.

SYNOPSIS 12–3 (*continued*)

- When a hearing loss comes on suddenly, medical treatment should be sought immediately to have the best chance of stabilizing or reversing the hearing loss with corticosteroid treatment by a physician. Sudden hearing loss may be caused by an autoimmune disorder, perilymph fistula, viral attack, or idiopathic causes. Hearing loss is usually unilateral but may occur later in the other ear.
- Bacterial infections (e.g., meningitis) or viral infections (e.g., mumps, measles, cytomegalovirus) often result in severe bilateral sensorineural hearing loss, especially in children.
- Temporal bone fractures from head injury can also result in hearing loss. A longitudinal fracture (sparing the otic capsule) usually produces a conductive loss. A transverse fracture (involving otic capsule) damages the cochlea and can cause a sensorineural hearing loss.
- Table 12–3 summarizes the auditory disorders of the inner ear covered in this chapter.

hearing loss can manifest as a conductive loss, sensorineural loss, or mixed loss depending on the extent and location of the fracture, some of which may spontaneously resolve within a week or so. In some cases, there is leakage of the cerebral spinal fluid, causing otorrhea and the risk of meningitis. Treatment depends on the type and extent of hearing loss. For those with permanent sensorineural loss, hearing aids and aural rehabilitation may be of benefit.

NEURAL DISORDERS

Hearing disorders of the 8th cranial nerve and the area around the nerve between the cochlea and the cochlear nucleus (cerebellar-pontine angle or CPA) are traditionally referred to as *retrocochlear* disorders. Although retrocochlear implies anything after the cochlea, disorders of the brainstem and cortical areas are usually considered central auditory disorders. The auditory nerve can be affected by a variety of factors, including tumors, vascular disorders, viral attacks, multiple sclerosis, diabetes, neural presbycusis, and a developmental abnormality, *auditory neuropathy spectrum disorder* (also called auditory neuropathy, or auditory

dyssynchrony). Acoustic neuroma and auditory neuropathy spectrum disorder are presented in more detail below.

Acoustic Neuroma

A benign tumor that involves the 8th cranial nerve and causes hearing loss and vestibular symptoms is called an *acoustic neuroma*. This tumor typically arises from the Schwann cells of the vestibular portion of the 8th cranial nerve, and is also called a *vestibular schwannoma* or an *acoustic schwannoma*. It is the most common type of tumor found in the CPA (Lustig & Jackler, 1997) and is most common in adults. As the tumor grows, it compresses or destroys the cochlear nerve; it can grow from the internal auditory canal into the CPA, where it can eventually involve the central auditory pathways. Although these tumors are benign and relatively slow growing, they need medical attention that generally involves surgical removal. The earlier the acoustic neuroma is identified and removed, the more likely that the hearing may be preserved. Many audiological tests (e.g., speech tests, acoustic reflexes, auditory brainstem responses [ABR]) have been developed to differentially diagnose

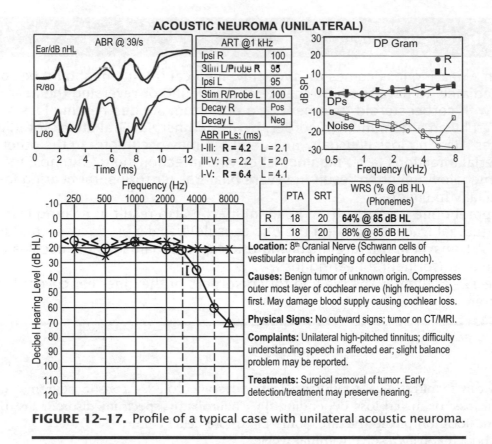

FIGURE 12–17. Profile of a typical case with unilateral acoustic neuroma.

acoustic neuroma disorders from cochlear disorders. The hearing loss associated with an acoustic neuroma is a unilateral, high frequency, progressive, sensorineural loss that can range from mild to severe. The higher frequencies are affected first because of the early pressure exerted on the outside of the cochlear nerve that originates from the more basal area of the cochlea. In some cases, hearing may be normal but the patient has unilateral tinnitus or difficulty with understanding speech. Acoustic reflexes may be absent or elevated beyond those considered for the amount of hearing loss. The speech recognition scores may also be poorer than would be predicted from the amount of hearing loss. A common symptom of an acoustic neuroma is a unilateral high-pitched tinnitus. Sometimes a patient reports dizziness or balance problems but this is not always a presenting symptom. Referral to a physician is warranted, especially when an asymmetrical, high frequency, sensorineural

hearing loss is present in an adult or there is unilateral tinnitus. Today, magnetic resonance imaging (MRI) and/or computerized tomography are quite sensitive in identifying acoustic neuromas, even when they are quite small. Figure 12–17 summarizes the features and audiologic profile of a case with an acoustic neuroma.

Auditory Neuropathy Spectrum Disorder (ANSD)

Auditory neuropathy spectrum disorders (ANSD), also known as auditory dyssynchrony, is a condition of the 8th cranial nerve in which the neurons do not fire with the normal synchrony (at the same time) necessary to transmit the neural output from the cochlea to the brainstem (Berlin, Morlet, & Hood, 2003; Sinninger, 2002; Starr, Picton, Sinninger, Hood, & Berlin, 1996). An ANSD

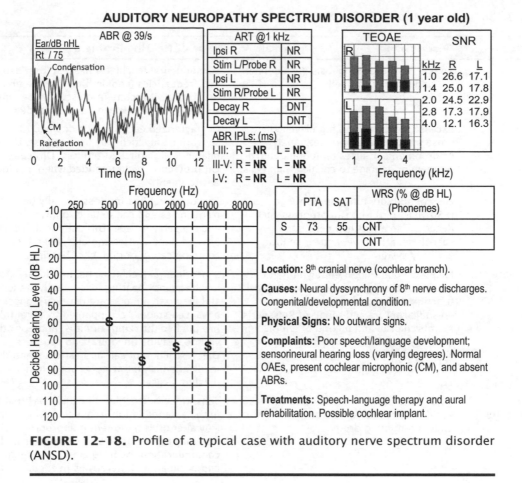

FIGURE 12–18. Profile of a typical case with auditory nerve spectrum disorder (ANSD).

is a developmental condition present at birth, the cause of which is not fully known. Although the cochlea appears to function normally, the 8th cranial nerve is somehow affected. The diagnosis of ANSD is often identified in newborns or young infants through newborn hearing screening programs using the auditory brainstem responses (ABRs). The classic diagnostic picture of ANSD is the absence or abnormality of the ABR and the presence of normal otoacoustic emissions (OAEs), as would be expected with normal outer hair cell function. In the ABR recording, there may be a *cochlear microphonic* present in the early part of the waveform coming from the outer hair cells, and which can be identified by recording with different polarity clicks (rarefaction and condensation). The source of the auditory neural dyssynchrony could be at the level of the inner hair cell, its synapse, or in the nerve itself. Audiometrically, any hearing loss would be sensorineural type; however, the severity can range from normal to profound. Patient's with ANSD also have absent acoustic reflexes beyond that expected for the degree of hearing loss, and they usually have difficulty understanding speech. The use of hearing aids as a treatment is not recommended; however, some success has been found with cochlear implants (Zeng & Sheng, 2006). Figure 12–18 summarizes the features and audiologic profile of a case with ANSD.

CENTRAL AUDITORY DISORDERS

Central auditory disorders are a general category that can include a variety of problems involving the central nervous system's auditory pathways and related auditory processing, both

TABLE 12–3. Summary of Auditory Inner Ear and 8th Nerve Disorders

Disorder	Description	Type of Hearing Problem
Cochlear otosclerosis	Toxins from otospongeosis invade inner ear and destroy hair cells.	Sensorineural (cochlear) hearing loss, usually mid frequencies (cookie bite). Can be unilateral or bilateral. Difficulty in noise. May benefit from sodium fluoride. Hearing aids if needed.
Noise induced hearing loss	Excessive exposure to high levels of noise in workplace or recreational environments. Causes temporary and/or permanent damage to cochlear hair cells.	Characterized early-on as a notched (3 to 6 kHz) sensorineural (cochlear) hearing loss. Usually bilateral. High-pitched tinnitus. Difficulty in noise. Ear protection recommended when in a loud environment.
Presbycusis	Loss of auditory function from age (>50 years old) that can progress each decade. Can affect hair cells, stria vascularis, 8th nerve, and/or central auditory system.	Sensorineural hearing loss; usually begins in high frequencies and can extend to lower frequencies and worsen with age. Difficulty in noise. High pitched tinnitus. Hearing aids when loss affects communication or quality of hearing.
Ménière disease	Excessive build-up of endolymph in the inner ear. Disrupts cochlear and hair cell function. Idiopathic origin. May have episodic rupture and repair of Reissner's membrane causing mixing of endolymph and perilymph.	Sensorineural (cochlear) hearing loss. Fluctuating low frequency hearing loss in early stages, stabilizing to a moderate flat hearing loss in more advanced stage. Accompanied by aural fullness, low pitched (buzzing) tinnitus, and episodic vertigo. May be unilateral and progress to bilateral. Diet restriction of salt and caffeine; anti-dizziness medication; shunt or nerve section in severe dizziness cases.
Ototoxicity (aminoglycoside)	Inner ear damage (cochlear and/or vestibular) resulting from treatment with infection-fighting drugs.	Sensorineural (cochlear) hearing loss that begins in the extended high frequency range. Bilateral. May alter drug treatment if appropriate. Hearing loss may move into lower frequencies and affect communication. Hearing aids, aural rehabilitation, and occupational therapy as needed.
Ototoxicity (loop diuretic)	Temporary alteration of stria vascularis (cochlea) during treatment with diuretics (loop of Henley), usually to treat edema from heart and lung, or renal disease.	Temporary mid frequency (cookie bite) sensorineural hearing loss during treatment. Bilateral. Hearing usually improves after treatment.
Meningitis/other infections	Systemic illness (usually bacterial) invades cochlea and destroys hair cells. Less frequent today due to vaccine given about age 2 years.	Severe to profound bilateral hearing loss possible. Trial period with hearing aids and consider cochlear implant. Aural rehabilitation and speech-language therapy if young child.
Sudden sensorineural	Idiopathic inner ear damage (most likely hair cells). Rule out Ménière disease and autoimmune inner ear disease.	Sensorineural hearing loss of sudden onset. Usually unilateral but may progress to bilateral. May have tinnitus. Not usually accompanied by dizziness. Medical treatment (corticosteroids?) as soon as possible to stabilize or restore hearing. Hearing aid(s) if needed.
Acoustic neuroma	Slow growing benign tumor or unknown cause. Grows from vestibular nerve and puts pressure on cochlear nerve. Can disrupt blood flow to inner.	Asymmetric sensorineural hearing loss first affecting the higher frequencies. Difficulty understanding speech in involved ear. Unilateral high-pitched tinnitus. May have some balance problem. Surgical treatment required. Early detection may preserve hearing. If hearing is damaged in involved ear, possible hearing aid (CROS).
Auditory neuropathy spectrum disorder (ANSD)	Dyssynchrony in firing of 8th nerves. Congenital origin.	Sensorineural hearing loss of varying degree. Difficulty with speech and language. Hearing aids probably not appropriate; however, some success has been seen with cochlear implants. Speech and language therapy.

Educational Audiology

The Educational Audiology Association (EAA) is a professional organization, established in 1985, for audiologists and related professionals who deliver a full spectrum of hearing services to all children, particularly those in educational settings. Educational audiology can be traced back to the eighteenth and nineteenth centuries when educators of the deaf eschewed sign language in favor of an aural approach. Before the advent of electronic amplification, intervention primarily involved training in lipreading (speechreading) and the use of speaking tubes or an amplifying chair. But even within the constraints of these limited resources, dedicated teachers in the classroom environment worked valiantly to develop communication skills in severely hearing-impaired children. In the modern era, one of the earliest educational audiologists was Moe Bergman, now a distinguished elder statesman of audiology at Tel Aviv University in Israel. In the 1930s, Bergman was employed in the New York City school system as a speech correctionist, and as part of a project to collect data on the prevalence of various speech disorders in the schools he began to use the newly developed Western Electric 6B portable audiometer to screen for hearing loss that fostered his interest in the educational needs of hearing impaired children. Ann Mulholland is credited as the first person to use the term "educational audiology" in 1965. The concept of educational audiology as a discipline began in 1966 when Frederick S. Berg generated the first known grant to train professionals to work with children with hearing losses in the public school system at Utah State University. During this period, Berg and Fletcher published *The Hard of Hearing Child* (1970), and Berg published *Educational Audiology: Hearing and Speech Management* (1976) which helped foster the concept of educational audiology on a national basis. Today educational audiologists work in school systems throughout the United States, and are involved with hearing assessment, hearing aid evaluation and management, communication training, educational evaluation and training, and environmental evaluation and adjustments.

at the brainstem and cortical levels. Some disorders of the central auditory system can be localized to a discrete area of the brain, such as those that might be caused by tumors or vascular lesions/strokes, or are more generalized, such as those that might be caused by developmental deficits, hereditary neuropathies, infections, presbycusis, chemicals, multiple sclerosis, or idiopathic causes. Depending on the source of the central disorder, there may be other more serious medical issues than hearing deficits. On the other hand, in some cases the disorder may only manifest as a subtle *auditory processing disorder* (APD), which may especially pose a problem with learning in school age children.

Disorders of the central auditory system do not typically affect hearing of pure tones or even basic speech measures because of the multiple neural pathways, including those that course through the brainstem along ipsilateral and contralateral routes (see Chapter 4). Even a stroke in the temporal lobe does not affect hearing per se but may affect receptive language abilities. Bilateral temporal lobe deficits are very rare but may result in deafness (Hood, Berlin, & Allen, 1994). Auditory deficits from central auditory disorders, if any, may show up on more complicated listening tasks, such as competing messages from the two ears, filtered speech, or time-compressed speech. Symptoms of central auditory disorders may include difficulty in noisy or reverberant environments, difficulty with complex directions, poor auditory memory, trouble localizing, distractibility, or inattentiveness. Specific audiologic tests for central auditory disorders are beyond the scope of this introductory text, and the interested reader is referred to other sources (Bellis, 2003; Musiek & Chermak, 2006; Stach, 2000).

NONORGANIC (FUNCTIONAL) HEARING LOSS

It is not uncommon to see patients who purposely feign or exaggerate their hearing loss, a situation that is labeled *nonorganic hearing loss, functional hearing loss, exaggerated hearing loss, pseudohypoacusis,* or *malingering.* In other words, these patients are "faking" their hearing loss. Most of these patients are fully aware of their actions; however, some may have underlying psychological problems for which the audiologist needs to make an appropriate referral to a psychiatrist or psychologist. The primary reason an adult patient might purposefully exaggerate hearing difficulty is for financial gain, including employee or military compensation or accident liability. There are many other reasons that a patient might feign a hearing loss. Some examples include military personnel who want to have a hearing test just for the distraction or to get out of an assignment, children who seek some attention or reward in their family or school environment, or students who believe they can use a hearing loss as an excuse for poor school performance or to get out of an assignment. Luckily, there are a variety of ways in which an audiologist can identify patients with functional hearing losses, and the audiologist can usually get the patient to provide fairly accurate test results. Testing these patients can often be challenging and interesting (or even entertaining). However, the audiologist should be cautious about how the results are presented to the patient, and avoid labeling them with any of the above terms. The audiologist's role is to end up with test results that are a reflection of the organic basis of the hearing loss and not be overly concerned about any underlying reason for the exaggeration (Martin, 2002).

Although it is beyond the scope of this text to present all the test strategies used by audiologists when suspecting a functional hearing loss, a few of them will be mentioned. First, otoacoustic emissions can often indicate that the patient has normal outer hair cell function suggesting good peripheral hearing, and if this is not in agreement with the initial behavioral thresholds obtained during pure-tone testing, the audiologist should suspect a functional hearing loss and proceed accordingly. In these situations, pure-tone threshold searches should start at the lowest level of the audiometer, and the audiologists should spend some time presenting tones less than 20 dB HL, and, yes, even deviate from the up-5-down-10 rule. For example, if patients do not respond at 20 dB HL, you might even decrease the level of the signal for a few trials, and then come up to 15 dB HL (they might then respond). The intent is to confuse them and wait them out; they may get nervous or they may even think you are testing at a higher level. Another strategy is to give them some instructions or make some comment through the earphones at a level equal to or less than the thresholds and see what they do. Of course, reinstructing patients as if they were not cooperating may also work well and/or act as if there is something wrong with the earphones, which you then proceed to "fix." You may also let them know that you are not getting consistent results and that you may need to do an auditory brainstem response test (where they do not have to do anything); often this will improve their cooperation. With most of these strategies, you are trying to give the patient a way out so that they then provide you with more truthful results.

There is also a very effective and easy test, the *Stenger test,* which can be used for patients who are feigning poorer thresholds in only one ear. The Stenger test takes advantage of the Stenger phenomenon, in which a tone (or word) presented simultaneously to both ears will only be heard in the ear where it is louder. In a clinical situation with a unilateral (or asymmetrical) hearing loss, the level of the tone (or word) is set at 10 dB above (louder than) the threshold in the better hearing ear, and the level of the same tone (or word) is set at 10 dB below (softer than) the threshold in the poorer hearing ear. The patient is not told that a signal will be in both ears. The signal is presented simultaneously to the two ears. If the patient is not feigning a hearing loss in the poorer ear, he or she should respond because the tone is above (louder than) the threshold in the good ear; however, if he or she is feigning a hearing loss in the poorer ear, he or she would not respond because he or she only perceives the tone in the poorer ear because it is louder than the tone in the good ear (he or she is not aware of the sound in the good ear). When the patient does not respond to the Stenger it is considered a positive Stenger and suggests that the patient's behavioral thresholds were being exaggerated. The Stenger should be used to verify any unilateral hearing loss. Of course, the ABR can be used as a more definitive test for objectively documenting thresholds in patients suspected of functional hearing loss, especially involving compensation cases.

In a case where a child may be exaggerating thresholds at first, after further testing the audiologist most likely will get the child to cooperate and provide true thresholds (e.g., normal hearing). In this case, it is usually sufficient to report to the parent that the child has normal hearing and leave it at that. When the audiologist is not confident that the hearing test results are an accurate reflection of a child's hearing abilities, this should be cautiously implied in the clinical report or in the discussion with the patient or family (e.g., "unable to get consistent responses"; "thresholds may be better than those obtained today"). Again, it is not useful to challenge the patient's behavior or motivation or label him or her with a functional hearing loss. In some cases, especially if unable to get accurate thresholds, it may be suggested that further testing is needed, including the possibility of an auditory brainstem response test.

TINNITUS

. . . my ears whistle and buzz continuously day and night. I can say I am living a wretched life. (Ludwig von Beethoven, 1801)

Tinnitus refers to auditory perceptions that are generated internally (within the head), without any externally applied stimulus. The word tinnitus (pronounced either "TIN-uh-tus" or "tin-EYEtus,") is derived from the Latin word *tinnire*, which means "tinkling" or "ringing." Tinnitus is not a disease but a symptom or consequence of many different types of disorders. It is estimated that about 15% of the general population (50 million Americans) has tinnitus, with increasing percentages with age. Of the 20 million people who seek medical attention for tinnitus, about 2 million are so affected by their tinnitus that they are unable to function on a daily basis (American Tinnitus Association, n.d.).

Tinnitus is typically divided into two general types, subjective (non-vibratory) and objective (vibratory). *Subjective tinnitus* is typically described by the patient as "ringing, hissing, or roaring" and is the type of tinnitus commonly encountered by audiologists due to its association with many types of hearing loss. *Objective tinnitus* is most often described by the patient as "whooshing" or "pulsing" sounds, and is the type of tinnitus usually associated with a non-auditory condition, such as a vascular problem in the head or neck that is transmitted internally as an auditory stimulus. An audiologist should be knowledgeable about both types of tinnitus so he or she can properly counsel patients and make appropriate medical referrals.

Subjective Tinnitus

Subjective tinnitus is much more common than objective tinnitus. Most patients with hearing loss, when asked, say that they have some type of ringing in their ears. In many cases, the patient seeks medical or audiologic services because of the tinnitus. Subjective tinnitus is most commonly reported as a high-pitched ringing or whistling in the head. Although the perceived level of the stimulus may be relatively loud, it is usually matched to the loudness of a tone (in an area of good hearing) less than 25 dB (Goodwin & Johnson, 1980) and is usually comparable to the frequency range where there is the greatest amount of hearing loss. Subjective tinnitus can be constant or intermittent, unilateral or bilateral, tonal or noise-like, temporary or permanent.

Historical Vignette

James Henry, of the National Center for Research in Auditory Rehabilitation (NCRAR) in Portland, Oregon, has traced the history of efforts to evaluate and treat tinnitus over the past several decades. He notes that, as early as 1821, Jean Marc Gaspard Itard, Chief Physician at the National Institute for Deaf Mutes in Paris, found that tinnitus could often be treated with a masking sound and that the pitch of the tinnitus was linked to the pitch of the most effective masking sound. As early as the 1930s, Edmund Prince Fowler (of audiogram fame) found that when patients were asked to match the loudness of their tinnitus to the intensity of a pitch-matched pure tone, the apparent sensation level of the match was in the 5 to 10 dB range. He concluded that tinnitus was an "illusion" that tended to be exaggerated by the patient. While some tinnitus sufferers hear a "ringing" tone, others hear a sound more accurately described as either a narrow or broadband noise; thus, matching to the pitch of a pure tone is not always feasible. Pioneers in tinnitus evaluation over the past 3 to 4 decades have included Victor Goodhill at UCLA, Jack Vernon, Robert Johnson, and Mary Meikle at the Oregon Health Sciences University Hearing Research Center, Richard Tyler at the University of Iowa, M. J. Penner, at the University of Maryland, and Aage Moller at the University of Texas at Dallas. In the continuing effort to quantify the actual handicap related to this elusive phenomenon, many investigators have turned to the development of questionnaires. Those in current use include the Tinnitus Handicap Questionnaire, developed by Kuk, Tyler, and Russell; the Tinnitus Handicap Inventory, developed by Newman and Jacobson; and the Tinnitus Cognitions Questionnaire, developed by Wilson and Henry. Harald Feldman, of Germany, is credited with the first observation that tinnitus could be relieved by purposely masking it with an external sound. He reported a success rate of 89% using a tinnitus masker. Subsequent research on this topic has demonstrated that either specific devices known as tinnitus maskers or actual hearing aids are helpful to many tinnitus sufferers. In recent years, treatment options for tinnitus have expanded dramatically, including drug treatments and cognitive therapies. Although investigators from many disciplines contribute to our understanding of tinnitus and its treatment, audiologists will play an increasing role in this area in the years to come.

Table 12–4 lists some disorders that are associated with subjective tinnitus. The most common cause of subjective tinnitus is noise exposure; up to 90% of tinnitus patients have some noise-induced hearing loss. High-pitched tinnitus is most often associated with high-frequency hearing loss; however, it can also occur without any measurable hearing loss. Unilateral high-pitched tinnitus is often the first symptom of acoustic neuroma. In Ménière disease, tinnitus is a primary symptom; however, it is usually low pitched and characteristically described as an "ocean roar" or "buzzing" sound. In some cases, the cause of the tinnitus is idiopathic. In any case, underlying history and/or medical examination should be included in the evaluation of tinnitus patients to help determine the type and cause of their tinnitus. One must also be aware that some patients may feign tinnitus, especially in cases involving compensation. Documentation of these functional cases is difficult to disprove.

The physiological mechanisms of subjective tinnitus are not well understood; most likely there are a variety of sensory, neural, autonomic, and psychological mechanisms associated with tinnitus, and one or more of these may play a role in different disorders. A confounding factor is the inherent differences that individuals have in their ability to cope with their tinnitus or even

TABLE 12–4. Disorders Associated with Subjective Tinnitus

Noise exposure	Otosclerosis
Presbycusis	Head injury
Ménière disease	Meningitis
Acoustic neuroma	Thyroid disorder
Ototoxic medications	Psychological
Sudden hearing loss	Depression
Central disorders	Anxiety

cope with stresses in their lives that may be exacerbating the tinnitus. Patients with depression or anxiety may have tinnitus; however, it may not be clear which came first. The source of the tinnitus can be in the peripheral auditory system, brainstem, or cortical areas. Regardless of the tinnitus's origin, its conscious perception has a cortical component, perhaps located in the prefrontal–temporal area associated with attention, emotion, and memory (Pederen, Johannsen, Ovesen, Stodkilde-Jorgensen, & Gjedde, 1999).

Fortunately, most patients learn to cope with their tinnitus when they are given information about how tinnitus is related to their hearing loss and how tinnitus is quite common and not a sign of some medical emergency. For those patients with more severe tinnitus or psychological reactions to their tinnitus, treatment options are available; however, these may have different levels of success and may vary depending on the individual. For more severe cases of tinnitus, a medical, psychological, and audiologic management approach is warranted.

A popular and comprehensive approach to tinnitus and its management comes from the work of Pawel Jastreboff and colleagues (Jastreboff & Hazell, 1993), commonly referred to as the *neurophysiological basis of tinnitus*. The Jastreboff model proposes that, in the more severe cases of tinnitus, the limbic (emotional) and autonomic (unconscious control and alerting system) play important roles, especially in the annoyance factor associated with tinnitus. The Jastreboff neurophysiological model has a tinnitus treatment program, known as *Tinnitus Retraining Therapy* (TRT), that has become clinically popular. The TRT is a comprehensive approach to tinnitus assessment and management based on Jastreboff's neurophysiological model, and includes a structured counseling component and a prescribed masking therapy (Henry, Jastreboff, Jastreboff, Schechter, & Fausti, 2002; Jastreboff, Gray, & Gold, 1996). In the TRT masking therapy, the patient learns to habituate to the tinnitus over several weeks whereby the patient listens to a noise that is set at a level that almost masks out the tinnitus. The idea is to allow the tinnitus to be audible, but to reduce the annoyance and/or focus on the tinnitus by presenting an external noise. Over time, the level of the noise is reduced, which results in an additional reduction in the patient's perception of the tinnitus. In successful cases, the patient "learns" not to perceive the tinnitus even during periods of time when the noise is removed. To use TRT as a treatment option, the therapy provider must attend TRT training workshops.

Another tinnitus treatment that uses sound therapy is called *Neuromonics*. This is a patented sound therapy technique discovered and developed at Western Australia's Curtin University of Technology by Dr. Paul Davis (http://www.neuromonics.com). The Neuromonics approach uses a specially designed Neuromonics Processor (about the same size and weight of a cell phone) for the sound therapy part of its comprehensive tinnitus treatment, which presents customized sounds to the patient through earphones. The stimulus is based on the patient's audiometric profile up to 12.5 kHz and can be different for each ear. The Neuromonics approach is to embed the customized stimulus into a music-like stimulus rather than listening to a noise-like stimulus as in TRT or other tinnitus masking methods, thereby presenting a more pleasant stimulus to the patient. This type of sound activates the auditory pathways, as well as the limbic and autonomic systems, and with time reduces the perception and/or annoyance associated with the tinnitus through desensitization (Davis, 2005). With the Neuromonics approach, the musical, time-varying sound stimulus is set to be above the patient's audiometric thresholds in the areas where he or she has a hearing loss, to provide auditory stimulation. During the treatment stage, the stimulus is adjusted so that there are times when the tinnitus is heard within the Neuromonics' musical stimulus. The goal of the Neuromonics treatment, similar to TRT, is to have the patient habituate or become desensitized to the presence of the tinnitus. According to the manufacturer, after about 6 months of wearing the device (2 hours per day), successful patients are no longer bothered by their tinnitus and can stop wearing the device for a period of time.

A variety of other treatment options are also available and have been used as traditional methods of treating tinnitus, including the use of: (a) background noise/music as a distraction, (b) tinnitus masking instruments that are housed in a casing similar to that of hearing aids, (c) hearing aids (with their inherent noise), (d) biofeedback or other stress management techniques, and (e) counseling. A detailed comparison of the underlying theories and sound therapy treatment methods of TRT compared with traditional tinnitus masking techniques is detailed by Henry, Schechter, Nagler, and Fausti (2002). In addition, a variety of drugs and herbs have been investigated for the treatment of subjective tinnitus, but thus far with limited success. The most common medications currently used include corticosteroids or anticoagulants (Mora et al., 2003); however, their success still needs more validation.

A detailed audiometric description of the tinnitus is also helpful. In addition to a careful questionnaire, the audiologist: (a) determines the extent and type of hearing loss, (b) documents if there is a retrocochlear disorder, and (c) provides a detailed description of the tinnitus that can be of help in diagnosing the problem but also in providing information that may be useful for the sound therapy approaches to tinnitus management. The audiometric description usually includes *tinnitus matching*, which includes documenting the general frequency range of the tinnitus to a pure-tone frequency or narrowband noise, as well as documenting the perceived loudness of the tinnitus by matching the tinnitus to different stimulus levels (at the perceived frequency). An additional measure, *tinnitus maskability*, documents how much of a narrowband

or white noise is needed to mask out the tinnitus (Mitchell, Vernon, & Creedon, 1993).

Objective Tinnitus

Objective tinnitus is much rarer than subjective tinnitus, especially in an audiological setting. Objective tinnitus is usually identified by a physician through a patient's medical visits, either because the patient is being treated for other related disorders or because the unusual sound in his or her head has caused some concern. However, audiologists should be familiar enough with objective tinnitus to be able to ask about it in the initial audiologic interview and to make the appropriate medical referral when encountered.

Objective tinnitus is caused by some vibration of tissues or structures within the head and neck region that are audible to the patient, and in most cases, audible to the examiner through a stethoscope (some cases have been reported where these sounds are loud enough to be heard in the room without a stethoscope). Objective tinnitus is usually caused by vascular abnormalities around the temporal bone, usually heard as a pulsing or whooshing sound, and is commonly referred to as *pulsatile tinnitus*. The most common sources of pulsatile tinnitus are the carotid artery and the jugular bulb. Glomus tumors of the middle ear are usually accompanied by objective tinnitus. These

TABLE 12–5. Disorders Associated with Objective Tinnitus

Glomus tumors
Arterial bruits
Misplaced or thin jugular bulb
Arterial/venous malformations
Benign intracranial hypertension
Anemia
Palatomyoclonus
Stapedial muscle spasm
Patulous eustachian tube
Temporal-mandibular joint
Paget disease
Pregnancy

vascular abnormalities can be caused by head injury, surgery, hypertension, or abnormal position of the jugular bulb (Crummer & Hassan, 2004).

Objective tinnitus can also originate from spasms in the middle ear muscles or palatal muscles brought on by neurological dysfunction (Fortune, Haynes, & Hall, 1999) and is typically described as a clicking or crackling sound. A patulous eustachian tube may also create objective tinnitus due to the patient hearing wind noise or breathing through the open tube. Sometimes muscular spasms or eustachian tube problems can show up as deflections superimposed on the tympanogram. The audiologist usually becomes aware of objective tinnitus through the patient's history or complaints. Anytime objective tinnitus is apparent, the audiologist should make a medical referral. Treatment for objective tinnitus is dependent on the origin and is handled by the physician. Sound therapy methods (TRT, *Neuromonics*, and tinnitus maskers), which are useful treatments for subjective tinnitus, are not useful for treating objective tinnitus. Table 12–5 provides a list of some causes of objective tinnitus.

SYNOPSIS 12–4

- The two most common 8th cranial nerve disorders that produce hearing loss are acoustic neuroma and auditory neuropathy spectrum disorder (ANSD). Acoustic neuroma is usually unilateral; ANSD usually occurs bilaterally. The use of acoustic reflexes, OAE, and ABR are important for identifying/differentiating these disorders. For example, auditory neuropathy spectrum disorder is characterized by normal OAEs and abnormal ABRs. See Table 12–3.
- Central pathologies do not produce any pure-tone hearing loss but are characterized by difficulty with other auditory processing tasks.
- Nonorganic (functional) hearing losses are those where the thresholds or hearing problems are exaggerated purposefully. Worker's compensation, military personnel, or children seeking attention may present with functional hearing loss. With careful attention to hearing test techniques, the patient eventually volunteers accurate results.
- Tinnitus is a symptom commonly associated with a variety of hearing disorders, and not a disease per se.
  - Subjective tinnitus (nonvibratory) is a perceived sound by the patient without any known source or internal source of vibration. It is often characterized as high-pitched ringing in most disorders, or an ocean roar common with Ménière disease.
  - Subjective tinnitus can be treated and/or alleviated with information or counseling, listening to background sounds, hearing aids, tinnitus maskers, or sound therapies, such as found with Tinnitus Retraining Therapy or Neuromonics tinnitus instruments. As of yet, drug treatments have shown only limited success.
  - Objective tinnitus (vibratory) is caused by some abnormal structure or restricted blood flow that causes an internal vibrational stimulus that is heard by the ear. Treatment is usually medical and/or surgical depending on the source of the objective tinnitus.
  - See Tables 12–4 and 12–5 for lists of some causes of tinnitus.

REFERENCES

American Tinnitus Association. (2007). About tinnitus; frequently asked questions; how many people have tinnitus? Retrieved from http:// www.ata.org/about tinnitus/patient_faq.php/.

Bellis, T. J. (2003). *Assessment and Management of Central Auditory Processing Disorders in the Educational Setting* Clifton Park, NY: Thomson Delmar Learning.

Bergemalm, P.-O., & Borg, E. (2001). Long-term objective and subjective audiological consequences of closed head injury. *Acta Otolaryngologica, 121,* 724–734.

Berlin, C. I., Morlet, T., & Hood, L. J. (2003). Auditory neuropathy/dyssynchrony: Its diagnosis and management. *Pediatric Clinics of North America, 50,* 331–340.

Brummett, R. E., Bendrick, T., & Himes, D. (1981). Comparative ototoxicity of bumetanide and furosemide when used in conjunction with kanamycin. *Journal of Clinical Pharmacology, 21,* 629–636.

Crummer, R. W., & Hassan, G. A. (2004). Diagnostic approach to tinnitus. *American Family Physician, 69,* 120–126.

Davis, P. B. (2005). Music and the acoustic desensitisation protocol. In R. Tyler (Ed.), *Tinnitus treatments* (pp. 146–160). New York, NY: Thieme.

Feeney, M. P., Grant, I. L., Marryott, L. P. (2003). Wideband energy reflectance measurements in adults with middle-ear disorders. *Journal of Speech, Language and Hearing Research, 46,* 901–911.

Fortune, D. S., Haynes, D. S., & Hall, J. W. I. (1999). Tinnitus. *Medical Clinics of North America, 83,* 153–162.

Gallagher, K. L., & Jones, J. K. (1979). Furosemide induced ototoxicity. *Annals of Internal Medicine, 91,* 744–745.

Goodwin, P. E., & Johnson, R. M. (1980). The loudness of tinnitus. *Acta Otolaryngologica, 90,* 353–359.

Henry, J. A., Jastreboff, M. M., Jastreboff, P. J., Schechter, M. A., & Fausti, S. A. (2002). Assessment of patients for treatment with Tinnitus Retraining Therapy. *Journal of the American Academy of Audiology, 13,* 523–544.

Henry, J. A., Schechter, M. A., Nagler, S. M., & Fausti, S. A. (2002). Comparison of tinnitus masking and Tinnitus Retraining Therapy. *Journal of the American Academy of Audiology, 13,* 559–581.

Hood, L. J., Berlin, C. I., & Allen, P. (1994). Cortical deafness: A longitudinal study. *Journal of the American Academy of Audiology, 5,* 330–342.

House, J. W. (1997). Otosclerosis. In G. B. Hughes & M. L. Pensak (Eds.), *Clinical otology.* New York, NY: Thieme.

Humes, L. (1996). Speech understanding in the elderly. *Journal of the American Academy of Audiology, 7,* 161–167.

Jastreboff, P. J., Gray, W. C., & Gold, S. L. (1996). Neurophysiological approach to tinnitus patients. *American Journal of Otology, 17,* 236–240.

Jastreboff, P. J., & Hazell, J. W. P. (1993). A neurophysiological approach to tinnitus: Clinical implications. *British Journal of Audiology, 27,* 7–17.

Joint Committee on Infant Hearing. (2007). Year 2007 position statement: Principles and guidelines for early hearing detection and intervention programs. *Pediatrics, 120,* 898–921.

Jordan, J. A., & Roland, P. S. (2000). Disorders of the auditory system. In R. J. Roeser, M. Valente, & H. Hosford-Dunn (Eds.), *Audiology diagnosis* (pp. 85–108). New York, NY: Thieme.

Kinney, W. C., Kinney, S. E., & Vidimos, A. T. (1997). Disorders of the auricle. In G. B. Hughes & M. L. Pensak (Eds.), *Clinical otology* (pp. 177–190). New York, NY: Thieme.

Lustig, L. R., & Jackler, R. K. (1997). Benign tumors of the temporal bone. In G. B. Hughes & M. L. Pensak (Eds.), *Clinical otology* (pp. 313–343). New York, NY: Thieme.

Martin, F. N. (2002). Pseudohypacusis. In J. Katz (Ed.), *Handbook of clinical audiology* (5th ed., pp. 584–596). Baltimore, MD: Lippincott Williams & Wilkins.

Martini, A., & Prosser, S. (2003). Disorders of the inner ear in adults. In L. Luxon (Ed.), *Textbook of audiological medicine* (pp. 452–475). London, UK: Martin Dunitz.

Mitchell, C. R., Vernon, J. A., & Creedon, T. A. (1993). Measuring tinnitus parameters: Loudness, pitch, and maskability. *Journal of the American Academy of Audiology, 4,* 139–151.

Monsell, E. M., Teixido, M. T., Wilson, M. D., & Hughes, G. B. (1997). Nonhereditary hearing loss. In G. B. Hughes & M. L. Pensak (Eds.), *Clinical otology* (pp. 289–312). New York, NY: Thieme.

Mora, R. M., Salami, A., Barbieri, M., Mora, F., Passali, G., Capobianco, S., Magnan, J. (2003). The use of sodium enoxaparin in the treatment of tinnitus. *International Tinnitus Journal, 9,* 109–111.

Musiek, F. E., & Chermak, G. D. (2006). *Handbook of (Central) Auditory Processing Disorders (Vol. 1). Auditory Neuroscience.* San Diego, CA: Plural.

Myerhoff, W. L., Marple, B. F., & Roland, P. S. (1997). Tympanic membrane, middle ear, and mastoid. In P. S. Roland, B. F. Marple, & W. L. Myerhoff (Eds.), *Hearing loss* (pp. 155–194). New York, NY: Thieme.

Nance, W. E., & Dodson, K. (2007). 2007 Marion Downs lecture, Part 1: How can newborn hearing screening be improved? *Audiology Today, 19*, 14–19.

National Institute for Occupational Safety and Health (NIOSH). (1998). Criteria for a recommended standard: Occupational noise exposure—Revised criteria. NIOSH Pub. No. 98-126. Cincinnati, OH: NIOSH.

Occupational Safety & Health Administration (OSHA). (1983). Occupational noise exposure (29 CFR 1910.95, May 29, 1971, vol. 36). Amended (March 8, 1983, Vol. 48, pp. 9776–9785). Washington, DC: Federal Register.

Pederen, M. F., Johannsen, P., Ovesen, T., Stodkilde-Jorgensen, H., & Gjedde, A. (1999). Positron emission tomography of cortical centers of tinnitus. *Hearing Research, 134*, 133–144.

Roland, P. S., & Marple, B. F. (1997). Disorders of inner ear, eighth nerve, and CNS. In P. S. Roland, B. F. Marple, & W. L. Myerhoff (Eds.), *Hearing loss* (pp. 195–256). New York, NY: Thieme.

Roland, P. S., & Rohn, G. N. (1997). History and physical examination. In P. S. Roland, B. F. Marple, & W. L. Myerhoff (Eds.), *Hearing loss* (pp. 107–131). New York, NY: Thieme.

Roush, J. E. (1985). Aging and hearing impairment. *Seminars in Hearing, 6*, 99–219.

Shambaugh, G. E. J. (1983). Adult fluoride therapy for otosclerosis (otospongiosis). *Archives of Otolaryngology, 109*, 353.

Shprintzen, R. J. (2001). *Syndrome Identification for Audiology*. San Diego, CA: Singular Thomson Learning.

Sinninger, Y. S. (2002). Auditory neuropathy in infants and children: Implications for early hearing detection and intervention programs. *Audiology Today, Special Edition, Update on Infant Hearing*, 16–21.

Stach, B. A. (2000). Diagnosing central auditory processing disorders in adults. In R. J. Roeser, M. Valente, & H. Hosford-Dunn (Eds.), *Audiology diagnosis* (pp. 355–379). New York, NY: Thieme.

Starr, A., Picton, T. W., Sinninger, Y. S., Hood, L. J., & Berlin, C. I. (1996). Auditory neuropathy. *Brain, 119*, 741–753.

Toriello, H. V., & Smith, S. D. (2013). *Hereditary Hearing Loss and Its Syndromes* (3rd ed.). New York, NY: Oxford University Press.

Woods, C. I., Strasnick, B., & Jackson, C. G. (1993). Surgery for glomus tumors: The Otology Group experience. *Laryngoscope, 103*(Suppl.), 65–72.

Zeng, F. G., & Sheng, L. (2006). Speech perception in individuals with auditory neuropathy. *Journal of Speech, Language, and Hearing Research, 49*, 367–380.

13 Screening for Hearing Loss

After reading this chapter, you should be able to:

1. List the principles and criteria established by the World Health Organization important for establishing early identification programs.

2. Understand the need for reliable and valid methods for screening.

3. Discuss the history and use of a high-risk register for hearing screening, and list some of the current high risk factors.

4. Describe the various methods used in screening newborns, school age children, and adults.

5. Discuss the pros and cons of OAE and AABR techniques for screening infants.

6. List the recommended fail and referral criteria for hearing screening of school age children.

7. List two hearing handicap inventories popular for hearing screening in adults.

8. Understand screening outcome matrices and how a specified screening criterion can affect the sensitivity and specificity.

9. Appreciate how the prevalence of a disorder can influence a test's predictive values.

Hearing screening is a process of identifying subpopulations of people with potential hearing disorders, using efficient and cost-effective methods. Hearing screening programs are sometimes referred to as *identification programs* for hearing loss. Screening programs essentially involve a pass or fail measure on a targeted population in order to separate those who most likely do not have the disorder (the passes) from those who may possibly have the disorder (the fails). Those who fail a screening should be referred for a more complete evaluation to determine if they actually have the disorder. In general, hearing screenings are conducted on groups of people who might not otherwise know they have a hearing problem or who are unable or reluctant to seek professional services.

Deciding to do a screening for a targeted disorder must include weighing a variety of factors before proactively taking it to the field to identify those who are not generally seeking any professional services. This is a different concept than developing diagnostic tests for those who come seeking professional services because of a perceived problem or symptom. For example, with regard to hearing disorders, newborns and young children will be unaware that they have anything wrong or may not be able to convey a complaint. Likewise, many elderly adults may discount or ignore hearing problems, or not realize that they are socially withdrawing due to unrecognizable changes in their hearing abilities. This chapter discusses some general components and issues common to any screening program, as well as some specific details and criteria used with different types of hearing screenings currently in use, including those for newborns, school age children, and adults.

HISTORICAL AND CURRENT PRACTICE GUIDELINES

The modern day principles of screening have their foundations established by the World Health Organization (WHO) with a commitment to early identification of several chronic diseases. Table 13–1 is a summary of some of the original WHO criteria for developing a screening test and en-

hancements of those criteria that occurred over the following 40 years (Andermann, Blancquaert, Beauchamp, & Déry, 2008).

One of the main considerations of a screening program is that it should target a disorder that is recognized as an important health issue. Hearing disorders have recognizable consequences on a person's ability to learn speech and language, as well as on many other important auditory listening functions per se. The absence or decline of hearing may lead to other associated social, academic, and/or behavioral problems. Implicit in the idea of screening is that it should be applied at an early stage in the development of the problem when consequences are minimal and benefit can be gained from early treatment.

A screening test should be reasonably safe, acceptable to society, and cost-effective. The positive benefits to the individuals and to society should outweigh any harm associated with the screening. It is also very important that there be adequate and appropriate follow up diagnostic tests, available facilities, and personnel or resources to diagnose and treat those who fail a screening test. You can have an excellent screening test, but if there is a lack of adequate follow up care, or if those who fail the screening are not motivated or monitored regarding their follow up, the screening test may not be appropriate or sustainable. Finally, any successful screening program will have scientific evidence of its effectiveness and benefits.

Effective screening tests should have good *reliability*, such that similar results should occur when applied several times to an individual and that different testers obtain similar results from the same individual. A screening test must also be designed to have good *validity* so you can be confident that the measure used is one that can provide the information sought. For example, if you want to identify central auditory processing disorders or middle ear disorders, you would not use a pure-tone hearing screening measure; other more appropriate measures should be used.

Screening is generally applied to populations that do not show or act upon symptoms of some disorder; however, there should be a significant probability of finding those with the disorder,

TABLE 13–1. World Health Organization Screening Criteria and Subsequent Enhancements

A. Classical screening criteria (Wilson & Jungner, 1968)
• The condition sought should be an important health problem.
• There should be an accepted treatment for patients with recognized disease.
• Facilities for diagnosis and treatment should be available.
• There should be a recognizable latent or early symptomatic stage.
• There should be a suitable test or examination.
• The test should be acceptable to the population.
• The natural history of the condition, including development from latent to declared disease, should be adequately understood.
• There should be an agreed-upon policy on whom to treat as patients.
• The cost of case finding (including diagnosis and treatment of patients diagnosed) should be economically balanced in relation to possible expenditure on medical care as a whole.
• Case finding should be a continuing process and not a "once and for all" project.
B. Synthesis of emerging screening criteria proposed over the past 40 years (Andermann et al., 2008)
• The screening program should respond to a recognized need. The objectives of screening should be defined at the outset.
• There should be a defined target population.
• There should be scientific evidence of screening program effectiveness.
• The program should integrate education, testing, clinical services, and program management.
• There should be quality assurance, with mechanisms to minimize potential risks of screening.
• The program should ensure informed choice, confidentiality, and respect for autonomy.
• The program should promote equity and access to screening for the entire target population.
• Program evaluation should be planned from the outset.
• The overall benefits of screening should outweigh the harm.

SYNOPSIS 13–1

- Hearing screenings are conducted on groups of people who might not know they have a hearing problem or who are unable or reluctant to seek professional services, and that there is a significant probability of finding those with the disorder, and/or that the disorder is considered to be important enough to identify in the larger population.
- Effective hearing screening programs (a.k.a. identification programs) should target subpopulations using efficient and cost-effective methods to identify people with potential hearing problems and have options for follow-up measures. Criteria for effective screening programs evolved from work of the World Health Organization (WHO) more than 50 years ago.
- Screening programs essentially involve a pass or fail measure to separate those who most likely do not have the disorder (the passes) from those who may possibly have the disorder (the fails).

> ### SYNOPSIS 13–1 (*continued*)
>
> - An effective screening test should have good reliability (similar results obtained each time) and validity (identifies what is intended).
> - A universal screening test is one that is applied to a relatively large population. A more cost-effective approach to screening is to do a targeted (or selective) screening. A targeted screening will have a higher prevalence rate of the disorder as compared with universal screening of the larger population.

and/or the disorder is considered to be important enough to screen a large population. A *universal screening* is one that is applied to a relatively large population, such as all newborns. A universal screening must consider the disorder to be of high significance, and must have personnel and equipment that make the screening feasible and cost-effective. It may, however, be more cost-effective to do a *targeted screening* test, in which case only a subgroup of the larger population is targeted for screening. A targeted screening will have a higher prevalence rate of the disorder compared with universal screening of the larger population, and may be more cost-effective. Obviously, the cost of a screening program should not be prohibitive in light of the significance of the disorder that is to be identified.

HEARING IDENTIFICATION PROGRAMS

We will now briefly discuss some details of hearing identification/screening programs, including screening for hearing loss in newborns, school age children, and adults. Following those sections, some issues regarding screening limitations, outcomes, and efficacy are presented.

Screening the Hearing of Newborns

Hearing screening of newborns, also referred to as *early hearing detection and intervention* (*EHDI*), has evolved over the past 50 years from not being very applicable when only behavioral hearing measures were available, to the use of auditory brainstem response (ABR) testing of infants in Neonatal Intensive Care Units (NICUs) and/or the use of high-risk registers, to today's approach of screening all newborns (universal newborn hearing screening) using otoacoustic emission (OAE) and/or automated auditory brainstem response (AABR) measures. In addition, the growing information about genetics has gained importance in hearing screening of newborns, especially as affordable DNA screening is becoming available (e.g., OtoSeq and OtoGenome) (see NCBI https://www.ncbi.nlm.nih.gov/gtr).

The primary goal of an EHDI program is to identify permanent and significant hearing loss that can affect and/or delay development of audition and speech-language abilities, which if left untreated would impact educational and psychosocial factors. Keep in mind that newborn hearing screening is only the beginning of a more comprehensive program that requires follow up confirmations of hearing loss by 3 months of age and appropriate intervention, including the goal of fitting hearing aids or cochlear implants before 6 months of age (Joint Committee on Infant Hearing [JCIH], 2007). Additionally, there must be close follow up care, rehabilitation, and counseling for those who are identified as having a hearing loss. This text will not review the early history of newborn hearing screening using behavioral methods; however, the interested reader may want to review some of the early work and research in this area (Downs & Sterritt, 1967; Durieux-Smith, Picton, Edwards, Goodman, & MacMurray, 1985; Ling, Ling, & Doehring, 1970; Northern & Downs, 2014; Thompson & Thompson, 1972). The limitations inherent in behavioral

TABLE 13–2. Risk Factors for Congenital and Delayed Onset Hearing Loss

* Caregiver concern§ regarding hearing, speech, language, or developmental delay.

* Family history§ of permanent childhood hearing loss.

* Neonatal intensive care of more than 5 days or any of the following regardless of length of stay: ECMO,§ assisted ventilation, exposure to ototoxic medications (gentamycin and tobramycin) or loop diuretics (furosemide/Lasix), and hyperbilirubinemia that requires exchange transfusion.

* In utero infections, such as CMV,§ herpes, rubella, syphilis, and toxoplasmosis.

* Craniofacial anomalies, including those that involve the pinna, ear canal, ear tags, ear pits, and temporal bone anomalies.

* Physical findings, such as white forelock, that are associated with a syndrome known to include a sensorineural or permanent conductive hearing loss.

* Syndromes associated with hearing loss or progressive or late-onset hearing loss,§ such as neurofibromatosis, osteopetrosis, and Usher syndrome; other frequently identified syndromes include Waardenburg, Alport, Pendred, and Jervell and Lange-Nielson.

* Neurodegenerative disorders,§ such as Hunter syndrome, or sensory motor neuropathies, such as Friedreich ataxia and Charcot-Marie-Tooth syndrome.

* Culture-positive postnatal infections associated with sensorineural hearing loss,§ including confirmed bacterial and viral (especially herpes viruses and varicella) meningitis.

* Head trauma, especially basal skull/temporal bone fracture§ that requires hospitalization.

* Chemotherapy.§

Note. Risk indicators that are marked with a "§" are of greater concern for delayed-onset hearing loss.
Source: Reproduced with permission from Joint Committee Infant Hearing (JCIH) (2007). Year 2007 position statement: Principles and guidelines for early hearing detection and intervention programs. *Pediatrics*, 120, 898–921. Copyright © 2007 by the American Academy of Pediatrics.

screening of newborns was an impetus for the development of more objective, physiological measures that would be more useful for detecting hearing loss in the newborn period. As discussed in earlier chapters, ABR and OAE have been accepted as objective (physiologic) measures of auditory function that can be effectively applied to screening of newborns. As these objective tests were being developed in the late 1970s to 1990s, others were establishing a list of neonatal conditions that were associated with hearing loss, called the *high-risk register*. For a more comprehensive review of newborn hearing screening, the interested reader is referred to other resources (Driscoll & McPherson, 2010; NCHAM, 2017; Tharpe & Seewald, 2017).

Screening High-Risk Infants

Targeted hearing screening of newborns and young infants has been advocated since the early 1970s through the use of a high-risk register (HRR) developed through the Joint Committee on Infant Hearing (JCIH).[1] The use of the HRR was a useful way to focus hearing screening and follow up testing on a subpopulation, especially before more cost-effective methods of universal screening became available. Today, the use of an HRR is quite useful in some circumstances. For example, there are some congenital disorders that have late onset or progressive hearing loss that could be missed if one relied solely on newborn hearing screening measures. Also, in developing countries without adequate resources for universal screening of newborns, the HRR allows more focused attention on those who are more likely to have a hearing problem. The risk factors that are on the HRR are periodically updated by the JCIH as new information becomes available. Table 13–2 lists the most current risk

---

[1]The JCIH was first formed in 1969 and includes members from the academies of Pediatrics, Ophthalmology and Otolaryngology, Council on Education of the Deaf, American Academy of Audiology, and the American Speech, Language, and Hearing Association.

factors for congenital deafness as developed by the JCIH (2007) and the U.S. Preventive Services Task Force (2008). Many of those infants with factors on the HRR will have been admitted to NICUs. For those in the NICU, and others on the HRR, hearing screening is generally performed using the ABR.

Even the most aggressive use of the HRR may fall short in identifying infants with hearing loss, as shown by a study in New Zealand (Project HEID, 2004), in which only 40% of children with significant permanent hearing loss would be identified by using the risk factor screening approach (Leigh, Taljaard, & Poulakis, 2010). The shortcomings of the HRR and the development of cost-effective objective measures for screening for auditory impairment have led to the implementation and acceptance of universal newborn hearing screening programs, as described more fully in the next section.

Universal Newborn Hearing Screening

Approximately 1.4 babies are found to have hearing loss for every 1000 babies screened in the United States (Center for Disease Control [CDC], 2014). Hearing screening of all newborns is now possible and widely implemented in most developed countries. In the United States, more than 96% of all babies born have their hearing screened by 1 month of age with OAEs and/or ABR. Of the babies screened, those who do not pass the screening (approximately 2% or 63,000 infants) must be evaluated for hearing loss (CDC, 2014). The acceptance of universal newborn hearing screening was made possible by the development of more cost-effective and valid screening measures of OAEs and/or AABR. Universal newborn hearing screening programs are very large-scale operations that involve the collaboration of many professionals, including physicians, nurses, audiologists, and trained screeners. Of course, the reason we want to screen all newborns is to be able to have early identification of those with hearing loss who do not have or who are not known to have any of the factors on the HRR, and to identify, diagnose, and treat those with significant hearing loss at the earliest possi-

ble age. Again, keep in mind that a comprehensive EHDI program includes an initial screening at birth, a follow up screening at birth or within 1 month, diagnostic testing of those who fail the screen by 3 months of age, and initiation of treatment for those confirmed to have a hearing loss by 6 months of age (referred to as the 1-3-6 rule). Also, those who pass the newborn hearing screenings should have follow up screening or a diagnostic hearing test between 24 and 30 months (JCIH, 2007), especially for those with risk factors for late onset of hearing loss. Since universal newborn hearing programs have been implemented, there has been a significant improvement in the average age of confirmation/initiation of treatment from about 20 months to less than 6 months (Leigh et al., 2010). Parents and pediatricians should monitor their child's hearing behavior and speech-language development, and follow up with any concerns. Table 13–3 provides a list of principles for EHDI programs developed by the JCIH (2007).

The initial screening of newborns occurs in the hospital before the baby is discharged. Because we are talking about screening all newborns, there is a need for adequate personnel and coordination of activities during the 1 to 2 days that babies are in the well-baby nurseries. Before the parents leave the hospital, they should know the results of their baby's hearing screening and any follow up recommendations needed. The hospital staff must also have a well-developed system for recording the information, and a plan to actively follow up on those who fail the hearing screenings or who have risk factors for late onset hearing loss to be sure the infant is seen for a diagnostic hearing test. Screening programs should also regularly evaluate the success of their procedures and outcomes, and make adjustments accordingly.

The two types of technologies used for hearing screening of newborns and young infants are otoacoustic emissions (TEOAEs and DPOAEs) and automated ABR (AABR). The basics of these physiological tests are described in Chapter 11. The AABR and/or OAE screening can be successfully performed in the well-baby nursery or in the overnight hospital room while the baby lies in his or her bassinet, as long as the baby is

TABLE 13–3. Principles of the Joint Committee Infant Hearing for Effective Early Hearing Detection and Intervention (EHDI) Program

1. All infants should have access to hearing screening using a physiological measure before 1 month of age.

2. All infants who do not pass the initial hearing screening and the subsequent rescreening should have appropriate audiologic and medical evaluations to confirm the presence of hearing loss before 3 months of age.

3. All infants with confirmed permanent hearing loss should receive intervention services before 6 months of age. A simplified, single point of entry into an intervention system appropriate to children with hearing loss is optimal.

4. The EHDI system should be family centered with infant and family rights and privacy guaranteed through informed choice, shared decision making, and parental consent. Families should have access to information about all intervention and treatment options and counseling regarding hearing loss.

5. The child and family should have immediate access to high-quality technology, including hearing aids, cochlear implants, and other assistive devices when appropriate.

6. All infants and children should be monitored for hearing loss in the medical home. Continued assessment of communication development should be provided by appropriate providers to all children with or without risk indicators for hearing loss.

7. Appropriate interdisciplinary intervention programs for deaf and hard-of-hearing infants and their families should be provided by professionals knowledgeable about childhood hearing loss. Intervention programs should recognize and build on strengths, informed choices, traditions, and cultural beliefs of the families.

8. Information systems should be designed to interface with electronic health records and should be used to measure outcomes and report the effectiveness of EHDI services at the community, state, and federal levels.

Source: Reproduced with permission from Joint Committee Infant Hearing (JCIH). (2007). Year 2007 position statement: Principles and guidelines for early hearing detection and intervention programs. *Pediatrics*, 120, 898–921. Copyright © 2007 by the American Academy of Pediatrics.

lying quietly. Although OAEs and AABR are used for universal newborn hearing screening, they provide only limited information about auditory function and are not measures of hearing in the complete sense. With this caveat in mind, the use of either or both of these technologies has been recommended for newborn screening by American Academy of Audiology (AAA) (2012) and by American Speech-Language-Hearing Association (ASHA) (n.d.), which meet the requirements of an adequate hearing screening program as outlined by the JCIH (2007). Each hospital needs to decide which one (or both) of the technologies they will incorporate into their newborn hearing screening program after careful consideration of their costs, training, logistics, and outcomes.

The AABR screening technology has been available since the early 1980s, and has been used by many hospitals for universal newborn hearing screening. An example of a newborn being tested with AABR is shown in Figure 13–1. The AABR uses quick-attaching disposable electrodes, a single preset click stimulus level (30 to 40 dB nHL), and incorporates an internal software algorithm to determine if specific criteria are met to consider the response a "pass." This automated decision eliminates the need to use an audiologist to make decisions based on recorded waveforms. The AABR has been found to be quick (about 10 min), reliable, and has acceptable outcomes, including referral (fail) rates and false positive rates of about 2% (Hall, 2007; Spivak, 2007).

The OAE technology received wider acceptance during the 1990s as OAE units were developed specifically for use with newborn screening programs. Figure 13–2 shows an automated OAE being conducted in the newborn's bassinet while asleep. Without the need for electrodes, the discovery that infants had large robust OAEs, along with a relatively low cost per test, made OAE screening a popular alternative to the AABR. Either TEOAEs or DPOAEs can be used for OAE screening. The TEOAEs are thought to be more sensitive to the 500 to 1000 Hz region than are DPOAEs, whereas DPOAEs are more sensitive in the higher frequencies (5000 to 8000 Hz) than TEOAEs. However, today's screening protocols typically do not include frequencies below

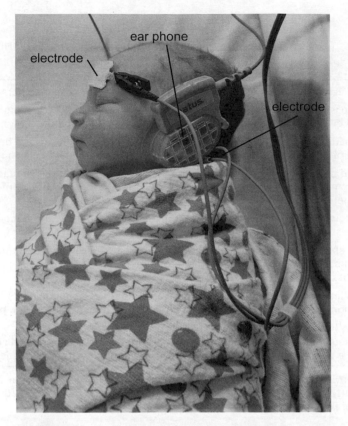

FIGURE 13–1. Automated ABR (AABR) being performed on a newborn. In this technique, the electrodes are attached to the forehead and nape of the neck. Clicks are presented to the ear through earphones coupled to the ear.

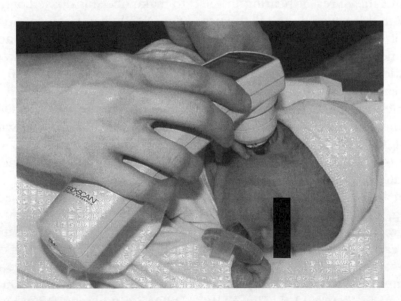

FIGURE 13–2. Newborn hearing screening using an otoacoustic emission screener. The infant needs to remain quite or asleep during the test to make the testing run faster.

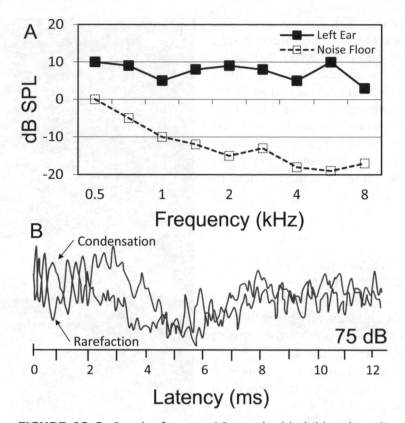

FIGURE 13–3. Results from an 18-month-old child with auditory neuropathy spectrum disorder (ANSD). (**A**) a normal DPOAE (emissions have a greater than 6 dB SNR) and (**B**) an abnormal ABR. The ABR waveform shows a cochlear microphonic (CM) but no other waves. The CM has a change in direction when the stimulus changes polarity from condensation to rarefaction.

1500 Hz due to problems with background noise where the testing takes place.

Like the AABR, the OAE screeners have built-in algorithms to determine if a baby meets the criteria for a pass. Initially, the false positive rate for OAE screening was quite high (10 to 20%), but with experience and the introduction of a two-stage screening procedure,[2] the false posi-

tive outcomes have been improved to less than 4% (Spivak, 2007; Vohr, Carty, Moore, & Letourneau, 1998). One limitation of OAE screening is that the response will be absent (infant will fail the OAE) when there is any outer or middle ear involvement, including middle ear fluid or vernix residue in the ear canal, which resolves after a day or two. In the near future, the use of wideband acoustic immittance (see Chapter 10) may become part of newborn hearing screening programs as a method to rule out conductive problems that may compromise the recordings of OAEs.

Another limitation of OAE screening is that it will miss infants with auditory neuropathy spectrum disorder (ANSD), characterized by normal OAEs and abnormal ABRs (Figure 13–3). It is

[2]One- and two-stage programs refer to the different technology used. In a one-stage screening program, only one technology (usually AABR) is used. In a two-stage program, the infant is screened with the less expensive OAEs and if they do not pass are immediately rescreened with an AABR. AABR is more tolerant of background acoustic noise and middle ear issues than is OAE.

estimated that ANSD may account for up to 10% of children with hearing loss (Sinninger, 2002). According to Sininger and Oba (2001), 80% of infants with ANSD will spend time in the Newborn Intensive Care Unit (NICU) and will most likely have ABR testing; however, the other 20% of infants with ANSD who would be in the well-baby nurseries would be missed if screening were done only with OAEs and not AABR. For more information about deciding on which system to use for newborn hearing screenings, see Leigh et al. (2010).

SCREENING THE HEARING OF SCHOOL AGE CHILDREN

Hearing screening of children has been around for about 60 years and was one of the earliest health screening initiatives in the United States. Guidelines for hearing screening of school age children have been developed by the American Academy of Audiology (AAA) (2011) and the American Speech-Language-Hearing Association (ASHA) (2017). These professional guidelines recommend that school age children have their hearing screened using earphones (air conduction) at a level of 20 dB HL, for frequencies of 1000, 2000, and 4000 Hz. Bone conduction screening is not done. Hearing screening should be done on all children in preschool through 3rd grade, in the 7th and 11th grades, and at any time there is a concern about a child's hearing, speech, or learning. School screening programs require close cooperation between the school administrators, teachers, parents, and personnel who are doing the screenings. The screening personnel should also be sure to visit the site and room to be used for the hearing screenings to be sure the background noise levels are acceptable,[3] the environment is relatively free of visual or other distractions, there are appropriate electrical outlets, and there are suitable tables and chairs. Portable screening audiometers (Figure 13–4) are avail-

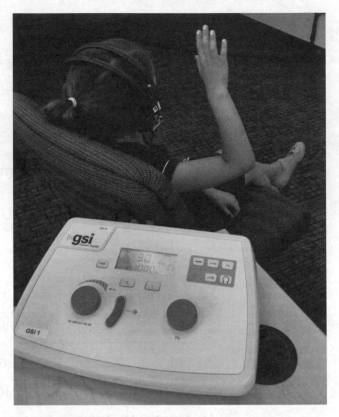

FIGURE 13–4. Screening a school age child with a portable screening audiometer.

able for use in school-based hearing screening programs. Hearing screening programs should be coordinated and/or supervised by an audiologist in order to ensure quality. The air conduction puretone hearing screenings per se can be performed with trained nurses, speech-language pathologists, supervised graduate students, or in some states by persons holding an audiometrist certificate. For tympanometry and otoscopy components of a screening program, an audiologist should be directly involved during the screenings.

The screening of school age children, especially those in preschool, should be done with conditioned-play audiometry techniques (see Chapter 6) when needed. For most of the children, raising their hand when hearing a tone suffices. Typically, two to three presentations are given at each frequency. A child fails the screening if he or she does not give an appropriate re-

---

[3]Allowable octave band acceptable noise levels based on ANSI S3.1-1999(R2013) and for screening at 20 dB HL are 41, 46, 54, and 57 dB SPL for 500, 1000, 2000, and 4000 Hz, respectively.

sponse at 20 dB HL for any of the three screening frequencies, for either ear. If a child fails the initial screening, it is recommended that he or she be rescreened again during the same day. A child who fails the pure-tone rescreening should be referred for a complete audiologic evaluation.

In addition to screening by air conduction, screening for outer and middle ear disorders is recommended. This can be done by otoscopic inspection, tympanometry, and/or through a brief questionnaire sent to the parents. A child should be referred for a medical examination if the screening finds drainage in the ear canal, structural abnormality, foreign object, impacted cerumen, infection, tympanic membrane abnormality, or perforation (e.g., flat tympanogram with large ear canal volume not due to pressure equalization tube). The AAA (2011) criteria for tympanogram failures are admittance at the tympanic membrane (Y_{tm}) < 0.2 mmho, tympanometric peak pressure (TPP) < –200 daPa, and/or tympanometric width (TW) > 250 daPa. Except for a perforation or foreign object, children who fail the tympanometry should be rescreened in 4 to 6 weeks. If tympanogram abnormalities are found on the rescreening, the child should be referred for a medical examination. If tympanometry is not included in a screening program, the addition of 500 Hz should be included with the pure-tone screening if the testing environment has acceptable background noise levels.

SCREENING THE HEARING OF ADULTS

Hearing screenings for adults has not received as much attention as screening of children. However, given that hearing disorders can be acquired during the adult years, and often progresses during the senior years, hearing screenings of adults may be the first place where an adult might feel comfortable finding out if they have a hearing problem. Screening is recommended every 10 years up to 50 years of age, and every three years above 50 years of age (AAA, 2011; ASHA 2017). Health fairs or senior centers are places where adult hearing screening might be conducted. Pure-tone air conduction screening

should be performed at 25 dB HL (ASHA, 2017) at 1000, 2000, and 4000 Hz. Otoscopic examination should also be included. A questionnaire is also helpful, and should include questions about any perceived hearing loss (one or both ears), its time course (sudden onset or gradual), ear drainage, ear pain, tinnitus, and/or dizziness. If any of these problems are identified, further medical and audiologic evaluations should be recommended. In addition, self-assessment communication scales of hearing disabilities have been developed and are available for screening adults. Some examples of valid, reliable, and normed hearing screening scales include the *Hearing Handicap Inventory for the Elderly-Screening* (Ventry & Weinstein, 1983) and the *Self-Assessment for Communication* (Schow & Nerbonne, 1982).

SCREENING OUTCOMES AND EFFICACY

Screenings are designed to separate those who have a high probability of having the targeted disorder from those who have a low probability of the targeted disorder. The pass or fail outcomes of a screening imply that there is a way to validate the results through some other follow up indicator, referred to as the *gold standard*, to determine whether those who fail the screening actually have the disorder, and whether those who pass the screening truly do not have the disorder. Results from a gold standard test are generally accepted as proof that the disorder or disease exists. For example, an acceptable diagnostic test to determine the amount of a sensorineural hearing loss is pure-tone audiometry. In the case of newborns or young infants, diagnostic ABRs might be a better gold standard. In the case of infant hearing screening, confirmation of a sensorineural loss might be delayed until pure-tone audiometry can confirm the results. On the other hand, it is possible that the outcome at the time of screening was valid, but the delayed outcome was different because the hearing problem resolved as in the case of middle ear problems, or the hearing loss developed between the time of the screening and the time that the gold standard audiometric testing was able to be performed.

Test Outcome	Disorder Present	Disorder Absent	TOTALS
FAIL (positive for disorder)	True positives (TP) HIT	False positives (FP)	TP+TP
PASS (negative for disorder)	False negatives (FN) MISS	True negatives (TN)	FN+TN
TOTALS	Total Present = TP + FN	Total Absent = TN + FP	TP+FP+ FN+TN

$$\text{SENSITIVITY} = \frac{TP}{TP + FN}$$

$$\text{SPECIFICITY} = \frac{TN}{TN + FP}$$

$$\text{Positive Predictive Value} = \frac{TP}{TP + FP}$$

$$\text{Negative Predictive Value} = \frac{TN}{FN + TN}$$

FIGURE 13–5. Screening test matrix showing test outcomes (Fail or Pass) and actual patient condition (Disorder Present or Disorder Absent). Calculation components are shown from which one can derive sensitivity and specificity, as well as positive predictive value and negative predictive value.

The usefulness of any test, including screening tests, depends on its validity, which is an indication of how well a test measures what it is supposed to measure. Figure 13–5 presents a commonly used matrix (2 × 2) for a screening test. There are typically four outcomes to any screening test:

1. *True positive (a hit)*. The test correctly identifies the targeted disorder.
2. *True negative*. The test correctly identifies the absence of the targeted disorder.
3. *False positive*. The test incorrectly identifies the targeted disorder (says the disorder is present, but the disorder turns out to be absent).
4. *False negative (a miss)*. The test incorrectly identifies the targeted disorder (says the disorder is absent, but the disorder turns out to be present).

With these four outcomes in mind, tests can be evaluated in terms of their:

1. *Sensitivity*. How well the test correctly identifies the targeted disorder (proportion of true positives).
2. *Specificity*. How well the test correctly identifies those without the targeted disorder (proportion of true negatives).
3. *Positive predictive value*. The percentage of true positives for the test (i.e., the level of confidence one has in the true positive outcome).
4. *Negative predictive value*. The percentage of true negatives for the test (i.e., the level of confidence one has in the true negative outcome).

Figure 13–6 shows an example of the screening matrix using numbers to show the calculations of the above four characteristics of a screening test. A screening test's sensitivity is the propor-

Test Outcome	Disorder Present	Disorder Absent	TOTALS
FAIL (positive for disorder)	4	30	34
PASS (negative for disorder)	2	180	182
TOTALS	6	210	216

SENSITIVITY =

$$\frac{4}{6} = 66.6\%$$

SPECIFICITY =

$$\frac{180}{210} = 85.7\%$$

Positive Predictive Value = $\frac{4}{34}$ = 11.7%

Negative Predictive Value = $\frac{180}{182}$ = 98.9%

FIGURE 13–6. Example of screening test matrix with hypothetical values to show how the various test parameters are calculated. See Figure 13–5 for help in understanding how the numbers are derived.

tion of the true positive (TP) outcomes to the total who actually have the disease (TP + FN), whereas the specificity is the proportion of the true negative (TN) outcomes to those who actually do not have the disease (TN + FP). Although sensitivity and specificity are measures of how well a specific test is able to separate those with and without the targeted disorder, in a clinical setting the positive and negative predictive values may be more meaningful when trying to decide if a screening procedure is worth the effort, or if one is interested in knowing the probability for those patients who fail the screening to actually have the disease. The positive predictive value is the proportion of the true positive (TP) outcomes to those who failed the test (TP + FP).

Predictive values are dependent on the *prevalence* of the targeted disorder, as can be seen in Table 13–4. A test could have an intrinsically good sensitivity, but may have a low positive pre-

dictive value if the targeted disorder is extremely rare (there is a very low prevalence within the population being screened). If most of the tested population is expected to pass (and very few expected to fail), then an important consideration of a test's predictive value would be related to its specificity (i.e., one might want a high negative predictive value). In other words, if one is screening for a low prevalence disorder within a population, it may be important to have a test with a high specificity so that there are not too many unnecessary referrals. Of course, if the rare disorder has significant health consequences, one may want to develop a screening test that would maximize sensitivity so that most of those with the disorder are identified; however, this may also result in a low specificity and high over-referral rate. Strategic targeting of the screening population and/or sequential screening programs will increase the prevalence as the "filter" is applied

TABLE 13–4. Example of How Prevalence Can Affect Positive Predictive Value (*PPV*)

Prevalence	Test Outcome	Has Disorder	No Disorder	Totals	+PPV
	Fail	95	1485	1580	
1%	Pass	5	8415	8420	95/1580 = 6%
	Totals	100	9900	10,000	
	Fail	475	1425	1900	
5%	Pass	25	8075	8100	475/1900 = 25%
	Totals	500	9500	10,000	

Note. For a test with 95% sensitivity and 85% specificity, based on testing 10,000 people.

and will have a corresponding effect on the predictive values.

Of course, ideally you would want a test with 100% sensitivity (it always detected the disorder when the disorder was present) and 100% specificity (it always identified those without the disorder). Unfortunately, this "super test" does not exist for hearing screening or any of the diagnostic hearing tests (nor is it ever likely to exist). Therefore, screening or diagnostic tests must set a measurement criterion at a point that maximizes sensitivity and specificity. A conservative (lax) measurement criterion could be set so that the screening is sensitive enough to get 100% of those with the disease; however, there will be a corresponding decrease in the specificity (due to a higher false positive rate). The higher false positive rate may not be acceptable because of the resources needed for following up a large number who really do not have the disorder. A more liberal (strict) measurement criterion could be set in order to reduce the false positive rate; however, there will be a corresponding decrease in the sensitivity, meaning you will miss more of those who have the disorder. This concept of manipulating the measurement criterion to change sensitivity and specificity, referred to as receiver operating characteristics (ROC), is beyond the scope of this text; the interested reader is referred to Swets (1988) and Hyde (2011).

SYNOPSIS 13–2

- Screening for hearing loss in newborns is now in widespread use. With the advent of OAEs, universal screening of all newborns is an accepted standard of care in the United States and in many other countries.
- The JCIH (2007) states that infants should be screened for hearing loss at birth (with a physiological testing method), hearing loss identified by 3 months of age, and those with significant hearing loss be fit with hearing aids or cochlear implants before 6 months of age. A screening program is just the first step of a comprehensive program, which must also include close follow-up care, rehabilitation, counseling, and appropriate social and educational services.
- Newborn hearing screening programs use OAEs (TEOAEs or DPOAEs) and/or AABR to screen all babies before they are discharged from the hospital. Upon failing the screen, an immediate rescreen is recommended to reduce the number of false positives. False positive rates are generally less than 5%.

SYNOPSIS 13–2 (*continued*)

- Auditory neuropathy spectrum disorder *(ANSD)*, also called auditory dyssynchrony disorder, may account for up to 10% of children with hearing loss, and may be missed by screening programs relying solely on OAEs (Sininger, 2002) because this disorder is characterized by normal OAE and abnormal ABR.

- Hearing screening is recommended for all preschool and school-aged children through the 3rd grade, and those in 7th and 11th grades.

- Pure-tone hearing screening of preschool and school-aged children should include air conduction frequencies of 1000, 2000, and 4000 Hz at 20 dB HL. If a child fails the initial screening, he or she should be rescreened the same day. A child who fails the rescreening should be referred for a complete audiological evaluation.

- Screening programs should also include a short history questionnaire, otoscopy, and tympanometry to identify middle ear disorders. A medical referral should be made if the screening finds drainage in the ear canal, structural abnormality, foreign object, impacted cerumen, infection, tympanic membrane abnormality, or perforation.

- The AAA (2011) criteria for tympanogram failures are $Y_{tm} < 0.2$ mmho, TPP < −200 daPa, and/or TW > 250 daPa. Children who show a flat tympanogram with normal ear canal volume or for those with an abnormally wide tympanogram should be rescreened in 4 to 6 weeks.

- Health fairs or senior centers are places where adult hearing screening might be conducted. In addition to otoscopy, audiometry, and tympanometry, adults are often screened through questionnaires designed for self-assessment of their communication and hearing abilities.

- Figure 13–5 presents a commonly used matrix of outcomes for a screening test resulting in true positives (a hit), true negatives, false positives, and false negatives (a miss).

- Sensitivity = how well a test correctly identifies the targeted disorder (proportion of true positives); specificity = how well a test correctly identifies those without the targeted disorder (proportion of true negatives).

REFERENCES

American Academy of Audiology [AAA]. (2011). Childhood hearing screening guidelines. Retrieved from http://audiology-web.s3.amazonaws.com/migrated /ChildhoodScreeningGuidelines.pdf_5399751c9 ec216.42663963.pdf

American Academy of Audiology [AAA]. (2012). American Academy of Audiology Clinical Practice Guidelines. (2012). Audiologic guidelines for the assessment of hearing in young infants and children [Guidelines]. Retrieved from www.audiology.org /resources/documentlibrary/Documents/201208 _AudGuideAssessHear_youth.pdf

American National Standards Institute [ANSI]. (1999). Maximum permissible ambient noise levels for audiometric test rooms *ANSI S3.1-1999*. New York, NY: Author.

American Speech-Language-Hearing Association [ASHA]. (n.d.). Expert panel recommendations on newborn hearing screening. Retrieved from http://www.asha

.org/Topics/Expert-Panel-Recommendations-on-Newborn-Hearing-Screening/#3

Andermann, A., Blancquaert, I., Beauchamp, S., & Dery, V. (2008). Revisiting Wilson and Jungner in the genomic age: A review of screening criteria over the past 40 years. *Bulletin of the World Health Organization, 86*(4), 317–319.

Center for Disease Control [CDC]. (2014). 2014 CDC EHDI Hearing Screening & Follow-up Survey (HSFS). Retrieved from https://www.cdc.gov/ncbddd/hearingloss/ehdi-data2014.html

Cooper, J. C., Gates, G. A., Owen, J. H., & Dickson, H. D. (1975). An abbreviated impedance bridge technique for school screening. *Journal of Speech and Hearing Disorders, 40*, 260–269.

Downs, M. P., & Sterritt, G. M. (1967). A guide to newborn and infant hearing screening programs. *Archives of Otolaryngology, 85*, 15–22.

Driscoll, C. J., & McPherson, B. (2010). *Newborn Screening Systems*. San Diego, CA: Plural.

Durieux-Smith, A., Picton, T., Edwards, C., Goodman, J. T., & MacMurray, B. (1985). The Crib-O-Gram in the NICU: An evaluation based on brain stem electric response audiometry. *Ear and Hearing, 6*, 20–24.

Hall, J. W. (2007). *New Handbook of Auditory Evoked Potentials*. Boston, MA: Pearson Education, Inc.

Hyde, M. (Ed.) (2011). *Principles and Methods of Population Hearing Screening in EHDI*. San Diego, CA: Plural.

Joint Committee on Infant Hearing [JCIH]. (2007). Position statement: Principles and guidelines for early hearing detection and intervention programs. *Pediatrics, 120*, 898–921.

Leigh, G., Taljaard, D., & Poulakis, Z. (2010). *Newborn Hearing Screening*. San Diego, CA: Plural.

Ling, D., Ling, A. H., & Doehring, D. G. (1970). Stimulus, response, and observer variables in the auditory screening of newborn infants. *Journal of Speech and Hearing Research, 13*(1), 9–18.

NCHAM. (2017). A Resource Guide for Early Hearing Detection & Intervention. Retrieved from http://infanthearing.org/ehdi-ebook/

Northern, J., & Downs, M. P. (2014). *Hearing in Children* (6th ed.). San Diego, CA: Plural.

Project HEID. (2004). *Improving Outcomes for Children with Permanent Congenital Hearing Impairment: The Case for a National Newborn Hearng Screening and Early Intervention Programme for New Zealand*. Auckland, New Zealand: National Foundation for the Deaf.

Schow, R. L., & Nerbonne, M. A. (1982). Communication screening profile: Use with elderly clients. *Ear and Hearing, 3*(3), 135–147.

Sininger, Y. S., & Oba, S. (2001). Patients with auditory neuropathy: Who are they and what can they hear? In Y. S. Sininger & A. Starr (Eds.), *Auditory neuropathy*. San Diego, CA: Singular.

Sininger, Y. S. (2002). Auditory neuropathy in infants and children: Implications for early hearing detection and intervention programs. *Audiology Today Special Edition*, 16–21.

Spivak, L. G. (2007). Neonatal hearing screening, followup and diagnosis. In R. J. Roeser, M. Valente, & H. Hosford-Dunn (Eds.), *Audiology diagnosis* (2nd ed., pp. 497–513). New York, NY: Thieme.

Swets, J. A. (1988). Measuring the accuracy of diagnostic systems. *Science, 240*, 1285–1293.

Tharpe, A. M., & Seewald, R. (2017). *Comprehensive Handbook of Pediatric Audiology* (2nd ed.). San Diego, CA: Plural.

Thompson, M., & Thompson, G. (1972). Response of infants and young children as a function of auditory stimuli and test methods. *Journal of Speech and Hearing Research, 15*(4), 699–707.

U.S. Preventive Services Task Force. (2008). *Universal Screening for Hearing Loss in Newborns; Topic Page*. Rockville, MD: Agency for Health Care Research and Quality.

Ventry, I. M., & Weinstein, B. (1983). Identification of elderly people with hearing problems. *ASHA, 25*, 37–47.

Vohr, B., Carty, L. M., Moore, P. E., & Letourneau, K. (1998). The Rhode Island hearing assessment program: Experience with statewide hearing screening. *Pediatrics, 139*, 353–357.

14 Hearing Aids

H. Gustav Mueller

After reading this chapter, you should be able to:

1. Describe the current status of dispensing hearing aids, and how the business of dispensing hearing aids has changed over the years.

2. Determine the current trends in hearing aids usage.

3. Explain the function of each of the basic components of hearing aids.

4. Provide a brief description of additional features of modern hearing aids.

5. Describe and differentiate the basic styles of hearing aids.

6. Identify basic earmold styles, along with their different functions and acoustic effects.

7. Identity at least four potential benefits of bilateral/binaural versus unilateral fittings of hearing aids.

8. Describe the importance of establishing an evidenced-based rationale for the fitting of hearing aids.

9. Describe what is meant by hearing aid verification, and explain real-ear (probe-microphone) measurements and why this is recommended to verify hearing aid performance.

10. Describe hearing aid validation, and how self-assessment inventories can be used to evaluate different domains.

The fitting of hearing aids is a key component to the overall treatment and rehabilitative audiology program for many patients with permanent hearing loss. While it is possible that simply obtaining some form of amplification is all that is needed (e.g., a consumer buys a pair of hearing aids on eBay), the audiologist has an important role in the comprehensive selection and fitting procedure, coupled with appropriate counseling at several stages before, during, and after the fitting of the hearing aids. Various types of auditory and acclimatization training may also be included for some patients. The general workflow for the treatment process involving hearing aids is shown in Table 14–1.

WHO DISPENSES HEARING AIDS

The term hearing aid dispenser may refer to either an audiologist or a hearing instrument specialist (non-audiologist), both of whom may legally dispense hearing aids if they have a professional license to do so in their state of practice. Audiologists in many states can dispense hearing aids as part of their audiology license; however, in some states, they must also hold a separate dispensing license. A hearing instrument special-ist must have a hearing aid dispenser's license. In addition to a state dispensing license, hearing aid dispensers may also choose to have special certifications. The most popular certification is the Board Certified in Hearing Instrument Services (BC-HIS). Board certification is not required for audiologists to dispense hearing aids; however, a state license is always required.

Following the American Speech-Language-Hearing Association (ASHA) change in ethics in 1977 that allowed audiologists to dispense/sell hearing aids, there was a sharp increase in the opening of audiology private practices with the purpose of dispensing hearing aids. The enthusiasm at the time was reflected in the name of a new audiology organization formed the same year, the Academy of Dispensing Audiologists (now the Academy of Doctors of Audiology). Today, most audiologists are involved with *hearing aids*, including selecting, fitting, testing, and dispensing/selling of the instruments. In addition, many audiologists are employed by hearing aid manufacturers in areas of research and development, consumer education, and as product representatives.

The hearing aid distribution channels, however, are changing, as Big Box stores have begun to dispense hearing aids in recent years. For example, it is estimated that Costco's market share of U.S. hearing aid sales is over 10%; many of

TABLE 14–1. Typical Workflow for the Selection and Fitting of Hearing Aids

- Step 1. Assessment: Determine the extent and cause of hearing loss. Determine candidacy for hearing aids based on pure-tone hearing loss, self-assessment inventories, and patient history.

- Step 2. Treatment Planning: Review the assessment results with the patient and/or family members. Identify areas of difficulty and explore different amplification options.

- Step 3. Selection: Determine the type of fitting (style, etc.). Decide on electroacoustic parameters and what special features are needed.

- Step 4. Verification: Determine that the hearing aids meet a set of standardized measures, including electroacoustic performance and patient's real-ear match to desired levels (presumably based on validated prescriptive targets). The hearing aids also should have good sound quality, be comfortable to wear, and have acceptable cosmetics.

- Step 5. Orientation: Counsel the patient on the use and care of the hearing aids. Discuss hearing aid adjustments and realistic expectations. Determine the need for a more comprehensive audiologic rehabilitation program.

- Step 6. Validation: Assess the effectiveness of the use of hearing aids in the patient's everyday environment, through the use of patient interview and/or formal self-assessment inventories of benefit and satisfaction. Readdress areas of need regarding the fitting.

Source: From Mueller and Hall, 1998. Copyright 1998 by Cengage.

their employees are audiologists. Also, more and more of the private audiology dispensing practices are being bought by the major manufacturers, and this has resulted in a serious decline in private audiology practices. Even when the hearing aid manufacturer does not own the business, in many cases the manufacturer has provided financing for the purchase, and indirectly, the audiologist is tied to that manufacturer's products. Finally, what may be the biggest game-changer in the distribution system is the current efforts to develop a new category of hearing aids that will be sold over-the-counter (OTC), often referred to as *Personal Sound Amplification Products (PSAPs)*.

ASHA's Change in Ethics

Although audiologists have always been involved in the process of selection and fitting of hearing aids, the actual business of "dispensing" (selling) hearing aids has changed over the years. Until the mid-1970s, once the appropriate hearing aids had been selected, the patient was referred by the audiologist to a licensed hearing aid dispenser to purchase the recommended hearing aids. The reason for using an outside dispenser as a middleman was that the selling of hearing aids was considered unethical by ASHA, although audiologists working in Veterans' Hospitals were allowed to dispense hearing aids free of charge. After the hearing aid dispenser fit and ordered the hearing aids, the patient usually would return to the audiologist for an evaluation or "approval" of the fitting. As one might guess, this practice often led to controversy, with the patient in the middle, as two professionals easily could disagree on what was "best" for a given patient. The ASHA ethical guidelines were changed around 1977 to allow audiologists to directly dispense hearing aids.

PSAPS and OTC Hearing Aids

Two slightly different but related issues facing the dispensing of hearing aids for audiologists to consider is the role of Personal Sound Amplification Products (PSAPs; pronounced "PEE-SAPs") and the over-the-counter (OTC) sale of hearing aids (or PSAPs, which may or may not be called hearing aids). The Food and Drug Administration (FDA) has issued guidance saying that a PSAP is not intended to make up for impaired hearing. Rather, they are intended for non-hearing-impaired consumers to amplify sounds in the environment—hunters, for example. The fact is, however, that many of the advanced PSAPs clearly are designed for individuals with hearing loss (you do not need 14 frequency channels, noise reduction, and directional microphones to hear a pheasant squawk!). It is, of course, possible that the OTC product of the future will be equal to the current products sold by audiologists. Or, audiologists will be selling OTC products. This is all very fluid, and by the time you read this, we may have seen changes.

CURRENT HEARING AID USAGE TRENDS

Data from the National Institute of Deafness and other Communication Disorders (NIDCD) suggest that approximately 15% of American adults (37.5 million) aged 18 and over report some trouble hearing. It is estimated that around 90 to 95% of hearing impaired individuals can be helped with hearing aids, at least for some listening conditions. For the current U.S. population, that would indicate that there are over 30 million people for whom hearing aids would be of some benefit. Yet, we know from other NIDCD data that among adults aged 70 and older with hearing loss who could benefit from hearing aids, fewer than one in three (30%) has ever used them. Even fewer adults 20 to 69 years of age (approximately 16%), who could benefit from wearing hearing aids, have never used them. This suggests that there may be an untapped market of 20 million or more individuals in the United States in need of hearing aids.

As reviewed by Mueller and Johnson (2014), some industry leaders believe that the untapped market is not as large as 20 million due to an overestimation of the pool of potential hearing aid consumers; just because a person has an admitted hearing loss does not mean a hearing aid is needed or that he or she is interested in using hearing aids. Data show that only about 1/3 of the people with admitted hearing loss perceive themselves as having significant need for hearing aids. This adjusted potential market for hearing aids, therefore, may be closer to about 11 million, based on the current estimate of people in the United States who have a hearing impairment (NIDCD, 2016).

According to recent data from the Hearing Industry Association (HIA), over 3.6 million hearing aids are sold each year in the United States (Strom, 2017). However, since about 80% of hearing aids are sold in pairs (for bilateral fittings), only about 1.62 million people actually purchase hearing aids each year. The unit volume of hearing aid sales has been slow to increase over time, considering that 1 million hearing aids were sold for the first time back in 1983. In 2004, the unit volume of hearing aid sales slowly climbed to about 2 million; however, sales have increased (up 5 to 7%) more rapidly in recent years, that is, 8.5% in 2016 (Strom, 2017), due mostly to increased purchases by the VA and large retail stores (Mueller et al., 2014).

Not surprisingly, the prevalence of hearing loss increases with increasing age; approximately 314 in 1000 people over age 65 have hearing loss, and 40 to 50% of people 75 and older have hearing loss. Although we know that decreased hearing sensitivity is part of the aging process, the majority (65%) of the 320 million people with hearing loss are under the age of 65. Hearing aid use within this younger majority is significantly less than the already disturbing low 20 to 25% figure mentioned earlier. And we know, of course, that individuals with hearing loss have problems understanding speech. But in addition to this obvious difficulty, we also know that hearing loss is associated with other serious negative consequences such as academic difficulties, various problems in the workplace, and psychosocial problems such as social isolation, depression, anxiety, loneliness, and lessened self-efficacy (see review by Mueller et al., 2014). Here are some general findings:

- Three in 10 people over age 60 have hearing loss.
- One in six baby boomers (ages 41 to 59), or 14.6%, have a hearing problem.
- One in 14 generation Xers (ages 29 to 40), or 7.4%, already have hearing loss.
- At least 1.4 million children (18 or younger) have hearing problems.

Untreated Hearing Loss Can Have Negative Consequences

Data from MarkeTrak9 (Abrams and Kihm, 2015) revealed that individuals who recently purchased hearing aids had known that they had a hearing loss for an average of 13 years. This delay in acting is important to consider when we view the negative consequences of untreated hearing loss:

- Irritability, negativism, and anger
- Fatigue, tension, stress, and depression
- Avoidance or withdrawal from social situations
- Social rejection and loneliness
- Reduced alertness and increased risk to personal safety
- Impaired memory and ability to learn new tasks
- Reduced job performance and earning power
- Diminished psychological and overall health

- It is estimated that 3 in 1000 infants are born with severe to profound hearing loss.

As discussed earlier, market penetration regarding hearing aid use is relatively poor. Why is this? As part of MarkeTrak VII, Kochkin examined some of the obstacles to hearing aid use for adults. One area that emerged as significant was the effects of age—that is, there is a perception that the use of hearing aids is probably okay for older people, but not okay for younger people. Konchkin (2007) found that, as expected, the use of hearing aids increases with the degree of loss for all age groups; however, age also has a strong influence. For example, in individuals with a moderate hearing loss, the hearing aid use rate is over 60% for individuals over 75 years of age, but only around 20% for those with moderate hearing loss in the 55 to 64 year age range. The 55 to 64 year age range group would have to be in the severe to profound hearing loss range before their hearing aid adoption would exceed 60%.

There are many other interwoven reasons to explain why hearing-impaired people are reluctant to use hearing aids. The leading reason is the type of hearing loss (Konchkin, 2007). Many individuals believe that there is something unique

Hearing Aids Can Lead to Positive Consequences

Research by the National Council on the Aging, on more than 2000 people with hearing loss, as well as their significant others, demonstrated that hearing aids clearly are associated with substantial improvements in the social, emotional, psychological, and physical well-being of people with hearing loss in all hearing loss categories from mild to severe. Specifically, hearing aid usage is positively related to the following quality of life issues:

- Earning power
- Communication in relationships
- Intimacy and warmth in family relationships
- Ease in communication
- Emotional stability
- Sense of control over life events
- Perception of mental functioning
- Physical health
- Group social participation

SYNOPSIS 14–1

- A comprehensive selection and fitting procedure should consist of the following steps (see Table 14–1 for details):
  - *Assessment* of hearing loss and candidacy for hearing aids
  - *Treatment* planning to review results and options with patient
  - *Selection* of hearing aid style, electroacoustic parameters, and any special features
  - *Development* of a formalized gold standard based on validated prescriptive algorithms
  - Verification that hearing aids meet expected performance standards and/or targets, both electroacoustically and with real-ear measures
  - *Orientation* on the use and care of the hearing aids, providing realistic expectations, and determining need for other rehabilitation
  - *Validation* measures to assess the patient's subjective satisfaction and benefit to determine any changes that might be needed

SYNOPSIS 14-1 (*continued*)

- Hearing aid selection and fitting have always been part of audiology practice; however, the actual selling of hearing aids by audiologists was not sanctioned by the profession until the late 1970s.
- There appears to be a large and growing untapped population who may benefit from hearing aids; however, the ability of the hearing aid industry to increase the penetration rate has remained relatively constant over the years.
- Hearing aid usage is only about 25% of people with a hearing loss. The primary reason for the relatively low penetration rate is that people think that hearing aids will not help them or that the cost is too high or that there is a social stigma attached to their use.

about their hearing loss that would make hearing aids not beneficial. Other factors include the cost and the social stigma associated with the use of hearing aids. Many simply believe that wearing hearing aids is a sign of "being old." It was believed by many that with all the currently available ear-level Bluetooth devices used by young people with normal hearing, these perceptions would change, but no data has emerged to show that this has happened.

Thus far, we have not presented very much good news, but here is something very important to remember—hearing aids work! Unfortunately, many prospective users simply are unaware of the fact that receiving early treatment for hearing loss has the potential to literally transform their lives. So, as professionals, we know that if we use the correct hearing aid selection and fitting procedures, good things will likely happen. We can only hope that these good things are passed along to other prospective users, and we begin to close the gap between those who need hearing aids and those who use them.

ASSESSMENT OF HEARING AID CANDIDACY AND TREATMENT PLANNING

The first step an audiologist needs to do before the selection and fitting of hearing aids is to determine if the patient is a suitable candidate for amplification. This decision typically begins with an assessment of the extent and cause of the hearing loss, and if there is any need for medical referral. When medical issues have been considered/resolved, there are several audiometric, personal, and psychological factors that have an impact on *hearing aid candidacy*. In many respects, the most straightforward factor is the hearing loss. In general, to be considered a candidate, the person should have a hearing loss (e.g., hearing thresholds of 25 dB or worse) in the frequency range of the key speech sounds (e.g., 500 to 4000 Hz). Because most hearing losses are downward sloping, a marginal candidate would be someone with normal hearing through 2000 Hz and a sloping hearing loss at 3000 Hz and above. If hearing is normal through 3000 Hz, the patient may or may not benefit with a hearing aid, and it is very unlikely that someone with normal hearing through 4000 Hz would be considered a candidate for hearing aids.

For the potential new hearing aid user, who still might be questioning the need for hearing aids, it might be necessary to illustrate how much of the average speech signal is *not* audible. For the experienced hearing aid user who is obtaining a new pair of hearing aids, it might be helpful to explain why the new hearing aids sound different from the old ones. For example, if more high frequency gain is being added, an explanation of the importance of these speech cues might encourage the user to be more accepting of this new amplification strategy. These visual demonstrations can also be very helpful for family members, who might be wondering why Mom can "hear but not understand."

There are several methods that utilize the patient's pure-tone audiogram for pre-fitting counseling. Some are more detailed than others, and the method selected often relates to the sophistication of the patient, the level of interest in learning about hearing loss, and how the loss might impact speech understanding. When we plot the *long-term average speech signal (LTASS)* on the dB HL scale, its outline more or less resembles a banana (refer to Chapter 8, Figure 8–3). This is commonly used for counseling patients regarding their hearing loss. Some audiologists have only the banana shaded on the audiogram, other audiograms or forms have symbols of common environmental sounds, or the various speech consonants/vowels displayed; this is a common option in the software of computer-based audiometers.

We have found the count-the-dot audiogram, shown in Figure 14–1, to be particularly helpful when counseling patients who are in denial

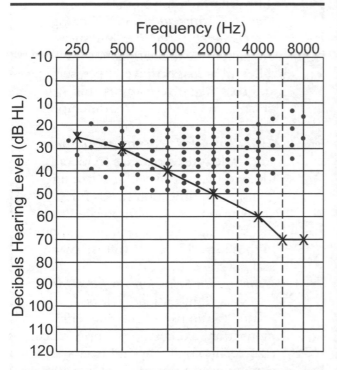

FIGURE 14–1. Count the dots audiogram displaying the 2010 Killion and Mueller count-the-dots SII speech spectrum with superimposed patient thresholds.

Pick Your Banana Carefully!

As mentioned, it is common to place the speech banana (average LTASS with percentiles) on the audiogram and use this for counseling. There have been several studies of defining average speech over the years, and LTASS findings do vary somewhat from study to study, but they are more or less in good agreement. So why is it then, that if we would do a Google image search on *Speech Banana* today, we find audiograms (apparently used in offices and clinics somewhere) with the 1000 to 2000 Hz frequency region of the LTASS ranging anywhere from 15 to 45 dB for the upper boundary and 40 to 70 dB for the lower boundary, with everything in between also used. A 25 dB difference! Since this is a fundamental concept of audiology, wouldn't it be nice if we all could get it right? We recently saw a speech banana in the software of a major hearing aid manufacturer that was plotted 10 to 15 dB too low on the audiogram.

Imagine if you took your three-year-old son in for testing, and the audiometric results revealed that he had a 35 dB loss (or is it really a loss?). If he were tested at Clinic A, where they use the 15 to 45 dB banana, you would be told that your son was missing about two-thirds of the important sounds of average speech. On the other hand, if he were tested at Clinic B, where the audiologists use the 40 to 70 dB speech banana, you would be told that all is well—he is hearing 100% of average speech! In our opinion, this borders on malpractice, as a child suffering from middle ear effusion, which often results in a hearing loss of 30 to 35 dB, might go untreated for months or years, simply because the parents were given the wrong counseling based on the wrong banana. In general, we recommend using a spectrum that has the soft components for the mid-frequencies around 20 to 25 dB HL, with the loud components of the LTASS at 50 to 55 dB HL.

regarding the degree of handicap that they might have (Killion & Mueller, 2010). Everyone can relate to the use of a percentage to make the point. Graphically, showing someone that they are missing 80% of average speech when they have just said they hear everything can be a convincing message. Patients often forget much of what we tell them during the pre-fitting counseling process, but they usually remember the percentage of dots they could (or could not) hear!

In Figure 14–1, you can see a typical sloping hearing loss plotted on the count-the-dots audiogram. To predict the SII, you would count the audible dots (above thresholds), which in this case there are 21 audible dots. In other words, this patient is only hearing 21% of average speech. Importantly, this is what he or she hears and not necessarily what is being understood, which depends on many other factors.

In addition to the pure-tone thresholds, it is useful to know the point where loud sounds become uncomfortable for the patient, referred to the patient's loudness discomfort level (LDL) or uncomfortable level (UCL). This is accomplished by presenting pure-tone signals at increasingly louder inputs until the rating of "Uncomfortably Loud" is reached—the patient is provided a 7-point chart of loudness anchors to assist in making the loudness perceptual judgments. These measured LDLs (usually conducted at two different frequencies) are then later used for programming the maximum power output (MPO) of the hearing aids at the time of the fitting. Results from speech-in-noise tests are also used in determining hearing aid candidacy. That is, a person may be having much greater speech communication difficulties in everyday situations than would be suggested by the audiogram alone. An audiologist must also consider whether a hearing loss is too severe for amplification using conventional hearing aids, in which case they must decide on whether to recommend a cochlear implant. There are guidelines available to help make these distinctions, and often the decision is based on a combination of factors, including degree of impairment and the benefit that can be obtained using conventional hearing aids, coupled with the desires of the patient.

Pre-fitting Self-Assessment Tools

There have been many pre-fitting inventories that have been introduced over the years. Here are some that we believe are useful, each of which provides unique information (from Mueller et al., 2014):

- *Hearing Handicap Inventory for the Elderly/Adult (HHIE/A)*. Measures the degree of handicap for emotional and social issues related to hearing loss.
- *Abbreviated Profile of Hearing Aid Benefit (APHAB)*. Provides the percentage of problems the patient has for three different listening conditions involving speech understanding (in quiet, in background noise, and in reverberation) and problems related to annoyance of environmental sounds (averseness scale) (http://harlmemphis.org/).
- *Expected Consequences of Hearing Aid Ownership (ECHO)*. Measures the patient's expectations for four different areas: positive effect, service and cost, negative features, and personal image (http://harlmemphis .org/).
- *Client Oriented Scale of Improvement (COSI)*. Requires patients to identify three to five very specific listening goals/communication needs for amplification. Can then be used to measure patients' expectations related to these specific goals (https://www .nal.gov.au/).
- *Hearing Aid Selection Profile (HASP)*. Assesses eight patient factors related to the use of hearing aids: motivation, expectations, appearance, cost, technology, physical needs, communication needs, and lifestyle.

The patient's opinions about the use of hearing aids, of course, are critical to determining candidacy. First, the patient must believe that the hearing loss is causing a problem: A mild high-frequency hearing loss could be a problem for a schoolteacher, but perhaps not a problem at all for a retired person living alone. Second, the patient must have a desire to obtain treatment (the wearing of hearing aids). Along with this comes the "ownership" of the hearing problem and the desire to make things better. It is common for family members to coax or even push a loved one into the audiologist's office for the fitting of hearing aids. To satisfy his or her family, these individuals often purchase hearing aids, but the chances are low that they will become satisfied hearing aid users. The prudent audiologist needs to pull together all the audiometric data and then carefully examine the thoughts and feelings of the patient when hearing aid candidacy is being decided. There are several self-assessment inventories that can be used to help determine a patient's readiness for hearing aid use. These inventories measure such things as motivation, expectations, and perceived handicap and disability.

SELECTION

Basic Hearing Aid Components and Technology

Other than miniaturization, the basic technology of a hearing aid has remained the same over the years, that is, the system must detect an acoustic signal, amplify it (which means a power source is needed), and then deliver it to the ear. While earlier instruments were based on analog amplification technology, today essentially all hearing aids use digital amplification technology. The basic components of a *digital hearing aid* are shown in Figure 14–2 and described in the following list:

- Microphone: An auditory transducer, which converts the acoustic signal from the sound field into an electrical signal that goes to the amplifier. Nearly all hearing aids today

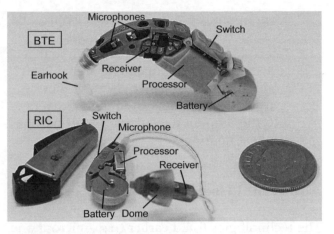

FIGURE 14–2. Two types of BTE hearing aids with their main components.

have two microphones, which allows for special directional processing.

- Digital conversion: The electrical signal is converted into digital information to allow for computerized signal manipulation and application of different processing algorithms. The digital signal is subsequently reconverted to an electrical signal that is sent to the receiver.
- Amplifier: The heart of the hearing aid circuitry where the input signal is increased in level and filtered in frequency, and then sent to the digital converter. This chip also includes algorithms for all special signal processing features of the hearing aid.
- Receiver: An auditory transducer (speaker) that converts the amplified signal from the hearing aid into an acoustical signal that is delivered to the patient's ear.
- Battery: Provides the power source for the hearing aid. Batteries come in different sizes to match the size and power requirements of the hearing aid. Some models have rechargeable batteries.
- Volume control: Many hearing aids have a volume control that can be a wheel or button on the aid itself or could be a function part of a remote-control device that also can be used to change the

programmed settings. Volume also may be controlled with smart phone apps.

- Telecoil: An alternative input source that converts the electromagnetic signal from a telephone, an assistive listening device or a wide-area loop system and delivers it to the amplifier; available on all but the smallest hearing aids.

Additional Hearing Aid Features

The technologies listed earlier (e.g., microphone, amplifier, etc.) are essential to provide basic amplification. Today's hearing aids, however, have many other features and algorithms designed to improve the amplified signal and to provide added audibility in different environments, more listening comfort, and easier operation for the patient. We will review a few of the features typically found on most of today's hearing aids:

- Multiple Channels: Digital hearing aids have between 4 and 48 frequency channels (frequency processing regions) allowing for adjustments in gain and output to be made in individual frequency regions that can compensate for a hearing loss. Although one might think that "more is better," and this is generally true, the differences are not as striking as they may seem.
- Multiple Memory Programs: A pushbutton or a remote control allows changes to the program settings. For example, they may have special programs for listening to music or listening in a car. For most situations, the hearing aid automatically selects the most optimum program for a given listening situation, as determined by the signal classification system.
- Signal Classification: Automatically and continually measures the input signal to determine overall level, spectrum of the signal (speech, noise, music, etc.), and azimuth of the signal in order to control features to automatically switch programs or to select the optimum processing for a given input signal. This classification

process is used to control gain and output, and to trigger noise reduction, directional microphones, or beam forming technologies.

- Compression (Automatic Gain Control): To prevent sounds becoming too loud to the listener there are two types of *compression*, *input* (AGCi or *wide dynamic range compression*, WDRC) and *output* (AGCo). These can be used together to provide different benefits to the patient. Input compression "repackages" the input signal so that it fits into the patient's useable dynamic range, whereas output compression assures that the "ceiling" of that dynamic range is not exceeded.
- Digital Noise Reduction: Based on the signal classification, different types of noise reduction are implemented, often simultaneously. Modulation-based tends to reduce over gain for a given channel when noise is the dominant signal in the channel. Fast filtering or spectral subtraction attempts to clean the signal and reduce noise in gaps. Most products also have an impulse noise reduction algorithm, designed to reduce annoying from harsh impulse sounds (e.g., clanking of dishes in a busy restaurant). Yet another type of noise reduction is for wind noise, which creates a unique turbulence at the input ports of the microphone, which make it easy to be classified by the hearing aid.
- Adaptive Feedback Reduction: Detects any acoustic *feedback* or "whistling" and reduces or eliminates the problem through phase cancellation. In most products, this allows the user an additional 5 to 15 dB of gain without feedback and is one of the most beneficial features introduced in hearing aids in recent years.
- Directional Microphone Technology: Reduces the output of the hearing aids for sounds from specific azimuth origins by using two omnidirectional microphones and creating phase delays between them. Sounds coming from the sides and back

or sides and front can be reduced without changing the output for sounds from the desired listening direction. For example, if the desired talker is in front, noise from the sides and back are reduced. On the other hand, if the desired speech is coming from the back (e.g., when listening to someone in the back seat while driving a car), this speech signal will be enhanced, while the sounds from the front and sides will be reduced.

- Linked Hearing Aids: Allows binaural hearing aids to "talk to each other" and share information through a type of near field magnetic induction transmission. This linking allows the patient to change a feature (e.g., volume) on one aid and the other aid will automatically equally change. The aid-to-aid communication has advanced to the point of allowing sharing of the audio signal between hearing aids.

- Binaural Beamformers (Bilateral Directional Microphone Technology): Bilateral hearing aids can share information from four microphones (two on each side) which allows for creating "beams of focus" for different azimuths. This gives a much narrower beam to the front than can be obtained with traditional directional technology. The focus of the beam will be in the "look direction" of the user.

- Frequency Lowering: This technology, using frequency compression or linear frequency transposition, takes the spectral speech energy available at higher frequencies and lowers it to a frequency region where the listener has better thresholds, increasing the likelihood that the speech signal (e.g., such as /s/ or /sh/) will be audible, albeit at a different frequency. This usually is applied when there is mild to moderate hearing loss in the low to mid frequencies, and a severe to profound loss in the high frequencies that is not usable for speech recognition with traditional amplification.

- Data Logging: Keeps a record of various listening situations experienced by the patient, such as the overall input level and signal-to-noise ratios for all listening situations, as well as the preferred attributes of the hearing aid function, such as volume control position and the listening program/memory setting. For example, after the patient has used the hearing aid for a period of time, the audiologist can read out (in the fitting software) the amount of time the aid (presumably on the patient's ear) was in different environments based on the data from the signal classification system.

- Trainable Hearing Aids: The ability to control or train the gain or output through direct patient control (patient-driven) or by the audiologist preprograming the device to make changes over time. Giving the patient some control allows him or her to become more vested in his or her hearing rehabilitation—getting the "best" fitting becomes a shared task between the patient and the audiologist. The hearing aid will "train" to the patient's favorite settings for a wide range of different listening situations. Audiologist-driven trainable hearing aids can be used to "auto acclimatize" the patient to the prescribed settings over the first several months of hearing aid usage—gain is slowly and automatically increased over time (several weeks or months).

- Wireless (Bluetooth) Connectivity: Wireless electromagnetic induction allows for binaural beamformers and linked hearing aids, and Bluetooth can be used to connect with smart phones, computers, personal audio players, and even navigations systems—this technology allows the patient to find a lost hearing aid with their smartphone. Additionally, the Bluetooth connectivity allows the audiologist to conduct remote hearing aid adjustments over the Internet.

FITTING STRATEGIES

As you now know, hearing aids today have some fascinating features, but these features are of little value if the hearing aids are not fitted appropriately. Potential hearing aid users are often asking what brand to buy. The truth is, the brands are all pretty much the same—what they should be asking is what audiologist is the best at fitting hearing aids, and providing post-fitting counseling. While a potential user could simply purchase a pair of hearing aids on eBay, it is the role of the audiologist to conduct a comprehensive individualized selection and fitting procedure, coupled with appropriate counseling at several stages before, during, and after the fitting of the hearing aids. Various types of auditory and acclimatization training may be included for some patients. We discuss specific fitting strategies later in this chapter, but we first need to address some fitting arrangement considerations.

Historical Vignette

The practice of audiology includes a wide range of areas and continues to expand. One area, however, which has been part of audiology practice from the beginning, is the selection and fitting of amplification devices called hearing aids. About the time that the word audiology was being coined in the mid 1940s, Dr. Raymond Carhart was involved with fitting returning World War II veterans with hearing aids at Deshon Army Hospital in Butler, Pennsylvania. This work prompted him to write an extensive hearing aid fitting protocol, and he carried this work experience on to his teachings at the first audiology program at Northwestern University. At the time, Northwestern University was a prominent training site for PhD audiologists, who subsequently went on to establish their own audiology training programs at universities across the United States. Portions of the original Carhart fitting protocol are still used in some clinics today.

Bilateral Hearing Aid Fittings

If you think of fitting hearing aids like fitting eyeglasses, then it would seem logical that two impaired ears would be fit with two hearing aids. Unfortunately, it is not quite that simple. Dispenser surveys reveal that in the United States, approximately 80% of patients are fitted bilaterally (Mueller et al., 2014). We know, however, that many of the people who purchase two hearing aids eventually become unilateral users. Although the monetary concerns of purchasing two versus one hearing aid are well understood (which partially accounts for the 20% who originally purchase one hearing aid), the decision to return or not use one of the hearing aids is not fully understood. It is difficult to identify the reason why these people do not obtain significant benefit with two hearing aids, but it may be related to the symmetry of the patient's hearing loss, the patient's central auditory processing capabilities, his ability to handle two instruments, as well as other unknown factors.

In theory, two hearing aids should provide more benefit than one for most individuals, and some of the common reasons cited for this are listed in Table 14–2. Given that most patients with relatively symmetrical hearing will benefit from a bilateral fitting, and the fact that it is difficult to identify those who will not benefit, it is generally recommended to start with a bilateral fitting arrangement; then, through follow-up visits, determine if the expected benefit is present.

CROS Hearing Aid Fittings

When the hearing loss in one ear is so severe that it is not able to use a hearing aid (unaidable), and the other ear has near normal hearing, the *contralateral routing of signals* (CROS) *hearing aid* fitting may be considered. The CROS arrangement transmits sounds that originate from the side of the head with the poor hearing ear over to the normal hearing ear. This involves placing a hearing aid on the poor hearing ear so that the

TABLE 14–2. Some Potential Benefits of a Bilateral versus Unilateral Hearing Aid Fitting

- Sound localization: Interaural cues for time, phase, intensity, and spectrum are required for localization in the horizontal plane.
- Speech understanding in noise: When inputs from both ears are compared in the central auditory system, there often is a "release" of noise, resulting in an improvement in the signal-to-noise ratio of 2 to 3 dB. Moreover, listening with two ears adds redundancy to the auditory system.
- Reduction of head shadow: When a hearing aid is worn on each ear, it is not necessary to position the head so the aided ear is near the talker.
- Loudness summation: At threshold, the summation effects for input from both ears are 2 to 3 dB. This effect can be as large as 5 to 8 dB at suprathreshold levels (less gain needed equals less feedback problems).
- Sound quality: When the input from two ears is balanced, and the perceived sound is "across the head," sound quality is rated higher than when the input is at an individual ear.

microphone can pick up the sounds on that side and transmit the electrical signals to the hearing aid receiver in the good ear. This gives the patient "two-sided" hearing, although not "two-eared" hearing. In other words, the sounds from the poor hearing side sound different than the sounds on the good hearing side because they are going through an electronic circuit. On the good hearing side, the sounds are more natural. If the good hearing ear also has a hearing loss, then a fitting called a *bilateral CROS* (BiCROS) may be used, in which a microphone is placed on both sides, and all sounds are amplified and channeled into the good ear.

As mentioned in the previous section, it is now possible to transfer full audio wirelessly from one hearing aid to another, and this is the preferred method to accomplish a CROS fitting today (years ago it was accomplished via a wire, or with FM transmission). It is also possible to use a *bone-anchored implantable* (BAI) hearing device to deliver a bone-conducted signal on the poor ear, which will be transferred to the cochlea of the good hearing ear (see Chapter 15 for more information). Although a CROS configuration with wireless transmission between conventional hearing aids works very well, some patients opt for this surgical approach.

SYNOPSIS 14–2

- Determining candidacy for hearing aids involves several factors. Generally, there should be some degree of hearing loss that involves the higher frequencies of the speech range. The decision should also include the needs, motivation, and abilities of the patient. Prefitting self-assessment questionnaires are available to assist in the process.
- The basic operation of a hearing aid involves components that detect an acoustic signal, amplify it, and then deliver it to the ear. Today, almost all hearing aids use some digital (computer chip) technology. The basic components of a hearing aid include: (a) microphone, (b) amplifier, (c) battery, (d) digital converter, (e) volume control, and (f) receiver. Some instruments include a *telecoil* for use with a telephone or loop system.
- Additional features and options available in hearing aids include: (a) multiple memory programs for different listening situations, (b) multiple frequency

---

SYNOPSIS 14–2 (*continued*)

channels, which can be individually adjusted to fit the hearing loss, (c) automatic gain control (AGC) on the input and output sides that limit the maximum levels to the patient and to adjust (compression) the gain depending on the level of sound, (d) signal classification, (e) directional microphone technology, (f) digital noise reduction circuits, (g) adaptive feedback reduction, (h) data logging of patient's real-world listening environment that can be used to train the hearing aid, and (i) linked hearing aids and wireless features.

- Bilateral fittings are generally recommended when there is a bilateral hearing loss, and about 80% of fittings are bilateral; however, some patients do not seem to obtain the expected benefit from two hearing aids, possibly due to asymmetric hearing loss, central auditory problems, difficulty handling the instruments, or other unknown reasons.
- CROS fittings are options for unilateral hearing loss. CROS hearing aids pick up sounds on the poorer hearing ear and transmit them to the better hearing ear. A BiCROS hearing aid arrangement is used when there also is a hearing loss in the "good" ear.

BASIC HEARING AID STYLES

Now that we have briefly reviewed the components and features of hearing aids, we will discuss the different styles that are available. There are five fundamental hearing aid styles. They are commonly referred to as: (1) body aid, (2) behind-the-ear (BTE or mini-BTE), (3) in-the-ear (ITE), (4) in-the-canal (ITC), and (5) completely-in-the-canal (CIC). These styles differ in size, in application, and in features and components. It is important not to confuse the hearing aid style with the technology contained within the hearing aid. Manufacturers have different models of hearing aids (with more features added for the more expensive models). However, a given product model will have the same digital processing chip across the various styles offered by a manufacturer, and, therefore, different styles of the same product model will tend to sound similar to the patient.

Body Hearing Aid

The *body aid* is seldom used in the United States today, but it is still commonly used in develop-

ing countries, as it is inexpensive to produce and does not require custom fitting. Simply described, it is a square or rectangular hearing aid worn on the body. The amplified signals are delivered to the ears by wires that connect to external receivers mounted in custom earmolds, headphones, or earbuds. From a design standpoint, these may look similar to an iPod or other digital music player. The main difference is that the hearing aid unit has a microphone to pick up environmental sounds, which are then amplified and sent to the earphones. Body aids typically do not have the sophisticated digital signal processing that is present in the other more common hearing aid styles.

Behind-the-Ear Hearing Aid (BTE)

The *behind-the-ear hearing aid*, called a BTE, is a hearing aid that is worn behind the ear (or one on each ear). The *traditional* BTE is a curve shaped unit that has a hard tube coming off the receiver end of the hearing aid, called the earhook, which rests on the helix of the auricle and helps keep the hearing aid unit in place behind

Earmolds

Earmolds come in various styles, ranging from large ones that fill the entire concha of the outer ear, to others that fit into the ear canal, or even some that are only a small piece of tubing or flexible tip that extends into the ear canal. The earmold's size, material, and other features (e.g., a small air vent) are determined by the audiologist when the earmold is ordered. Regardless of style, earmolds attach to the *earhook* of a traditional BTE via tubing and serve to route sound into the ear canal. With mini-BTEs, the thin tubing or the wire connector of the RIC attaches directly to the hearing aid. In general, the greater the hearing loss, the larger and tighter fitting the earmold needs to be to reduce the likelihood of feedback (whistling) that is related to the high gain requirements, and also to obtain the often necessary low-frequency amplification (e.g., low frequency sounds leak out of the ear when there is an open fitting).

the ear. The amplified sound from the hearing aid's receiver is delivered through the earhook and through a flexible tube attached from the earhook to a custom-made *earmold* that fits into the concha and/or ear canal. Different styles of ear molds are shown in Figure 14–3. Today, the traditional earhook and tubing usually are replaced with a one-piece thin tubing, or a wire that has the receiver at the end. There are two general categories of BTE, the traditional BTE and the mini-BTE.

Traditional BTE

The traditional BTE style (Figure 14–4) continues to be used for fitting some individuals with severe to profound hearing losses, individuals with visual or dexterity issues, and young infants and children with hearing loss. For severe to profound hearing losses, the BTE offers the benefit of increased gain and output compared with smaller hearing aid styles. In addition, the increased receiver-to-microphone distance separation is useful in reducing feedback (whistling) that can occur when high amounts of gain are required. The traditional BTE style is often selected for those with visual and dexterity issues because the hearing aid components (e.g., volume control and battery) are larger and more accessible than on smaller custom styles, and the hearing aid is easier to remove. The BTE style is also appropriate for an infant or young child because the outer ear will continue to grow for many years. In this situation, the earmold will need to be replaced every 6 months to 1 year due to the developmental changes. Purchasing a new earmold for a BTE is much easier and less expensive than the replacing required for some of the other models, where all the hearing aid components are housed within the custom shell casing. In addition, the child would not have to be without the hearing aid while the new earmold is being made, unlike the other styles where the entire hearing aid must be sent to the manufacturer for recasing. Because the traditional BTE is larger, it might have some features that are not available on the smaller instruments. One of these, important for children, is the ability for connectivity with remote FM systems—an excellent method to improve audibility and improve the signal-to-noise (SNR) ratio.

Mini-BTE (Receiver-in-the-Canal)

BTE style began losing market share with the development of smaller in-the-ear (ITE) instruments (see next section). This was, in part, due to the BTE's bulkiness, requirement for a separate earmold, and its overall cosmetic visibility. However, this trend began to turn around, beginning around 2003, with the advent of *mini-BTE hearing aids*.

One type of mini-BTE hearing aid has all the hearing aid components (microphone, amplifier, receiver, and battery) housed within the hearing aid casing, the same as for a traditional BTE, but the casing is typically smaller. In addition, the sound from the receiver is sent to the ear through a much thinner and smaller diameter tube (nearly invisible) than that used with

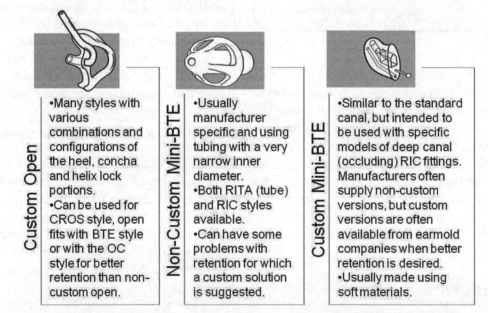

Full Shell
- Often used for more severe to profound hearing losses and younger children
- Canal portion can be made thicker (better seal), thinner (for better cosmetics), fitted with a snap ring instead of tubing (for body aid, powered stethoscopes, etc.), or the top portion of the canal can be removed (half shell).
- Can be difficult to insert if tight fitting.

Skeleton
- One of the more common styles used with traditional BTE hearing aids.
- Can be used with a wide range of hearing loss.
- Sometimes modified to remove the middle portion of the "ring" that fills the concha bowl (semi-skeleton).

Canal
- Not usually fit as tight, so it is more suitable for mild-moderate loss. Appropriate for some patients with severe hearing loss using soft materials. Retention can be a problem, though easier insertion than many styles.
- Can be modified with a "concha lock" or by hollowing out the canal (sometimes combined with soft material for a comfort fit for patients with large changes in earcanal size with jaw movement).

Custom Open
- Many styles with various combinations and configurations of the heel, concha and helix lock portions.
- Can be used for CROS style, open fits with BTE style or with the OC style for better retention than non-custom open.

Non-Custom Mini-BTE
- Usually manufacturer specific and using tubing with a very narrow inner diameter.
- Both RITA (tube) and RIC styles available.
- Can have some problems with retention for which a custom solution is suggested.

Custom Mini-BTE
- Similar to the standard canal, but intended to be used with specific models of deep canal (occluding) RIC fittings. Manufacturers often supply non-custom versions, but custom versions are often available from earmold companies when better retention is desired.
- Usually made using soft materials.

FIGURE 14–3. Advantages and limitations to a few common earmolds. This information is particularly useful when deciding on an earmold style within the constraints of individual patient differences, cosmetics, and gain requirements. *Source*: From Mueller, Ricketts, & Bentler, 2014, p. 299. Copyright 2014 by Plural Publishing, Inc.

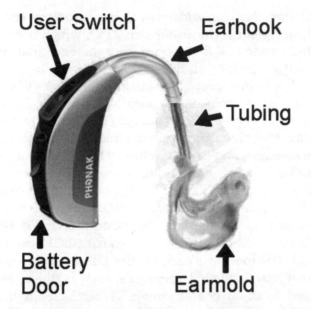

FIGURE 14–4. External features of a traditional BTE hearing aid with tubing and earmold attached. *Source*: Photo courtesy of Phonak, LLC and Westone® The In-Ear Experts®.

traditional BTEs. A second type of mini-BTE, by far the most popular, does not house the receiver in the casing, but instead places the receiver in the earmold (often simply a soft plastic sleeve), which is connected to the casing via an electrical wire encased in thin tubing (Figure 14–5). By removing the receiver from the hearing aid, the overall size of hearing aid can be reduced. This type of mini-BTE is usually called a receiver-in-the-canal or simply an RIC.

The mini-BTE RIC style hearing aid has become quite popular today because of its small case, thin tube, and open ear canal fitting. The open ear canal fitting is one in which the end of the tubing or the receiver is loosely inserted into the ear canal and held in place by an open earmold or tip made of a flexible, thin material that comes premade in a variety of sizes, thus allowing for more natural sound quality, a more comfortable feel, and no need for a custom earmold (see Figure 14–3; note small fitting tips on end). As we stated, these tend to be more comfortable than the standard earmold, but the downside is that they might not be tight enough if considerable gain is needed (too much leakage), they tend to work themselves out of the ear, and they

often need to be replaced after several months (something that patients can do themselves). Modern-day mini-BTE products are very light and can easily fall off the ear if the user bends over, and therefore, the eartip must also serve as a retention anchor. For these reasons, many audiologists continue to use a custom earmold with the mini-BTE.

The open fitting is only suitable for high frequency hearing losses. However, high frequency hearing losses are typical of those who are in the untapped market of potential hearing aid users that was discussed earlier. Recent marketing efforts of hearing aid manufacturers have redirected professionals and patients to products specifically promoted as mini-BTE open fittings. With the renewed interest brought about by mini-BTEs, the BTEs comprise about 80% of hearing aid sales as compared with 10 years ago when they represented only 20 to 25% of all sales. However, the increased popularity of the mini-BTE RIC style hearing fittings has only resulted in reduced sales of other hearing aid styles (e.g., the ITE, ITC, and CIC) instead of bringing more new consumers into the hearing aid market.

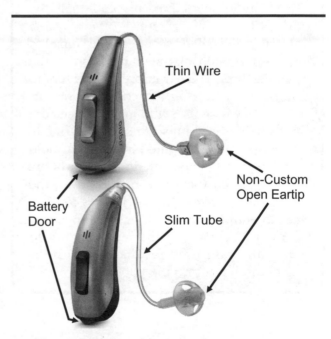

FIGURE 14–5. Two examples of mini-BTE hearing aids. The upper instrument is an RIC, and the lower instrument is an RITA configuration. *Source*: Photos courtesy of Sivantos GmbH.

Making an Impression

All hearing aids require some method to channel sound into the ear canal and to help retain the hearing aid to the ear, this is typically done with some type of earmold or shell, which is custom made to fit into each patient's ear. The earmold/shell is created by taking an ear impression made of special materials, which when mixed together form a solid impression after 2 to 3 minutes. To make the *earmold impression*, a foam or cotton plug with an attached string that remains outside the ear, is inserted deeply into the ear canal to prevent the material from going too far down the canal. The impression material is mixed and inserted relatively quickly into the ear canal, the concha, and part of the auricle. Taking a good impression of the ear is an art that must be learned by the audiologist. Bad impressions result in bad earmolds or shells, which result in bad fittings and unhappy patients. After the impression material solidifies, it is removed from the ear. Some audiologists box up and mail the impression itself, whereas others use a specially designed scanner and email a scanned version of the impression to the manufacturer. The ear impression is sent to the selected hearing aid company or earmold lab, which uses it to make the custom hard shell or custom soft material earmold. For BTEs, tubing is glued into the earmold to allow it to be connected to the ear hook. For all the custom style hearing aids, the audiologist makes the ear impression (either the impression itself or a scanned version) and sends it to the manufacturer to create the case used for the custom hearing aid to be fit into the patient's ear.

Custom In-the-Ear Hearing Aid (ITE)

Hearing aids that have the components inside the earmold casing are generally referred to as *custom hearing aids*. The largest custom style hearing aid is the *in-the-ear* (ITE), which uses a full casing that fills a portion of the ear canal, as well as most or all the concha. The ITE hearing aid was first produced in the late 1950s when transistors replaced vacuum tubes for the hearing aid amplifier components (Dillon, 2001). Today, the digital integrated circuit has replaced transistors, and this has allowed hearing aid sizes to be reduced to the point where all the hearing aid components can be fit into a customized case that fits into the ear canal. Discussed more fully below, the smallest of the custom styles is referred to as completely-in-the-canal (CIC) hearing aid. For the most part, all the latest technology that is available in larger BTEs, such as Bluetooth and bilateral beamforming, is available in the larger custom instruments, with the exception of some FM accessibility features. The smallest CICs may not be able to offer very many options due to space limitations.

In-the-Ear Hearing Aid

The *in-the-ear* (ITE) hearing aid has all the hearing aid components built inside of the customized casing (made from the ear impression), and the hearing aid is placed in the concha portion of the auricle with the receiver portion extending a little way into the ear canal (Figure 14–6). There are three general variants of the ITE style, the full shell, the low profile, and the half shell. The full-shell ITE fills the entire concha portion of the outer ear. The low-profile ITE fills the inner half of the concha, but does not protrude outward as much as the full-shell ITE. The half-shell ITE only fills the lower half of the concha (see family of custom products in Figure 14–7).

In-the-Canal Hearing Aid (ITC)

Like the ITE, the *in-the-canal* (ITC) hearing aid has all the hearing aid components built inside of the customized casing (Figure 14–7). The ITC hearing aid only partially fills the lower approximate one quarter of the concha; thus, the ITC is even smaller than the half-shell ITE. With the smaller size of the ITC there is a tradeoff of less

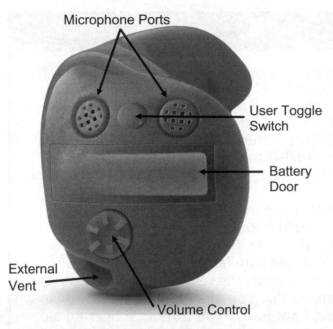

FIGURE 14–6. External features of a full-concha ITE hearing aid. *Source*: Photo courtesy of Sivantos GmbH.

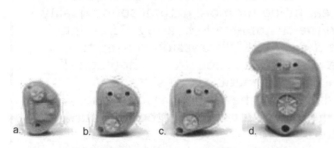

FIGURE 14–7. Four examples of traditional custom hearing aids ranging in size from ITC to full-sized ITE. *Source*: From Mueller, Ricketts, & Bentler, 2014, p. 256. Copyright 2014 by Plural Publishing, Inc.

amplifier gain. For this reason, the selection of an ITC may be most appropriate for those with some cosmetic concerns regarding hearing aids, and who have less severe hearing loss and relatively good manual dexterity. The ITC is also the smallest hearing aid style that can accommodate the space needed for directional microphone technology (e.g., appropriate spacing for two microphone ports). Also, for patients who want to have controls for volume, or changing programs, and do not want to use a remote, the ITC often is the smallest custom hearing aid that can accommodate this.

Completely-in-the-Canal Hearing Aid (CIC)

The *completely-in-the-canal* (CIC) hearing aid is the smallest of the custom style hearing aids, and resides completely in the ear canal of the patient (Figure 14–8). The CIC is often selected by the patient who is looking for the "invisible" hearing aid. If the patient has a large enough ear canal, and the hearing aid can be fitted fairly deeply in the ear canal, the CIC is, indeed, barely noticeable. In case you are wondering, there is a small, clear filament that sticks out from the hearing aid that the patient can grasp to remove the aid (see Figure 14–8).

Traditionally, the CIC has not offered enough amplification for patients with moderate to severe hearing losses. However, there are some new high powered CICs with advanced electronic feedback reduction systems; these newer models have been challenging the longstanding belief that CICs cannot be fit to individuals with severe hearing losses. One disadvantage of the CIC style is that the repair rate is higher than for other hearing aid styles; thus, the patient will be without his or her hearing aid more often during times when the hearing aid is returned to the manufacturer for a repair. Repairs are more frequent with CICs because components contained within the casing are more susceptible to perspiration and cerumen due to their deeper placement in the ear canal.

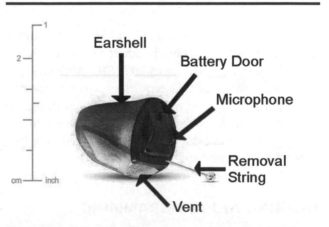

FIGURE 14–8. Latest generation of smaller CIC hearing aid. *Source*: From Mueller, Ricketts, & Bentler, 2014, p. 258. Copyright 2014 by Plural Publishing, Inc.

SYNOPSIS 14–3

- There are five basic styles of hearing aids: (a) body aid, (b) behind-the-ear (BTE), (c) in-the-ear (ITE), (d) in-the-canal (ITC), and (e) completely-in-the-canal (CIC).
- The major manufacturers typically provide all the different styles of hearing aids. A manufacturer may have different models of hearing aids (e.g., entry level, mid-level, premier) that have different features or options; however, for a given model the same processing chip usually is used in each style.
- Body aids are not used much in the United States but may be used in developing countries.
- Body aids and BTEs have an earmold that is separate from the hearing instrument. The dispenser makes an earmold impression for a patient's ear that is sent to the manufacturer along with the request for the hearing aid. Generally, more output power can be obtained with larger instruments like a body aid or BTE; however, a good fitting earmold is essential to avoid feedback. BTEs are appropriate for young children, so that only the earmold needs to be replaced as children grow and they would not have to be without a hearing aid when the earmold is being remade.
- Mini-BTEs have become popular recently and have some of the advantages of the traditional BTE, with additional advantages of being smaller and having a very thin tube connecting to the ear canal. The mini-BTE often is used for high frequency hearing losses with an open ear fitting for more natural sound quality.
- ITEs have all the components built into the custom-made hearing aid casing. There is no need for an earmold, since the earmold impression is used to create the ITE custom hearing aid. The ITEs were a product of technological miniaturization and became very popular for cosmetic reasons.
- ITCs and CICs are smaller versions of the ITE and have a less visible case. While these may be cosmetically appealing, they have limitations in their output levels and special features. Newer technology is being developed to reduce the feedback issue of CICs allowing an increase in the output levels and increasing the fitting range.

A variant of the CIC is what is sometimes called the mini-CIC. This product fits even deeper into the ear than the standard CIC. Moreover, at least one model of this type needs to be inserted and removed by the audiologist, and is designed for extended wear (several months) without removing. These products are indeed invisible when placed in the ear canal.

HEARING AID PROGRAMMING

Today, the audiologist clicks on handles or buttons in the computer software to change the hear-ing aid settings. The hearing aid settings are programmed digitally between the computer and the digital hearing aid circuit. The programmed settings can be saved to the hearing aid's memory and to a patient database in the software and stored on either a local hard drive or network server. With digital hearing aids, it is now possible to make changes on 20 or more different parameters for a single hearing aid. Moreover, the changes are significant, for example, changes in gain of up to 70 dB are achievable.

The computer software for hearing aids is nearly always manufacturer specific, that is, each manufacturer develops and maintains ongoing versions of a software application for fitting its hearing aid products. These software applications may either be stand-alone or may be programming modules within a larger, more universal computer software platform called *Noah*. Stand-alone software programs are installed and assessed much like other software programs on a computer. Noah, on the other hand, is a software system that has programming modules from different manufacturers, and a dispenser may see a wide variety of patients fit with different brands of hearing aids; thus, nearly all software programming modules need to be available. The downside to multiple stand-alone software applications is the difficulty it imposes on maintaining one central patient database, as each standalone application has its respective patient database. In contrast, Noah allows for execution of many different manufacturer software modules, and uses only one central patient database.

As we mentioned, there are thousands of adjustments possible on today's hearing aids, and for programming efficiency, audiologists usually only fit one or two brands of hearing aids. However, even within these brands there may be 10 or so different models with different programming features, and manufacturers add new products and software updates every year. It would be impossible (and unnecessary) for an audiologist to be proficient in programming all brands of hearing aids. It is not uncommon to have a patient walk into your clinic with Brand X hearing aids that need to be reprogrammed, but you only fit Brand Y; therefore, you simply send him down the street to an audiologist you know who fits Brand X.

PRESCRIPTIVE FITTING METHODS

In the preceding section, "programming" of the instruments was mentioned. A reasonable question might be: "What do we program them to do?" Desired hearing aid gain and output for the patient is first selected using a validated *prescriptive fitting method* (for review, see Mueller et al., 2017). This is a mathematic model of selecting gain and output, based on the patient's hearing loss, that has been shown to provide the best outcome. Ear canal gain and output target levels are

used as the prescription; the goal of the fitting is to have the optimal frequency-specific gain and output for soft, average, and loud speech inputs. Additionally, the maximum power output (MPO) of the hearing aid cannot exceed the patient's loudness discomfort levels (LDLs). Although the exact prescriptive targets may not be the ideal fitting for all patients, it has been shown that they will optimize the fitting for the average patient. Given the large variety of hearing aid settings, it is important to have a good starting point. Two fitting methods that are currently used are:

- National Acoustic Laboratories' (NAL) NonLinear method v.2 (NAL-NL2). See http://www.nal.gov.au
- Desired Sensation Level method v.5 (DSLv5.0). See http://www.dslio.com

In general, most audiologists use the NAL method with adults and the DSL method with children. However, in Australia, where the NAL-NL2 method was developed, it is also used with children; in Canada, where the DSLv5 was developed, it remains popular for adult hearing aid fittings. In essence, the methods are appropriate for both populations and ongoing comparison work between the two methods continues.

Quality Control: The 2-cc Coupler Assessment

All hearing aids must meet certain performance requirements based on an *electroacoustic analysis*. There are standards from the American National Standards Institute (ANSI) (2014) that describe how hearing performance is measured. In general, this involves attaching the hearing aid to a 2-cc metal coupler, and using sweep tones and noise signals to test the aid in an isolated sound enclosure (normally referred to as a test box). When new products are developed, detailed specifications are established. These specifications (e.g., the gain and output results from the test box evaluation) are used for quality control when each product is manufactured. In other words, the product is not shipped to the audiologist unless it meets the specifications.

In addition to the specifications and testing by the manufacturers, the measurement of hearing aids using the 2-cc coupler also is commonly conducted by audiologists, and most clinics have a "test box." This small test chamber is often part of the probe-microphone equipment, as similar test signals for both measures are used (see Figure 14–9). The standard 2-cc coupler may either be a HA-1 or HA-2 style. With a HA-1 coupler, the receiver of the hearing aid is placed into a large opening, and putty-like material is placed around the case of the hearing aid to seal off the opening. A HA-2 coupler can be used for attaching to a BTE hearing aid, by using an additional snap-on earmold tubing attachment, and a standard length of tubing. In general, audiologists use 2-cc coupler measures for three reasons:

- To assess the performance of the hearing aid when it arrives from the manufacturer to assure that it is performing according to specifications.
- To assist with the fitting process, that is, corrections are made to the 2cc coupler findings to predict performance in the patient's ear. This approach is commonly used with infants and young children in cases where direct probe-microphone verification is not possible.
- To troubleshoot a patient complaint of a faulty hearing aid, or to simply conduct an annual check of the hearing aid's performance.

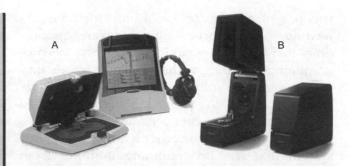

FIGURE 14–9. A and B. Two examples of hearing instrument test chambers for analyzing hearing aids. **A.** Audioscan Model Verifit. **B.** Otometrics Model AURICAL HIT. *Source*: Photos courtesy of Audioscan (Dorchester, Ontario) (A) and Otometrics/Audiology Systems (B).

verify that the prescriptive fitting method produces the appropriate ear canal output when the hearing aids are actually being worn by the patient. In other words, just because prescriptive targets are met on the simulated version shown on the computer fitting screen does not assure that the SPL values are correct in the individual's ear. In fact, there is considerable evidence that what the manufacturer has displayed in the fitting software as "simulated real-ear output" often deviates by 10 dB or more from the true real-ear output (Mueller et al., 2017). Real ear *verification* is essential, and not to do so is considered unethical practice by some.

Verification of prescriptive targets is accomplished using probe-microphone *real-ear measures*. A thin silicone tube is placed in the ear canal and is attached to a measurement microphone, which measures the aided ear canal levels for externally produced signals such as speech. The preferred method is to deliver calibrated real speech at input levels ranging from soft to loud. This procedure is often referred to as "speech mapping."

HEARING AID VERIFICATION

As mentioned in the preceding section, hearing aids typically are programmed according to a prescriptive fitting method that is appropriate for the patient's hearing loss. It is important to

Speech Mapping

As mentioned, the primary verification method is to use probe-microphone measures (assessing SPL near the tympanic membrane) for a calibrated real-speech input signal. Using this ap-

Speech Testing for Verification?

Because the patient usually enters the hearing aid fitting process due to difficulty understanding speech, particularly speech in background noise, it seems logical that the verification procedure should measure his or her ability to understand aided speech. Although this seems logical, because of the poor sensitivity of most speech material, it is difficult to use outcomes of speech testing in clinical practice for selecting the best hearing aid frequency response or signal processing strategy—the probe-microphone measures must be used for this. However, in some cases, speech testing can provide useful information as to the suitability of the hearing aids. In other words, is wearing the hearing aids better than not wearing the hearing aids, as determined by scores on unaided versus aided clinical speech measures? Although this is not useful for selecting the best hearing aid setting or arrangement, it may be useful in demonstrating to the patient the benefits of amplification. The aided speech results, especially when background noise is included, add useful information for counseling.

If you're new to using an SPL-O-Gram, the common "upward sloping" audiogram takes some getting used to because it seems upside down compared to the traditional HL audiogram, but it is well worth the effort.

Shown in Figure 14–10 is a typical fitting screen from the probe-microphone equipment using the REAR for verification. The example here is for a real-speech 65 dB SPL input—the complete verification process would also include a soft and loud input signal (e.g., 55 and 75 dB SPL). The dB HL audiometric thresholds and the patient's LDLs have been converted to ear canal SPL (the equipment does this for us using average correction factors). In this example, we are looking at the NAL-NL2 fitting targets. The shaded area represents the amplitude range of the amplified signal (30th to 99th percentiles), with the LTASS as the dark line near the middle. The goal, accomplished very nicely here, is to make the LTASS equal to the prescriptive targets. The amplitude range of the amplified speech signal also provides some insights regarding compression (discussed earlier); note that the range is smaller for the higher frequencies, where compression is the greatest (e.g., 500 Hz versus 4000 Hz).

proach, we attempt to place the LTASS at a level that matches the mathematically derived fitting targets that we discussed earlier (e.g., the fitting goals of the NAL-NL2). The most commonly used signal today is the International Speech Test Signal (ISTS), which was derived to resemble average speech of an international speech spectrum. When you verify the fitting using probe-microphone measures and real speech, the procedure used is referred to as the *real-ear aided response*, or the REAR. Using the REAR to verify the fitting is quite logical, as everything is referenced to ear canal SPL, and you can easily visualize the portion of the speech signal that is audible for individual patients in their own ear. The SPL-O-Gram format (see Figure 14–10) means that louder outputs indeed fall above softer outputs.

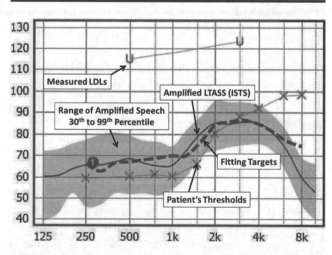

FIGURE 14–10. Example of typical REAR fitting screen. Thresholds are converted from dB HL to dB SPL in the ear canal. The amplified speech (65 dB SPL input) is shown both as the average LTASS and as the range (30th to 99th percentile). The patient's thresholds, LDLs, and fitting targets also are displayed. *Source*: From Mueller, Ricketts, & Bentler, 2017, p. 123. Copyright 2017 by Plural Publishing, Inc.

All about the ISTS

The International Speech Test Signals (ISTS) was created by segmenting (into 500 ms units) and then splicing back together the recordings of female speakers reading the internationally known passage, "The North Wind and the Sun," in six different languages (American English, Arabic, Chinese, French, German, and Spanish). Because of splicing and segmentation, the ISTS is largely unintelligible. The final reassembled signal was then filtered to match the average female LTASS as described by Byrne et al. (1994). The resulting ISTS has been lauded for its speech-like characteristics including a realistic 20 to 30 dB dynamic range, as well as having relatively natural combinations of voiced and voiceless speech segments.

Ratings of Loudness

A general goal of the fitting process is to make soft sounds audible, average sounds comfortable, and loud sounds loud—but not too loud. It is useful, therefore, to conduct some aided loudness measures as part of the verification procedure. In general, when wearing the hearing aids, inputs of around 45 dB SPL should be rated soft, inputs around 65 dB SPL should be rated average (comfortable), and inputs around 85 dB SPL should be rated loud, but not uncomfortably loud (see Mueller, 1999). Gain and compression can be adjusted to assure that these ratings are appropriate. The fitting software from different manufacturers also has several different types of speech and real-world environmental sounds that can be used for this testing. An important measure, using environmental sounds, is to ensure that high level inputs do not exceed the patient's loudness discomfort level. Protocols for this testing are also available (Mueller et al., 2017).

HEARING AID ORIENTATION

Following the verification of hearing aid performance, the patient then receives a *hearing aid orientation* involving extensive counseling and hands-on instruction on the use and care of the new hearing aids. This portion of the fitting process cannot be slighted, as the first few weeks of ownership are critical regarding hearing aid use and acceptance (estimates are that as many as 10% of people who own hearing aids do not use them). Many times, the hearing aids are not used simply because the patient becomes frustrated with the basic operation and handling of the instruments during those first few days. The best circuitry in the world does not help much if the patient is unable to properly fit the hearing aid in the ear. Frequent follow-up phone calls and clinic visits are essential. Some clinics offer group classes for new hearing aid users that are very helpful.

VALIDATION OF HEARING AID BENEFIT

The next step in the fitting process is to conduct some measure of validation. By validation we mean one or more measures to determine if the fitting was successful during real-world use by the patient. Typically, validation involves using a *self-assessment inventory*, which is a questionnaire completed by the patient. There are many of these types of questionnaires available; some are rather informal and others have been researched extensively. One reason there are so many different questionnaires is that there are many ways to measure success with hearing aids. Normally, we are interested in both benefit and satisfaction, although you could have one without the other. Hearing aid use is highly correlated with satisfaction, so this is an important area of interest, too. We also, of course, would like to know if the hearing aids improved the patient's social and emotional well-being; and maybe most importantly, did the intervention improve his or her quality of life?

One easy to use and well-researched questionnaire that incorporates many of the domains related to success is the International Outcome

Verification Versus Validation?

If you look up dictionary definitions of verification and validation, you may be hard pressed to discriminate between the two words, which mean essentially the same thing. However, in the world of quality control, there has been a great deal of discussion on the topic, and several industries have provided definitions for these two words that are specific to their work. In most cases, verification is used when discussing if specific goals (i.e., design or manufacturing) were met. In contrast, validation is used to describe whether the end user/target audience obtains what they wanted or needed. Stated simply:

- Verification: Are we building the system right?
- Validation: Are we building the right system?

Applied to the selection and fitting of hearing aids, hearing aid *verification* often refers to the process of ensuring that the hearing aid meets specific criteria (are we building the system right?) on the day of the fitting such as did we achieve our target prescriptive gain and output and verify that aided loudness does not exceed threshold of discomfort? In contrast, hearing aid *validation* is the process of ensuring we meet the goals set forth in the communication needs assessment (are we building the right system?). This is usually accomplished with post-fitting self-assessment inventories.

the validation process is to assure that the fitting is beneficial and that the patient is satisfied. If low scores are observed, the patient should be targeted for more counseling, and in some cases, adjustments to the fitting should be considered.

While the IOI-HA covers many domains, the main focus of many self-assessment inventories is hearing aid benefit. Two commonly used scales for this are:

- Client Oriented Scale of Improvement (COSI): Measures early and final abilities for specific communication situations important to the patient; used as a pre-test to define goals and to plan management and quantify expectations, and as a post-test to assess the success of the management in meeting the patient's goals. This is popular among audiologists, as the patient more or less creates his or her own questionnaire by nominating his or her personal listening situations for improvement. This facilitates counseling, and adds important personalization to the fitting process. In Figure 14–11, we see an example of a completed COSI for a new hearing aid user after three weeks of hearing aid use. Notice that he nominated five different listening situations that were important to him and then later rank ordered them. In general, we would consider these ratings suggestive of a "good" outcome (https://www.nal.gov.au/).
- Abbreviated Profile of Hearing Aid Benefit (APHAB): Provides the "percent of problems" the patient has for three different listening conditions involving speech understanding (in quiet, in background noise, and in reverberation) and problems related to annoyance of environmental sounds (averseness scale). These values can be obtained as a pre-fitting or unaided measure, as an aided measure, or—by looking at the aided to unaided difference score—as a benefit measure. The advantage of the APHAB is that it is supported with considerable normative data, which makes it easy to compare your patient's findings to expected performance (http://harlmemphis.org/).

Inventory for Hearing Aids (IOI-HA) (http://harlmemphis.org/). It is displayed in Table 14–3. This inventory is relatively easy to administer and score and is available in several languages. An advantage of this scale is that it addresses many of the different areas of "hearing aid success" that we have mentioned. Again, the purpose of

TABLE 14–3. International Outcome Inventory—Hearing Aids (IOI-HA)

- Think about how much you used your present hearing aid(s) over the past two weeks. On an average day, how many hours did you use the hearing aid(s)?

none	less than 1 hour a day	1 to 4 hours a day	4 to 8 hours a day	more than 8 hours a day
□	□	□	□	□

- Think about the situation where you most wanted to hear better, before you got your present hearing aid(s). Over the past two weeks, how much has the hearing aid helped in that situation?

helped not at all	helped slightly	helped moderately	helped quite a lot	helped very much
□	□	□	□	□

- Think again about the situation where you most wanted to hear better. When you use your present hearing aid(s), how much difficulty do you STILL have in that situation?

very much difficulty	quite a lot of difficulty	moderate difficulty	slight difficulty	no difficulty
□	□	□	□	□

- Considering everything, do you think your present hearing aid(s) is worth the trouble?

not at all worth it	slightly worth it	moderately worth it	quite a lot worth it	very much worth it
□	□	□	□	□

- Over the past two weeks, with your present hearing aid(s), how much have your hearing difficulties affected the things you can do?

affected very much	affected quite a lot	affected moderately	affected slightly	affected not at all
□	□	□	□	□

- Over the past two weeks, with your present hearing aid(s), how much do you think other people were bothered by your hearing difficulties?

bothered very much	bothered quite a lot	bothered moderately	bothered slightly	bothered not at all
□	□	□	□	□

- Considering everything, how much has your present hearing aid(s) changed your enjoyment of life?

worse	no change	slightly better	quite a lot better	very much better
□	□	□	□	□

English Version

Translations of the International Outcome Inventory for Hearing Aids (IOI-HA)	Cox/Stephens/Kramer	9

SYNOPSIS 14–4

- The frequency and output settings, as well as other special features, are programmed by a computer (to which the hearing aid is attached). Noah is a computer platform that has many of the manufacturers' software packages installed for easy access.
- The dispenser programs a digital hearing aid using accepted prescriptive algorithms, which have been validated by research to provide the best gain across the frequencies for a range of speech inputs for a particular hearing loss. These prescriptive algorithms provide targets that the programmer tries to meet

SYNOPSIS 14–4 *(continued)*

to optimize the hearing aid fitting for a particular patient. The two most popular prescriptive fitting methods are the NAL-NL2 (National Acoustics Laboratory Nonlinear method) used mostly for adults and the DSLv5.0 (Desired Sensation Level v5.0) used mostly for children.

- Electroacoustic analyses are obtained in a hearing aid test box with the hearing aid attached to a small (2-cc) coupler, to see if it meets certain standards (ANSI). This is not a verification procedure, but can be used to predict real-ear output when probe-microphone measurements are not possible (infants and young children).
- In the verification step, the audiologist determines if the prescriptive fittings are actually achieved and are acceptable to the patient. The verification is conducted using real-ear probe microphone measures obtained from the patient's ear canal while he or she is wearing the hearing aid.
- In the validation step, the audiologist is interested in the patient's opinion on the benefits he or she is obtaining from the hearing aids, and how satisfied the patient is with their use. These opinions are obtained using various self-assessment inventories, such as the International Outcome Inventory for Hearing Aids (IOI-HA), the APHAB, or the COSI.

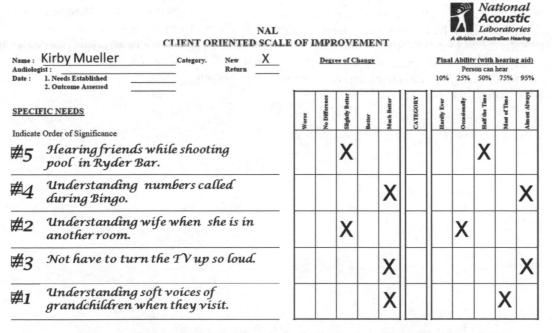

FIGURE 14–11. The post-fitting COSI for a patient. Prior to the fitting, the patient selected five areas for improvement and rated them in priority. Shown here are the patient ratings of benefit obtained with the hearing aids for each communication situation. *Source*: From Mueller, Ricketts, & Bentler, 2017, p. 234. Copyright 2017 by Plural Publishing, Inc.

SUMMARY

As the discipline of audiology has evolved and progressed over the years, the evaluation and fitting of hearing aids has been a constant companion. As we have outlined in this chapter, there are several important steps in the overall fitting process. The digital technology of today's hearing aids has improved to the extent that it is not so much what the hearing aid can do, but rather, does the audiologist have the skills to program this technology to make the hearing aid perform at its maximum for a given patient? The theoretical fitting algorithms and real-ear verification techniques allow a tailoring of the hearing aid fitting that was not possible only a few years ago. Of course, it is critical to involve the patient in the decision-making along the way, and to provide the post-fitting counseling that is necessary for optimum benefit and satisfaction. Properly fitted hearing aids can change a person's life, and the audiologist is the person to make this happen.

REFERENCES

Abrams, H. B., & Kihm, J. (2015). An introduction to MarkeTrak IX: A new baseline for the hearing aid market. *Hearing Review. 22*(6):16.

American National Standards Institute [ANSI]. (2014). Specification of hearing aid characteristics. *ANSI S3.22-2014*. New York, NY: Author.

Byrne, D., Dillon, H., Tran, K., Aringer, S., Wilbraham, K., Cox, R., & Ludvigsen, C. (1994). An international comparison of long-term average speech spectra. *Journal of the Acoustical Society of America. 96*(4), 2108–2120.

Dillon, H. (2001). *Hearing Aids*. Turramurra, Australia: Boomerang Press.

Dillon, H. (2012). *Hearing Aids* (2nd ed.). New York, NY: Thieme Medical Publishers.

Killion, M., & Mueller, H. G. (2010). Twenty years later: A new count-the-dots method. *Hearing Journal, 63*(1): 10–17.

Kochkin, S., Mason, P., & Tharpe, A. M. (2007). Hearing loss in America being left behind? *Hearing Review, 14*(10), 10–34.

Mueller, H. G., & Johnson, E. E. (2014). Hearing aid amplification. In *Introduction to Audiology*, 2nd ed. Kramer, S. (Ed.). San Diego, CA: Plural. Pp. 292–325.

Mueller, H. G., Ricketts, T. A., & Bentler R. (2014) *Modern Hearing Aids: Pre-Fitting Testing and Selection Considerations*. San Diego, CA: Plural.

Mueller, H. G., Ricketts, T. A., & Bentler, R. (2017). *Speech Mapping and Probe Microphone Measurements*. San Diego, CA: Plural.

Mueller, H. G. (1999). Just make it audible, comfortable and loud but okay. *Hearing Journal, 52*(1), 10–17.

National Institute of Deafness and Communication Disorders. (2016). Quick statistics about hearing. Retrieved from www.nidcd.nih.gov.

Strom, K. (2017). US hearing aid unit sales increased by 8.7% in 2016. *Hearing Review*. www.hearingreview.com

15 Implantable Devices

After reading this chapter, you should be able to:

1. Describe two different categories of bone-anchored implants and give an example of each.
2. Explain the candidacy criteria for bone-anchored implants.
3. Explain the difference between percutaneous and transcutaneous devices.
4. Define when to use a Softband with a bone-anchored implant.
5. Describe the design and function of a middle ear implant.
6. Explain how middle ear implants are categorized.
7. Compare and contrast piezoelectric and electromagnetic transduction.
8. Describe the candidacy rules for a middle ear implant.
9. Describe the design and function of a cochlear implant.
10. Explain the function of each of the basic components of a cochlear implant.
11. Describe the speech coding strategies and list some common strategies.
12. Describe the components of an audiologic and medical evaluation for a cochlear implant.

SPECIALIZED HEARING AIDS AND AUDITORY IMPLANTS

Rather than being fit with a conventional hearing aid, sometimes a patient will perform better with the use of a different type of hearing device, which could be recommended as a treatment option depending upon the individual patient characteristics. In these types of patients, the audiologist would generally work with an otologist or neurotologist when managing the patient's case. There are four such specialized auditory devices; the bone-anchored implant (BAI); the middle ear implant (MEI); the cochlear implant (CI), and the auditory brainstem implant (ABI). Each of these devices fits a specific type of hearing loss or meets the need of a certain type of patient. The BAI can be used with patients who have a conductive or mixed hearing loss or for those with single-sided deafness (unilateral hearing loss). The MEI is typically used with patients who have an intact middle ear system but have a mild to severe-to-profound sensorineural hearing loss. A CI and ABI are a different type of hearing device, whereby the acoustic signals are delivered to electrodes that are implanted into either the cochlea or brainstem: The CI is inserted in the cochlea and requires an intact 8th cranial nerve, whereas the ABI is placed along the surface of the dorsal or ventral cochlear nucleus. Each of these types of hearing devices are discussed in the following sections.

BONE-ANCHORED IMPLANT (BAI)

A bone-anchored implant (BAI) is a class of hearing device that is surgically implanted by an otologist into the mastoid area behind the ear. These *osseointegrated* hearing implant systems are different from cochlear implants and, therefore, have a different classification. The Food and Drug Administration (FDA) has approved BAIs as a Class II medical device, which puts them in the same category as powered wheelchairs, surgical drapes, and x-ray equipment. Class II devices are a higher risk than Class I devices, which means they require greater regulatory control so that the public can be assured that the device is safe and effective (FDA, n.d.).

The BAI is similar to a bone conduction oscillator, which means that it can transmit a signal to the cochlea and bypass the outer and middle ears. By missing the conductive parts of the ear, the sound can be passed directly to the cochlea via mechanical vibrations. Prior to the development of the BAI, patients with conductive losses had only one option when it came to amplification, a bone-conducted hearing aid. A conventional bone-conducted hearing aid had a clinical type of bone vibrator that was held in place on the head with either a metal headband or wig tape. In the past 20 years, a number of other devices have entered the marketplace to fill the need of patients who wanted a bone conduction device that was more comfortable and provided better sound quality. The users of this newer technology usually have a bilateral conductive or mixed hearing loss, but some have found benefit with a unilateral hearing loss, which is a type of CROS fitting (see Chapter 14). With the BAI, the sound is transduced to the cochlea in a way similar to other bone conduction transducers, such as the ones used for bone conduction audiometry. Acoustic signals are picked up by the BAI's microphone and transduced into vibrations that stimulate the skull, thus creating the normal vibratory energy in the normal hearing cochlea.

In order for the BAI to function, it must transmit the auditory signal to the cochlea via bone conduction; it does this by permanently attaching the device to the skull through a process called *osseointegration*. Osseointegration is the connection between living bone and the surface of a load-carrying implant. In other words, it is the method by which the implant adheres to the bone. This connection is formed by the use of titanium as the transitional metal, which allows for a strong and stable implant-to-tissue interaction giving a structural and functional contact between the implant and the bone (Kuhn & Perez, 2015). When the surgeon implants an abutment or magnet, he or she utilizes a titanium screw. After drilling a hole into the skull, the surgeon threads the screw into bone. Due to osseointegration, the bone creates a fibrous layer around the screw and then the bone begins to weave

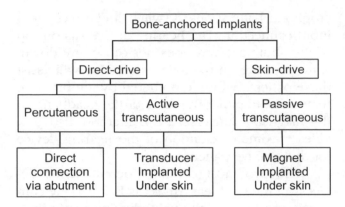

FIGURE 15–1. Classification of bone-anchored implants. *Source*: Modified from Reinfeldt, Hakansson, Taghavi, Jansson, & Eeg-Olofsson, 2015.

itself into the implant creating a solid integration of the implant, which usually takes about 4 to 6 weeks.

Bone-anchored implants can be either transcutaneous or percutaneous. A transcutaneous device has a magnet attached to the skull under the skin and the hearing device can then be held on with another magnet so that they attract to each other across the skin. A percutaneous device has an abutment with a screw attached that is osseointegrated into the skull, a post is attached to the abutment, which penetrates through the skin, the hearing device is then attached to the post. Figure 15–1 shows a chart that you can use to categorize the different types of bone-anchored implant devices. Essentially there are two methods, direct-drive or skin-drive, in which to categorize the different types of devices that are currently or coming onto the market. Direct-drive refers to devices in which there is no tissue in-between the hearing device and the skull and skin-drive refers to devices in which there is a layer of skin that may absorb or change the signal prior to vibrating the skull. Although not an implantable device, the conventional air-conduction hearing device connected to a bone vibrator (bone conduction hearing aids) could be considered a type of skin-drive device because it has to transmit the vibration across the skin prior to vibrating the skull. The BAI devices offer some benefits to these conventional bone conduction hearing

aids including elimination of feedback, headband pressure and stability of the position of the vibrator, improved high frequency gain, and reduced distortion (Gelfand, 2016). These different type of devices give both the audiologist and the user options to choose the best device for the user's hearing loss and lifestyle.

Candidacy for BAI

As described in Table 15–1, patients would be considered candidates for a bone-anchored implant if they fall into one of two categories: (1) have a conductive or mixed hearing loss, or (2) have a unilateral hearing loss. Candidacy for a BAI is set by each manufacturer according to the audiometric criteria they reported to the FDA. In general, the candidacy requirements are similar for both those patients with conductive/ mixed hearing loss and those with single-sided deafness. Patients with a conductive hearing loss must have a conductive component with at least a 30 dB air-bone gap. Patients with a mixed hearing loss must have a conductive component with at least a 30 dB air-bone gap and a mild to moderate sensorineural component. Currently patients with single sided deafness (SSD) must have normal hearing in the better hearing ear

TABLE 15–1. Candidacy Considerations for a Bone-Anchored Implant

Conductive/Mixed Loss	Unilateral Hearing Loss
Atresia – bilateral	Atresia – unilateral
Abnormal ear canal structure	Acquired unilateral conductive/mixed hearing loss
Chronic ear drainage	
Stapedectomy	Congenital or acquired profound unilateral loss
Failed middle ear surgery	Tumors of the conductive pathway
Unable to use air conduction hearing aid	
Hypersensitivity to earmolds	Autoimmune inner ear disease
Severe dermatitis of the ear canal	Meniere disease
Severe otitis externa	

(a PTA <20 dB HL by air-conduction) and a profound SNHL (a PTA > 90 dB HL) in the poor ear but research is showing that patients with less of a loss are also showing benefit (Zeitler, Snapp, Telischi, & Angeli, 2012). In addition to these audiometric criteria, there are some surgical contraindications that need to be observed for both pediatric and adults when undergoing any surgical procedure. In addition, children are not considered to be candidates until they are at least 5 years of age due to the thickness of the temporal bone, which must have a minimum bone thickness of 2.5 mm (Kuhn & Perez, 2015).

Direct-Drive

Percutaneous

Percutaneous BAIs penetrate through the skin connecting the hearing device on the outside with a direct coupling to the skull on the inside, as shown in Figure 15–2. The fixture or abutment (Panel A) that penetrates the skin is used to connect to the hearing device and acts as a breakaway point should an external force be applied to it. Panel B shows the hearing device attached to the abutment, with the microphone on the face. As with other amplification devices, it contains a mi-

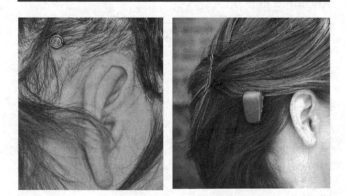

FIGURE 15–2. An example of a direct-drive percutaneous device—the Baha® percutaneous abutment is shown (**A**) with the Baha® device attached to the abutment (**B**). *Source*: Images courtesy of Cochlear Americas, © 2017.

crophone, battery, on-off switch, and direct audio input connection. The hearing device sits on top of the abutment and does not cause any downward pressure on the skin tissue. This will assist those patients who are bothered by the pressure that is due to either the force of the headband or the magnets. Conversely, this method also provides maximum retention of the hearing device for those active patients.

The two most common percutaneous devices are the Cochlear Americas Baha® bone conduction system and the Ponto by Oticon Medical. The Baha received its FDA clearance for adult use in 1996, making it one of the first BAI to be available to patients who had either a conductive or a mixed hearing loss. Three years later it was cleared for children, 5 years of age and older. In 2001, it could be fit bilaterally and a year later, it was made available as a treatment to those patients who had single-sided deafness. The Ponto bone-anchored hearing system is designed to transfer sound via bone conduction to the cochlea. Like the Baha, it consists of three parts: (1) a small 3 to 4 mm titanium implant that is implanted in the temporal bone just posterior to the auricle, (2) the abutment that connects to the hearing device to the temporal bone, and (3) the sound processor with a microphone that is attached on the outside of the skin.

The advantages of percutaneous devices are: they provided a mean threshold improvement in the mid to high frequencies, and; they use a lower force level when compared to transcutaneous. Disadvantages are that patients must be diligent about cleaning around the abutment or risk causing skin infections because of poor hygiene for this open wound that they will have for life (Hodgetts, 2017).

Active Transcutaneous

Active transcutaneous devices are a newer class of direct-drive devices where the transducer is implanted under the skin and allows the vibrations to be transmitted from the transducer directly to the temporal bone. It is, however, a transcutaneous device because the implant receives an electromagnetic signal from the sound processor located outside the skin. The processor transmits the signal through the skin via an inductive link instead of as vibrations, which would be the case in typical transcutaneous devices. Retention magnets are used on the sound processor to attach it to the implant under the skin (Reinfeldt, Hakansson, Taghavi, & Eeg-Olofsson, 2015). Currently no active transcutaneous devices are available in the United States but these devices are available elsewhere around the world. Results from studies on this technology have shown that these type of devices could provide patients with an improvement in gain of 26 to 31 dB, speech recognition threshold in quiet improved as much as 27.0 dB, and WRS in quiet and in noise improved 21 to 50% (Reinfeldt, Hakansson, Taghavi, Jansson, & Eeg-Olofsson, 2015; Schmerber, S., Deguine, O., Marx, M., Van de Heyning, P., Sterkers, O., Mosnier, I., Garin, P., Godey, B., Vincent, C., Venail, F., Mondain, M., Deveze, A., Lavieille, J. P. & Karkas, A., 2017).

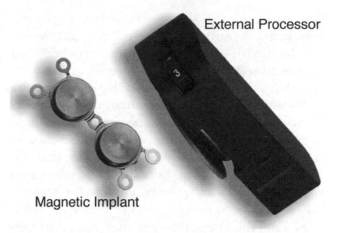

FIGURE 15–3. An example of a skin-drive passive transcutaneous device with an implanted magnet and external hearing device—the Sophono™ Alpha 2 MPO™ Bone Conduction Hearing Device. *Source*: Courtesy of Medtronix, Jacksonville, FL.

Skin-Drive

Passive Transcutaneous

Transcutaneous BAIs do not penetrate through the skin but instead connect to a magnet that is osseointegrated into the skull with a sound processor outside the skin. The hearing device on the outside is held in place via magnetic attraction to the magnet on the inside, as shown in Figure 15–3. As with other magnetic devices, should an external force be applied, the device will detach from the scalp without trauma or injury to the user. This may be important for users who are active and play contact sports. The hearing device itself contains a microphone, battery, and vibrating source to transmit the signal to the magnet under the skin. Due to the attraction of the two magnets (outside and under the skin), there is some pressure on the skin tissue that lies between the two components. This will assist those patients who are bothered by the pressure that is due to the force of the headband with a conventional bone conducted hearing aid. There is minimal risk of skin infections since it is transcutaneous and there is no open wound.

This is especially important for patients who are unable to care for their site or have poor personal hygiene.

There are two transcutaneous bone-anchored devices; the Sophono bone-anchored hearing system and the Cochlear Attract bone conduction system. The Sophono system received its FDA clearance in 2010 and the Baha Attract does not currently have FDA clearance for use in the United States. Both of these bone-anchored hearing systems are designed to transfer sound from the processor outside of the skin to the cochlea via bone conduction. These units have two parts: (1) the internal magnet, and (2) the external sound processor with a microphone, battery, vibrator, and magnet. The internal magnet is osseointegrated to the skull and the two magnets couple together across the skin holding the external processor in place and function similarly to a traditional bone conduction vibrator.

The advantages of transcutaneous devices are that they provide an improvement in threshold especially in the low frequencies. Disadvantages are that as the vibrations travel through the skin they lose energy compared to percutaneous devices, gain drops off in the high frequencies and patients may experience minor complications because of the pressure on the skin between the two magnets (Kohan, 2015; Hodgetts, 2017).

In certain situations, a patient may not want a surgical solution, in which case there is an option that still allows them to utilize either a Baha or Ponto device. The Baha Softband allows these devices to be connected to the mastoid and held in place with an elastic headband. The Softband is considered a passive skin-drive device that can allow a child to receive benefit of auditory input while they are waiting to be eligible for surgery. When they become old enough and have sufficient skull thickness, they can then have the abutment implanted and continue to use their device without the Softband.

MIDDLE EAR IMPLANT (MEI)

A *middle ear implant* (MEI) is a specialized type of hearing device that is different from conventional types of hearing aids. Patients who use these devices are ones who would be considered unsuccessful hearing aid users, whose lifestyle would be hampered by the use of or are medically unable to wear conventional hearing aids. These device should not be considered new as the concept of MEI has been around since the experiments of the Finnish scientist, Alvar Wilska in the 1930s (Stach, 2014), with the first commercially available device being produced in 1984. The partially implantable hearing aid (Rion Ehime) had

SYNOPSIS 15–1

- There are four specialized auditory devices: (1) the bone-anchored implant (BAI); the middle ear implant (MEI); the cochlear implant (CI), and the auditory brainstem implant. Each fits a specific type of hearing loss or meets the need of a certain type of patient.
- BAI (bone-anchored implant) is a special type of hearing aid that is surgically implanted into the mastoid bone and can provide good bone conduction hearing in cases with conductive or mixed hearing losses or single-sided deafness.
- The middle ear implanted hearing device (MEI) is typically used with patients who have an intact middle ear system but have a mild to severe-to-profound sensorineural hearing loss.
- Cochlear implants and auditory brainstem implants are a different type of hearing device, in which the acoustic signals are delivered to electrodes that are implanted into either the cochlea or brainstem.
- In order for the BAI to function, it must transmit the auditory signal to the cochlea via bone conduction; it does this by permanently attaching the device to the skull through a process called osseointegration. Osseointegration is the connection between living bone and the surface of a load-carrying implant.
- Patients are considered candidates for a BAI if they fall into one of two categories: (1) have a conductive or mixed hearing loss, or (2) have a unilateral hearing loss.
- There are two categories of BAI: Direct-drive and skin-drive. Direct-drive implant can be either percutaneous or active transcutaneous and skin-drive implants are passive transcutaneous.
- In certain situations, a patient may not want a surgical solution. The Baha Softband becomes an option allowing them to utilize either a Baha or Ponto device and connected them to the mastoid with an elastic headband.

a microphone, induction coil, and battery on the outside and the internal component had a coil in the middle ear space connect to a piezoelectric transducer in the mastoid and was fixed to the stapes. Other devices have been developed such as the totally implantable cochlear amplifier (TICA), the SOUNDTEC, Vibrant Soundbridge, Esteem, and others (Channer, Eshraghi, & Lui, 2011). These devices are implanted in the middle ear and coupled to the ossicles bypassing the ear canal, thus the ear canal is left unoccluded and are more cosmetically appealing to patients (Achar, 2013). In 1998, the Vibrant Soundbridge was released in Europe and in 2000, it became the first MEI to receive FDA clearance in the United States. The Esteem device received FCA clearance for use in the United States in 2010. Although MEIs are available on the market, they make up only a small number of the hearing aids fit annually in the United States.

The MEI is a device that is categorized either by its implant status (partially or fully implanted) or on the type of transducer used in the device (Channer, Eshraghi, & Lui, 2011). MEIs are surgically placed in the middle ear and depending on the device can be attached to the ossicular chain, oval window, or round window or as a method of treating sensorineural hearing losses (Bassim & Fayad, 2010; Gifford, 2017). Most transducers used in MEIs are either piezoelectric and electromagnetic transduction mechanisms (Kuhn & Perez, 2015). The piezoelectric implementation uses an external microphone placed by the ear or under the skin in the ear canal to detect sounds around the listener. From this, an electrically encoded signal is sent to an implanted middle ear crystal placed on the ossicular chain. The crystal moves in response to stimulation from the sound transduction and propagates this electrical activity onto the cochlea, where it is processed by the remaining hair cells and 8th cranial nerve fibers. Piezoelectric devices are smaller and use less power than electromagnetic devices. The electromagnetic implementation is larger than the piezoelectric version; therefore, it is only partially implantable. Most of the electromagnetic implants have an external coil that is connected to a microphone and an amplifier. The amplified signal is sent to an implanted magnet located at or near the incus–stapedial joint of the ossicular chain

and oscillates as electromagnetic waves move past the magnet; thus, the electromagnetic energy is converted to mechanical energy (ossicular movement). The electromagnetic devices have greater gain and output but they are offset by a greater power consumption and larger size compared to the piezoelectric transducers (Channer, Eshraghi, & Lui, 2011).

Candidacy for MEI

Given the number of different devices that are or have been on the market over the years, the audiological criteria are very similar. Candidacy for a MEI is set by each manufacturer according to the audiometric criteria they reported to the FDA. In general, MEIs are designed for patients with a stable sensorineural hearing loss in the moderate to severe range ($\leq$65 to 70 dB HL). Word recognition scores need to be greater than 40 to 60% (Achar, 2013; Kuhn & Perez, 2015). Candidates must be medically stable and not have any preexisting medical conditions.

MEI Devices

Examples of currently available devices include the Vibrant Soundbridge and the Esteem. The Vibrant Soundbridge is an electromagnetic device that consists of the SAMBA external sound processor (hearing device) and the vibrating ossicular prosthesis (VORP). The VORP includes a magnet for attaching the external device, an internal coil, a demodulator for receiving and converting the electrical signals from the processor and the floating mass transducer (FMT), which attaches to and vibrates the ossicles. Studies have demonstrated that the FMT can also show benefit when attached to either the stapes or oval window (Kuhn & Perez, 2015).

The Esteem is a two channel analog device that uses a different approach and does not have an external processor or microphone (Figure 15.4). The device, including the battery, is totally implanted within the temporal bone and the middle ear space. A piezoelectric transducer or

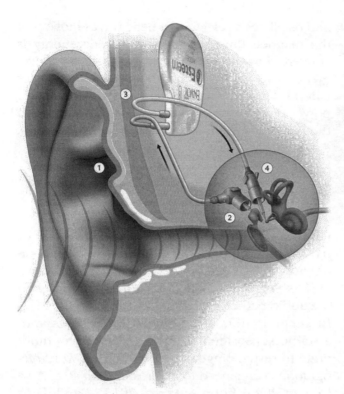

FIGURE 15–4. An example of a middle ear implant—the Esteem. (1) An electronic microphone is not used, instead the external ear funnels the sound waves down the ear canal to the tympanic membrane causing it to vibrate and acts as the microphone. (2) The sensor is connected to the incus and receives the mechanical vibrations, converting them to an electrical signal and forwarding them to the processor. (3) The processor implanted in the temporal bone amplifies the signal. (4) The driver is coupled to the stapes footplate and converts the enhanced signal back to mechanical energy for transfer into the cochlea. *Source*: Courtesy of Envoy Medical Corporation, White Bear Lake, Minnesota.

MEI Outcomes

Middle Ear Implants have been shown have slightly better thresholds, and speech-in-noise performance compared to conventional hearing aids (Truy, Philibert, Vesson, Labaassi, & Collet, 2008). In a number of studies, results have reported an overall improvement in patient satisfaction. However, more importantly patients have reported benefit with MEI in terms of reduced problems with feedback, the occlusion effect, reverberation, and sound distortion (Kuhn & Perez, 2015). For these patients, MEI serves a purpose and allows many of them who would otherwise not use amplification to gain auditory benefit.

COCHLEAR IMPLANT (CI)

A *cochlear implant (CI)* is a biomedical device that bypasses the middle ear, the traveling wave, and the sensory cells on the basilar membrane, and electrically stimulates neurons of the cochleovestibular nerve. The purpose of a cochlear implant is to provide people with substantial hearing losses hearing improvement beyond that which can be offered by conventional hearing aids. Even individuals with severe to profound hearing losses have some functional auditory nerve fibers that can be stimulated electrically through a cochlear implant. Much like a hearing aid, a cochlear implant can provide reasonably good detection and correct identification of environmental and speech sounds. A simulation showing how cochlear implants work can be found on the Internet at http://ecs.utdallas.edu/loizou/cimplants/children/.

Cochlear implants are regulated by the Food and Drug Administration (FDA), and considered a Class III medical device along with implantable pacemakers and implanted neuromuscular stimulators. The process for clearance for cochlear implants requires data on the safety and efficacy in clinical trials. Examples of safety data include prevalence of facial nerve paralysis, infection, device migration, and implant failure necessitating another implant. Efficacy data include studies on the benefits of the implant related to speech understanding as well as promoting the devel-

sensor is connected to the incus and moves with motion of the tympanic membrane. It receives the mechanical vibrations from the incus and converts them to electrical signals, which are sent to a sound processor implanted in the temporal bone. The sound processor filters and amplifies the signal, and sends the processed signal to the driver (another piezoelectric transducer) coupled to the stapes footplate. At the driver, the electrical signal is converted back to mechanical energy, which moves the stapes in and out of the oval window, transmitting the signal to the cochlea.

SYNOPSIS 15–2

- A middle ear implant (MEI) is a specialized type of hearing device that has been commercially available since 1984.
- MEI is surgically placed into the middle ear, where the normal middle ear transduces mechanical activity into electrical stimulation of remaining hair cells and nerve fibers in the inner ear.
- The MEI is a device that is categorized either by its implant status (partially or fully implanted) or on the type of transducer used in the device. MEIs are surgically placed in the middle ear and depending on the device can be attached to the ossicular chain, oval window, or round window or as a method of treating sensorineural hearing losses.
- MEI transducers are either piezoelectric or electromagnetic transduction mechanisms. Piezoelectric devices are smaller and use less power than electromagnetic devices. Electromagnetic devices have greater gain and output but they are offset by a greater power consumption and larger size.
- MEIs are designed for patients with a sensorineural hearing loss in moderate to severe range (≤65 to 70 dB HL). These thresholds need to have been stable for the past two years. Word recognition scores need to be greater than 40 to 60%.
- MEIs are useful devices for a certain segment of people with hearing loss who would otherwise not use amplification.

opment of language and speech production. Approval from the FDA is directly related to coverage of cochlear implants by health insurance programs. The FDA approved the use of CIs for adults with postlingual deafness in 1984 and for children in 1989. At that time, CIs were devices that only provided sound awareness and were an aid to speech-reading. Cochlear implants function differently and provide an input that is different than normal hearing.

Often, the actual success and the functional level obtained with a cochlear implant depend on many factors. Some of these factors include time of onset of hearing loss, length of deafness prior to implantation, residual function of auditory neurons, appropriate programming of the implant, and consistent use of the implant. Some limitations to cochlear implants include surgical risk (complications less than 1%), implanted electrode array may destroy some of the remaining functional hair cells, expense (~$40,000), the need to travel to and from a CI center for remapping and/or programming and checks, and

unpredictable benefits and outcomes before surgery. Fortunately, the cost associated with cochlear implants, including the surgery, device, and programming visits, is covered by most medical insurances. Multichannel, multielectrode cochlear implants available in the United States may be found at the following cochlear implant manufacturers' websites: http:// www. advanced bionics.com, http://www.cochlearamericas.com, or http://www.medel.com/.

A cochlear implant may be conceptualized as a device divided into external and internal components (Figure 15–5). The external components consist of a microphone, speech processor, and external transmitter (headpiece). As with all amplification devices, the microphone changes the acoustic energy into electrical energy. The signal is sent to the speech processor for processing and analyzing, and then it is band-pass filtered, creating frequency bands of electric stimulation. The external transmitter receives these signals via radio frequency and sends them to the internal implant. The implant consists of a magnet, receiving coil, circuitry, and an electrode array. The external transmitter is attached to the implant via a magnet. The signal from the external transmitter is sent to the receiving coil and then to the electrode array. In this way the signal bypasses the ear canal, middle ear, and cochlear hair cells, and the electrical impulses stimulate the cochlear portion of the 8th cranial nerve.

After the sound is converted to an electrical signal, it is changed into a speech strategy specific electrical code. Cochlear implants have several different ways to process speech, called speech coding strategies. These strategies are the way in which the cochlear implant changes the sounds into patterns of electrical signals delivered to the cochlea needed to convey frequency, intensity, and duration information. Three common processing strategies used in cochlear implants are the simultaneous analog stimulation (SAS), continuous interleaved sampler (CIS), and spectral PEAK extraction (SPEAK). Some more recent developments have incorporated parts of

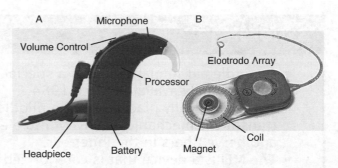

FIGURE 15–6. Components of a cochlear implant. (**A**) External device with the processor and coil that attaches to the internal magnet. (**B**) Implant with the electrode array. *Source*: Images courtesy of Advanced Bionics LLC, © 2017.

these strategies to form hybrid speech strategies; these include advanced combination encoders (ACE) and multiple pulse sample (MPS). Then, the external transmitter coil of a cochlear implant sends the coded electrical signal to internal components.

The internal receiver coil picks up the carrier signal from the transmitter and sends an electrical code along to the electrode array (e.g., 22 channels of electrodes). As shown in Figure 15–6, the electrode array is attached to the implant. The electrode array is surgically inserted into the scala tympani of the cochlea and the nerve fibers are activated in accordance with the electrical code arising from the output of the speech processing strategy.

CI EVALUATION

Two important criteria for cochlear implant referrals are: (1) the patient must have a severe to profound bilateral sensorineural hearing loss (some corner audiograms may be considered even when hearing thresholds at 250 and 500 Hz are less severe), and (2) more importantly, little or no benefit from hearing aids. An evaluation by a team of medical professionals is required for consideration of a cochlear implant. The cochlear implant team at a minimum consists of the surgeon and audiologist. When a child is con-

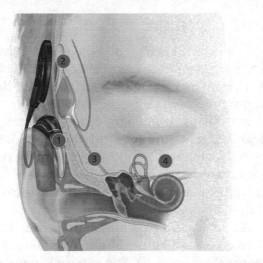

FIGURE 15–5. Cochlear implant with placement of external and internal CI components. (1) The microphone on the sound processor picks up and converts the sound into digital information. (2) This information is transferred through the coil to the implant located under the skin. (3) The implant sends electrical signals down the electrode into the cochlea. (4) The auditory nerve fibers in the cochlea pick up the electrical signals and conduct them up the auditory pathway to the auditory cortex. *Source*: Image courtesy of Cochlear Americas, © 2017.

sidered for implantation, a speech-language pathologist, psychologist, social worker, and educator may also be involved. The entire cochlear implant team usually participates in the evaluation and final decision on whether a patient is appropriate to receive a cochlear implant.

A medical evaluation includes a CT scan to determine the presence of a cochlea and auditory nerve, as well as an assessment of the patient's ability to cope physically with surgery. The audiology evaluation includes air conduction and bone conduction thresholds (or ABR thresholds for children too young to be tested behaviorally), tympanometry, acoustic reflex thresholds, speech reception thresholds, word recognition ability under insert earphones, and, last, aided word recognition in the sound field. A speech-language pathology evaluation will include a determination of current speech and language development.

As mentioned before, cochlear implants are approved for both children and adults. Typically, the earlier the age of implantation and/or the sooner the implantation after the onset of hearing loss, the better the prognosis for outcomes will be for the patient. Since the cochlea is adult size at birth and infant temporal bone growth

can be compensated for by lengthening the electrode array, cochlear implant surgeries may be completed as early as 1 year of age.

Once a patient is determined to be eligible for a cochlear implant, surgery is scheduled. In general, for experienced surgeons cochlear implant surgery is a relatively uncomplicated. The surgery can be completed in less than 3 hours under general anesthesia. The cochlear implant is programmed by an audiologist 3 to 6 weeks after the surgery (after time to heal). The programming visit is often referred to as *cochlear implant mapping*. The cochlear implant is programmed utilizing a computer, a device-specific software program developed by the manufacturer of the implant, and an interface box. The electrical thresholds for soft inputs and the upper limit of comfort thresholds are established at the initial visit, as well as the speech processing strategy to be used. It is often common to turn off the electrodes in which stimulation causes pain, facial twitches, and/or no improvement in hearing sensitivity. The patient will return multiple times within the first 6 months to 1 year for additional cochlear implant mapping sessions in order to fine-tune the cochlear implant.

SYNOPSIS 15–3

- A cochlear implant (CI) is a biomedical device that bypasses the middle ear, the traveling wave, and the sensory cells on the basilar membrane, and electrically stimulates neurons of the 8th cranial nerve.
- CIs provide people an improvement in their hearing beyond that offered by conventional hearing aids. Even individuals with severe to profound hearing losses have some functional auditory nerve fibers that can be stimulated electrically through a cochlear implant. A CI can provide reasonably good detection and correct identification of environmental and speech sounds.
- Cochlear implants are composed of an array of electrodes that are implanted into a nonfunctioning cochlea and a processor on the side of the skull. The processor transduces acoustic signals into electrical signals along the electrode array to stimulate auditory nerve fibers.
- A candidate for a cochlear implant must have a severe/profound hearing loss and only marginal benefit from traditional amplification.

SYNOPSIS 15–3 (continued)

- After the sound is converted to an electrical signal, it is changed into a speech strategy specific electrical code. CIs have different ways to process speech, called speech coding strategies that change the sounds into patterns of electrical signals delivered to the cochlea needed to convey frequency, intensity, and duration information.
- Common processing strategies are the simultaneous analog stimulation (SAS), continuous interleaved sampler (CIS), spectral PEAK extraction (SPEAK), advanced combination encoders (ACE), and multiple pulse sample (MPS).
- Criteria for CI referral are: (1) patient must have a severe to profound bilateral sensorineural hearing loss and (2) little or no benefit from hearing aids.
- The CI is programmed by an audiologist 3 to 6 weeks after the surgery at a cochlear implant mapping. CIs are programmed utilizing a computer, a device-specific software program developed by the manufacturer of the implant, and an interface box. The electrical thresholds for soft inputs and the upper limit of comfort thresholds are established at the initial visit, as well as the speech processing strategy to be used.
- Outcome performance is negatively correlated with the duration of deafness and age. After implantation, individuals will need counseling regarding realistic expectations, additional training with communication strategies, speech-language therapy, academic support, continued instruction, and additional fine-tuning of the cochlear implant.

Most adults with postlingually acquired hearing loss show significant improvements in speech recognition abilities after implantation. The speech recognition abilities appear to improve and plateau for most individuals within the first 3 months and may continue to improve up to 1 year post-implant.

Outcome performance is negatively correlated with the duration of deafness and age. Following a cochlear implant, prelingually deafened children vary substantially with respect to their final communication mode. Most implanted children will use spoken language only, although some will use spoken language with continued used of sign language, or rely heavily on sign language as their primary means of communication. After implantation, children will require significant rehabilitation to obtain maximum outcomes. Individuals and their families need counseling regarding realistic expectations, additional training with communication strategies, speech-language therapy, academic support, continued instruction, and additional fine-tuning of the cochlear implant.

REFERENCES

Bassim, M. K., & Fayad, J. N. (2010). Implantable middle ear hearing devices: a review. *Seminars in Hearing*. 31(1): 28–36.

Channer, G. A., Eshraghi, A. A., & Lui, X. Z. (2011). Middle ear implant: Historical and futuristic perspective. *Journal of Otology*, 6(2): 10–18.

Food and Drug Administration (n.d.). What does it mean for FDA to "classify" a medical device? https://www.fda.gov/aboutfda/transparency/basics/ucm194438.htm

Gelfand, S. A. (2016). *Essentials of Audiology*. New York, NY: Thieme.

Gifford, R. H. (2017). The future of auditory implants. In A. M. Tharpe & R. Seewald, *Comprehensive Handbook of Pediatric Audiology* (2nd ed.). San Diego, CA: Plural.

Hodgetts, B. (2017). Other hearing devices: Bone conduction. In A. M. Tharpe & R. Seewald, *Comprehensive Handbook of Pediatric Audiology* (2nd ed.). San Diego, CA: Plural.

Kohan, D. (2015). Implantable Auditory Devices. A paper presented at the Ultimate Colorado Midwinter Meeting, Vail, CO.

Litovsky, R. Y., Colburn, H. S., Yost, W. A., & Guzman, S. J. (1999). The precedence effect. Review and tutorial paper. *Journal of the Acoustical Society of America*, 106: 1633–1654.

Kuhn, J. J., & Perez, A. J. (2015). Implantable hearing devices. In M. L. Pensak & D. I. Choo, *Clinical Otology* (4th ed.). New York, NY: Theime.

Reinfeldt, S., Hakansson, B., Taghavi, H., & Eeg-Olofsson, M. (2015). New developments in bone-conduction hearing implants: a review. *Medical Devices (Auckl)*. 8: 79–93.

Reinfeldt, S., Hakansson, B., Taghavi, H., Jansson, K. F., & Eeg-Olofsson, M. (2015). The bone conduction implant: Clinical results of the first six patients. *International Journal of Audiology 54*(6): 408–416.

Schmerber, S., Deguine, O., Marx, M., Van de Heyning, P., Sterkers, O., Mosnier, I., Garin, P., Godey, B., Vincent, C., Venail, F., Mondain, M., Deveze, A., Lavieille, J. P., & Karkas, A. (2017). Safety and effectiveness of the Bonebridge transcutaneous active direct-drive bone-conduction hearing implant at 1-year device use. *European Archives of Otorhinolaryngolgy 274*(4): 1835–1851.

Stach, B. A. (2014, September). 20Q: Advances in middle ear implant amplification. *AudiologyOnline*, Article 12947. Retrieved from: http://www.audiology online.com

Truy, E., Philibert, B., Vesson, J.F., Labaassi, S., & Collet, L. (2008). Vibrant Soundbridge versus conventional hearing aid in sensorineural High-frequency hearing loss: a prospective study. *Otol Neurotol* 29: 684–687.

Zeitler, D. M., Snapp, H. A., Telischi, F. F., & Angeli, S. I. (2012). Bone-anchored implantation for single-sided deafness in patients with less than profound hearing loss. *Otolaryngol Head Neck Surg*. 147: 105–111.

16 Vestibular System

After reading this chapter, you should be able to:

1. Identify and name the five vestibular structures and how they are oriented in the skull in relation to the auditory structures. Describe the main types of body motions to which each structure responds.

2. Identify and name the parts of the sensory organs of the semicircular canals. Describe where these sensory organs are located within the semicircular canals.

3. Identify and name the parts of the sensory organs of the utricle and saccule. Describe how the hair cells are oriented with regard to the striola for the utricle and saccule.

4. Describe the inferior and superior vestibular parts of the 8th cranial nerve, and from which parts of the vestibular system they innervate.

5. Explain what happens in the vestibular organs for different types of head movements and how the two sides work as pairs.

6. List the four vestibular nuclei and the components of the two main vestibular pathways (VSR and VOR).

7. Explain how nystagmus occurs, as well as how it is recorded and categorized based on its slow and fast phases.

8. Describe a variety of vestibular disorders, including the underlying cause (pathophysiology) and common symptoms/ complaints.

9. Describe and differentiate between the methods of ENG and VNG recordings.

10. List several subtests of VNG/ENG battery and briefly described how they are performed.

11. Describe rotary chair, computerized platform posturography, and VEMP methods of assessing the vestibular system.

The vestibular system is important for maintaining one's balance. The integration of neural activity of the vestibular, visual, somatosensory, and cerebellar systems allows you to maintain an upright posture, perform coordinated complex movements, and maintain a visual target while moving (Goebel & Hanson, 1997). Disorders in one or more of these systems may cause a patient to feel dizzy. *Dizziness* is a general term that patients might use to describe unsteadiness, lightheadedness, and/or a spinning sensation, called *vertigo*. Vertigo is a symptom of a peripheral vestibular disorder, whereas other dizziness or balance problems may be related to central nervous system involvement, other medical conditions, and/or psychological factors. It is estimated that 40% of people in the United States will have some dizziness and/or balance problem sometime in their lifetime (National Institute on Deafness and Other Communication Disorders [NIDCD], 2014). Vestibular disorders also occur in the pediatric population (Rine, 2009) with estimated prevalence ranging from 8 to 18% (American Speech-Language-Hearing Association [ASHA], 2004, n.d.).

The vestibular system operates, for the most part, without conscious control; you are not generally aware of its importance until it is affected by disease or by other atypical stimulations such as the reflexive action that occurs when you lean back in your chair just a little too far, or motion sickness that may occur in a boat bobbing in the waves, a spinning amusement park ride, or when riding in a car on winding roads. Understanding and controlling for motion sickness is also an important issue for astronauts and jet pilots. Another example of an atypical stimulation of the vestibular organs occurs when too much alcohol has been consumed resulting in vertigo and nausea.

The peripheral sensory organs of the vestibular system are housed within the inner ear, and several of the auditory disorders you have learned about can have associated involvement of the vestibular system, and vice versa. In addition, there are a number of vestibular disorders without any associated hearing problems. Vestibular screening, assessment, and some forms of management for both adult and pediatric patients are part of the scope of practice for audiologists (ASHA, 2004). The audiologist interacts with physicians (e.g., primary care doctors, otologists, neurologists, cardiologists, ophthalmologists) and other professionals (e.g., physical therapists, occupational therapists, psychologists) in the assessment and rehabilitation of patients with balance or dizziness problems. Fortunately, the vestibular system is remarkably adaptive and many vestibular disorders spontaneously recover or undergo central nervous system reorganization, known as *vestibular compensation* (Vidal, de Waele, Vibert, & Mühlethaler, 1998). This chapter provides an introductory look at the anatomy and physiology of the vestibular system, common vestibular disorders, and basic tests used to assess the vestibular system. For more detailed descriptions of the vestibular system, the reader is referred to other references (e.g., Barin, 2009; Desmond, 2011; Holt, Lysakowski, & Goldberg, 2010; Schubert & Shepard, 2016).

ANATOMY AND PHYSIOLOGY OF THE VESTIBULAR SYSTEM

In general, the vestibular organs provide neural information to the central nervous system that signals changes in the position of the head, as well as changes in the body's orientation relative to gravity. In other words, the vestibular organs respond to accelerations and decelerations of the head. The vestibular structures are located within the petrous portion of the temporal bone (bony labyrinth) along with the auditory structures, often collectively called the inner ear (refer to Chapter 4, Figure 4–2 for a general orientation). Figure 16–1A provides a closer look at the bony labyrinth and nerves of the inner ear. There are five separate structures that make up the peripheral vestibular system of the inner ear; three *semicircular canals*, superior (also called anterior), posterior, and horizontal (also called lateral), and two *otoliths*, *saccule* and *utricle*, housed inside the vestibule. As with the cochlea, there are bipolar afferent neurons that carry information from the vestibular hair cells to the brain, and a much smaller number of efferent neurons carrying input from the central nervous system to the ves-

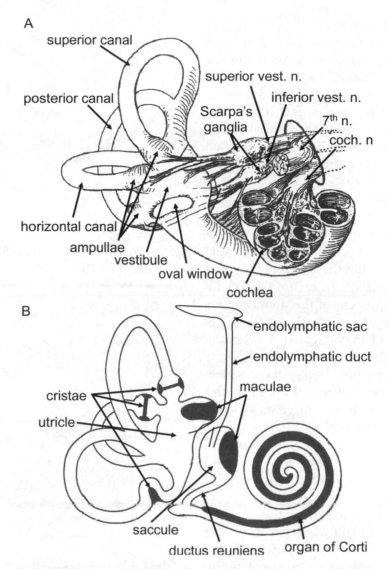

A

superior canal

superior vest. n.

inferior vest. n.

posterior canal

Scarpa's
ganglia

7th n.

coch. n

horizontal canal

ampullae

vestibule

oval window

cochlea

B

endolymphatic sac

endolymphatic duct

maculae

cristae

utricle

saccule

ductus reuniens

organ of Corti

FIGURE 16–1. A AND B. General orientation of the peripheral vestibular system. **A.** Bony labyrinth and 8th nerve. **B.** Membranous labyrinth showing locations of the sensory organs within the inner ear. *Source*: (A) Republished with permission of Oxford University Press, from Baloh, R. W., & Honrubia, V. H. (2001). *Clinical Neurophysiology of the Vestibular System.* New York, NY: Oxford University Press. p. 11; permission conveyed through Copyright Clearance Center, Inc. (B) From Bloom & Fawcett, 1962. Copyright 1962 by W.B. Saunders.

tibular hair cells. Less is known about the efferent vestibular system, but in general it is thought that it modulates some of the afferent vestibular neuron activity (Holt, Lysakowski, & Goldberg, 2010). The cell bodies for the bipolar peripheral vestibular afferent neurons are gathered together in *vestibular ganglia*, also known as *Scarpa's*

ganglia, located just peripheral to the internal auditory canal. The afferent neurons from the posterior semicircular canal and part of the saccule form the *inferior branch* of the vestibular nerve, whereas the afferent neurons from the other two semicircular canals, the utricle, and the remaining part of the saccule form the *superior branch* of the vestibular nerve. The vestibular branches of the 8th cranial nerve course through the internal auditory canal, along with the cochlear branch of the 8th cranial nerve and the 7th cranial nerve. Figure 16–1B shows the membranous labyrinth of the inner ear that is suspended within the bony labyrinth. The membranous labyrinth of the vestibular system is filled with endolymph and is continuous with the endolymph in the cochlea through the ductus reuniens (see also Chapter 4, Figure 4–14). As with the auditory system, perilymph is in the bony labyrinth outside the membranous labyrinth of the vestibular system. Each semicircular canal has a sensory organ within the membranous labyrinth, the *crista ampullaris* or *crista*. Each crista is located in an enlargement of the membranous (and bony) labyrinth, the *ampulla*, at the anterior end of each semicircular canal nearest the vestibule. The saccule and utricle each have a sensory organ, the *macula*. Unlike the cochlea, where the sensory cells continue along the entire length of the coiled cochlea, the crista of each semicircular canal is localized to a patch of cells within each ampulla rather than continue around the semicircular canal. The maculae are situated along one edge of the saccule and utricle.

Figure 16–2 is a diagram of a crista. A crista is composed of hair cells that have their stereocilia embedded into a gelatinous membrane, the *cupula*, which extends above the hair cells and completely seals off the semicircular canal within the ampulla. Remember, there is a separate crista for each semicircular canal. Figure 16–3 is a diagram of a macula. A macula is comprised of sensory hair cells distributed along one side of the saccule or utricle. The stereocilia of the hair cells within each macula are embedded in a gelatinous *otolith membrane*; however, the macula also has a layer of dense calcium carbonate crystals, *otoconia*, on top of the otolith membrane, which adds mass to the otolith membrane.

As with the inner and outer hair cells of the organ of Corti, each of the vestibular organs has two types of hair cells, type I and type II. As seen in Figure 16–4, a type I hair cell is more flask shaped, and a type II hair cell is more cylinder shaped. The stereocilia of the hair cells in a crista are arranged in two or three rows with increas-

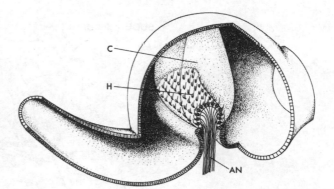

FIGURE 16–2. A crista within the ampulla of a semicircular canal. C, cupula; H, hair cells; AN, afferent nerves. *Source*: From Barber & Stockwell, 1976, p. 22. Copyright 1976 by Mosby.

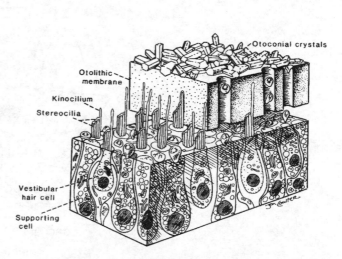

FIGURE 16–3. A macula of the otolith organ showing the otoconia crystals on the surface of the gelatinous otolithic membrane. *Source*: Republished with permission of Oxford University Press, from Furman, J. M., & Cass, S. P. (1996). *Balance Disorders: A Case-Study Approach*. Philadelphia, PA: F. A. Davis. p. 6; permission conveyed through Copyright Clearance Center, Inc.

ing heights, and each hair cell has a single large cilium, *kinocilium*, adjacent to the tallest row of stereocilia. The kinocilium has a functionally relevant orientation for the direction of stereocilia bending during head movements that produce distinct physiological responses, discussed in more detail later in the chapter. As you may recall, the hair cells of the organ of Corti do not have a visible kinocilium; however, each of the

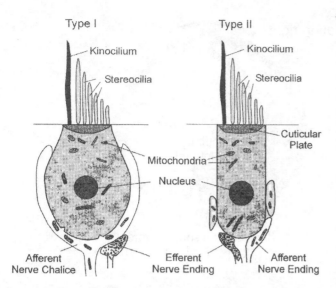

FIGURE 16–4. Diagram of type I and type II vestibular hair cells. *Source*: Republished with permission of Lippincott Williams & Wilkins, from Barin, K. (2009). Clinical neurophysiology of the vestibular system. In J. Katz, L. Medwetsky, B. Burkard, & L. Hood (Eds.), *Handbook of Clinical Audiology* (6th ed., pp. 431–466). Baltimore, MD: Lippincott Williams & Wilkins. p. 436; permission conveyed through Copyright Clearance Center, Inc.

hair cells in the organ of Corti has a rudimentary base of a kinocilium embedded in the top surface of the hair cell adjacent to the tallest row of stereocilia, and which also provides functionally relevant orientations for the direction of stereocilia bending as part of the ear's physiological response to sound vibrations. A type I vestibular hair cell synapses with a relatively large afferent neuron surrounding the cell body (calyx). There are also efferent neurons that synapse on the afferent neuron as it leaves the type I hair cell (similar to IHCs of the cochlea). The type II vestibular hair cell synapses with both afferent and efferent neurons directly with the body of the hair cell (similar to OHCs of the cochlea). The proportion of type I and type II vestibular hair cells varies among species and among the different vestibular organs. Functional relevance of having two types of hair cells within the vestibular organs is not as distinct as for the IHCs and OHCs of the organ of Corti. Hair cell transduction within the vestibular organs occurs similarly to cochlear

hair cells, whereby stereocilia tip-links open and close potassium ion (K+) channels, effecting depolarization and hyperpolarization phases of transduction. Vestibular hair cells have been shown to have motility that might influence the stereocilia as part of an active process (Takumida, Hironori, Miyawaki, Arishige, Harada,1994; Baloh, Honrubia, & Kerber, 2011).

Function of the Semicircular Canals

The semicircular canals are responsive to rotational (angular) accelerations and decelerations of the head. Each of the three semicircular canals is most sensitive to rotation in a particular orthogonal plane of motion, including head rotations left and right (*x*-axis), forward and backward (*y*-axis), or tilted toward each shoulder (*z*-axis). More than one semicircular canal may respond when head rotations occur in more complicated directions of head rotation that typically occur in everyday patterns of movement. For example, the horizontal semicircular canals are most responsive to rotation of the head left and right, whereas the posterior and inferior semicircular canals are most responsive for forward and backward (pitch) and tilting left or right (yaw) rotations. In a normal system, semicircular canals on both sides of the head work together in functional pairs: The horizontal semicircular canal on the left side is paired with the horizontal semicircular canal on the right side; the superior semicircular canal on the left side is paired with the posterior semicircular canal on the right side; and the posterior semicircular canal on the left side is paired with the superior semicircular canal on the right side. Direction of head rotation is signaled by an increase in the neural discharge rate (above the resting discharge rate) on one side and a decrease (below the resting discharge rate) on the other side (Baloh, 1998).

During head movement, the direction that the stereocilia bend determines excitation or inhibition; bending toward the kinocilium increases the neural discharge rate (excitation) and bending away from the kinocilium decreases the neural discharge rate (inhibition). The kinocilia of the hair cells within a crista are oriented away from

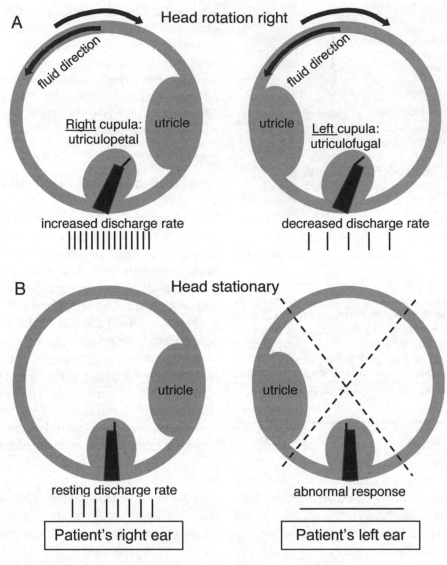

FIGURE 16–5. A AND B. Illustration of how semicircular canals from each side of the head work to provide information to the central nervous system. **A.** Normal vestibular system. When the head rotates to the right, the bending of the stereocilia on the right side is utriculopetal that produces an increase in the neural discharge rate relative to the resting rate; bending of the stereocilia on the left side is utriculofugal that produces a decrease in the neural discharge rate relative to the resting rate. **B.** The left canal is damaged. Without rotating the head, there is an imbalance in the neural discharges from the two sides (acting as if the head rotates to the right) giving rise to the sensation of movement (dizziness). May also be accompanied by spontaneous nystagmus.

the utricle for the superior and posterior canals, and oriented toward the utricle for the horizontal semicircular canals. During head accelerations, there is centrifugal force developed and the movement of the fluid in the semicircular canal lags behind the canal movement due to its viscous and inertial properties, which results in a deflection of the cupula. Within the functional pairs of canals, the deflection of the cupula on one side is toward the utricle, *utriculopetal*, and the stereocilia bend toward the kinocilium (excitation); the deflection of the cupula on the other side is away from the utricle, *utriculofugal*, and the stereocilia bend away from the kinocilium (inhibition). As Figure 16–5A illustrates, for head acceleration to the right, the cupula on the right side causes the stereocilia to bend toward the kinocilium (utriculopetal), producing an increase in the neural discharge rate on the right side: At the same time on the left side, the cupula causes the stereocilia to bend away from the kinocilium (utriculofugal), producing a decrease in the neural discharge rate. The vestibular nuclei in the brainstem integrate the neural information from the two sides in order to signal the direction of head rotation. Similar events take place for other directions of head movement involving the functional pairs of superior and posterior canals. When head rotation reaches a steady velocity, the stereocilia return to their resting state and the neural activity is once again in balance; however, additional accelerations or decelerations will result in renewed stimulation. Figure 16–5B illustrates what happens with a damaged semicircular canal on one side of the head. In this case, even when the head is stationary, the disruption/abnormality in neural information from the damaged left side, compared to the resting neural discharge rate from the normal side, signals a neural imbalance from the two sides that gives rise to the sensation of head turning, causing one to experience vertigo and imbalance.

Functions of the Utricle and Saccule

The utricle and saccule respond to linear accelerations and decelerations of the head, as well as maintain the body's orientation relative to gravity. The stereocilia of the maculae are covered by otoconia, a gelatinous mass covered with calcium carbonate crystals. These calcium carbonate crystals have a higher specific gravity than the surrounding fluid, making them responsive to head position relative to gravity, as well as to changes that occur during linear head accelerations and decelerations. The utricle is primarily responsive to linear motions in the horizontal plane (forward and backward, or left and right), whereas the saccule is primarily responsive to linear motions in the vertical plane (up and down).

Linear movements in other directions produce responses from combinations of these organs. The utricle and saccule on one side of the head work together with the utricle and saccule on the other side of the head to signal the direction of head movement by comparing which organ has increased its neural discharge rate and which has decreased its neural discharge rate. As with the semicircular canals, when the stereocilia are bent toward the kinocilium there is an increase in neural discharge rate above the spontaneous rate (excitation), and when they are bent away from the kinocilium there is a decrease in neural discharge rate (inhibition). However, the directional polarization of the kinocilia in the maculae is more complex than in the semicircular canals. Figure 16–6 illustrates the functional arrangements of the hair cells in the macula of the saccule and utricle. The hair cells within each macula are separated into two orientations based on the position of their kinocilia. The dividing line between the two different orientations of hair cells is called the striola that lies near the middle of the macula. In the utricle, the kinocilia of the hair cells on each side of the striola are oriented toward the striola. In the saccule, the kinocilia of the hair cells on each side of the striola are oriented away from the striola. During accelerations of the head, the hair cells in one group increase their neural discharge rate (deflection of stereocilia is toward the kinocilia) and the hair cells in the other group decrease their neural discharge rate (deflection of stereocilia is away from the kinocilia). Once the head movement reaches a steady velocity, the discharge rates are back in balance and ready for additional accelerations or decelerations.

CENTRAL PATHWAYS INVOLVED IN BALANCE AND MOVEMENT

As mentioned earlier, maintaining your balance and making coordinated movements involves the integration of information from several sensory and motor systems. Figure 16–7 summarizes the components and pathways of the balance systems. The vestibular and auditory portions of the 8th cranial nerve enter the brainstem at the pontine level of the brainstem; however, instead of synapsing with the cochlear nucleus as

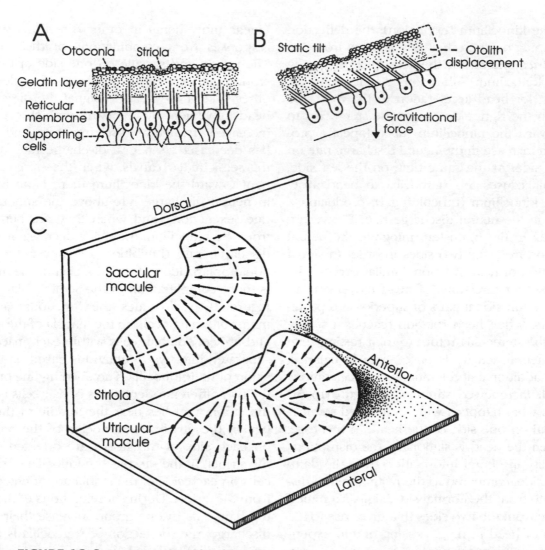

FIGURE 16–6. A–C. Functional polarization of the maculae in the utricle and the saccule. In the saccule, there are two groups of hair cells, functionally separated by the striola, and the kinocilia are directed away from the striola. In the utricle, there are also two groups of hair cells, also functionally separated by the striola; however, the kinocilia are directed toward the striola. *Source*: From Barber & Stockwell, 1976. Copyright 1976 by Mosby.

do the auditory neurons, the vestibular neurons synapse with cells within specialized vestibular nuclei within the brainstem and a small number go directly to the cerebellum. There are four vestibular nuclei, superior, medial, lateral, and spinal, on each side of the brainstem. The vestibular neurons of the 8th cranial nerve first synapse with vestibular nuclei on the ipsilateral (same) side as the sensory organs. However, as with the auditory nuclei, there are interconnections between the vestibular nuclei on the left and right sides of the brainstem. In addition to the small

number of connections to the cerebellum, there are two main vestibular pathways, the *vestibulo-ocular reflex* (VOR) and the *vestibulospinal reflex* (VSR).

Vestibulo-Ocular Reflex (VOR)

The vestibular neural pathway has connections within the brainstem to neurons that reflexively control the muscles of the eyes so that a clear vi-

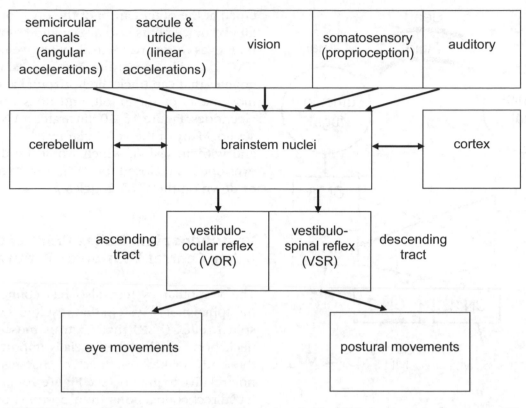

FIGURE 16–7. Overview of the components involved with balance and movement. Different sensory systems are processed by the brainstem, with connections to the cerebellum and cortex, to control eye movements, posture, and coordinated movements.

sual image can be automatically maintained during head movement (Wright & Schwade, 2000). This ascending neural pathway is called the *vestibuloocular reflex* (VOR). The VOR involves connections from parts of the vestibular nuclei to the oculomotor nuclei through the medial longitudinal fasciculus or indirectly through the reticular formation. The VOR reflexively controls the relevant muscles of the eyes as needed. The VOR results in eye movements that are equal and opposite to the direction of head movements (Barber, 1984). As an example, the VOR for the horizontal semicircular canals involves afferent neurons from the vestibular nerve to the vestibular nucleus on the same side. From the vestibular nucleus on each side, there are connections to the contralateral nucleus of the 6th cranial nerve (abducens nerve) that contracts the lateral rectus muscle of the eye on that side and the medial rectus (via 3rd cranial nerve) of the other eye. As Figure 16–8 shows, for a head turn

to the right, the excitatory input from the right semicircular canal (and inhibitory input from the left semicircular canal) causes contraction of the lateral rectus muscle of the left eye and contraction of the medial rectus muscle of the right eye, which makes the eyes move to the left. For a head turn to the left, the excitatory input from the left semicircular canal (and inhibitory input from the right) causes contraction of the lateral rectus muscle of the right eye and contraction of the medial rectus muscle of the left eye, which makes the eyes move to the right. Because the eyes can only move a small distance in the orbit, there is an additional neural connection from the reticular formation that quickly brings the eyes back to the center (Wright & Schwade, 2000).

Nystagmus

Observing and/or recording eye movements under different conditions is very useful for assessment

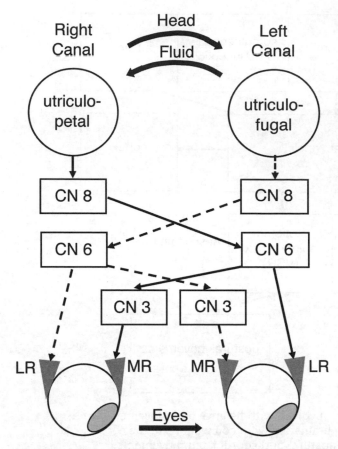

FIGURE 16–8. The vestibulo-ocular reflex pathway. In this example for a head turn to the right, the right ear horizontal canal is excitatory and causes the eye muscles from each side to work together to move the eyes to the left. CN, cranial nerve; LR, lateral rectus; MR, medial rectus.

taped at the outer canthi of the eyes for horizontal eye movements and above and below one or both eyes to record vertical eye movements. The VNG is a video recording method using special goggles that can track the horizontal and vertical movements of the pupil, and does not require electrodes. Figure 16–10 illustrates a VNG testing set-up. Many of the vestibular tests are done with and without vision, which would be done with eyes open and closed for ENG, or with a visor up or down on the VNG goggles.

Vestibulospinal Reflex (VSR) and Other Central Vestibular Pathways

The vestibular system also has connections to the spinal motor system that result in a vestibulospinal reflex (VSR) that controls muscles in the neck, body, and limbs, especially important when the body makes unexpected changes in position relative to gravity (see Figure 16–7). The VSR has direct connections from portions of the vestibular nuclei to motor neurons in the spinal cord (vestibulospinal tracts) and indirect connections through the reticular formation (reticulospinal tract), which act to reflexively control the

of many vestibular disorders. The slow (vestibular) and fast (reticular formation) components of reflexive eye responses during head rotation as described above is called *nystagmus*, which continually repeats during head rotation. Figure 16–9 shows a repeated pattern of nystagmus for a head turn to the right. Nystagmus can be induced through vestibular clinical tests or may be abnormally present in certain vestibular disorders.

Videonystagmography (VNG) and *electronystagmography (ENG)* are two methods used to monitor eye movements and record nystagmus during a vestibular evaluation. The ENG has traditionally been used, whereas VNG is a newer method that has become increasingly popular. The ENG measure changes in the *corneoretinal potential* of the eye through surface electrodes

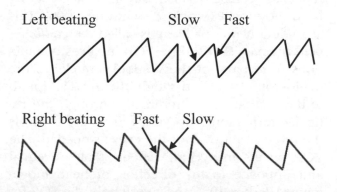

FIGURE 16–9. An example of nystagmus. Because the eyes can only move so far during a head turn, there is a central component that continually brings them back to center. Nystagmus has a slow phase due to the semicircular canal response and a fast phase due to the central (reticular formation) response. These responses can be observed by measuring (with electrodes around the eyes) how the corneoretinal potential changes with eye movements (ENG), or by video recording of eye movement (VNG).

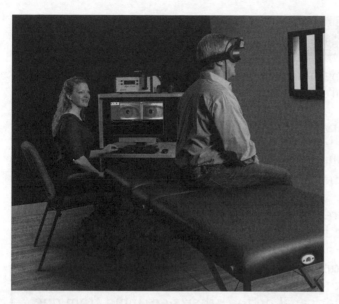

FIGURE 16–10. Illustration of a typical VNG testing arrangement. *Source*: Photo courtesy of Micromedical Technologies, 10 Kemp Drive, Chatham, IL 62629.

relevant skeletal muscles as needed. The vestibular system also has connections with the reticular formation of the autonomic nervous system, which influences respiration and gustatory or visceral reflexes. These latter vestibular pathways account for a person's nausea or vomiting from motion sickness, excessive alcohol, or other vestibular disorders.

VESTIBULAR DISORDERS

In this section, you will be introduced to some vestibular disorders (listed alphabetically). For each disorder, there is a brief description of the underlying cause and pathophysiology, as well as typical complaints. Many audiologists are involved with assessment of the vestibular system (see next section for vestibular tests) from physician referrals.

Alcohol Overconsumption

Consuming too much alcohol (which dilutes the blood) can alter the specific gravity of the cupula of the semicircular canals which makes it lighter than the surrounding endolymph and causes it

to become more sensitive to rotational acceleration or may even produce a sensation of spinning while standing or lying still. In addition, too much alcohol may result in vomiting that could result in vertigo as a symptom of dehydration.

Benign Paroxysmal Positional Vertigo (BPPV)

Benign paroxysmal positional vertigo (BPPV) occurs when some of the calcium carbonate crystals of the otoconia within the macula of a utricle become dislodged and fall into one or more of the semicircular canals. This is one of the most common vestibular disorders, and occurs most frequently in the elderly with no specific cause, or may occur following trauma to the head. The inappropriate accumulation of the crystals affects the normal fluid movement of the semicircular canals, resulting in incorrect neural information being sent to the central vestibular system that gives the sensation of spinning (vertigo). These periodic/rapid (paroxysmal) episodes of vertigo are often triggered when the head moves or gets into a certain position.

Bilateral Vestibular Hypofunction

Bilateral vestibular hypofunction is a loss/reduction of vestibular function on both sides as a secondary affect to either a known disorder such as ototoxicity or vestibular neuritis, or from an unknown cause (idiopathic). The loss of vestibular function causes a generalized feeling of being off-balance (as opposed to spinning vertigo attacks) or may cause difficulty walking, especially when other sensory input is not able to be effectively used, such as in the dark or on irregular surfaces.

Endolymphatic Hydrops/ Ménière's Disease

Endolymphatic hydrops is a condition resulting from excessive build-up of endolymph within the inner ear. Symptoms typically include vertigo, hearing loss, aural fullness, and low-pitched

SYNOPSIS 16–1

Vertigo is an abnormal balance sensation mediated by the peripheral vestibular system in which there is a perception that things are spinning.

- The vestibular system relies on sensory information from the peripheral vestibular organs, as well as from the visual and proprioceptive systems, which is integrated in the brainstem, cerebellum, and cerebral cortex to control eye movements, posture, and limb movements in certain situations that change the position of the head.
- The semicircular canals are primarily responsive to rotational (angular) accelerations and decelerations of the head. Each of the three semicircular canals is most sensitive to rotation in a particular orthogonal plane of motion: The horizontal semicircular canal on one side is paired with the horizontal semicircular canal on the other side; the superior semicircular canal on one side is paired with the posterior semicircular canal on the other side. Input from one side of the head works with input from the other side to maintain balance and control during movement.
- The utricle and saccule maintain the body's orientation relative to gravity, and are also responsive to linear accelerations and decelerations of the head. The utricle is primarily responsive to linear motions in the horizontal plane (forward and backward or left to right), whereas the saccule is primarily responsive to linear motions in the vertical plane (up and down). The utricle and saccule on one side of the head work together with the utricle and saccule on the other side of the head to signal the direction of head movement by comparing which organ has increased its neural discharge rate and which has decreased its neural discharge rate.
- Bending of the stereocilia within the peripheral vestibular organs is accomplished by head movement that displaces the gelatinous mass that covers the tops of the stereocilia. In the crista, this is accomplished by the cupula; in the otoliths by the otoconia.
- The vestibular neural pathways within the brainstem have connections to the motor neurons of the cranial nerves that are involved with control of the extraocular muscles of the eyes, called the vestibulo-ocular reflex (VOR), so that a clear visual image can be automatically maintained during head movement.
- Observing and/or recording eye movements, nystagmus, under different conditions is very useful for assessment of many vestibular disorders. Nystagmus is a rapid involuntary movement of the eyes, characterized as a sawtooth recording in which there is a slow phase in the opposite direction from the perceived direction of head movement (due to vestibular input) and a fast phase that resets the eye back toward center (due to a central nervous system).
- Nystagmus can be measured through videonystagmography (VNG) or through electronystagmography (ENG) with electrodes mounted next to the eyes that can record changes in the electrical potential, called the *corneoretinal potential*, as the eyes move.

SYNOPSIS 16–1 (*continued*)

- The vestibular system has central brainstem connections to the spinal motor system that result in vestibulo-spinal reflexes (VSR) to control muscles in the neck, body, and limbs when the body makes unexpected changes in position relative to gravity.
- The vestibular system also has connections with the reticular formation of the autonomic nervous system and can influence respiration and gustatory or visceral reflexes, as with motion sickness.

tinnitus. When the cause is known, such as an autoimmune disorder, head trauma, or allergies, the disorder is called endolymphatic hydrops; when the cause is unknown (idiopathic), the disorder is called *Ménière's disease*. The condition is usually unilateral, but can occur or progress to a bilateral condition. Ménière's disease is more prevalent in the 2nd to 5th decades of life. The increased pressure from the build-up of endolymph produces a sensation of aural fullness and may eventually rupture the inner ear membrane (thought to occur in Reissner's membrane). When the membrane ruptures, there is a mixing of perilymph with the endolymph that has a temporary (at least initially) toxic effect on the hair cells. The hair cells become hyperactive and produce the sensation of vertigo. The toxic effects may also cause a fluctuating low frequency hearing loss, initially, but may end up as a permanent, relatively flat, sensorineural loss. A low frequency (buzzing/ocean roar) tinnitus is also a common symptom. The ruptured membrane can repair itself, returning the fluids to a more normal balance, and the hair cells may regain normal function but the cycle may repeat.

Enlarged Vestibular Aqueduct (EVA)

An *enlarged vestibular aqueduct (EVA)* is a developmental malformation. The vestibular aqueduct is normally a very narrow bony canal in which the endolymphatic duct is located that ends in the endolymphatic sac. An enlarged endolymphatic duct and sac may lead to abnormal

inner ear function causing a sensorineural hearing loss, or the hereditary factor that caused the EVA may in itself be responsible for the hearing loss. The hearing loss can be syndromic or non-syndromic, can be present at birth or with a later onset, and may progress over time. Vestibular symptoms are less common, but may include problems with coordination or balance.

Labyrinthitis/Vestibular Neuritis

Labyrinthitis or vestibular neuritis is an infection (commonly viral) of the inner ear labyrinth and/or vestibular nerve. The infection causes temporary disruption of vestibular function producing dizziness/vertigo, balance problems, nausea, and/or hearing and vision problems. Function typically returns to normal when the infection is resolved; however, there can also be permanent neural degeneration of the vestibular nerve or sensory cells of the inner ear.

Motion Sickness

Motion sickness is caused by getting mixed signals from different sensory systems. It occurs when the vestibular system senses movements, but the other sensory systems do not have the same sensation or are not able to counteract the sensation of movement. This can happen when the body is moving, but the eyes cannot adjust to the movement. It can also happen if the eyes see movement (e.g., during a video game), but the body does not sense movement. Vertigo is also a relatively big problem for astronauts because they have to adapt to changes in gravitational forces that may give an incorrect spacial orientation.

Perilymph Fistula (PLF)

Perilymph fistula (PLF) is a rupture or defect in the oval window or round window membranes (most often from head trauma) that causes some of the perilymph of the inner ear to leak into the middle ear. A PLF may result in a feeling of unsteadiness, vertigo, and/or nausea, especially during changes in middle ear pressure or when in certain positions. In some cases, there may be hearing loss, aural fullness, and/or tinnitus. The symptoms of PLF are similar to those of Meniere's disease. In addition, when perilymph leaks into the middle ear, CSF levels around the brain may be reduced and can cause a mild headache. Symptoms often worsen with changes in altitude or from increased CSF pressure when bending over, coughing/sneezing, or during heavy lifting.

Persistent Postural Perceptual Dizziness (PPPD)

Persistent postural perceptual dizziness (PPPD), also called chronic subjective dizziness (CSD), is a long-lasting (at least three months) dizziness that is usually the sequela of some other event that caused acute vertigo or balance problems (e.g., Ménière's disease, BPPV). It can also occur following whiplash, concussion, or a panic attack. The main symptom of PPPD is a persistent (every day or two) sensation of unsteadiness, described as rocking or swaying, without vertigo. Anxiety and/or depression may contribute to or exacerbate PPPD.

Superior Canal Dehiscence (SCD)

Superior canal dehiscence (SCD) is a small opening in the bony labyrinth of the superior semicircular canal. This opening acts like a third window of the inner ear (the other two are the oval window and the round window), and allows the membranous portion of the superior semicircular canal to be displaced during sound or increased pressure. It is thought that SCD begins as a thinner than normal section of bone of the superior canal due to a developmental abnormality, but typically does not manifest itself until the bone completely wears away during the 3rd or 4th decade of life. Symptoms include vertigo and oscillopsia (apparent motion of stationary objects) that can be caused by loud noises and/or by pressure changes of middle ear or intracranial pressures from coughing, sneezing, or straining. Additionally, there may be an increased sensitivity/increase in the perceived volume of the person's own voice, and hypersensitivity to bone-conducted sounds. Many patients experience a low frequency conductive hearing loss that occurs because some of the energy of the vibrations entering the middle ear are "diverted" to the 3rd window and less energy is routed through the normal pathway to the cochlea.

Vestibulotoxicity/Ototoxicity

Vestibulotoxicity (ototoxicity) refers to "poisoning" of the vestibular organs and/or vestibular nerve from drugs or chemicals. The generic term ototoxicity refers to toxic damage to the auditory and/or vestibular senses. Some drugs are more vestibulotoxic, while others are more cochleotoxic. The amount of damage depends on the drug/chemical involved, and can be temporary or permanent. Symptoms will vary, but typically vestibulotoxicity causes dizziness and balance problems; when there is damage to the auditory system, hearing loss and tinnitus occur.

Vestibular Schwannoma/ Acoustic Neuroma

Vestibular schwannoma, also known as an acoustic neuroma, is a benign, non-hereditary, slow-growing tumor that arises from an overproduction of Schwann cells of the 8th cranial nerve fibers (usually from the vestibular branch). These tumors generally occur in the 3rd to 5th decade of life from an unknown cause. As the tumor grows, it compresses the 8th nerve causing a unilateral hearing loss, tinnitus (high-pitched), aural fullness, reduced speech understanding, and/or balance problems. Relatively large tumors can also impinge on the facial nerve, causing facial numbness. Over time, if left unchecked, the tumor may produce severe pressure on the brainstem and cerebellum. There is a genetic version of this disorder, called neurofibromatosis (NF2), where a tumor occurs in both ears (and other places in the body), which can lead to deafness if the tumors are not removed.

ASSESSING VESTIBULAR DISORDERS

Audiologists are often involved in the assessment of vestibular disorders as part of an interdisciplinary team that includes otologists and neurologists. Vestibular screening, diagnostics, and some forms of management are in the audiology scope of practice (American Academy of Audiology [AAA], 2004; American Speech-Language-Hearing Association [ASHA], 2004). The reader is also referred to ASHA's practice guidelines regarding balance system disorders and assessment (ASHA, n.d.).

Case History

As with most clinical assessments, the case history is an important component and can be useful when screening or diagnosing vestibular and balance disorders. Some basic case history questions to ask the patient include:

- What is the nature of the dizziness (e.g., vertigo, disorientation, imbalance)?
- Are there other associated symptoms (e.g., hearing loss, tinnitus, aural fullness, vision)?
- When did the problem start and how often/when do the symptoms occur?
- Are there specific factors/actions that precipitate or alleviate the symptoms?
- What prescription or over-the-counter medications are you taking?

Additionally, you should consider having the patient complete one or more of the available questionnaires/inventories to characterize the patient's dizziness and balance problems, such as the Dizziness Handicap Inventory (Jacobson & Newman, 1990) or about the effects of the problem on the patient's quality of life. A comprehensive description of some of these assessment scales can be found in Jacobson, Newman, and Piker (2016).

Screening for Vestibular Disorders

Office or bedside screening of vestibular and balance problems can be done with very little equipment; however, these screening techniques should only be done by those who are qualified. Abnormalities in these measures would necessitate referral for further testing. Basic screening methods may include the following:

- Tracking of static eye movements, including shifting gaze back and forth, up and down (saccades), and following a moving target (smooth pursuit).
- Observation of static spontaneous nystagmus (eyes open) with and without fixation.
- Observation of dynamic nystagmus after shaking head back and forth for about 30 seconds (Head Shake Test).
- Inability to maintain visual fixation on a target after short rapid head thrusts in different planes (Head Thrust Test).
- Comparison of static and dynamic visual acuity. Patient first reads an eye chart with head stationary to find where about 50% of characters are identifiable, and then again while rotating head left and right to see how many lines (if any) are lost.
- Dix–Hallpike maneuver for BPPV. Observe if there is nystagmus with the maneuver for head down and to the right and/or head down and to the left.

The VNG/ENG Test Battery

Saccade/Ocular Dysmetria

The saccade/ocular dysmetria test should always be done before any of the other tests in order to calibrate the recording instrument and to be sure the patient has the ability to perform saccades. Saccades are quick movements of the eye that occur when trying to refixate on a target that is quickly moved from one point to another. A light bar or video projection is used to intermittently present visual spots or flashing lights at 10 to 30 degrees in the horizontal and vertical planes. The patient is instructed to follow/find the target as quickly as possible without moving the head. The equipment should be calibrated to a scale of 20 degrees of eye movement = 20 mm. A normal result would show that the eye movements pretty closely match the movements of the target. Undershooting or overshooting of the target is called ocular dysmetria. If saccades are not able to be performed accurately (e.g., delayed onset, dysmetria, and/or too slow), the patient most likely has a cerebellar or other central disorder rather than a peripheral vestibular disorder.

Spontaneous Nystagmus

The spontaneous nystagmus test is looking for nystagmus that is not induced by vestibular testing. The nystagmus can be observed with eyes closed during the VNG/ENG exam. It can also be observed with Frenzel lenses or the VNG googles in which the tester can see the patient's eyes magnified but the patient cannot see out. Testing for spontaneous nystagmus is typically performed with the head/body in several positions. A normal finding would have no nystagmus, even when vision is denied. Spontaneous nystagmus is present when found in at least three body/head positions. In some cases, spontaneous nystagmus can be present with vision during an acute stage of peripheral vestibular insult. The presence of horizontal spontaneous nystagmus, without vision, is a sign of a peripheral vestibular disorder, such as with a vestibular schwannoma. Vertical spontaneous nystagmus is usually a central disorder.

Gaze

The gaze test assesses the patient's ability to maintain visual fixation, without moving the head, on a spot or finger positioned in the center posi-

tion (same as testing for spontaneous nystagmus), then at 30 degrees left and right (horizontal plane), and 30 degrees up and down (vertical plane). The patient is asked to maintain fixation on each spot for at least 20 to 30 seconds with vision and then without vision while performing some simple arithmetic task to maintain alertness. A normal result would be that the patient can maintain fixation (no nystagmus) at the target points with vision and without vision (but may have a slow drift back toward center without vision). A peripheral vestibular abnormality (e.g., vestibular neuritis) would typically show horizontal gaze nystagmus that is larger when tested without vision compared to when tested with vision. Gaze-induced nystagmus beats toward the side that has the more active neural activity. For example, with vestibular neuritis in the left ear there would be a large right-beating gaze nystagmus because the right ear would be more neurally active compared to the decreased (abnormal) neural activity from the left ear. Vertical gaze nystagmus may be a sign of central disorders.

Optokinetic

The optokinetic test induces nystagmus by having the patient look at bars of light that are projected onto a curved surface (or black and white stripes on a revolving drum). The bars/stripes move right to left or left to right across the patient's field of vision at a slow and fast velocity (20 to 60 degrees/second). The patient is asked to not follow/track the bars/stripes, but instead should watch/count them as they go past, thus inducing nystagmus. A normal response should show presence of nystagmus with the fast phase directed away from the direction of the stimulus movement. In addition, the velocity of the slow phase is compared to the velocity of the stimulus, and referred to as optokinetic velocity gain. A normal response would have the velocity of the slow phase at least 50% of the velocity of the stimulus and be relatively symmetrical for both directions. An abnormal result would show asymmetry for the two directions of stimulation, that is, slow phase velocity is reduced in one of the directions and the asymmetry is more pronounced when tested at the higher velocity. Another abnormal result would show normal nystagmus at the slower stimulus velocity, but significantly weaker nystagmus when tested at the higher stimulus velocity. An optokinetic asymmetry is often due to a central disorder when accompanied by abnormal saccades and/or smooth pursuit; however, without these signs, the asymmetric results suggest reduced peripheral vestibular function. It is also possible to have asymmetry with intense peripheral vestibular nystagmus that may cause the optokinetic induced nystagmus to appear weaker in the direction opposite to the peripheral induced nystagmus.

Paroxysmal Nystagmus (for BPPV)

The paroxysmal nystagmus test (a.k.a. positioning test) is used to evaluate benign paroxysmal positional vertigo (BPPV). In patients with BPPV, the displaced otoconia within the posterior semicircular canal can cause vertigo and rotary nystagmus (eyes rotate about the visual axis) when moved. With the patient in a sitting position, the tester rapidly moves the patient's head backward while rotating the head to the right or the left to hang off the table (supported by the tester) in order to stimulate the posterior semicircular canal (Dix–Hallpike or the modified Hallpike maneuver). In a normal individual, there may be a brief episode of nystagmus during movement, but that quickly subsides after the movement. Patient's with BPPV show a slightly delayed burst of strong rotary nystagmus after the movement is completed when the involved ear is facing down, then there is a period with a build-up in intensity, and then the nystagmus slowly dissipates over 10 to 15 seconds. The response can easily fatigue; therefore, this test should be done before the positional test.

Positional

The positional test looks for nystagmus in different stationary positions of the head/body, that is, monitoring effects of linear gravitational forces on the otolith organs (saccule and utricle). Positional testing should be done after the paroxysmal nystagmus (Dix–Hallpike) test. Positional testing is done without vision (20 seconds) and with vision (20 seconds). A normal finding would not show any nystagmus in any of the positions, with or without vision. If nystagmus is present without vision, this would suggest a peripheral or central disorder; however, if nystagmus is present with vision, this would be a sign of a central disorder.

Caloric

The caloric test is the main part of the VNG/ENG battery focused on the assessment of peripheral vestibular organ abnormality. The caloric test induces nystagmus with warm and cold (bithermal) stimulations of the ear canal to affect, indirectly, the vestibular organs by induction through the skull. The caloric test is done independently on each ear and then compared to each other. The main piece of equipment is an irrigation system that delivers either water or pressurized air at the different temperatures into the ear canals. To perform the test, the patient lies on a table with the table/head raised 30 degrees in order to orient the horizontal canals in a vertical position (perpendicular to the ground). The patient should have his or her eyes closed during most of the caloric test and is asked to perform simple mental arithmetic to maintain alertness. Each irrigation should last 30 to 60 seconds, and the induced nystagmus is recorded during stimulation as well as after stimulation until the nystagmus is no longer present.

The caloric (warm and cold) stimulation (water or air) indirectly, through convection, alters the density of the endolymph that causes the endolymph to flow, thus causing stimulation of the crista within the canal. The warm stimulus decreases the density of the endolymph at the end of the canal closest to the stimulus causing the endolymph to flow toward the ampulla (ampullopetal) producing an excitatory neural response: The cold stimulus increases the density of the endolymph at the end of the canal closest to the stimulus causing the endolymph to flow away from the ampulla (ampullofugal) producing an inhibitory neural response. The nystagmus beats away from the stimulated ear with cold stimulation (e.g., right beating nystagmus for left ear stimulation) and beats toward the stimulated ear with warm stimulation (e.g., right beating nystagmus for right ear stimulation). The acronym COWS is useful to remember the direction of the beats, that is, "cold opposite, warm same."

After the nystagmus reaches its peak amplitude (about 60 to 90 seconds after the start of irrigation) the patient is asked to visually fixate on a spot for about 10 to 15 seconds and then asked to close eyes again; recording continues until nystagmus disappears (2 to 3 minutes after beginning of irrigation). During visual fixation, a normal vestibular system should be able to suppress the nystagmus, whereas an abnormal vestibular system would not be able to suppress the nystagmus (called failure of fixation suppression).

To evaluate the caloric-induced nystagmus, the velocity of the slow phase for each of the stimulations for each ear is calculated by taking the mean of several of the strongest beats. The following measures of the slow phase velocity (degrees/second) are made of the caloric responses from the two irrigations in each ear (computerized VNG or ENG systems can calculate these measures automatically):

1. Bilateral weakness (BW): Looks at the average amplitude of the peak nystagmus (speed of the slow phase component) from each ear. RW = right warm; RC = right cold; LW = left warm; LC = left cold:

   Right ear total = RW + RC (ignore the sign and use absolute values)

   Left ear total = LW + LC (ignore the sign and use absolute values)

Note: BW is present if each of the above is less than 12 degrees/second. If BW is present, then the rest of the caloric testing may not be valid and is not usually performed. Bilateral weakness suggests a bilateral vestibular disorder (e.g., from vestibulotoxic drugs, autoimmune disorder, head trauma) or from cerebellar or other central abnormality.

2. Unilateral weakness (UW): Compares right ear responses to left ear responses.

$$\frac{(RW + RC) - (LC + LW) \times 100}{RW + RC + LC + LW} = X \text{ (unilateral weakness)};$$

Note: A negative total value in the above calculation indicates right weakness; positive number indicates left weakness. If the absolute value of the unilateral weakness is greater than about 20 to 30%, it is usually considered abnormal involvement of the peripheral vestibular organs or nerve on the side of the weakness.

3. Directional preponderance (DP): Compares right beating responses to left beating responses

$$\frac{(RW + LC) - (RC + LW) \times 100}{RW + LC + RC + LW} = X \text{ (directional preponderance)}$$

Note: DP is according to the direction of the stronger response. A negative total value in the above calculation indicates a DP to the left; a positive number indicates a DP to the right. If the absolute value of the DP is greater than about 30%, it is usually considered abnormal involvement of either the peripheral or central system.

4. Fixation index (failure of fixation suppression): Measured during the stage of peak nystagmus. Compares the nystagmus amplitude (slow phase velocity) during visual fixation to the nystagmus amplitude without visual fixation. If the nystagmus disappears entirely with fixation, the fixation index would be 0%; if it does not reduce at all, it would be 100% (same as without fixation). If the fixation index is 60% or higher, it suggests abnormal involvement of the central system.

Rotary Chair Testing

Rotary chair testing requires relatively expensive equipment comprised of a chair that can

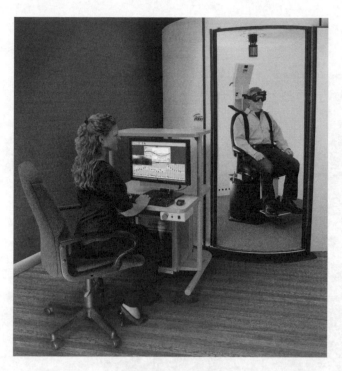

FIGURE 16–11. Illustration of a typical rotary chair testing arrangement. *Source*: Photo courtesy of Micromedical Technologies, 10 Kemp Drive, Chatham, IL 62629.

Posturography

Posturography requires relatively expensive equipment comprised of a calibrated force sensitive platform inside a movable enclosure, all under computer control and computer analyses. Figure 16–12 shows a photo of a dynamic computerized posturography set-up. Computerized posturography is able to assess a patient's functional balance and interactions of vestibular, visual, and somatosensory inputs. The Sensory Organization Test (SOT) measures patient's postural stability with stationary and moving surface with eyes open and closed and makes comparisons to normative data. The Motor Control Test (MCT) monitors patient's postural stability/control and recovery with unexpected linear movements of the surface. The Adaptation Test (ADT) measures the patient's ability to correct for changes when the surface is tilted so that the toes are up or down to simulate irregular walking surfaces.

Vestibular Evoked Myogenic Potential (VEMP)

The vestibular evoked myogenic potentials (VEMPs) are short-latency myogenic (muscle) potentials that can be elicited by relatively high intensity air-conduction or bone-conduction stimuli. The concept of the VEMP has been around since 1929, when Pietro Tullio, studying pigeons, showed that the birds experienced balance issues when he played his flute into tiny holes drilled into their semicircular canals (McCaslin & Jacobson, 2016). However, it was not until the 1960s that Bickford and colleagues recorded short latency electrical responses from the surface of the scalp to loud tone bursts (Bickford, Jacobson, & Cody, 1964).

VEMP recordings are done using surface-mounted electrodes and signal averaging (similar to auditory brainstem response measures), and are characterized by a negative polarity peak (N1) followed by a positive polarity peak (P1). The VEMP can be recorded with electrodes positioned around the area of the cervical muscles (cVEMP) or the ocular muscles (oVEMP). The cVEMP assesses vestibular function through the vestibulocollic reflex (VCR), whereas the oVEMP

be rotated in calibrated oscillations at different frequencies. The patient's head is properly secured so that the head rotations are in sync with the chair rotations. Figure 16–11 shows a photo of a rotary chair set-up. Rotary chair tests both ears simultaneously using a more natural type of stimulus. The testing may include (1) sinusoidal harmonic acceleration test by oscillating the clockwise and counterclockwise at varying frequencies. Measurements are made using VNG or ENG to monitor eye movement (VOR) gain, phase, and symmetry during chair rotations in the dark (to eliminate fixation) as compared to the chair (head) movement; (2) visual-vestibular interaction test to see if there are any changes to the VOR gain with the patient following objects on the wall during rotation or fixating on an object during rotation; and (3) step velocity test that included a rapid acceleration and deceleration of the chair in one direction and rotation of the chair at a constant speed for about 1 minute. The time it takes for the induced nystagmus to decay is measured and compared to normative data.

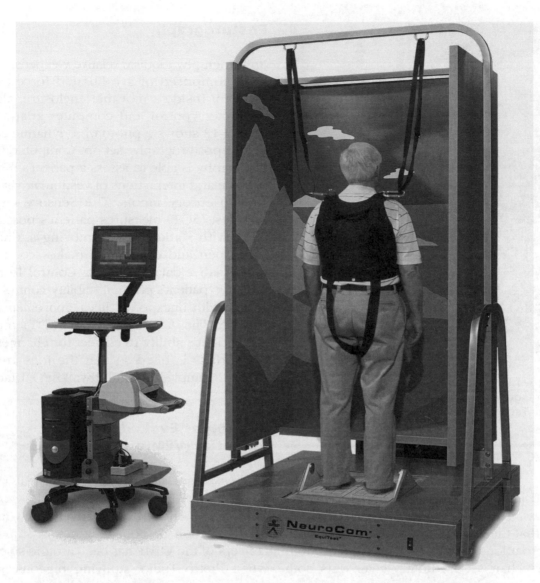

FIGURE 16–12. Illustration of computerized dynamic posturography testing arrangement. *Source*: Photo courtesy of Natus Medical Incorporated.

assesses vestibular function through the vestibulo-ocular reflex (VOR). The cVEMP is recorded from the sternocleidomastoid muscle on the neck, which is activated through the descending vestibular neural pathway from the inferior vestibular nerve, and mostly involves the saccule. To record the cVEMP, the patient lifts his or her head off the table unsupported to activate the sternocleidomastoid muscle. Patients are instructed to tense the muscle during the recording runs of acoustic stimulation, and to relax the muscle between runs. The oVEMP is recorded from the eye muscles, which are activated through the ascending vestibulo-ocular neural pathway from the superior vestibular nerve, and mostly involves the utricle. With oVEMP, the goal is to record the muscle activity from the inferior oblique muscle (under the eye) by having the patient look upward during the recording runs of acoustic stimulation, and to relax between runs.

SYNOPSIS 16–2

- Vestibular disorders include:
  - Alcohol overconsumption
  - Benign paroxysmal positional vertigo (BPPV)
  - Bilateral vestibular hypofunction
  - Endolymphatic hydrops/Ménière disease
  - Enlarged vestibular aqueduct
  - Labyrinthitis/vestibular neuritis
  - Motion sickness
  - Perilymph fistula
  - Persistent postural perceptual dizziness
  - Superior canal dehiscence
  - Vestibulotoxicity
  - Vestibular (acoustic) neuroma
- The VNG/ENG battery consists of the following subtests:
  - Saccade/ocular dysmetria
  - Spontaneous nystagmus
  - Gaze
  - Optokinetic
  - Dix–Hallpike (Paroxysmal nystagmus) for BPPV
  - Positional
  - Caloric
- The caloric test induces nystagmus with warm and cold (bithermal) stimulations of the ear canal to affect, indirectly, the vestibular organs by induction through the skull.
  - Direction of nystagmus depends on temperature of stimuli; cold opposite, warm same (COWS).
  - Bilateral weakness (BW): Looks at the average amplitude of the peak nystagmus (speed of the slow phase component) from each ear.
  - Unilateral weakness (UW): Compares right ear responses to left ear responses.

$$\frac{(RW + RC) - (LC + LW) \times 100 =}{RW + RC + LC + LW} \quad X \text{ (unilateral weakness);}$$

  - Directional preponderance (DP): Compares right beating responses to left beating responses

$$\frac{(RW + LC) - (RC + LW) \times 100 =}{RW + LC + RC + LW} \quad X \text{ (directional preponderance)}$$

SYNOPSIS 16–2 (*continued*)

- Rotary chair and computerized dynamic posturography and advance vestibular tests require specialized (more expensive) equipment.
- VEMP are myogenic responses using loud auditory stimuli to assess the saccule and inferior vestibular nerve central connections. oVEMP involves the ocular muscles; cVEMP involves the sternocleidomastoid muscle.

REFERENCES

American Academy of Audiology [AAA]. (2004). Scope of practice. Retrieved from https://www.audiology.org/publications-resources/document-library/scope-practice.

American Speech-Language-Hearing Association [ASHA]. (2004). Scope of practice in audiology [Scope of Practice]. Retrieved from www.asha.org/policy

American Speech-Language-Hearing Association [ASHA]. (n.d.). Balance system disorders. Retrieved from http://www.asha.org/PRPSpecificTopic.aspx?folderid=8589942134&section=Assessment

Baloh, R. W. (1998). *Dizzyness, Hearing Loss, and Tinnitus*. Philadelphia, PA: F. A. Davis.

Baloh, R. W., Honrubia, V., & Kerber, K. A. (2011). *Clinical Neurophysiology of the Vestibular System* (4th ed.). New York, NY: Oxford University Press.

Barber, H. O. (1984). Vestibular neurophysiology. *Otolaryngology—Head and Neck Surgery, 92*(1), 55–58.

Barin, K. (2009). Clinical neurophysiology of the vestibular system. In J. Katz, L. Medwetsky, B. Burkard, & L. Hood (Eds.), *Handbook of Clinical Audiology* (6th ed., pp. 431–466). Baltimore, MD: Lippincott Williams & Wilkins.

Bickford, R. G., Jacobson, G. P., & Cody, D. T. R. (1964). Nature of average evoked potentials to sound and other stimuli in man. *Annals of the New York Academy of Sciences, 112*, 204–218.

Bloom, W., & Fawcett, D. W. (1962). *A Textbook of Histology*. Philadelphia, PA: W. B. Saunders.

Desmond, A. (2011). *Vestibular Function*. New York, NY: Thieme.

Goebel, J. A., & Hanson, J. M. (Eds.). (1997). *Clinical Otology* (2nd ed.). New York, NY: Thieme.

Holt, J. C., Lysakowski, A., & Goldberg, J. M. (2010). The efferent vestibular system. *Auditory and Vestibular Efferents*, 135–186.

Jacobson, G. P., & Newman, C. W. (1990). The development of the Dizziness Handicap Inventory. *Archives of Otolaryngology-Head and Neck Surgery, 116*, 424–427.

Jacobson, G. P., Newman, C. W., & Piker, E. G. (2016). Assessing dizziness-related quality of life. In G. P. Jacobson & N. T. Shepard (Eds.), *Balance Function Assessment and Management* (2nd ed.). San Diego, CA: Plural.

McCaslin, D. L., & Jacobson, G. P. (2016). Vestibular-evoked myogenic potentials (VEMPs). In G. P. Jacobson & N. T. Shepard (Eds.), *Balance Function, Assessment, and Management*. San Diego, CA: Plural.

National Institute on Deafness and Other Communication Disorders [NIDCD]. (2014). *NIDCD Fact sheet: Balance disorders* [NIH Pub. No. 09-4374]. Retrieved from http://www.nidcd.nih.gov/staticresources/health/balance/NIDCD-Balance-Disorders.pdf

Rine, R. M. (2009). Growing evidence for balance and vestibular problems in children. *Audiological Medicine, 7*, 138–142.

Schubert, M. C., & Shepard, N. T. (2016). Practical anatomy and physiology of the vestibular systems. In G. P. Jacobson & N. T. Shepard (Eds.), *Balance Function Assessment and Management* (2nd ed., pp. 1–16). San Diego, CA: Plural.

Takumida, M., Miyawaki, H., Arishige, S., & Harada, Y. (1994). Motile responses of isolated vestibular hair cells. *Auris Nasus Larynx, 21*, 209–214. Retrieved from https://doi.org/10.1016/S0385-8146(12)80082-4

Vidal, P. P., de Waele, C., Vibert, N., & Mühlethaler, M. (1998). Vestibular compensation revisited. *Otolaryngology—Head and Neck Surgery, 119*, 34–42.

Wright, C. G., & Schwade, N. D. (Eds.). (2000). *Anatomy and Physiology of the Vestibular System*. New York, NY: Thieme.

Glossary

Academy of Doctors of Audiology (ADA) professional organization for audiologists in private practice or those who wished to establish a private practice.

acoustic equivalent volume measurement of the volume of ear canal.

acoustic feedback "whistling" heard from a hearing aid when the sound leaks back into the microphone from the receiver.

acoustic neuroma (or acoustic schwannoma) benign tumor involving the 8th cranial nerve; also known as vestibular schwannoma due to its common origin being on the vestibular portion of the 8th cranial nerve.

acoustic reflex involuntary contraction of the stapedius muscle and tensor tympani muscle when stimulated by loud sounds that reduce the vibration of the ossicles; also called the middle ear reflex or the stapedial reflex (because the stapedius muscle is mostly involved in humans).

acoustic reflex decay (ARD) inability of the acoustic reflex to sustain contraction during a 10-s tonal stimulation at 10 dB above the acoustic reflex threshold; abnormal acoustic reflex decay is defined as more than 50% return of the acoustic reflex toward baseline within 5 s, and is suggestive of an 8th nerve tumor.

acoustic reflex threshold (ART) lowest intensity level (in 5 dB steps) of a reflex eliciting tone that produces a repeatable acoustic reflex (e.g., greater than or equal to 0.02 mmhos).

acoustics study of the physical properties of sounds in the environment and how they travel through air.

acquired hearing loss hearing loss that occurs due to injury or disease that is not of genetic or congenital origin.

active cochlear process physiological process present in a healthy normal cochlea related to the motility of the outer hair cells, and which is responsible for enhanced displacement of the traveling wave, good sensitivity, and relatively sharp frequency selectivity (tuning).

acute disorder disease that is in its initial stage; usually comes on suddenly and lasts a relatively short duration.

acute otitis media inflammation (infection) of the fluid in the middle ear.

admittance (Y) amount of applied energy that flows through a system; measured in millimhos (mmhos); reciprocal of impedance.

admittance of the middle ear (Y_{tm}) measure of admittance during tympanometry that is representative of the middle ear (after removing the admittance due to the ear canal); the difference between overall admittance (Y) and the ear canal admittance (V_{ea}); also called peak compensated static acoustic admittance.

afferent auditory neurons nerve fibers that carry impulses from the sensory organs (peripheral) toward the brain (central); approximately 31,000 afferent auditory neurons come from each cochlea.

affricates type of speech sound created by the transition of a stop into a fricative.

air–bone gap difference in pure-tone threshold obtained by air conduction (AC) and bone conduction (BC); represents amount of hearing loss related to involvement of the conductive parts of the ear (outer and middle).

air conduction (AC) testing mode of sound presentation through earphones; stimulates the entire auditory system.

American Academy of Audiology (AAA) professional organization of audiologists; offers accreditation to academic programs (ACAE) and professional certification for audiologists (ABA certification).

American Board of Audiology (ABA) Certification professional certification available for audiologists through the American Academy of Audiology.

American National Standards Institute (ANSI) a committee of specialists that develops standards; responsible for standards related to audiologic test

383

equipment and recommended procedures for hearing testing.

American Speech-Language-Hearing Association (ASHA) professional organization of audiologists and speech-language pathologists; offers accreditation to academic programs (CAA) and professional certification for audiologists and speech-language pathologists.

aminoglycosides antibiotic drugs that are associated with hearing loss (cochleotoxic) and/or balance disorders (vestibulotoxic).

amplitude characteristic of a waveform that is related to its magnitude or size.

ampulla (plural = ampullas) bulbous region near the anterior end (near the vestibule) of each semicircular canal; houses the crista ampullaris.

anotia complete absence of the auricle.

antihelix ridge of cartilage that runs along the central portion of the auricle; parallel to the helix.

antimalarial drugs used to prevent malaria, for example, quinine and chloroquine.

antinodes property of resonance whereby two interacting tones combine.

antitragus small cartilaginous flap at the top of the earlobe and at the end of the antihelix; opposite to the tragus.

aperiodic vibration sound wave in which the pattern of vibration does not regularly repeat itself over time; also known as noise.

apex (of cochlea) narrow tip region of the coiled cochlea. Most responsive to low frequencies.

area ratio advantage one of the middle ear mechanical amplification methods due to the larger size (area) of the tympanic membrane compared with the oval window.

articulation or audibility index (AI) prediction of the amount of the acoustic information (scale of 01) of speech that is available to the listener; basic principle is that as less of the speech spectrum becomes audible (by externally filtering or by the presence of a hearing loss) speech intelligibility gets poorer in a predictable way; later revised and renamed the speech intelligibility index (SII).

articulators oral and nasal components of movement during shaping of speech sounds (e.g., tongue, lips, velum, jaws).

ascending threshold procedure thresholds are obtained by raising the level from inaudible to audible; opposite of descending method.

aspect ratio size relationship between the *y*-axis and the *x*-axis on an audiogram so that a 20 dB change along the *y*-axis corresponds to a doubling of frequency (octave change) along the *x*-axis.

asymmetric audiogram description in which the thresholds are different between the two ears.

atresia (atretic ear) congenital absence of an external auditory canal.

attenuation rate amount that a filter reduces certain frequencies; slope of the curve in a filter above and below the cutoff frequencies, specified as dB per octave.

AuD see **Doctor of Audiology** degree designator commonly used for the professional doctorate in audiology; minimum degree needed to practice clinical audiology.

audiogram graph used in audiometry to plot the patient's pure-tone thresholds.

audiologist professional who has the appropriate degree and license in his state to practice audiology; typically certified by a professional board (American Academy of Audiology and/or American Speech-Language-Hearing Association).

audiology discipline that focuses on the scientific study and clinical practice related to hearing and hearing disorders.

audiometer electronic or computer-based instrument used for many of the behavioral hearing tests performed in audiometry.

audiometric pertaining to measures made with audiometry.

audiometry assessment of a person's responses to sounds.

auditory brainstem response (ABR) physiological objective test used in audiology for documenting auditory sensitivity in difficult-to-test populations or for assessment of 8th nerve tumors; series of auditory evoked potentials from the 8th nerve and brainstem auditory pathways that occur within the first 10 ms after stimulus onset and measured with small disk electrodes placed on the surface of the head.

auditory (8th) cranial nerve portion of the 8th cranial nerve consisting of nerve fibers from (afferent neurons) and to (efferent neurons) the cochlea.

auditory dyssynchrony see auditory neuropathy spectrum disorder (ANSD).

auditory evoked responses electrical potentials evoked by sound; include the auditory brainstem responses, middle latency responses, late latency responses, and otoacoustic emissions; used to assess and screen for auditory function in difficult-to-test populations and/or to differentially diagnose type and locations of some hearing disorders.

auditory neuropathy spectrum disorder (ANSD) congenital hearing disorder in which the 8th nerve neurons do not fire with normal synchrony; characterized by the absence of auditory brainstem responses and the presence of normal otoacoustic emissions. Also known as auditory neuropathy or auditory dyssynchrony. See **auditory dyssynchrony**.

auditory processing disorder (APD) reduced ability to process or use auditory information when it is presented in more degraded types of listening situations; pure-tone thresholds are typically normal; sometimes called central auditory processing disorders (CAPD).

aural fullness reported sensation of pressure in the ear; can occur with inner or middle ear disorders.

auricle cartilaginous portion of the outer ear that is attached to the lateral surface of the temporal bone.

auricular pertaining to the auricle.

auricular hematoma internal bleeding within the auricle; like a bruise.

automatic gain control (AGC) circuitry that automatically maintains the level of a signal; used to maintain immittance probe tone at 85 dB SPL in the ear canal; used in hearing aids to adjust the gain depending on the changes in signal level.

band-pass filter filter that transmits (passes) a range of frequencies between some selected high and low frequency cutoffs (at 3 dB down points), and excludes those above and below the cutoff frequencies at a specified attenuation rate.

band-reject filter filter that excludes (rejects) a range of frequencies between some selected high and low frequency cutoffs (at 3 dB down points), and transmits (passes) those above and below the cutoff frequencies at a specified attenuation rate.

barotrauma middle ear disorder caused by sudden change in external air pressure; results in a mismatch in pressure between that in the ear canal and that in the middle ear spaces.

base (of cochlea) the wider part of the coiled cochlea closest to the vestibule. Most responsive to high frequencies.

basilar membrane portion of the membranous labyrinth that supports the organ of Corti; attaches from the osseous spiral lamina to the outer wall of the bony labyrinth; separates scala media from scala tympani; important for the transduction of sound in the cochlea through the generation of the basilar membrane traveling waves.

behind-the-ear hearing aid (BTE) curved hearing aid that is worn behind the ear (or one on each ear) and coupled to the earmold in the ear through a tube.

Bel unit of sound intensity or pressure expressed as the logarithm of a ratio scale relative to a specified reference value; Bels are too large for use in hearing measures (see decibel).

benign paroxysmal positional vertigo (BPPV) vestibular disorder caused by some of the calcium carbonate crystals of the otoconia within the macula of a utricle become dislodged and fall into one or more of the semicircular canals. Most commonly found in the elderly.

BiCROS (bilateral CROS) bilateral CROS type of hearing aid fitting used when one ear has poor hearing and the better ear has a mild to moderate hearing loss; a microphone is placed on the poorer hearing ear and a complete hearing aid is placed on the better hearing ear; all sounds are amplified and channeled into the better hearing ear.

bilateral pertaining to both sides or to both ears.

Bilateral vestibular hypofunction a vestibular disorder characterized by a loss/reduction of vestibular function on both sides as a secondary affect to either a known disorder such as ototoxicity or vestibular neuritis, or from an unknown cause (idiopathic).

binaural hearing simultaneous use of both ears in hearing.

binomial distribution statistically derived table of probabilities, made popular by Thornton and Raffin (1978), to interpret critical differences (95% confidence intervals) between two-word recognition scores; reflects the variability (standard deviation) of scores as a function of the number of test items.

biochemical transduction stage of energy transduction that occurs in the hair cells.

body aid a relatively large square or rectangular hearing aid worn on the body; the sounds are delivered by an electrical cord to the receiver/earmold, which is placed in the ear.

bone-anchored implant (BAI) hearing aid that is surgically implanted by an otologist into the mastoid area behind the ear; useful for hearing losses with good bone conduction thresholds.

bone conduction (BC) testing mode of sound presentation through a bone oscillator used in pure-tone audiometry; delivers vibration directly to the inner ear through vibrations in the temporal bone, which essentially bypasses the conductive (outer and middle ear) portions of the auditory pathway; provides a measure of the sensorineural component of a hearing loss.

bone conduction vibrator transducer which has a hard plastic casing that is set into vibration by pure tones; used in pure-tone audiometry for bone conduction (BC) testing, and usually placed behind the ear on the mastoid portion of the temporal bone; also called a bone conduction oscillator.

bony labyrinth series of canals within the petrous portion of the temporal bone that houses the inner ear.

broadly tuned loss of frequency selectivity in damaged ears; loss of tip region of tuning curve.

carboplatin antineoplastic cancer-treating chemical agent; can cause hearing loss.

Carhart's notch mild decline in the bone conduction threshold at 2000 Hz often seen with otosclerosis.

carrier phrase short sentence, such as, "Say the word _____," often used prior to the test word in word recognition score testing.

case history information obtained from the patient regarding pertinent background and conditions about their hearing health.

center frequency frequency at the center of a filter where the maximum sound is delivered.

central auditory disorders pathologies and/or processing that involve the central auditory system.

central auditory (or vestibular) system part of the auditory system that includes the neural pathways and nuclei in the brainstem and cortical areas; excludes the peripheral auditory structures.

central masking small elevation in threshold of the test ear when masking is put into the nontest ear at levels that are less than the interaural attenuation. Due to some central nervous system effect.

Certificate of Clinical Competence in Audiology (CCC-A) professional certification available for audiologists through the American Speech-Language-Hearing Association.

cerumen waxy substance produced by glands in the external auditory canal that helps protect, lubricate, and clean the canal; also called earwax.

characteristic frequency the frequency where the basilar membrane or auditory nerve fiber is most sensitive; most sensitive point of a tuning curve.

chase part of the plateau method of masking when masking is insufficient; prior to reaching the masking plateau.

chemotherapeutic (neoplastic) agents cancer-treating chemical drugs.

chirp a broad-band sound (made up of a wide range of frequencies) used as a stimulus in evoked potentials and WAI.

cholesteatoma benign tumor-like mass that invades middle ear space; formed by deposits of squamous epithelia that become keratinized and infected; often secondary to retracted tympanic membrane from poor eustachian tube function.

chronic disorder persistent condition over a long period of time.

chronic otitis media persistent middle ear condition with thickening fluid remaining in the middle ear for an extended time; infections may reoccur and hearing loss may be present.

cisplatin cancer-treating chemical agent; can cause hearing loss.

Claudius cells support cells within the organ of Corti; located next to the Hensen cells along the outer edge of the organ of Corti.

clinical masking process of putting noise into the nontest ear while measuring thresholds in the test ear.

closed-head injury nonpenetrating trauma to the skull.

closed-set speech materials in which patients select from a list with which they are familiarized or is visually available to them.

cochlea part of the inner ear involved with hearing; houses the organ of Corti.

cochlear aqueduct narrow bony canal of the inner ear that connects the perilymph of the bony labyrinth with the cerebrospinal fluid.

cochlear implant (CI) biomedical device with an electrode array inserted into a nonfunctional cochlea to electrically stimulate neurons of the cochlear nerve.

cochlear implant mapping computer software, designed by manufacturers of cochlear implants, and used by audiologists to maximize the patient's use of the electrode array for communication.

cochlear microphonic an early response in the ABR waveform that reverses polarity when the click used to generate the waveform is reversed; waveforms generated by rarefaction clicks produce a response in one direction and waveforms generated by condensation clicks produce a response in the opposite direction.

cochlear nerve portion of the 8th cranial nerve consisting of nerve fibers from the cochlea.

cochlear nucleus (CN) collection of cell bodies in the lateral pontine region of the brainstem that connects to the 8th cranial nerve fibers associated with the cochlea.

cochlear otosclerosis a type of otosclerosis (otospongiosis) in which the bony growth invades the inner ear and destroys hair cells.

collapsed canals temporary closing off of the ear canal that can occur in some individuals with reduced elasticity in the cartilaginous portion of the external ear canal and due to pressure exerted by supra-aural earphones.

commissure nerve fibers that provide interconnections between two sides of the brain; as in commissure of Probst and commissure of the inferior colliculi of the auditory pathways in the brainstem.

compensated tympanogram tympanogram whereby the instrument automatically removes the component of admittance related to the ear canal (as measured at +200 daPa) and only graphs the admittance characteristics of the middle ear.

completely-in-the-canal (CIC) hearing aid in which all the components reside in a casing that fits completely in the ear canal; smallest of the custom hearing aids.

complex periodic vibration nonsinusoidal sound wave in which the vibratory pattern is composed of more than one tone and which repeats itself as a function of time; also known as complex periodic tone.

compression nonlinear amplifier gain that is part of most hearing aids; adjusts the gain dependent of the amount of input.

computer-based audiometry audiometric hearing tests in which a computer is used to generate and control the signals; can also record patients' responses, automatically analyze and print the results, and track patient databases.

concha the bowl-shaped indentation of the auricle just before the entrance (meatus) to the external auditory canal.

condensation phase of a waveform that is associated with an increase in the density of air molecules, which corresponds to an increase in sound pressure or intensity.

conditioned-play audiometry audiometric technique used for testing children 2 to 4 years old; procedure employs play techniques such as putting a toy in a bucket when they hear the sound.

conductive hearing loss hearing loss due to involvement of the outer and/or middle ear; characterized by an air–bone gap of more than 10 dB and bone conduction thresholds within normal range.

congenital hearing loss hearing loss present at birth due to prenatal or perinatal events.

connexin-26 genetic protein mutation during embryologic development; common cause of congenital hearing loss.

continuous spectrum amplitude spectrum that involves a continuous line to indicate that there are infinite frequencies that are present over the specified range.

contralateral acoustic reflex acoustic reflex obtained from the ear on the opposite side from the ear being stimulated; due to the contralateral pathway of the bilateral acoustic reflex.

corneoretinal potential electrical potential from the eyes; surface electrodes around the eyes are used to measure eye movements (nystagmus) during vestibular testing with electronystagmography.

coronal plane divides the structure into anterior (front) and posterior (back) parts also known as frontal plane.

corpus callosum prominent band of nerve fibers that connects the two hemispheres of the cortex.

count-the-dots audiogram simpler method to represent the acoustic weightings from the articulation/speech intelligibility index as dots on an audiogram; a specified number of dots are used to represent the speech banana, weighted more heavily at 2000 and 4000 Hz regions; useful tool to let patients know how much of the speech sounds they may be missing.

crista (plural = cristae) sensory organ of the semicircular canals that responds to angular accelerations of the head; located in the ampulla within the membranous labyrinth of each semicircular canal; also called crista ampullaris.

critical differences table used to compare two-word recognition scores to determine if they are significantly different from each other (95% confidence interval), based on a binomial distribution.

CROS (contralateral routing of signals) hearing aid type of hearing aid fitting used as an option with unilateral hearing loss; a microphone is placed on the poorer hearing ear and the sounds are channeled into the better hearing ear fit with an open-fitting-type earmold.

cross hearing amount of a signal presented to one ear that can be heard in the other ear when the interaural attenuation is exceeded.

cross-links microfilaments that interconnect the stereocilia of each inner and outer hair cell; well-developed cross-links of the outer hair cell stereocilia keep them well organized and rigid.

cubic difference tone most prominent distortion product tone associated with the nonlinearity of the basilar membrane; occurs at frequencies equal to $2f_1 - f_2$.

cupula gelatinous membrane within the crista; stereocilia and kinocilium of the sensory hair cells are embedded in the cupula and are bent with deflections of the cupula during angular accelerations.

curved membrane advantage one of the middle ear mechanical amplification methods resulting from the cone shape of the tympanic membrane, which tends to focus its movement in such a way that it moves the malleus with more force than if the tympanic membrane was flat.

custom hearing aids hearing aids worn in the concha or ear canal that have all the components built inside of the earmold, for example, in-the-ear (ITE), in-the-canal (ITC), and completely-in-the-canal (CIC).

cutoff frequency upper and/or lower frequencies where the filter begins to be attenuated; defined as the frequency that is 3 dB less than the frequency with the highest amplitude.

cycle pattern of movement as an object goes through its full range of motion one time.

cytomegalovirus (CMV) a common viral infection with mild flu-like symptoms; primary cause of congenital progressive hearing loss when fetus is exposed to virus in utero.

damage risk criteria industrial standards that limit the amount of noise exposure workers can be exposed to in a 24-hour period without the risk of noise-related hearing loss.

Davis Battery Theory cochlear function theory, first postulated by Davis (1965), stating that the 120 to 140 mV electrical potential between the endolymph and the inside of the hair cells acts like the voltage of a battery, and this serves as the force that drives the ionic current into the hair cell that is modulated by changes in resistance due to the bending of the stereocilia.

decibel (dB) unit of sound intensity or pressure that is 1/10 of a Bel.

decibel hearing level (dB HL) decibel scale in which the reference value is the minimum sound pressure level standards for normal hearing as a function of frequency, where 0 dB HL at any frequency represents the lowest level for normal hearing.

decibel intensity level (dB IL) intensity (in dB) of a sound that is referenced to the standard reference value for intensity (10^{-12} w/m^2); dB IL implies that 10^{-12} w/m^2 is in the denominator of the dB formula for intensity measures.

decibel sensation level (dB SL) decibel scale in which the reference value is the patient's own threshold.

decibel sound pressure level (dB SPL) pressure (in dB) of a sound that is referenced to the standard reference value for pressure (20 µPa); dB SPL implies that 20 µPa is in the denominator of the dB formula for pressure measures.

degree of hearing loss one of the parameters used in describing audiograms; refers to the amount of hearing loss; slight, mild, moderate, moderately severe, severe, and profound.

Deiter cells support cells within the organ of Corti that have outer hair cells sitting on top of them; each Deiter cell also has a phalangeal process that extends to the upper surface of the outer hair cells

and fills in the gaps; also called outer phalangeal cell.

depolarization changes in the intracellular potential of the hair cells that occurs during the excitatory phase resulting in release of neurotransmitter substance at the synapse between the hair cell and the afferent neurons.

diagnostic (clinical) audiometer electronic or computer-based instrument capable of performing a variety of tests, including pure-tone audiometry (with masking), speech, and other special tests; must conform to standards of operation as specified by American National Standards Institute (ANSI).

differential diagnosis analyses of different tests to determine the type and/or location of a disorder (determine which part or parts of the ear are affected).

digital hearing aid hearing aid that uses computer-based technology (digital) to process sounds.

disarticulation separation of the ossicular chain or break in one of the ossicles; also called ossicular discontinuity.

discharge rate number of discharges per second that a neuron produces in response to a specified sound.

distortion product additional tones generated in the cochlea that were not present in an externally applied stimulus; due to nonlinearities of the ear.

distortion product otoacoustic emissions (DPOAEs) type of otoacoustic emissions evoked by two closely spaced pure tones (f_2/f_1 = 1.22) to produce distortion tones in the cochlea, the largest of which is the cubic difference tone ($2f_1 - f_2$); measured by signal averaging of the acoustic signals generated by the ear and picked up by a sensitive microphone in the ear canal.

dizziness a general term to describe unsteadiness, lightheadedness, or spinning related to the central nervous system or other medical or psychological factors.

Doctor of Audiology (AuD) professional doctorate which is the entry-level degree to practice clinical audiology.

ductus reuniens small channel connecting the membranous labyrinth of the vestibular organs and the cochlea.

dynamic range difference in decibels between the patient's hearing threshold and an uncomfortable listening level for tones or speech.

earlobe noncartilaginous lower portion of the auricle; traditional location for decorative earrings.

early hearing detection and intervention (EHDI) synonymous with hearing screening and implies a comprehensive strategy of detection and follow up.

early-onset genetic hearing loss hearing loss due to genetic factors that manifests during the infant–toddler stage.

earmold custom-made earpiece that is attached to a behind-the-ear (BTE) hearing aid.

earmold impression ingredients are mixed and inserted partially into a patient's ear to form a custom shape for the hearing aid or earmold; the impression is sent to the manufacturer to form the permanent earmold or casing for the hearing aid.

Educational Audiology Association (EAA) professional membership organization of audiologists and related professionals who deliver a full spectrum of hearing services to all children, particularly those in educational settings.

effective masking levels calibrated amount of narrowband noise that provides a threshold shift to a corresponding dB HL for a tone centered within the noise.

efferent neurons nerve fibers that carry impulses from the brain (central) toward the sensory organs (peripheral).

effusion accumulation of fluid into a cavity; middle ear effusion occurs from the extraction of fluid from the mucous lining of the middle ear cavity.

electroacoustic analysis measurements of a hearing aid in a special test box to determine whether the hearing aid meets certain performance requirements, set by the American National Standards Institute (ANSI).

electronystagmography clinical tests of vestibular function based on recordings of the corneoretinal potential and nystagmus that is induced by various conditions.

endocochlear potential (EP) 80 mV electrical potential (charge) in the endolymph of the scala media due to the high concentration of potassium (K+); maintained by the stria vascularis.

endolymph fluid in the membranous labyrinth that has a relatively high potassium (K) concentration and low sodium (Na) concentration; ionic composition similar to that of intracellular fluid; therefore, endolymph is unique as an extracellular fluid.

endolymphatic duct narrow canal arising from the area of the saccule that is part of the membranous labyrinth, and which ends in a flattened sac located in the subarachnoid space lining the brain tissues within the temporal bone; thought to control the buildup of endolymph; may be compromised in Ménière disease.

endolymphatic hydrops vestibular disorder due to excessive buildup of endolymph in the scala media and vestibular labyrinth; characterized by episodes of vertigo, fluctuating hearing loss, low-pitched tinnitus, and fullness. When cause is known, such as an autoimmune disorder, head trauma, or allergies, the disorder is called endolymphatic hydrops; when the cause is unknown (idiopathic), the disorder is called Ménière's disease.

endolymphatic sac part of the membranous labyrinth, which is a flattened sac located in the subarachnoid space lining the brain tissues within the temporal bone.

endolymphatic shunt operation to redirect or relieve the flow of endolymph as a treatment option for Ménière disease.

enlarged vestibular aqueduct (EVA) a vestibular disorder due to a developmental malformation in which the vestibular aqueduct is enlarged resulting in an enlarged endolymphatic duct/sac that may lead to a sensorineural hearing loss.

envelope of the traveling wave an outline of the amplitudes associated with the traveling wave along the basilar membrane for a specified frequency.

epitympanic recess the upper portion of the middle ear cavity

equal loudness contours representations of dB SPL as a function of frequency that are judged to be equal in loudness; expressed as phons, such that 40 phons is equivalent to the loudness of a 40 dB, 1000 Hz pure tone, according to which all other frequencies are judged.

equal pitch contours representation of how pitch is affected by changes in intensity for different frequencies.

equivalent volume of the ear canal (Vea) the ear canal volume as calculated by the admittance measurement at +200 daPa in tympanometry.

eustachian tube connects the middle ear to the nasopharynx; comprised mostly of cartilage that is normally closed, and is opened by action of the tensor veli palatini muscle during chewing and swallowing to equalize air pressure in the middle ear to that of the surrounding environment.

eustachian tube dysfunction condition whereby the eustachian tube is unable to equalize middle ear pressure; common cause of middle ear effusion.

evoked responses electroacoustic and neuroelectric measures of auditory function, for example, OAEs and ABRs; physiologic objective measures of auditory system.

excitatory phase transduction process in the cochlea associated with bending of stereocilia toward the tallest row of stereocilia (away from the modiolus); increase in the discharge rate of an auditory nerve fiber.

exostosis (exostoses) bony outgrowths in the external auditory canal caused by repetitive irritation from cold water; also known as surfer's ear.

extended high-frequency (EHF) or circumaural earphones are used to evaluate hearing above 8000 Hz.

external auditory canal (EAC) canal leading from the auricle to the tympanic membrane; part of the outer ear.

externship full-time clinical experience at an approved clinical site during the last year of an audiology doctoral program.

facial nerve 7th cranial nerve. In the auditory system, the stapedial branch innervates the stapedius muscle of the middle ear.

false positive patient responds in the absence of a presented sound; also, term used in a screening matrix for those who are incorrectly identified as have the disorder.

false negative patient reluctant to respond during the presence of a sound that is expected to be audible; also, term used in a screening matrix for those who truly have the disorder, but are identified as not having the disorder (miss).

far-field electrical potential measured at a relatively far distance from the source (e.g., ABRs measured from the scalp).

fast Fourier transform (FFT) mathematical relationship showing that any complex sound is a predictable combination of different pure tones; FFT instruments are available that will produce the spectrum of any complex sound.

feedback whistling-type sound produced by hearing aids due to the amplification of sounds from the receiver reaching the microphone and being re-amplified.

filtering process in which certain frequencies are excluded and certain frequencies are passed.

final masking level (FML) highest level of masking noise used in the non-test ear during clinical masking.

footplate part of the stapes that connects to the oval window.

foreign objects unnatural items found in the ear canal, for example, cotton swabs, insects, food.

formant concentrations of energy for bands of frequencies of periodic speech sounds, for example, F1, F2 frequencies.

formant transitions dynamic changes (rising or falling) in the frequencies of the formants during connected speech.

frequency number of cycles of a vibration that occur in 1s, measured in hertz (Hz).

frequency counter electronic instrument used to determine the frequency of pure tones.

frequency range of audibility for humans 20 to 20,000 Hz.

frequency selectivity/tuning representation of how different measures of the auditory system respond to frequency by intensity combinations, often represented by tuning curves; description of how well the auditory system can differentiate frequencies.

frequency theory theory of frequency coding based on the processing of discharge patterns in the afferent auditory nerve fibers.

FRESH (FREquency Specific Hearing) noise a test stimulus that uses a better narrowband noise that has results closer to pure-tone thresholds.

fricatives noise-like sounds produced by passing air through the oral cavity with turbulence caused by positioning of the articulators.

functional hearing loss exaggerated or feigned hearing loss, often for financial or psychological reasons; hearing loss with no organic basis; also called nonorganic hearing loss or malingering.

fundamental frequency (f_0) lowest frequency component in a complex periodic vibration.

gain an increase in amplitude from one level to another.

genetic hearing loss hearing loss caused by alterations in the genes during embryological development.

glomus jugulare type of glomus tumor that is associated with the jugular bulb along the floor of the middle ear.

glomus tumor benign slow-growing tumor of the middle ear.

glomus tympanicum type of glomus tumor that is associated with nerves coursing through the middle ear, especially near the promontory.

gold standard an acceptable test for a disorder in which other tests can be compared to judge their validity.

graded potential variable electrical gradient in nerve fibers prior to excitation; dependent on amount of available neurotransmitter substance at neural synapse.

habenula perforata regularly spaced holes in the osseous spiral lamina through which the afferent nerve fibers leave the organ of Corti and enter the modiolus.

half-power points (3 dB down-point) term for filter cutoff frequency that is 3 dB down from the maximum.

half-wave resonator condition of resonance whereby the fundamental frequency is equal to a halfwavelength, for example, for a tube open at both ends.

harmonics integer multiples of the fundamental frequency (f_0), for example, $1f_0$, $2f_0$, $3f_0$, and so on, where f_0 = fundamental (lowest) frequency.

head shadow attenuation of sound by the head in the ear farther away from the sound source; occurs for sounds whose wavelengths are equal to or less than the size of the head.

hearing aid electronic device for amplifying sounds for patients with hearing loss.

hearing aid candidacy process of determining whether a patient would potentially benefit from hearing aids.

hearing aid orientation part of the hearing aid fitting process in which the patient is instructed on the use, care, and expectations of new hearing aids.

hearing conservation program industrial hearing care program that monitors noise levels, educates employees about noise-induced hearing loss, and provides hearing protection devices and strategies.

Hearing Handicap Inventory for the Elderly-Screening self-assessment scale of hearing disability generally used with adult hearing screening.

hearing protection devices noise-reduction devices worn over the ear or inside the ear canal in work or recreational settings with high noise levels.

helicotrema space at the apex of the coiled bony labyrinth in the cochlea where the scala tympani and scala vestibuli are continuous with each other due to the ending of the scala media.

helix ridge of cartilage that runs around the outer border of the auricle.

Hensen cells support cells in the organ of Corti that lie on the outer margin of the outer cells.

hertz (Hz) unit of measure for frequency that represents cycles per second.

Heschl's gyrus ridge along the upper surface of the temporal lobe that is the primary auditory reception area of the cortex.

high frequency slope part of a tuning curve that shows a steep slope for frequencies higher than the center frequency.

high-pass filter type of filter that transmits (passes) all frequencies above its cutoff frequency and attenuates those below the cutoff frequency.

high-pass masking physiological masking paradigm used in auditory brainstem responses recordings to provide more frequency-specific information about the function of the cochlea; the cutoff frequency of a high-pass filtered noise is systematically changed to desynchronize some parts of the cochlea to observe responses from other regions.

high-risk register (HRR) factors known to have a high association with hearing loss; recommendations made periodically by a Joint Committee on Newborn Hearing.

hydromechanical vibrations (and events) vibrations that occur in the fluid filled inner ear during the transduction process, including the vibratory energy in the cochlear fluids, followed by the movements of the basilar membrane, and bending of the stereocilia by the tectorial membrane.

hyperpolarization changes in the intracellular potential of the hair cells that occurs during the inhibitory phase resulting in a decrease in the release of neurotransmitter substance at the synapse between the hair cell and the afferent neurons.

identification program program designed to screen for hearing loss.

idiopathic disorder with an unknown cause.

immittance term used to encompass both admittance and impedance.

immittance test battery of middle ear measures, including tympanometry and acoustic reflexes.

impacted cerumen abnormal buildup of earwax (cerumen) that completely blocks off the ear canal.

impedance (Z) total opposition to the flow of energy in an acoustic/mechanical system; measured in units of ohms.

impedance mismatch situation in which two systems have different impedances so that there is an inefficient transfer of energy, for example, vibrations in air are not efficiently transferred to fluid.

incus second of the three middle ear ossicles; consists of a body, short process, long process, and lenticular process; the body articulates with the malleus, and the lenticular process articulates with the head of the stapes.

inferior branch of vestibular nerve portion of the 8th cranial nerve that innervates the posterior semicircular canal and part of the saccule. See also **superior branch of vestibular nerve**.

inferior colliculus (IC) auditory nucleus located in the upper brainstem.

inhibitory phase transduction process in the cochlea associated with bending of stereocilia away from the tallest row of stereocilia (toward the modiolus); decrease in the discharge rate of an auditory nerve fiber.

initial masking level (IML) masker level first applied to the nontest ear using the plateau method of clinical masking; for air conduction the IML = 10 dB above AC threshold; for bone conduction the IML = 10 dB above AC threshold plus the amount of any occlusion effect.

inner ear includes the cochlea and vestibular systems.

inner hair cells (IHCs) auditory sensory hair cells within the organ of Corti; approximately 3500 IHCs arranged in a single row.

inner pillar cells support cells in the organ of Corti that form the inner "leg" of the triangular shaped tunnel of Corti; also called inner rods of Corti.

inner radial fibers afferent nerve fibers originating from the inner hair cells; approximately 95% of afferent fibers come from inner hair cells.

inner support (phalangeal) cells cells within the organ of Corti that surround the inner hair cells and provide support.

input compression (AGCi) changing the incoming signal to correspond to the reduced dynamic range of the hearing aid user also known as wide dynamic range compression (WDRC).

input–output (I/O) function measure of how the output of a system changes as a function of the input, for example, the discharge rate of an auditory nerve fiber as a function of stimulus intensity.

insert earphone air conduction transducer used in audiology that is placed within the ear canal; electroacoustic diaphragm is housed in a small case, which then sends an acoustic signal through a small tube held in place with a disposable foam cuff; common model, ER-3A.

instantaneous phase phase of a pure tone at any point in time (usually how a cycle relates to degrees around a circle).

intensity measure of power distributed over an area in units of watts/cm² or watts/m² depending on the system of measurement being used (MKS or CGS); also, generically used to describe the relative level of a sound.

interaural attenuation (IA) difference in intensity between the stimulus delivered to the test ear and the amount that crosses over (by bone conduction) to the nontest ear; the amount of sound level (dB HL) needed to vibrate the skull for different transducers. Minimum IA for supra-aural earphones is 40 dB HL; for insert earphones minimum IA is 55 dB HL; for bone conduction minimum IA is 0 dB HL.

interaural intensity differences localization cue that is dependent on the different intensities of sounds at the two ears.

interaural time differences localization cue that is dependent on the different arrival times of sounds at the two ears.

intermittent disorder pathologic condition that comes and goes or reoccurs often.

internal auditory canal opening in the posterior wall of the petrous part of the temporal bone through which the vestibulocochlear (VIII) nerve and facial (VII) nerve exit.

interpeak latency interval calculated differences in the latencies between ABR waves, especially, I-III, III-V, and I-V.

interspike intervals (ISIs) time intervals that occur between discharges of an auditory nerve fiber.

in-the-canal (ITC) type of custom hearing aid that has all the hearing aid components built inside the casing, and which partially fills the lower approximate one-quarter of the concha with the receiver portion extending a short distance into the ear canal.

in-the-ear (ITE) type of custom hearing aid that has all the hearing aid components built inside the casing, and which fills most of the concha with the receiver portion extending a short distance into the ear canal.

intracellular potential electrical potential that is present inside the cochlear hair cells; –40 mV for inner hair cells and –60 mV for outer hair cells.

inverse square law decrease in a sound's intensity with distance, expressed by the equation: Intensity $(I) = 1/D^2$ or Pressure $(P) = 1/D$; where $D = d1/d2$.

ipsilateral acoustic reflex acoustic reflex obtained from ear on the same side as the ear being stimulated; due to the ipsilateral pathway of the bilateral acoustic reflex.

kilohertz (kHz) 1000 cycles; kilo = 1000.

kinocilium single large cilium adjacent to the tallest row of stereocilia on each hair cell in the crista; oriented away from the utricle for the anterior and posterior canals, and toward the utricle for the horizontal semicircular canal.

labyrinthectomy surgical operation to destroy the vestibular organs.

labyrinthitis infection (commonly viral) of the inner ear labyrinth and/or vestibular nerve that may cause temporary disruption of vestibular function producing dizziness/vertigo, balance problems, nausea, and/or hearing and vision problems. Also called vestibular neuritis.

late latency response (LLR) auditory evoked response occurring in the post-stimulus latency range of 100 to 300 ms reflecting activity of auditory events at the cortical level; later latency than auditory brainstem response and the middle latency response.

latency time it takes for a response to occur relative to the onset of an abrupt auditory stimulus; in auditory evoked responses, latency is measured in milliseconds.

latency-intensity (L-I) function plot of response latency as a function of stimulus level; often used for interpretation of auditory brainstem responses.

late-onset genetic hearing loss hearing loss due to genetic factors that manifests during childhood or adult stages.

lateral lemniscus (LL) auditory nucleus of the lower brainstem; prominent nerve fiber bundle formed by ascending auditory fibers.

lenticular process slightly enlarged ring at the end of the long process of the incus that articulates with the head of the stapes.

lever advantage one of the middle ear mechanical amplification methods that is due to the fact that the manubrium of the malleus is longer than the long process of the incus in the ossicular chain.

light reflex reflection of an otoscope light off the curved tympanic membrane; also called the cone of light.

line spectrum amplitude spectrum that plots vertical lines at discrete frequencies present in periodic vibrations.

localization ability to determine the direction from which a sound originated.

longitudinal fracture temporal bone fracture that runs parallel along the edge of the petrous portion; generally results in conductive loss.

longitudinal wave type of wave movement that involves increases and decreases in pressure in the direction of the vibrating object.

long-term average speech signal (LTASS) a speech signal used in the prescription and evaluation of hearing aid fittings

loop diuretics drugs used to treat edema in patients with heart or lung disease.

loudness psychological correlate of intensity.

low frequency tail part of a tuning curve that shows a relatively wide range of across frequencies lower the center frequency that can produce a response when stimulated at moderate to high intensities.

low-pass filter type of filter that transmits (passes) all frequencies below its cutoff frequency and attenuates those above the cutoff frequency.

macula (plural = maculae) sensory organ of the saccule and utricle that is responsive to linear accelerations of the head; also called macula utriculi or macula sacculi.

malleus first and largest of the middle ear ossicles, consisting of a manubrium, neck, anterior or lateral process, and head; the manubrium is attached to the tympanic membrane, and the head articulates with the body of the incus.

manubrium handle (or long process) of the malleus that is attached to the tympanic membrane; visible through the tympanic membrane with otoscopy.

masked thresholds thresholds obtained in the test ear when masking was used in the nontest ear.

masker noise that is used to elevate or make inaudible a test signal; noise that is presented in the nontest ear during clinical masking.

masking elevation in threshold of a test signal by the presence of another sound, called the masker.

masking dilemma unable to find true threshold due to overmasking. Minimum amount of masking in nontest ear exceeds the interaural attenuation and the masker is heard in the test ear causing an elevation of the true threshold.

mechanical vibrations back-and-forth movements of an object; action of the middle ear ossicles in the transduction process; bone conduction audiometry sets up mechanical vibrations in the skull that stimulate the inner ear.

medial geniculate body (MGB) auditory nucleus at the level of the thalamus; receives ascending fibers from the inferior colliculi and sends fibers to the ipsilateral auditory cortex.

medial superior olive (MSO) collection of cell bodies in the brainstem (pontine level) that is involved with auditory processing. First location where neural information for both ears in integrated.

mel unit used to establish a pitch scale; assigns a standard reference value of 1000 mels to the pitch associated with 1000 Hz (at a loudness of 40 phons), to which other frequencies are judged to be some multiple of 1000 mels.

membranous labyrinth fluid filled membrane system that is suspended within the bony labyrinth; filled with endolymph; houses the organ of Corti in the cochlea, and the cristae and maculae in the vestibular organs.

Ménière disease (see **endolymphatic hydrops**)

meningitis inflammation of the meninges (membranous sheets covering the brain).

microtia abnormally small or malformed auricle.

middle ear the area between the eardrum (tympanic membrane) and the oval window includes the ossicles.

middle ear implant (MEI) hearing aid that is surgically placed in the middle ear and operates using piezoelectric and electromagnetic transduction mechanisms.

middle ear reflex see **acoustic reflex**.

middle latency response (MLR) auditory evoked response occurring in the post-latency range of 12 to 80 ms reflecting activity of auditory events at the thalamus and cortical level; later latency than the auditory brainstem response and earlier latency than the late latency response.

millimhos (mmhos) unit of measurement for admittance; 1/1000 of a mho.

milliseconds (ms) unit of time; one-thousandth of a second (0.001 s).

mini-BTE hearing aids smaller version of the traditional behind the ear (BTE) style, with smaller tubing; can be worn with a more open canal fitting without custom earmold.

minimum masking level lowest level of masker introduced to the nontest ear when using the plateau method of clinical masking that is sufficient to keep the nontest ear from hearing the test tone.

mixed hearing loss type of hearing loss in which there is a sensorineural component and a conductive component at a particular frequency; audiogram shows an elevation in bone conduction threshold (BC > 25 dB HL) and air–bone gap greater than 10 dB HL.

modiolus porous bony core of the cochlea, where the nerve fibers from the cochlear hair cells come together to form the cochlear portion of the 8th cranial nerve, which then exits the cochlea through the internal auditory canal.

monitored live voice method of presenting speech stimuli through the audiometer by speaking into a microphone; to insure proper calibration, the level of the speech is adjusted to peak the VU meter at zero.

monomere (monomeric tympanic membrane) healed area of the tympanic membrane that is thinner than the rest of the membrane due to absence of the fibrous tissue layer.

morphology the overall shape of an evoked potential waveform.

most comfortable loudness level (MCL) dB HL of a tone or speech that is judged to be at a comfortable (preferred) level to listen.

motility movement (elongations and contractions) of the outer hair cells that is a normal component of cochlear transduction; responsible for the active process of the cochlea that is necessary for good sensitivity and frequency tuning.

mucoid otitis media chronic middle ear disorder in which the fluid in the middle ear becomes thick or puss-like; also called purulent otitis media or glue ear.

multifrequency tympanometry tympanometric measures that record susceptance (B) and conductance (G) tympanograms as a function of probe-tone frequency (226–2000 Hz) to determine the resonant frequency of the middle ear to differentiate mass from stiffness disorders.

myringotomy surgical procedure to drain middle ear fluid by making a small incision in the tympanic membrane and extracting the fluid with a needle-type syringe; may be combined with placement of pressure equalization (PE) tubes.

narrowband noise bandpass filtered noise concentrated around a center frequency; used in clinical pure-tone masking because it allows efficient masking over a wider intensity range than wideband noise; also called narrowband maskers.

nasals speech sounds resulting from opening the velopharyngeal port sending air flow through the nasal cavity.

nasopharynx an area above the tonsils in the upper part of the oral cavity/throat.

National Student Speech Language Hearing Association (NSSHLA) student membership organization for those preparing to be speech-language pathologists and/or audiologists; associated with the American Speech-Language-Hearing Association.

negative predictive value percentage of true negatives for a screening test (level of confidence identifying the true negatives).

neural synchrony relatively large number of auditory neurons firing simultaneously.

neural transduction energy change that occurs in the nerves (or synapses).

neuroelectric electrical potentials in the body activity generated from neural conduction.

Neuromonics type of tinnitus treatment using sound therapy.

neurophysiological basis of tinnitus comprehensive theory of tinnitus and treatment approach established by Pawel Jastreboff and colleagues.

Noah computer software platform that contains programming modules for digital hearing aids of different manufacturers.

nodes property of resonance where two interacting tones cancel each other out.

noise aperiodic vibrations that are produced by a combination of many pure tones with random starting phases; unwanted potentials obtained from movement or electrical sources in evoked potential measures.

noise floor inherent background signals in electronic equipment or otoacoustic emission measures, which the signal of interest must exceed.

noise-induced hearing loss (NIHL) hearing loss resulting from excessive exposure to loud sounds; also called acoustic trauma; see also **noise notch**.

noise notch sensorineural hearing loss in the 3 to 6 kHz region typical of excessive exposure to high noise levels.

noncompensated tympanogram tympanogram whereby the display includes the admittance due to the ear canal (V_{ea} at 200 daPa) and the middle ear (Y_{tm}).

nonorganic hearing loss see **functional hearing loss**.

notched noise masking physiological masking paradigm used in auditory brainstem response recordings to provide more frequency-specific information about the function of the cochlea; the noise is notch filtered to desynchronize part of the cochlea to observe responses from other regions.

nucleus is used to identify a location within the brainstem where there is a collection of specialized cell bodies.

nystagmus involuntary horizontal eye movements resulting from neural connections between the vestibular and ocular systems; characterized by a slow (vestibular) component in the opposite direction of perceived head movement and a fast (visual) component that brings eyes back to center; recorded by monitoring the corneoretinal potential during electronystagmography.

objective tests measures that do not require patients' subjective judgments or responses, for example, tympanometry, acoustic reflexes, otoacoustic emissions, evoked potentials; usually independent of age, level of consciousness, and sedation.

objective tinnitus relatively rare type of sound in the ear due to some vibratory source in the ear, head, or neck; may be audible to an external listener; often described as whooshing, pulsing, or clicking; usually has an underlying medical condition.

occluded ear that has a supra-aural earphone on the ear or an ear with an insert earphone or hearing aid in the ear; blocked.

occlusion effect (OE) improvement in the bone conduction thresholds as a result of covering the nontest ear with a supra-aural earphone or wearing some hearing aids; originates from vibrations of the cartilaginous portion of the external auditory canal resulting from bone conducted sounds. OE is greatest as 250 Hz and lessens at 500 and 1000 Hz; OE is negligible above 1000 Hz. OE is offset (not a factor) when there is an air–bone gap in the nontest ear.

octave doubling or halving of frequency.

ohm unit of measurement for impedance; also used for electrical resistance.

olivocochlear bundle (OCB) band of efferent auditory nerve fibers that originate in the superior olivary complex region and travel to the organ of Corti through the modiolus; approximately 800 to 1200 crossed (originate on contralateral side of brainstem) and uncrossed (originate on ipsilateral side of brainstem) efferent neurons comprise the OCB.

one-third octave band-pass filter that is one-third octave wide at the 3 dB down points; narrowband noises used in clinical masking are one-third octave wide.

open-set speech materials in which the patient does not have any prior familiarization or set of choices visually available.

organ of Corti sensory organ of hearing that lies within the scala media along the basilar membrane from the base to apex of the cochlea; composed of receptor cells (inner and outer hair cells), support cells, spaces filled with perilymph, and the tectorial membrane.

osseointegration connection between living bone and the surface of a load-carrying implant.

osseous spiral lamina shelf of bone that extends from the modiolus and winds (like threads of a screw) along the cochlea from the base to the apex of the cochlea; serves as the inner attachment of the basilar membrane.

ossicles group of three bones of the middle ear—the malleus, incus, and stapes—which articulate with each other to transduce mechanical vibrations from the tympanic membrane to the inner ear; see also **ossicular chain**.

ossicular chain middle ear ossicles, collectively; see also **ossicles**.

ossicular disarticulation a separation of the ossicular chain or a break in one of the ossicles, typically a dislocation of the long process of the incus from the stapes; also called *ossicular discontinuity*.

ossiculoplasty surgical procedure to repair middle ear ossicles and/or replace with a prosthetic component.

osteoma benign single pearl-shaped bony growth in the ear canal.

otalgia pain in the ear.

otitis externa inflammation of the tissues lining the external auditory canal, usually caused by bacterial infection; also called swimmer's ear.

otitis media inflammation or accumulation of fluid in the middle ear; also called otitis media with effusion; can be acute, chronic, intermittent; can be fluid free of bacteria (serous otitis media) or infected with bacteria (purulent).

otoacoustic emissions (OAEs) low-intensity acoustic vibrations measured in the ear canal that originate from energy produced by the motility of the outer hair cells, with reverse transmission of this activity along the basilar membrane and through the middle ear to the ear canal; widely used in newborn hearing screening programs and basic diagnostic tests of auditory function; see also transient otoacoustic emissions and distortion product otoacoustic emissions.

otoconia layer of dense calcium carbonate crystals on top of the otolithic membrane in the maculae.

otoliths term used to refer to the saccule and utricle, sac-like sensory organs of the vestibular system; part of the membranous labyrinth located in the vestibule region of the inner ear.

otologists appropriately trained and licensed/certified medical physicians specializing in disorders and surgery related to the ears, also called neuro-otologists, otolaryngologists, or ear, nose, and throat (ENT) specialists.

otology medical specialty related to the ears, practiced by appropriately trained and certified otologists.

otorrhea fluid draining into external auditory canal from the middle ear.

otosclerosis caused by outgrowth of bony wall (otospongiosis) around the stapes footplate; commonly causes middle ear conductive hearing loss when stapes is immobilized; less commonly, toxins may invade the cochlea and cause a sensorineural hearing loss; also called otospongiosis.

otoscope lighted instrument used to examine external auditory canal and tympanic membrane.

otoscopy a method to visually inspect the ear canal and tympanic membrane.

otospongiosis see **otosclerosis**.

ototoxicity hearing loss due to poisonous side effects from some therapeutic drugs or environmental toxins.

outer ear includes the auricle and external ear canal.

outer hair cells (OHCs) auditory sensory hair cells within the organ of Corti; approximately 12,500 OHCs arranged in three rows; have a motoric function (see motility) that is part of the active cochlear process responsible for good hearing sensitivity and frequency.

outer spiral fibers afferent nerve fibers that cross the tunnel of Corti and connect to the outer hair cells (less than 5% of afferent neurons are outer spiral fibers).

output compression (AGCo) uses a type of automatic gain compression on the output signal in hearing aids to prevent sounds from becoming too loud to the listener.

oval window oval-shaped opening into the cochlea (scala vestibuli) to which the stapes footplate is attached; normal route for transmission of vibrations to the inner ear.

overmasking situation that may arise in clinical masking in which the level of the masker is sufficient to exceed the interaural attenuation and the noise masker crosses over to the test ear that interferes with establishing the true threshold.

pars flaccida small region at the superior margin of the tympanic membrane that is thinner and more flaccid due to the absence of the fibrous tissue layer; also called Shrapnell's membrane.

pars tensa major part of the tympanic membrane that is fairly rigid due to the presence of a fibrous tissue layer between the skin lining the external ear canal and the mucous lining of the middle ear space.

passive cochlear process the process of cochlear transduction that is related to the physical parameters of the basilar membrane (e.g., narrower and stiffer at the base), which produce the tonotopic traveling waves well documented by Békésy; when measured without the active process of the outer hair cells, the passive process is more broadly tuned and less sensitive.

patent open, usually referring to an unoccluded PE tube or abnormally open eustachian tube.

PB$_{max}$ patient's maximum speech recognition score, usually in reference to percent correct of phonemically balanced words used in word recognition score tests; also used as one of the values in the calculation of a rollover ratio from performance intensity functions (PI–PB functions).

PB$_{min}$ the word recognition score at high intensities, beyond PB$_{max}$, that is used in the calculation of the rollover ratio.

PB words single-syllable words that are phonetically or phonemically balanced.

peak amplitude (A$_p$) amplitude of a waveform as measured from baseline to one of the peaks.

peak-to-peak amplitude (A$_{p-p}$) amplitude of a waveform as measured from the most positive point to the most negative point.

perforation hole in the tympanic membrane.

performance-intensity function for PB words (PI–PB function) method to characterize a patient's word recognition score as a function of presentation level; useful for determining a patient's best word recognition ability (PBmax) and to calculate a rollover ratio; see **PI–PB rollover**.

perilymph fluid in the bony labyrinth, but outside the membranous labyrinth, that has relatively high sodium (Na+) and low potassium (K+) concentrations.

perilymph fistula rupture in the oval window or round window membrane leaking perilymph fluid into the middle ear.

perinatal conditions or situations occurring during birth.

period description used to characterize sound waves that refers to the time (seconds or milliseconds) it takes to complete one cycle; reciprocal of frequency.

period histogram recording of the firing pattern from a neuron, displayed as a function of the period of the stimulus.

periodic vibration sound waves in which the vibratory pattern repeats itself at regular intervals.

peripheral auditory (or vestibular) system refers to auditory and vestibular structures and nerves that are located outside the central nervous system.

permanent threshold shifts (PTS) hearing loss due to excessive exposure to noise that does not recover; also called noise-induced hearing loss (NIHL).

persistent postural perceptual dizziness (PPPD) vestibular disorder defined as a long-lasting (at least three months) dizziness; usually the sequela of some other event that caused acute vertigo or balance problems. Also called chronic subjective dizziness (CSD).

Personal Sound Amplification Products (PSAP) a wearable electronic device intended to amplify sounds in the environment not to compensate for hearing loss.

petrous part of the temporal bone that is directed medially into the skull and houses the middle ear and inner ear structures.

phalangeal process fingerlike process coming from the Deiter cells, which extends up to the upper surface of an adjacent outer hair cell and fills in what would have been a space between the outer hair cells at the upper surface.

phase-locking characteristic pattern of neural discharges in which they always fire during the same phase of the stimulus.

phon unit used to describe a scale of loudness judgments that are judged equal across frequency; a phon is equal to the dB HL of a 1000 Hz tone, for example, 40 phons is equal to the loudness associated with a 1000 Hz tone at 40 dB HL; see **equal loudness contours**.

phoneme score a way of analyzing word recognition score performance that counts the number of correctly identified phonemes for each word (each phonemically balanced [PB] word has three phonemes), and reports the score as a percentage of the total available phonemes across the entire list of words (e.g., a 25-item PB word list has 75 phonemes).

phonemically balanced (PB) words lists of single-syllable words in which the consonant-**phonemic**

regression WRS can be poorer than one would expect based on the audiometric configuration.

pillar cells support cells in the organ of Corti that form the tunnel of Corti, which separates the inner hair cells from the outer hair cells.

PI–PB rollover performance intensity function for phonemically balanced words, which demonstrates a measured decrease in the word recognition score at high presentation levels; rollover is calculated as PBmax – PBmin/PBmax; rollover ratios greater than 0.35 are suggestive of 8th nerve disorder.

pitch psychological correlate of frequency.

place theory theory of frequency coding based a tonotopic arrangement along the basilar membrane for sounds of different frequencies.

plateau term used in clinical masking that represents a range of noise increases in the non-test ear that are not accompanied by any change in the threshold in the test ear.

plateau method commonly used masking method, first described by Hood (1960), in which a masking plateau is established; see also **plateau**.

positive predictive value percentage of true positives for a screening test (confidence in identifying true positives).

preauricular appendage or tag small skin growth anterior to the tragus due to embryologic alterations.

preauricular pit or sinus small dimple just anterior to the tragus due to embryologic alterations.

precepted/precepting/preceptor being supervised by someone with authority who has the needed experience and knowledge to model, teach, and facilitate the learning of new skills by a **preceptee**.

prenatal conditions or situations occurring prior to birth.

presbycusis hearing loss related to aging.

prescriptive fitting method strategy for fitting hearing aids that has been shown to provide the best outcome; uses a mathematical model of selecting gain and output based on the patient's hearing loss.

pressure measure of force distributed over an area; units of dynes/cm^2, newton/m^2, or micropascals (µPa) depending on the system of measurement being used.

pressure equalization (PE) tube small polyethylene tube inserted into the tympanic membrane to permit (maintain) ventilation of middle ear; allows equalized air pressure on both sides of tympanic membrane in cases of persistent otitis media and poor eustachian tube function.

prevalence epidemiology term to refer to the number of new and old cases of a disorder present within a specified period of time.

primary tones two externally applied tones (f_1 and f_2) used to generate the distortion product tone ($2f_1 - f_2$) during distortion product otoacoustic emission (DPOAE) testing.

probe microphone verification see **real-ear measures**.

probe tone tone used in immittance testing that is applied through the probe in the ear canal, and which is used to monitor changes in admittance; standard probe tone is 226 Hz at 85 dB SPL; higher frequency probe tones are sometimes used; see **multiple component** or **multiple frequency tympanometry**.

promontory bony wall on the medial surface of the middle ear that lies between the round window and oval window; used as a site for cochlear stimulation in cochlear implant assessments and transtympanic electrocochleography.

propagation (propagate) sound waves moving within a medium such as air, water, solids.

psychoacoustics science concerned with how humans perceive sound; study of the psychological correlates of physical properties of sound.

pulsatile tinnitus type of objective tinnitus generally described as a pulsing or whooshing sound; related to the rhythm of blood flow/heartbeat.

pure-tone audiometry basic hearing test that involves finding a patient's thresholds (in dB HL) for different pure tones presented by air conduction and bone conduction; used to describe type and degree of hearing loss.

pure-tone average (PTA) average threshold calculated from the air conduction thresholds at 500, 1000, and 2000 Hz.

pure tones simple sound waves that have only one frequency of vibration; also called sinusoids or sine waves.

quarter-wave resonator a condition of resonance whereby the fundamental frequency is equal to a quarter wavelength, for example, for a tube open at one end.

rarefaction phase of a waveform that is associated with a decrease in the density of air molecules, and which corresponds to a decrease in sound pressure or intensity.

real-ear aided response (REAR) a method to verify a hearing aid fitting using probe-microphone measures and real speech.

real-ear measures hearing aid verification step process in which measures are made of the output of the hearing aid at the tympanic membrane of the hearing aid user; requires the placement of a thin silicone tube in the ear canal, which is attached to a measurement microphone, to obtain patient-specific information relative to the ear canal characteristics while it is being worn by the patient.

recorded speech materials speech materials that are on some recorded media such as tape or compact disk; used for speech testing.

recruitment abnormal growth of loudness in an ear with a cochlear hearing loss.

reference equivalent threshold dB SPL (RETSPLs) reference levels for pure tones and speech, set by ANSI, that correspond to the average normal thresholds; calibration values used for audiometers for dB hearing level, the most recent of which should appear on the y-axis of an audiogram.

reference level for intensity lowest average intensity needed to hear a sound as provided by accepted standards (ANSI); current standard is 1.0×10^{-12} w/m².

reference level for pressure lowest average pressure needed to hear a sound as provided by accepted standards (ANSI); current standard is 20 Pa.

reflex eliciting tones the stimulus tones (500, 1000, and 2000 Hz) used to test for acoustic reflexes; may be presented ipsilaterally or contralaterally.

Reissner's membrane surface of the membranous labyrinth (scala media) in the cochlea that separates scala media from scala vestibuli.

rejection rate see **attenuation rate**.

reliability description of a test's ability to obtain the same results when repeated across sessions or multiple testers.

reproducibility value correlation between two channels of otoacoustic emission recordings; calculated for different frequency components and displayed as a percentage for each frequency band.

resonance property of an object or cavity that produces a maximum vibratory response at a particular frequency (resonant frequency) that is dependent on its size and shape.

reticular lamina upper surface of the organ of Corti, formed by the tight mosaic of the tops of all the cells, including the phalangeal processes, tops of the pillars, and the cuticular plates of the hair cells; boundary between endolymph above the reticular lamina and perilymph below the reticular lamina (in the spaces of the organ of Corti).

retraction pocket abnormal condition of the tympanic membrane in which the pars flaccida region of the tympanic membrane is drawn into the middle ear due to the negative middle ear pressure; early sign of eustachian tube dysfunction.

retrocochlear pertaining to the 8th cranial nerve and cerebellar-pontine angle.

rollover ratio ratio of the greatest amount of decline (PB_{min}) of word recognition score that occurs at intensities higher than the PBmax: rollover ratio = (PB_{max} – PB_{min})/PB_{max}; rollover ratio greater than 0.35 suggests retrocochlear disorder; also called rollover index.

root-mean-square (RMS) amplitude (A_{rms}) average amplitude (dB SPL) of a waveform integrated over a period of time; obtained by squaring each of the instantaneous amplitudes, averaging the squared values, and taking the square root of the average; equivalent to 0.707 times the peak amplitude for pure tones; measured with sound level meters.

Rosenthal's canal channel that coils from the base to the apex located in the bony core of the cochlea just prior to the osseous spiral lamina; location of the spiral ganglia.

round window membrane-covered round-shaped opening between the middle ear and the cochlea (scala tympani); allows for vibrations to enter the fluid-filled cochlea through reciprocal action with the oval window.

saccule one of the sensory organs (otoliths) of the vestibular system, located in the vestibule of the inner ear; houses the macula, which responds to linear accelerations of the head and orientation relative to gravity; see also **utricle**.

sagittal plane divides the anatomical structure into right and left sections.

salicylates group of anti-inflammatory drugs, such as aspirin; can cause temporary sensorineural hearing loss.

sawtooth waveform complex periodic waveform that is composed of a fundamental frequency and its harmonics; produces a buzzing type of tonal sound.

scala media membranous labyrinth within the cochlea; filled mostly with endolymph and houses the organ of Corti; divides the bony labyrinth of the cochlea into its three chambers (scala media, scala vestibuli, and scala tympani); one edge of the scala media is called the basilar membrane and the other edge is called Reissner's membrane.

scala tympani lowermost section of the bony labyrinth next to the basilar membrane of the scala media; filled with perilymph; joins the scala vestibuli at the helicotrema.

scala vestibuli uppermost section of the bony labyrinth next to Reissner's membrane of the scala media; filled with perilymph; joins the scala tympani at the helicotrema.

Scarpa's ganglion see **vestibular ganglion**.

scope of practice documents developed (separately) by the American Academy of Audiology (AAA) the American Speech-Language-Hearing Association (ASHA) that describe the services that are considered appropriate for audiologists.

screening audiometer a small portable device that only uses pure tones to assess hearing.

Self-Assessment for Communication self-assessment of hearing disability generally used with adult hearing screenings.

self-assessment inventory is a patient questionnaire used in validation of a hearing aid fitting.

semicircular canals three orthogonally oriented canals of the vestibular system that respond to angular accelerations of the head; superior (anterior), posterior, and horizontal (lateral).

sensitivity how well a test identifies the targeted disorder (proportion of true positives).

sensorineural hearing loss type of hearing loss described from pure-tone audiometric results that is caused by disorders in the inner ear or neural pathways; characterized by elevation of both bone conduction and air conduction thresholds, with air–bone gaps less than or equal to 10 dB.

serous otitis media fluid in the middle ear is clear and not infected.

shape of hearing loss one of the parameters used in describing audiograms; refers to the amount configuration of the thresholds across frequency, for example, sloping, flat, notched, rising.

sharply tuned tuning curves with a relatively narrow (sharp) tip region, as occurs with normal hearing; good frequency selectivity.

Shrapnell's membrane see **pars flaccida**.

signal-averaging computer specialized computer that averages synchronous neural responses; typically used in measurement of evoked potentials; response is time-locked to the onset of the stimulus to enhance the response of interest and reduce the random noise signals (improves the signal-to-noise ratio).

signal-to-noise-ratio (S/N ratio) relationship between the level of a sound or evoked potential and a background noise, that is either purposefully presented or is inherent in the evoked response recording.

simple periodic vibration vibratory pattern repeats itself at regular intervals wave.

sine waves see **simple vibration**.

sinusoids see **simple vibration**.

sone loudness scale where one sone is defined as the loudness of a 1000 Hz tone at 40 dB SPL (or 40 phons).

sound-field testing presentation of test materials using loudspeakers; also called free-field testing.

spaces of Nuel spaces surrounding the outer hair cells of the organ of Corti; filled with perilymph.

speaker (or loudspeaker) electroacoustic transducer that converts electrical energy to acoustic energy; used in audiometry during sound-field testing.

specificity how well a test correctly identifies those without the targeted disorder.

spectral splatter spread of energy across a relatively wide frequency range, as occurs with brief signals (transient).

spectrogram graphic output of a spectrograph displaying frequencies (y-axis) as function of time (x-axis); intensity can be represented by the darkness of the displayed frequencies.

spectrograph instrument used to measure the spectra of speech sounds.

spectrum (plural = spectra) representation of complex vibrations that determines the individual amplitudes as a function of frequency (frequency spectrum) and/or the starting phases as a function of frequency (phase spectrum); see also **fast Fourier transform (FFT)**.

specula disposable end of the otoscope that is place into the ear canal for viewing.

speech audiometry method used in clinic to evaluate how well a patient can hear and understand specific types of speech stimuli.

speech banana representation of how different speech sounds are distributed on the audiogram; term comes from the general outline of the distribution.

speech detection threshold (SDT) speech audiometry test that determines the lowest level at which a patient indicates he is aware that a sound was presented, but does not require the patient to repeat the word; also called speech awareness threshold (SAT).

speech intelligibility index (SII) see **articulation index**.

speech-language pathologist professional who has the appropriate degree and license in their state to practice speech-language pathology; typically certified by the American Speech-Language-Hearing Association (ASHA).

speech noise masker masking noise used in speech audiometry that is filtered to resemble the range of frequencies representative of those in the speech spectrum.

speech recognition threshold (SRT) speech audiometry test that determines the lowest level at which a patient can correctly identify words at least 50% of the time; used to be called speech reception threshold procedure; also called speech reception threshold.

speech threshold lowest level at which a patient is able to respond to speech at least 50% of the time; see **speech recognition threshold**.

speed of sound (in air) how fast sound travels; in air 343 m/s or 1126 feet/s at 68° F at sea level. Slightly different speeds occur at different temperatures.

spike nerve impulse or action potential.

spiral ganglion (plural ganglia) collection of cell bodies of the afferent auditory neurons; located in Rosenthal's canal within the modiolus of the cochlea from base to apex.

spiral limbus connective tissue cell within the organ of Corti that lies just above the edge of the osseous spiral lamina; serves as the attachment point for the medial end of the tectorial membrane.

spondee words two-syllable (compound) words with equal stress on each syllable, used to obtain the speech recognition threshold (SRT).

standing waves interaction of pure-tones that results in cancellation.

stapedectomy surgical procedure that replaces part of the stapes with a prosthetic device that connects the incus to the oval window; a treatment for otosclerosis.

stapedial branch (of the 7th cranial nerve) branch of the facial nerve that innervates the stapedius muscle of the middle ear; involved in the acoustic reflex.

stapedial reflex involuntary contraction of the stapedius muscles when the ear is stimulated by loud sounds as part of the acoustic reflex; innervation through the stapedial branch of the 7th cranial nerve; stimulation of either ear results in a bilateral stapedial reflex; also called acoustic reflex.

stapedius muscle small middle ear muscle that arises from the medial wall of the middle ear cavity and attaches to the head (neck) of the stapes; the muscle is innervated by the stapedial branch of the 7th cranial nerve.

stapedotomy surgical procedure in which a prosthesis is inserted into a hole drilled in the stapes footplate; a treatment for otosclerosis.

stapes third and smallest of the middle ear ossicles, consisting of a head (neck), anterior crus, posterior crus, and footplate; the head is attached to the incus at the lenticular process, and the footplate is attached to the oval window at the entrance to the inner ear.

stapes fixation bony growth (otospongiosis) in otosclerosis that encapsulates the stapes and prevents its vibration in the oval window.

starting phase position in a waveform's cycle where the vibration begins, expressed in degrees relative to the angle around the circle.

Stenger test audiometric test for unilateral nonorganic (functional) hearing loss.

stenosis (stenotic ear) abnormal narrowing of the external auditory canal.

stereocilia bundles of hair-like microvilli that project from the tops of inner and outer hair cells; stereocilia on each hair cell are arranged in three to four rows with increasing heights and joined to each other by tip links and cross links; stereocilia arrangement looks like a "W" on outer hair cells and a crescent on inner hair cells; bending of stereocilia opens ionic channels that alter the ionic flow to the hair cell.

stops parts of speech in which there is a brief period in which airflow is blocked followed by a burst of airflow when articulators are opened; can be voiced or unvoiced. Blockage can occur as bilabial stops, alveolar stops, or velar stops.

stria vascularis highly vascularized system of cells along the outer wall of the scala media in the cochlea that maintains the ionic charge of the endolymph.

Student Academy of Audiology (SAA) national student membership organization devoted to audiology education, student research, professional requirements, and networking of students enrolled in audiology doctoral programs; associated with the American Academy of Audiology.

styloid process is part of the temporal bone that interfaces with non-auditory structures and is the connection point for muscles used in speech production.

subjective tests tests that require the patient to make a judgment; based on one's perceptions; opposite of objective tests.

subjective tinnitus perception of sounds in the ear commonly reported with a variety of hearing losses, and which are not audible to others; typically described by patients as a ringing, hissing, or roaring sound; also known as nonvibratory tinnitus.

sudden sensorineural hearing loss (or sudden hearing loss) hearing loss with a rapid onset (within a few hours).

superior branch of vestibular nerve part of the 8th cranial nerve that innervates superior and horizontal semicircular canals, the utricle, and part of the saccule. See also **inferior branch of vestibular nerve**.

superior canal dehiscence (SCD) vestibular disorder dur to a small opening in the bony labyrinth of the superior semicircular canal that acts as a third window of the inner ear (the other two are the oval window and the round window), and allows the membranous portion of the superior semicircular canal to be displaced during sound or increased pressure.

superior olivary complex (SOC) auditory nucleus located in the lower brainstem.

supra-aural earphone air conduction transducer that is placed on the auricle; converts electrical energy to acoustic energy; commonly used model, TDH-50.

suprathreshold decibel level that is above the patient's hearing threshold.

tactile (vibrotactile) response pure-tone threshold that occurs due to the patient feeling the vibrations (sense of touch) rather than hearing them; may occur with bone conduction testing at 250 and 500 Hz between 40 and 60 dB HL; also called vibrotactile responses.

targeted screening screening of a subgroup of the larger population; targeted screening will have a higher prevalence rate of the disorder compared with screening the larger population.

tectorial membrane thin membrane overlying the stereocilia of hair cells in the organ of Corti; attached medially to the spiral limbus and laterally to the Hensen cells; stereocilia of the outer hair cells are embedded in the undersurface of the tectorial membrane, whereas those of the inner hair cells are not embedded.

telecoil alternative input source to a hearing aid that converts the electromagnetic signal from a telephone or assistive listening device and delivers it directly to the amplifier.

temporal bone lateral part of the skull in which the auditory and vestibular structures are found; divided into four main parts, squamous, mastoid, tympanic, and petrous (where most of the middle and inner structures are located).

temporal integration relationship between the threshold of audibility and the duration of a sound; thresholds for a pure tone generally increase as the duration decreases below 200 ms.

temporal lobe part of the cortex on the lateral side, above the temporal bone and below the lateral sulcus; location in the cortex of the primary auditory reception area of the cortex (Heschel's gyrus).

temporary threshold shift (TTS) non-permanent hearing loss that can occur from exposure to high levels of noise, but recovers within several hours after exposure; occurs at noise levels lower than those that can cause permanent threshold shift.

tensor tympani muscle small middle ear muscle that arises from the bony wall above the eustachian tube and its tendon attaches to the manubrium of the malleus; innervated by the 5th cranial nerve; may have some involvement in the acoustic reflex, but in humans it does not play much of a role; see **stapedius muscle**.

tensor veli palatini muscle in the nasopharynx that is responsible for opening the eustachian tube; innervated by the 5th cranial nerve.

threshold the lowest level of a pure tone that a person reliably responds to at least 50% of the time for a specified number of trials.

threshold of audibility curve graphical representation of the average dB SPL for normal hearing human listeners across the frequency range of hearing.

time-domain waveform representation of a vibration's amplitude as a function of time; see also **waveform**.

time-locked term used in signal averaging to indicate that the physiological response of interest is recorded relative to the onset of each stimulus and is enhanced with signal averaging; random noise is not time-locked and is reduced during signal averaging.

tinnitus auditory perceptions in the absence of externally presented sounds, commonly reported with a variety of hearing disorders; often called ringing in the ears; see also **objective tinnitus** and **subjective tinnitus**.

tinnitus maskability audiometric assessment of how much narrowband noise is needed to mask a patient's tinnitus.

tinnitus matching audiometric matching of a patient's tinnitus to a pure-tone or narrowband noise.

tinnitus retraining therapy (TRT) sound therapy treatment approach for tinnitus that is based on a neurophysiological/psychological basis of tinnitus made popular by Pawel Jastreboff.

tip links microfilaments that interconnect the tops of stereocilia of each inner and outer hair cell; thought to be the source of the ion channels that open and close with bending of the stereocilia.

tip region of the tuning curve narrow range of frequencies with the best sensitivities as displayed by a tuning curve; the tip represents the characteristic frequency of the tuning curve.

tone bursts short-duration tonal stimuli, with a relatively rapid onset (rise time), used for evoked potential testing.

tonotopic relation between location and different frequencies.

tragus flap of cartilage on the auricle that protrudes anterior to the entrance of the external auditory canal.

transducer instrument that converts energy from one type to another; an earphone is a transducer that converts electrical energy to acoustic energy, and a microphone is a transducer that converts acoustic energy into electrical energy.

transduction change in sound energy from one form to another.

transfer function experimental measurements that document changes in pressure as a function of frequency that occur between the one point and another point; for example, middle ear transfer function measures changes from tympanic membrane and the oval window membrane.

transient evoked otoacoustic emissions (TEOAEs) type of otoacoustic emissions that are evoked by a series of brief clicks (transients) and measured by signal averaging of the acoustic signals generated by the ear and picked up by a sensitive microphone in the ear canal.

transient brief acoustic signals with nearly instantaneous onset and offset and broad frequency spectrum; used to achieve neural synchrony in evoked response measures of the auditory system.

transverse plane the section that divides a structure into superior and inferior parts also known as horizontal plane.

transverse fracture temporal bone fracture that is perpendicular to the long axis of the petrous portion of the temporal bone; often causes sensorineural hearing loss due to damage to the inner ear.

traveling wave displacement pattern along the basilar membrane that is essential in sound processing, characterized by initial displacements near the base and progressing to its maximum displacement (see **traveling wave peak**) at the location corresponding to its characteristic frequency; peaks of the traveling waves occur tonotopically, in which high frequencies produce peaks at the base and low frequencies produce peaks at the apex.

traveling wave peak location where the maximum amplitude (displacement) of the basilar membrane occurs for any given pure tone, represented by the peak of the traveling wave envelope.

triangular fossa indentation formed between the antihelix and the helix on the auricle.

trigeminal nerve 5th cranial nerve. In the auditory system, a branch innervates the tensor tympani muscle of the middle ear.

true negative term used in screening matrix to indicate that the test correctly identified the absence of a disorder.

true positive (hit) term used in screening matrix to indicate that the test correctly identified the disorder.

tuning curve representation of the frequency selectivity of the auditory system, generated for a variety of physiologic and psychoacoustic measures; shows the different intensity by frequency combinations that produce some criterion threshold response; characterized by a tip region (around the characteristic frequency), a low frequency tail, and a steep high frequency slope.

tuning fork handheld metal instrument (two pronged) designed to produce a tone when struck; used by otologists during hearing exams.

tunnel of Corti space in the center of the organ of Corti, formed by the inner and outer pillar cells, which separates the inner and outer hair cells; filled with perilymph.

tympanic membrane membrane that separates the ear canal from the middle ear; has a fibrous tissue layer throughout most of the membrane (pars tensa), but is devoid of the fibrous tissue layer in the superior margin (pars flaccida); transduces acoustic vibrations entering the ear canal into mechanical vibrations of the middle ear ossicles.

tympanic ring outer rim of the tympanic membrane which is embedded into an indentation (tympanic sulcus) of the tympanic portion of the temporal bone, to hold the tympanic membrane in place; also called the tympanic **annulus**.

tympanic sulcus indentation in the tympanic portion of the temporal bone where the tympanic annulus of the tympanic membrane is embedded.

tympanogram graph used for tympanometry to display how the admittance in mmhos (y-axis) changes as a function of applied air pressure in daPa (x-axis).

tympanometric peak pressure (TPP) pressure (in daPa) where the peak admittance of the tympanogram occurs.

tympanometric width (TW) measure (in daPa) to describe the shape of a tympanogram; determined by the absolute difference between the two pressure values (on the x-axis) that are associated with the intersections of a horizontal line across the tympanogram at half of its height.

tympanometry part of the clinical immittance test battery that measures how the admittance changes as a function of applied air pressure (above and below atmospheric pressure), and how this func-

tion is affected by different conditions of the middle ear; produces a graph called a tympanogram.

type A tympanogram normal tympanogram, characterized by a peak admittance of the middle ear (Y_{tm}) in the expected normal range, a tympanometric peak pressure (TPP) at 0 daPa, and a normal tympanometric width.

type A$_d$ tympanogram abnormal tympanogram, characterized by a peak admittance of the middle ear (Y_{tm}) that is higher than the expected normal range, a tympanometric peak pressure at 0 daPa, and a normal tympanometric width (if measurable); suggests a highly flaccid tympanic membrane or a disarticulation of the ossicles.

type A$_s$ tympanogram abnormal tympanogram, characterized by a peak admittance of the middle ear (Y_{tm}) that is lower than the expected normal range, a tympanometric peak pressure at 0 daPa, and a normal tympanometric width; suggests a reduced mobility stiffening of the tympanic membrane that is often seen with otosclerosis.

type B tympanogram abnormal tympanogram, characterized by a flat (no change) admittance across the pressure range; seen with middle ear fluid, impacted cerumen, or perforation of the tympanic membrane differentiated by the measured ear canal equivalent volume (V_{ea}).

type C tympanogram abnormal tympanogram, characterized by a peak admittance of the middle ear (Y_{tm}) that occurs with a tympanometric peak pressure that is more negative than normal range; may have normal or reduced peak admittance of the middle ear and normal or abnormally wide tympanometric width; suggests negative middle ear pressure associated with poor eustachian tube function.

type of hearing loss one of the parameters used in describing audiograms; type of loss can be either conductive, sensorineural, or mixed for any frequency.

umbo central location on the tympanic membrane where the tip of the manubrium of the malleus is attached.

uncomfortable loudness level (UCL) intensity level where the patient finds speech or tones to cause discomfort; also called loudness discomfort level (LDL).

undermasking levels used in clinical masking that are not sufficient to eliminate cross hearing in the non-test ear (not yet on the plateau); initial masking level to where the plateau begins; also called "the chase."

unilateral to one side; hearing loss affecting only one side.

universal screening screening test applied to a large population.

unmasked threshold audiometric threshold obtained without masking in the other (nontest) ear.

unoccluded without earphone on or in the ear; open.

up-5-down-10 procedure threshold search procedure used in audiometry; performed by increasing the level in 5 dB steps when the patient does not respond, and decreasing the level in 10 dB steps when the patient responds.

utriculofugal deflection of the cupula away from the utricle.

utriculopetal the deflection of the cupola when it moves toward the utricle.

utricle one of the sensory organs (otoliths) of the vestibular system, located in the vestibule of the inner ear; houses the macula which responds to linear accelerations of the head and orientation relative to gravity; see also **saccule**.

validation part of the hearing aid fitting process that obtains information, usually through subjective questionnaires, about how well the hearing aid is working for the patient and the benefit he is receiving.

validity reflection of a test's ability to measure what it purports to measure.

verification part of the hearing aid fitting process to obtain confirmation through some measure (e.g., real-ear measures) that a hearing aid fitting has maximized the audibility and speech understanding, has good sound quality, and appropriate loudness perceptions, and is "acceptable" to the patient.

vertigo type of dizziness that originates in the vestibular organs of the inner ear, generally described as a sensation of "the room is spinning" or "motion sickness."

vestibular compensation ability of the vestibular system to adapt to vestibular disorders through reinterpretation of the abnormal input by the central nervous system; may improve spontaneously or through vestibular rehabilitation.

vestibular ganglion (ganglia) cell bodies for the vestibular peripheral neurons; located within the internal auditory canal; also called Scarpa's ganglion.

vestibular nerve portion of the 8th cranial nerve consisting of nerve fibers from the semicircular canals, saccule, and utricle that form the inferior and superior branches of the nerve.

vestibular nerve section surgical procedure in which the vestibular portion of the 8th cranial nerve is cut to alleviate vertigo in patients with serious vestibular disorder.

vestibular neuritis (see **labyrinthitis**).

vestibular schwannoma (see **acoustic neuroma**).

vestibule is part of the inner ear between the cochlea, and the semicircular canals that contains the utricle and saccule.

vestibulocochlear nerve 8th cranial nerve, composed of the vestibular nerve and the cochlear (or auditory) nerve; also called cochleovestibular nerve.

vestibulo-ocular reflex (VOR) eye movements that are equal and opposite to the direction of head movements, induced through the vestibular neural pathway and its connections with the cranial nerves that control the extraocular muscles of the eyes.

vestibulospinal reflex (VSR) body-orienting reflexes, induced through the vestibular neural pathway and its connections with reticular formation and spinal tract nerves that control skeletal muscles.

vestibulotoxicity vestibular damage/disorder due to poisonous side effects from some therapeutic drugs or environmental toxins.

videonystagmography (VNG) clinical tests of vestibular function based on video recordings of eye movements and nystagmus that is induced by various conditions.

visual reinforcement audiometry (VRA) technique used to test children 6 months to 2 years of age using visual reinforcements in a conditioning paradigm.

VU meter (volume unit meter) monitoring meter to adjust the input level of signals so that the output is set to be in calibration with the audiometer intensity (dB HL) dial.

warble tones tone in which the frequency is modulated with small rapid changes; used in sound-field testing to reduce standing waves (where two waves come together and reduce the amplitude).

wave I earliest positive wave in an auditory brainstem response recording; source is the more peripheral (distal) portion of the 8th cranial nerve; occurs with a latency around 1.5 to 2.0 ms at moderately high stimulus levels.

wave V most prominent positive deflection in an auditory brainstem response recording; occurs with a latency around 5.5 to 6.0 ms at moderately high stimulus levels; most common wave peak used for assessment of objective auditory thresholds; origin in the contralateral lateral lemniscus/inferior colliculus regions of the brainstem.

waveform pattern of movement of a sound wave displayed with amplitude as a function of time; also, is used in reference to evoked responses (otoacoustic emissions or evoked electrical potentials) to describe how the response amplitude varies as a function of time; also called time-domain waveform.

wavelength (λ) distance a sound wave travels in one cycle, measured in units of length; the distance between the same points on two successive cycles of a pure tone; λ = c/f, where c is the speed of sound in air and f is the frequency.

white noise noise with an infinite number of frequencies with random phases and equal amplitudes over the entire frequency range.

whole word score method of reporting the word recognition score (WRS) that reflects the percentage of correctly identified words.

wideband acoustic immittance (WAI) measures the stimulus power that is either absorbed by (absorbance) or reflected from (reflectance) the middle ear (tympanic membrane) for a variety of applied frequencies.

wide dynamic range compression (WDRC) type of input compression used in hearing aids that prevents sounds from becoming too loud to the listener also referred to as input automatic gain control (AGCi).

word recognition Score (WRS) a supra-threshold speech test using single-syllable word lists (e.g., Northwestern University [NU-6]) that are phonemically balanced (PB) words to determine the percentage of correctly identified words.

zygomatic process a part of the temporal bone that interfaces with non-auditory structures and is the connection point for muscles used in speech production.

Index

Note: Page numbers in **bold** reference non-text material